Transcultural Concepts in Nursing Care

● Seventh Edition

Margaret M. Andrews, PhD, RN, CTN-A, FAAN
Director and Professor of Nursing
School of Health Professions and Studies
University of Michigan-Flint
Flint, Michigan

Joyceen S. Boyle, PhD, RN, MPH, FAAN
Adjunct Professor of Nursing
College of Nursing
University of Arizona
Tucson, Arizona
Adjunct Professor of Nursing
College of Nursing
Georgia Regents University
Augusta, Georgia

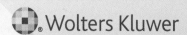 Wolters Kluwer

Philadelphia • Baltimore • New York • London
Buenos Aires • Hong Kong • Sydney • Tokyo

Acquisitions Editor: Christina C. Burns
Product Development Editor: Christine Abshire
Development Editor: Elizabeth Connolly
Editorial Assistant: Cassie Berube
Marketing Manager: Dean Karampelas
Production Project Manager: Joan Sinclair
Design Coordinator: Joan Wendt
Illustration Coordinator: Jennifer Clements
Manufacturing Coordinator: Karin Duffield
Production Service: SPi Global

7th edition

Copyright © 2016 by Wolters Kluwer

Two Commerce Square
2001 Market Street
Philadelphia, PA 19103 USA
LWW.com

Printed in China

Library of Congress Cataloging-in-Publication Data
Transcultural concepts in nursing care / editors, Margaret M. Andrews, Joyceen S. Boyle. — Seventh edition.
      p. ; cm.
   Includes bibliographical references and index.
   ISBN 978-1-4511-9397-8
   I. Andrews, Margaret M., editor. II. Boyle, Joyceen S., editor.
   [DNLM: 1. Transcultural Nursing. 2. Culturally Competent Care.   WY 107]
   RT86.54
   362.17'3—dc23

2015015790

Contributors

Margaret M. Andrews, PhD, RN, CTN-A, FAAN
Director and Professor of Nursing
School of Health Professions and Studies
University of Michigan-Flint
Flint, Michigan

Martha B. Baird, PhD, APRN/CNS-BC, CTN-A
Assistant Professor
School of Nursing
University of Kansas Medical Center
Kansas City, Kansas

Joyceen S. Boyle, PhD, RN, MPH, FAAN
Adjunct Professor of Nursing
College of Nursing
University of Arizona
Tucson, Arizona
Adjunct Professor of Nursing
College of Nursing
Georgia Regents University
Augusta, Georgia

Joanne T. Ehrmin, PhD, RN, CNS
Professor
Department of Health Promotion
College of Nursing
University of Toledo
Toledo, Ohio

Patricia A. Hanson, PhD, RN, APRN-BC, GNP
Professor
College of Nursing and Health
Madonna University
Livonia, Michigan

Jana Lauderdale, PhD, RN, FAAN
Assistant Dean for Cultural Diversity
School of Nursing
Vanderbilt University
Nashville, Tennessee

Patti Ludwig-Beymer, PhD, RN, CTN-A, NEA-BC, FAAN
Vice President and Chief Nursing Officer
Edward Hospital and Health Services
Naperville, Illinois

Margaret A. McKenna, PhD, MPH, MN
Clinical Associate Professor
Department of Health Services
University of Washington
Seattle, Washington

Margaret Murray-Wright, MSN, RN
Associate Director, Undergraduate Programs and Clinical Assistant Professor of Nursing
University of Michigan-Flint
Flint, Michigan

Dula F. Pacquiao, EdD, RN, CTN-A, TNS
Cultural Diversity Consultant
Education, Research and Practice
Lecturer, University of Hawaii
Hilo School of Nursing
Hilo, Hawaii

Maureen J. Reinsel, MA, MSN, APRN, AGPCNP-C
Technical Writer for Patient and Program Monitoring
Improving Data for Decision-Making in Global Cervical Cancer Programs (IDCCP)
Jhpiego Corporation
Baltimore, Maryland

Barbara C. Woodring, EdD, CPN, RN
Professor Emerita
Byrdine F. Lewis School of Nursing and Health Professions
Georgia State University
Atlanta, Georgia

I am pleased for the opportunity to write the Foreword to Drs. Margaret Andrews and Joyceen Boyle's seventh edition of their book, which illuminates the historical and theoretical foundations and evolution of transcultural nursing emerging from the disciplines of nursing and anthropology. I have been asked to "fill the shoes" of our mentor and colleague, the late Dr. Madeleine Leininger, who wrote the previous Forewords to their book. Dr. Leininger, the first nurse anthropologist and the "mother" of transcultural nursing, passed away in 2012 leaving us a legacy of transcultural nursing scholarship and a body of knowledge that has accelerated exponentially from its earliest beginnings in Cincinnati, Ohio, in the 1950s to its adoption in most nations of the world. Leininger addressed the human condition through knowledge of what it means to be human, caring, understanding, and open to all cultural traditions by creating the discipline of transcultural nursing. At the outset of the programmatic development of the discipline of Transcultural Nursing, Joyceen Boyle and I were asked by Dr. Leininger to become her first two doctoral students in 1977 at the University of Utah, College of Nursing, Salt Lake City, Utah. Both of us had backgrounds in public health or anthropology and a great interest in the study of diverse cultures. As friends and students, Joyceen and I felt privileged to be pioneers as Dr. Leininger put into motion her beliefs, and values of transcultural nursing, focusing on nursing and human science, caring science, theory development, anthropology, culture, and transcultural nursing. Leininger advanced her theoretical understanding developing The Worldwide Nursing Theory of Culture Care Diversity and Universality and her Ethnonursing methodology. Her transcultural beliefs and values have been infused into nursing program objectives for education, research, administration, and practice and were the foundation for the development of *standards of practice* for culturally competent care for individuals, groups, local and global communities, and organizations. Dr. Andrews teamed up early in her scholarly career with her mentor, Dr. Joyceen Boyle and they, with other major contributors, wrote one of the earliest textbooks, *Transcultural Concepts in Nursing Care* published first in 1989 who also was influenced by Dr. Leininger.

Because of their long history of knowledge generation in transcultural nursing, this work of Andrews and Boyle is very comprehensive and shows the depth of their scholarship in terms of culture, theory development and application, research, and their commitment to the delivery of culturally competent care in practice. Rapid changes in science, technology, genetics, health care, economics, geopolitics, transportation, demographics, migration and immigration, religious ideologies, unrelenting wars, and global issues including human rights and social justice have challenged nurses to understand new ways of engaging with clients and families, and also professional colleagues in terms of transcultural nursing. By means of the new sciences of complexity and the generation of enormous quantities of research of every affiliation, and diverse philosophical, political, and religious perceptions, we can see the interconnectedness of everything in the universe and the necessity for discernment and evaluation of what is really happening in the world. Theoretical and experiential knowledge about our responsibilities to one another thus is growing and impacts the need for intense communication to examine and solve problems both locally and globally. Continuing to identify relevant issues to promote health, human safety, and

improve the quality of life of all people is a major goal of thoughtful national and international health care professionals. For example, we can explore, within the United Nations Millennium Development Goals for 2015 and beyond, the framework for the world community. These developments are now shaping Andrews' and Boyle's paradigmatic thinking in the seventh edition and their interest in addressing the challenges of the interconnectedness of all by their **Transcultural Interprofessional Practice (TIP) Model** with a theoretical foundation. Their model illuminates the necessity for increased collaboration and communication with clients and multiple health care and folk participants to address complex approaches to transcultural issues in the provision of culturally congruent, safe, and competent care.

The beginning chapters in their book highlight foundational and evolutionary knowledge of the concepts of culture, subculture, race, ethnicity, context, communication including digital communication—the Internet and social media—evidence-based practice and problem solving, culture-specific nursing care, interprofessional collaboration and best practices, transcultural nursing, genetics, and theory development. The chapters focus on culturally competent nursing care by highlighting transcultural nursing across the life span, multicultural health care settings including the culture of organizations, the delivery of mental health care, a focus on family and community, a spotlight on the cultural diversity of the workforce, and the challenges in transcultural nursing (religion, ethics, and international nursing). Each chapter follows with a set of review questions and learning activities that illuminate what students, faculty, and clinical practitioners will have integrated into their plan of care to meet mutual goals presented in the chapter case studies. The seventh edition reflects many of the changes in the concept of the culture-at-large, especially genetics. While giving attention to Leininger's theory in Chapter 1, what is significant in this seventh edition, as stated, is the development of their *own* theory, the Andrews and Boyle **Transcultural Interprofessional Practice (TIP)**

Model. The key concepts identified in the TIP model are *context, interprofessional health care team, communication,* and *problem-solving process.* The cultural *context* (health-related beliefs and practices that weave together environmental, economic, social, religious, moral, legal, political, educational, biophysical, genetic, and technological factors), the *interprofessional health care team* (nurses, physicians, social workers, therapists, pharmacists, and others), *cross-cultural communication* among client, family, and significant others, and members of the interprofessional health care team including folk and traditional healers, and religious and spiritual healers facilitate the foundation of the problem-solving process that has five steps. These five steps include comprehensive holistic client assessment, mutual goal setting, planning, implementation of the plan of action and interventions, and evaluation of the plan for effectiveness to achieve the stated goals, and desired outcomes; provide culturally congruent and competent care; deliver quality care that is safe and affordable; and ensure that the care is evidence based with best practices.

As I reflect on the work of my colleagues, Andrews and Boyle, not only within the pages of this book but also what each of them has accomplished over many years as leaders, teachers, researchers, online educators, and as Presidents of the Transcultural Nursing Society, what comes to mind is their *deep dedication and devotion* to the discipline and profession of Transcultural Nursing. Through their intellectual astuteness and creative actions, they have been and are role models and mentors to students and other leaders who have spread and broadened transcultural care knowledge worldwide. They are committed to the primary goal of transcultural nursing to facilitate culturally congruent knowledge and care so that people of the world are understood and their health care needs can be met within the dynamics of their cultures and cultural understanding. A seventh edition of a book attests to the fact that students, faculty, and other practitioners find within its pages relevant and challenging information to learn about cultures and

ethnic groups, know how to relate and serve them, conduct research, facilitate the solving of problems, and "making things work." Today *collaboration and communication* are the key. Margaret Andrews and Joyceen Boyle have captured that essence in their Transcultural Interprofessional Practice (TIP) theory and model, which is presented in this work. I wholeheartedly endorse this new edition. I am most proud to call these authors not only my colleagues but also my friends as they move forward in the evolution of what can be termed authentic transcultural nursing by means of collaboration and interprofessionalism. Nursing students, faculty, other health care professionals, and practitioners of every health care and anthropological discipline will be stimulated by the theory and the content expressed by the authors and the many contributors in this new edition to improve the health of and help people of diverse cultures worldwide.

Marilyn A. Ray, RN, PhD, CTN-A, FSfAA, FAAN
Colonel (Retired), United States Air Force, Nurse Corps
Professor Emeritus
The Christine E. Lynn College of Nursing
Florida Atlantic University
Boca Raton, Florida

Preface

Given the large number of cultures and subcultures in the world, it's impossible for nurses to know everything about them all; however, it is possible for nurses to develop excellent cultural assessment and cross-cultural communication skills and to follow a systematic, orderly process for the delivery of culturally competent care.

The Andrews/Boyle Transcultural Interprofessional Practice (TIP) Model, which we are introducing in this seventh edition of *Transcultural Concepts in Nursing Care* and describe in more detail in Chapters 1 and 2, emphasizes the need for effective communication, efficient, client- and patient-centered teamwork, and collaboration among members of the interprofessional health care team.

The TIP Model has a theoretical foundation in transcultural nursing that fosters communication and collaboration between and among all members of the team and enables multiple team members to manage complex, frequently multifaceted transcultural care issues, moral and ethical dilemmas, challenges, and care-related problems in a collegial, respectful, synergistic manner.

The process used in the TIP Model is an adaptation and application of the classic scientific problem-solving method used to deliver nursing and health care to people from different national origins, ethnicities, races, socioeconomic backgrounds, religions, genders, marital statuses, sexual orientations, ages, abilities/disabilities, sizes, veteran status, and other characteristics used to compare one group of people to another.

The Commission on Collegiate Nursing Education, the American Association of Colleges of Nursing's Essentials of Baccalaureate Education for Professional Nursing Practice, the National League for Nursing, most state boards of nursing, and other accrediting and certification bodies require or strongly encourage the inclusion of cultural aspects of care in nursing curricula. This, of course, underscores the importance of the purpose, goal, and objectives for *Transcultural Concepts in Nursing Care*, Seventh Edition.

Purpose: To contribute to the development of theoretically based transcultural nursing knowledge and the advancement of transcultural nursing practice.

Goal: To increase the delivery of culturally competent care to individuals, families, groups, communities, and institutions.

Objectives:

1. To apply a transcultural nursing framework to guide nursing practice in diverse health care settings across the lifespan.
2. To analyze major concerns and issues encountered by nurses in providing transcultural nursing care to individuals, families, groups, communities, and institutions.
3. To expand the theoretical bases for using concepts from the natural and behavioral sciences and from the humanities to provide culturally competent nursing care.
4. Provide a contemporary approach to transcultural nursing that includes effective cross-cultural communication, team work, and interprofessional collaborative practice.

We believe that cultural assessment skills, combined with the nurses' critical thinking abilities, will provide the necessary knowledge on which to base transcultural nursing care. Using this approach, nurses have the ability to provide culturally competent and contextually meaningful care for clients—individuals, groups, families, communities, and institutions.

The editors and chapter authors share a commitment to:

- Foster the development and maintenance of a disciplinary knowledge base and expertise in culturally competent care.
- Synthesize existing theoretical and research knowledge regarding nursing care of different ethnic/minority/marginalized and other disenfranchised populations.
- Identify and describe evidence-based practice and best practices in the care of diverse individuals, families, groups, communities, and institutions.
- Create an interdisciplinary and interprofessional knowledge base that reflects heterogeneous health care practices within various cultural groups.
- Identify, describe, and examine methods, theories, and frameworks appropriate for developing knowledge that will improve health and nursing care to minority, underserved, underrepresented, disenfranchised, and marginalized populations.

Recognizing Individual Differences and Acculturation

We believe that it is tremendously important to recognize the myriad of health-related beliefs and practices that exist within the population categories. For example, the differences are rarely recognized among people who identify themselves as Hispanic/Latino: this group includes people from along the U.S.–Mexico border, Puerto Rico, Mexico, Spain, Guatemala, or "little Havana" in Miami, as well as other Central and South American countries, who may share some similarities (speaking Spanish, for example) but who may also have distinct cultural differences.

We would like to comment briefly on the terms *minority* and *ethnic minorities*. These terms are perceived by some to be offensive because they connote inferiority and marginalization. Although we have used these terms occasionally, we prefer to make reference to a specific subculture or culture whenever possible. We refer to categorizations according to race, ethnicity, religion, or a combination, such as ethnoreligion, but we make every effort to avoid using any label in a pejorative manner. We do believe, however, that the concepts or terms *minority* or *ethnicity* are limiting, not only for those to whom the label perhaps applies but also for nursing theory and practice. We believe that concept of *culture* is richer and has more theoretical usefulness. In addition, we all have cultural attributes while not all are from a minority group or claim a particular ethnicity.

Critical Thinking Linked to Delivering Culturally Competent Care

We believe that cultural assessment skills, combined with the nurse's critical thinking ability, will provide the necessary knowledge on which to base transcultural nursing care. Using this approach, we are convinced that nurses will be able to provide culturally competent and contextually meaningful care for clients from a wide variety of cultural backgrounds, rather than simply memorizing the esoteric health beliefs and practices of any specific cultural group. We believe that nurses must acquire the skills needed to assess clients from virtually any and all groups that they encounter throughout their professional life.

Many educational programs in nursing are now teaching transcultural nursing content across the curriculum. We suggest that *Transcultural Concepts in Nursing Care* can be used by faculty members to integrate transcultural content across the curriculum in the following manner: Chapters 1 to 4 in the first clinical courses when students are learning how to conduct health histories, health assessments, and physical examinations; Chapters 10 and 11, mental health nursing and family and community nursing, in the appropriate specialty nursing courses; Chapters 5 to 8, which include nursing care across the lifespan, in courses that focus on the nursing care of the childbearing family, children, adults, and older adults; Chapters 9, 12, and 14, which concern culturally competent organizations, diversity in the

multicultural health care workforce, and competence in ethical decision making, in courses that focus on nursing leadership and management; Chapter 13, which examines religion, culture, and nursing, an excellent resource throughout the curriculum; and Chapter 15 in courses that focus on global health/community health nursing.

New to the Seventh Edition

All content in this edition was reviewed and updated to capture the nature of the changing health care delivery system, new research studies, and theoretical advances, emphasis on effective communication, team work, and collaboration, and to explain how nurses and other health care providers can use culturally competent skills to improve the care of clients, families, groups, and communities. In writing the seventh edition, we have been impressed with the developments in the field of transcultural nursing. The Transcultural Nursing Society and the American Academy of Nursing (AAN) have moved ahead with developing Standards of Practice for Culturally Competent Care that nurses around the world are using as a guide in clinical practice, research, education, and administration. In addition, a special task force from the Transcultural Nursing Society has developed a Core Curriculum for Transcultural Nursing that is being used as a basis for certification in transcultural nursing and for instructional purposes by faculty and students in educational programs. The recognition of the Standards of Practice and Core Curriculum for transcultural nursing enhances the development of cultural competence in nursing, thus improving the care of clients. Lastly, the Andrews/Boyle Transcultural Interprofessional Practice Model is introduced in recognition of the need to put the client or patient first and of the changing complexion of the health care workforce.

New Chapter Contributors

We welcome two new colleagues in the seventh edition, both from the University of Michigan-Flint School of Health Professions and Studies. Margaret (Margie) Murray-Wright, Associate Director of Undergraduate Programs and Clinical Assistant Professor of Nursing, infused state-of-the art content on genetics and genomics and coauthored Chapter 3, Cultural Competence in the Health History and Physical Examination. An Adult-Gerontology Nurse Practitioner, Maureen J. Reinsel has extensive experience in global public health and international development in Asia, Africa, and Europe. In addition to her nursing background, Maureen earned her MA degree in International Affairs from the Johns Hopkins University School of Advanced International Studies. She wrote Chapter 15, Nursing and Global Health, which is available online.

Chapter Pedagogy

Learning Activities

All of the chapters include review questions as well as learning activities to promote critical thinking. When relevant web-based information is available to supplement the chapter content, references are provided on thePoint®. In addition, each chapter includes chapter objectives and key terms to help readers understand the purpose and intent of the content.

Evidence-Based Practice

Current research studies related to the content of the chapter are presented as Evidence-Based Practice boxes. We have included a section in each box describing clinical implications of the research.

Case Studies

Case Studies based on the authors' actual clinical experiences and research findings are presented to make conceptual linkages and to illustrate how concepts are applied in health care settings. Case studies are oriented to assist the reader to begin to develop cultural competence with selected cultures.

Text Organization

Part One: Foundations of Transcultural Nursing

This first section focuses on the foundational aspects of transcultural nursing. The development of transcultural nursing frameworks that include concepts from the natural and behavioral sciences are described as they apply to nursing practice. Because nursing perspectives are used to organize the content in *Transcultural Concepts in Nursing Care*, the reader will not find a chapter purporting to describe the nursing care of a specific cultural group. Instead, the nursing needs of culturally diverse groups are used to illustrate cultural concepts used in nursing practice. Chapter 1 provides an overview of the theoretical foundations of transcultural nursing, and Chapter 2 introduces key concepts associated with cultural competence using the Andrews/Boyle Transcultural Interprofessional Practice Model as the organizing framework. In Chapter 3, we discuss the domains of cultural knowledge that are important in cultural assessment and describe how this cultural information can be incorporated into all aspects of care. Chapter 4 provides a summary of the major cultural belief systems embraced by people of the world with special emphasis on their health-related and culturally based values, attitudes, beliefs, and practices.

Part Two: Transcultural Nursing: Across the Lifespan

Chapters 5 through 8 use a developmental framework to discuss transcultural concepts across the lifespan. The care of childbearing women and their families, children, adolescents, middle-aged adults, and the elderly is examined, and information about cultural groups is used to illustrate common transcultural nursing issues, trends, and concerns.

Part Three: Nursing in Multicultural Health Care Settings

In the third section of the text (Chapters 9 through 12), we explore the components of cultural competence in mental health and in family and community health care settings. We also examine cultural competence in health care organizations and cultural diversity in the health care workforce, two very critical and current topics of concern. The clinical application of concepts throughout this section uses situations commonly encountered by nurses and describes how transcultural nursing principles can be applied in diverse settings. The chapters in this section are intended to illustrate the application of transcultural nursing knowledge to nursing practice.

Part Four: Contemporary Challenges in Transcultural Nursing

In the fourth section of the text, Chapters 13 to 15, we examine selected contemporary issues and challenges that face nursing and health care. In Chapter 13, we review major religious traditions of the United States and the interrelationships among religion, culture, and nursing. Recognizing the numerous moral and ethical challenges in contemporary health care as well as within the transcultural nursing, Chapter 14, available on thePoint®, discusses cultural competence in ethical and moral dilemmas from a transcultural perspective. Chapter 15, available on thePoint®, provides a global perspective of what is occurring in the international areas to promote human and health. This chapter is slightly different from the rest of the chapters as it highlights the field of international nursing and the ways in which nurses can contribute to the global efforts to improve the health status of people across the world.

Instructor Resources

The following tools to assist you with teaching your course are available upon adoption of this text on thePoint®:

- The **Test Generator** lets you generate new tests from a bank of NCLEX-style questions to help you assess your students' understanding of the course material.
- **PowerPoint Presentations** provide an easy way for you to integrate the textbook with your

students' classroom experience, either via slide shows or handouts.

- **Instructor's Guide for Teaching Transcultural Concepts** includes activities and discussion topics to help you engage students in the material.

Student Resources

Students who have purchased *Transcultural Concepts in Nursing Care*, Seventh Edition have access to the following additional resources:

- Chapter 14, **Cultural Competence in Ethical Decision Making**, discusses cultural competence in ethical and moral dilemmas from a transcultural perspective.
- Chapter 15, **Nursing and Global Health,** discusses the field of international nursing and the opportunities available for nurses who would like to practice internationally.
- **Journal Articles** corresponding to book chapters offer access to current research available in Wolters Kluwer journals.

Lippincott RN to BSN Online

Lippincott RN to BSN Online, a full curriculum online course solution aligned with *The Essentials of Baccalaureate Education for Professional Nursing Practice* and *Quality and Safety Education for Nurses Competencies*, uniquely features self-paced multimedia modules that foster experiential, active learning. Lippincott RN to BSN Online capitalizes on the "flipped classroom" pedagogy trend by integrating quality textbook content, assessments, and remediation with interactive modules. At its core is its exceptional instructional design strategies—storytelling, modeling, case-based, social, and collaborative learning. These innovative student and instructor resources take RN to BSN courses to the next level by featuring a guiding framework derived from the Cognitive Learning Theory and the best practices for e-learning from the Next Generation Learning Initiative. For more information, go to http://thepoint.lww.com/rntobsn.

Acknowledgments

We are pleased to acknowledge the assistance and support of our families, friends, and colleagues in once again making this book possible. We also appreciate the help of the many nursing faculty members, practitioners, and students who have offered helpful comments and suggestions. We have found it very gratifying to be able to call upon many of our colleagues for help and advice in this new edition.

We would like to gratefully acknowledge and thank Elizabeth Connolly, Development Editor, Wolters Kluwer Health, for her helpful recommendations on ways to strengthen the seventh edition, her careful attention to detail, her flexibility, her invaluable input on the Andrews/Boyle Transcultural Interprofessional Practice Model, her assistance in locating suitable digital images, and the long hours that she spent reviewing and rereviewing the chapters and appendices.

We gratefully acknowledge the support of our friends, too numerous to list by name, who wrote encouraging e-mails or phoned to express their interest and encouragement. We thank all of our colleagues who have purchased our book in the past and the many who have expressed interest in the seventh edition. We are always appreciative of their support.

Last of all, we would once again like to thank each other for what has been a lifetime of friendship that has withstood the test of time and now seven editions of this book! Through it all, we have found our professional endeavors in transcultural nursing and the friends that we have made along the way to be both satisfying and rewarding.

Margaret M. Andrews, PhD, RN, CTN-A, FAAN
Joyceen S. Boyle, PhD, RN, MPH, FAAN

For a list of the reviewers of this book and the accompanying Test Generator questions, please visit the**Point**® at http://thepoint.lww.com/Andrews7e.

Contents

Part Four: Contemporary Challenges in Transcultural Nursing

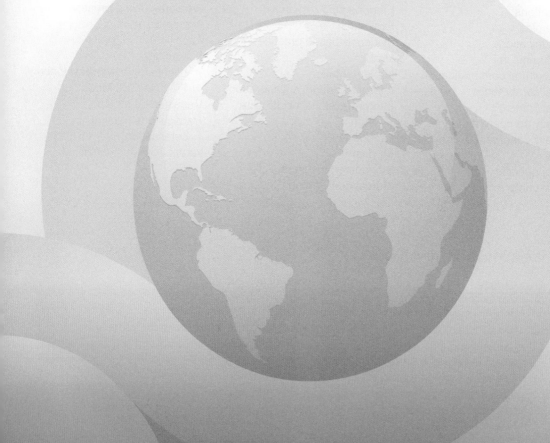

Part One

Foundations of Transcultural Nursing

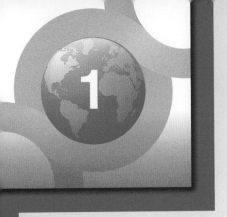

1

Theoretical Foundations of Transcultural Nursing

● Margaret M. Andrews and Joyceen S. Boyle

Key Terms

Anthropology
Assessment
Assumptions
Chronemics
Communication
Core Curriculum
Cross-cultural communication
Cultural competence
Cultural context
Culturally competent care
Culturally congruent nursing
  care
Cultural-specific
Cultural universals

Culture
Culture-specific nursing care
Culture-universal nursing care
Ethnicity
Ethnonursing research
Evaluation
Evidence-based practice
Hijab
Implementation
Interprofessional collaboration
Interprofessional health care
  team
Language
Modesty
Monochronic culture
Mutual goal setting

Nonverbal communication
Paralanguage
Personal space
Polychronic culture
Problem-solving process
Proxemics
Race
Subculture
Transcultural Interprofessional
  Practice (TIP) Model
Transcultural nursing
Transcultural nursing
  certification
Verbal Communication

Learning Objectives

1. Explore the historical and theoretical foundations of transcultural nursing.
2. Critically examine the relevance of transcultural nursing in addressing contemporary issues and trends in nursing.
3. Analyze Leininger's contributions to the creation and development of transcultural nursing as a theory and evidence-based formal area of study and practice within the nursing profession.
4. Critically examine the contributions of selected transcultural scholars to the advancement of transcultural nursing theory and practice.
5. Discuss key components of the Andrews/Boyle Transcultural Interprofessional Practice (TIP) Model.

Introduction to Transcultural Nursing

In her classic, groundbreaking book titled "Nursing and Anthropology: Two Worlds to Blend," Leininger (1970) analyzed the ways in which the fields of anthropology and nursing are interwoven and interconnected (c.f., Brink, 1976; McKenna, 1985; Osborne, 1969). Leininger used the term **transcultural nursing (TCN)** to describe the blending of nursing and anthropology into an area of specialization within the discipline of nursing. Using the concepts of culture and care, Leininger established TCN as a theory and evidence-based formal area of study and practice within nursing that focuses on people's culturally based beliefs, attitudes, values, behaviors, and practices related to health, illness, healing, and human caring (Leininger, 1991, 1995; Leininger & McFarland, 2002, 2006).

TCN is sometimes used interchangeably with cross-cultural, intercultural, and multicultural nursing. The *goal* of TCN is to develop a scientific and humanistic body of knowledge in order to provide **culture-specific** and **culture-universal nursing care** practices for individuals, families, groups, communities, and institutions of similar and diverse cultures. *Culture-specific* refers to particular values, beliefs, and patterns of behavior that tend to be special or unique to a group and that do not tend to be shared with members of other cultures. *Culture-universal* refers to the commonly shared values, norms of behavior, and life patterns that are similarly held among cultures about human behavior and lifestyles (Leininger, 1978, 1991, 1995; Leininger & McFarland, 2002, 2006; McFarland & Wehbe-Alamah, 2015a). For example, although the need for food is a culture-universal, there are culture-specifics that determine what items are considered to be edible; acceptable methods used to prepare and eat meals; rules concerning who eats with whom, the frequency of meals, and gender- and age-related rules governing who eats first and last at meal time; and the amount of food that individuals are expected to consume.

Given that culture is the central focus of anthropology and TCN, we begin this chapter by introducing, defining, and describing the concept of culture. We'll then discus the historical and theoretical foundations of TCN, including its relevance in contemporary nursing practice and the significant contributions of Leininger and other TCN scholars, leaders, and clinicians to the global advancement of TCN research, theory, education, and clinical practice. In the remainder of the chapter, we examine the Transcultural Interprofessional Practice (TIP) Model as a framework for delivering client-centered, high-quality nursing and health care that are culturally congruent and competent, safe, affordable, and accessible to people from diverse backgrounds across the lifespan. The term client is used throughout the book because nursing concerns not only the care of people who are ill but also those who strive for optimum health and wellness in their lives.

Anthropology and Culture

To understand the history and foundations of TCN, we begin by providing a brief overview of **anthropology**, an academic discipline that is concerned with the scientific study of humans, past and present. Anthropology builds on knowledge from the physical, biological, and social sciences as well as the humanities. A central concern of anthropologists is the application of knowledge to the solution of human problems. Historically, anthropologists have focused their education on one of four areas: sociocultural anthropology, biological/physical anthropology, archaeology, and linguistics. Anthropologists often integrate the perspectives of several of these areas into their research, teaching, and professional lives (American Anthropological Association, n.d.; Council on Nursing and Anthropology, n.d.). One of the central concepts that anthropologists study is **culture**. A complicated, multifaceted concept, culture has numerous definitions. The earliest recorded definition comes from a 19th century British pioneer in the field of anthropology named Edward Tylor, who defines

culture as the complex whole that includes knowledge, beliefs, art, morals, law, customs, and any other capabilities and habits acquired by members of a society (Tylor, 1871). Influenced by her formal academic preparation in anthropology (Meade, 1937), Leininger defines culture as the "learned, shared, and transmitted values, beliefs, norms, and lifeways of a particular group of people that guide thinking, decisions, and actions in a patterned way.... Culture is the blueprint that provides the broadest and most comprehensive means to know, explain, and predict people's lifeways over time and in different geographic locations" (McFarland & Wehbe-Alamah, 2015a, p. 10).

Culture influences a person's definition of health and illness, including when it is appropriate to self-treat and when the illness is sufficiently serious to seek assistance from one or more healers outside of the immediate family. The choice of healer and length of time a person is allowed to recover, after the birth of a baby or following the onset of an illness, are culturally determined. How a person behaves during an illness and the help rendered by others in facilitating healing also are culturally determined. Culture determines who is permitted, or expected, to care for someone who is ill. Similarly, culture determines when a person is declared well and when they are healthy enough to resume activities of daily living and/or return to work. When someone is dying, culture often determines where, how, and with whom the person will spend his or her final hours, days, or weeks. Although the term culture sometimes connotes a person's racial or ethnic background, there are also many other examples of *nonethnic cultures*, such as those based on *socioeconomic status*, for example, the culture of poverty or affluence and the culture of the homeless; *ability or disability*, such as the culture of the deaf or hearing impaired and the culture of the blind or visually impaired; *sexual orientation*, such as the lesbian, gay, bisexual, and transgender (LGBT) cultures; *age*, such as the culture of adolescence and the culture of the elderly; and *occupational* or *professional* cultures, such as nursing (American Nurses Association, 2013; International Council of Nurses, 2013) (see Figure 1-1), medicine,

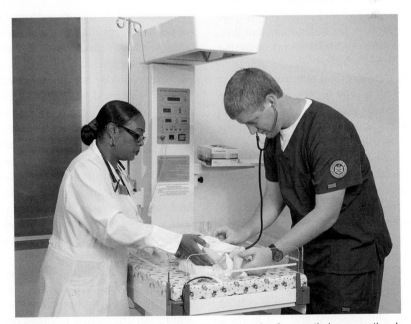

Figure 1-1. The profession of nursing is an example of a nonethnic occupational culture. The faculty member on the left is transmitting the requisite knowledge and skills from one generation to the next by mentoring the nursing student on the right.

and other professions in health care, business, education, and related fields.

In a classic study of culture by the anthropologist Edward Hall (1984), three levels of culture are identified: primary, secondary, and tertiary. The *primary level* of culture refers to the implicit rules known and followed by members of the group, but seldom stated or made explicit, to outsiders. The *secondary level* refers to underlying rules and assumptions that are known to members of the group but rarely shared with outsiders. The primary and secondary levels are the most deeply rooted and most difficult to change. The *tertiary level* refers to the explicit or public face that is visible to outsiders, including dress, rituals, cuisine, and festivals.

The term **subculture** refers to groups that have values and norms that are distinct from those held by the majority within a wider society. Members of subcultures have their own unique shared set of customs, attitudes, and values, often accompanied by group-specific language, jargon, and/or slang that sets them apart from others. A subculture can be organized around a common activity, occupation, age, ethnic background, race, religion, or any other unifying social condition. In the United States, subcultures might include the various racial and ethnic groups. For example, Hispanic is a panethnic designation that includes many subcultures consisting of people who self-identify with Mexican, Cuban, Puerto Rican, and/or other groups that often share Spanish language and culture (Morris, 2015).

Ethnicity is defined as the perception of oneself and a sense of belonging to a particular ethnic group or groups. It can also mean feeling that one does not belong to any group because of multiethnicity. Ethnicity is not equivalent to race, which is a biological identification. Rather, ethnicity includes commitment to and involvement in cultural customs and rituals (Douglas & Pacquiao, 2010). In the United States, ethnicity and race are defined by the federal Office of Management and Budget (OMB) and the U.S. Census Bureau; they provide standardized categories, which are used in the collection of census information on racial and ethnic populations and are also often used by biomedical researchers. There are six officially recognized ethnic and racial categories: White American, Native American, and Alaska Native; Asian American, Black, or African American; Native Hawaiian and other Pacific Islander; and people of two or more races; a race called "some other race" is also used in the census and other surveys but is not official. The Census Bureau also classifies Americans as "Hispanic or Latino" and "Not Hispanic or Latino," which identifies Hispanic and Latino Americans as a racially diverse *ethnicity*.

In the traditional anthropological and biological systems of classification, **race** refers to a group of people who share such genetically transmitted traits as skin color, hair texture, and eye shape or color. Races are arbitrary classifications that lack definitional clarity because all cultures have their own ways of categorizing or classifying their members (Hesmondhalgh & Sala, 2013; Hunt, Truesdel, & Kreiner, 2013). Some define race as a geographically and genetically distinct population, whereas others suggest that racial categories are socially constructed (Zimitri, 2013). The most current scientific data indicate that all humans share the same 99.1% of genes; the remaining 0.1% accounts for the differences in humans (National Human Genome Institute, 2014).

Historical and Theoretical Foundations of Transcultural Nursing

More than 60 years ago, Madeleine Leininger (1925 to 2012; see Figure 1-2) noted cultural differences between patients and nurses while working with emotionally disturbed children. This clinical nursing experience piqued her interest in cultural anthropology. As a doctoral student in anthropology, she conducted field research on the care practices of people in Papua New Guinea and subsequently studied cultural similarities and differences in the culture care perceptions and expressions of people around the world.

At the same time that Leininger (Leininger, 1978, 1991, 1995, 1997, 1998, 1999; Leininger & McFarland, 2002, 2006) was establishing TCN,

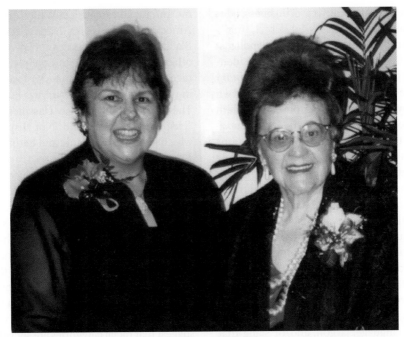

Figure 1-2. Author, Dr. Margaret Andrews *(left)*, and Transcultural Nursing Foundress, Dr. Madeleine Leininger *(right)*, at a meeting of the American Academy of Nursing.

other anthropologists, nurse–anthropologists, and nurses who were studying, teaching, and writing about ethnicity, race, diversity, and/or culture in nursing used terms such as cross-cultural nursing, *ethnic nursing care* (Orque, Bloch & Monrroy, 1983), or referred to *caring for people of color* (Branch & Paxton, 1976). The term *transcultural nursing* is used in this book, in recognition of the historical, research, and theoretical contributions of Leininger (1978), who used this term in her research and other scholarly works.

Leininger cites eight factors that influenced her to establish TCN as a framework for addressing 20th-century societal and health care challenges and issues, all of which remain relevant today:

1. A marked increase in the migration of people within and between countries worldwide
2. A rise in multicultural identities, with people expecting their cultural beliefs, values, and ways of life to be understood and respected by nurses and other health care providers
3. An increase in health care providers' and patients' use of technologies that connect people globally and simultaneously may become the source of conflict with the cultural values, beliefs, and practices of some of the people receiving care
4. Global cultural conflicts, clashes, and violence that impact health care as more cultures interact with one another
5. An increase in the number of people traveling and working in different parts of the world
6. An increase in legal actions resulting from cultural conflict, negligence, ignorance, and the imposition of health care practices
7. A rise in awareness of gender issues, with growing demands on health care systems to meet the gender- and age-specific needs of men, women, and children
8. An increased demand for community- and culturally based health care services in diverse environmental contexts (Leininger, 1995)

TCN exists today as an evidence-based, dynamic area of specialization within the nursing profession because of the visionary leadership of its founder, Madeleine Leininger, and many other nurses committed to the provision of care that is consistent with and "fits" the cultural beliefs and practices of those receiving it. This section explores the contributions of Leininger and then examines the ways in which other nursing scholars contributed to the development and advancement of TCN theory, research, practice, education, and administration globally.

Leininger's Contributions to Transcultural Nursing

Leininger's Theory of Culture Care Diversity and Universality describes, explains, and predicts nursing similarities and differences in care and caring in human cultures (Leininger, 1991). Leininger uses concepts such as worldview, social and cultural structure, language, ethnohistory, environmental context, and folk and professional healing systems to provide a comprehensive and holistic view of factors that influence culture care. Culturally based care factors are recognized as major influences on human experiences related to well-being, health, illness, disability, and death. After conducting a comprehensive cultural assessment based on the preceding factors, the three modes of nursing decisions and actions—culture care preservation and/or maintenance, culture care accommodation and/or negotiation, and culture care repatterning and/or restructuring—are used to provide **culturally congruent nursing care** (Leininger, 1991, 1995; Leininger & McFarland, 2002, 2006). Culturally congruent nursing care "refers to those cognitively based assistive, supportive, facilitative, or enabling acts or decisions that are mostly tailor-made to fit with an individual's, group's or institution's cultural values, beliefs, and lifeways in order to provide meaningful, beneficial, satisfying care that leads to health and well-being" (Leininger, 1991, p. 47). Cultural congruence is central to Leininger's Theory of Culture Care Diversity and Universality.

Among the strengths of Leininger's theory is its flexibility for use with individuals, families, groups, communities, and institutions in diverse health systems. To help develop, test, and organize the emerging body of knowledge in TCN, Leininger recognized that it would be necessary to have a specific conceptual framework from which various theoretical statements are developed. Leininger's Sunrise Enabler (Figure 1-3) depicts components of the Theory of Cultural Care Diversity and Universality, provides a visual representation of these components, and illustrates the interrelationships among the components. As the world of nursing and health care has become increasingly multicultural, the theory's relevance has increased as well.

While creating TCN as a respected and recognized nursing specialty and developing her theory, Leininger also had the foresight to establish the Transcultural Nursing Society (TCNS), generate the TCNS Newsletter, and create the Journal of Transcultural Nursing (JTN), for which she served as the founding editor. The TCNS holds regional and annual conferences, disseminates the newsletter, and collaborates with a publishing company to produce a quarterly journal, all of which provide forums for the exchange of TCN knowledge, research, and evidence-based, best practices relative to the provision of culturally congruent and culturally competent nursing and health care. To integrate TCN into the curricula of schools of nursing, Leininger established the first master's and doctoral programs in nursing with a theoretical and research focus in TCN and provided exemplars for TCN courses and curricula suitable for all levels of nursing education (undergraduate and graduate) through her lectures, publications, and consultations. Leininger also created a new qualitative research method called **ethnonursing research** to investigate phenomena of interest in TCN (Leininger, 1995; Leininger & McFarland, 2002, 2006; McFarland, Mixer, Webhe-Alamah, & Burk, 2012; McFarland & Wehbe-Alamah, 2015). Hundreds of studies have been conducted using ethnonursing research, which is the first research methodology developed by a nurse for

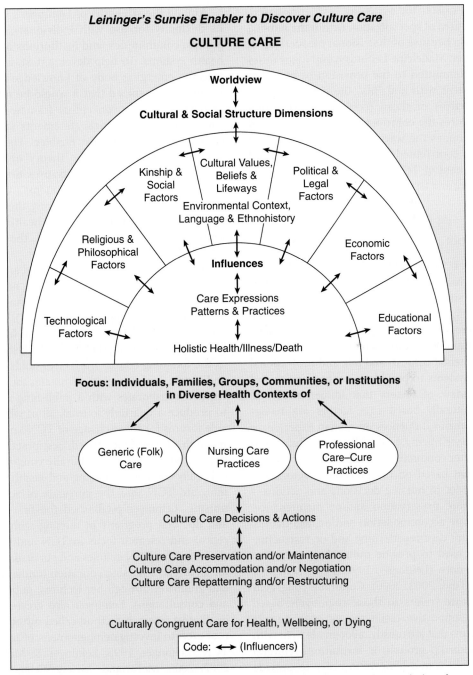

Figure 1-3. Leininger's Sunrise Enabler to discover culture care. (Reprinted by permission of McFarland, M. R., & Wehbe-Alamah, H. B. (2015). Leininger's sunrise enabler. In M. R. McFarland & H. B. Wehbe-Alamah (Eds.), *Culture care diversity and universality: A worldwide nursing theory* (3rd ed., p. 25). Burlington, MA: Jones and Bartlett Learning.)

use in studying topics relevant to nursing. Ray and colleagues studied caring, complexity science, and transcultural caring dynamics in nursing and healthcare (Davidson & Ray, 2011; Ray, 2010; Ray, Turkel, & Cohn, 2011). Lastly, Leininger's contributions to TCN rapidly gained global and interprofessional recognition as many health care professionals from medicine, physical therapy, occupational therapy, social work, and related disciplines learned about the Theory of Cultural Care Diversity and Universality and either adopted or adapted it to fit their respective disciplines.

As nursing and health care have become increasingly multicultural and diverse, TCN's relevance has increased as well. There also is heightened societal awareness that people of all cultures deserve to receive nursing and health care that are culturally congruent and culturally competent. **Cultural competence** refers to the complex integration of knowledge, attitudes, values, beliefs, behaviors, skills, practices, and cross-cultural encounters that include effective communication and the provision of safe, affordable, quality, accessible, evidence-based, and efficacious nursing care for individuals, families, groups, and communities of diverse and similar cultural backgrounds. Cultural competence is discussed in detail in Chapter 2.

Advancements in Transcultural Nursing

In addition to Leininger, many other TCN scholars and leaders around the world have made, and continue to make, significant contributions to the body of transcultural knowledge, research, theory, and evidence-based practices that guide nurses in the delivery of culturally congruent and culturally competent care for people from similar and diverse cultures (Clark, 2013; Courtney & Wolgamott, 2015; deRuyter, 2015; Eipperle, 2015; Larson, 2015; McFarland & Wehbe-Alamah, 2015a & b;McFarland, et al., 2015; Mixer, 2015; Raymond & Omeri, 2015). While the authors of this textbook have chosen to emphasize the research and theory generated by Leininger, there are many different ways to conceptualize TCN and deliver culturally congruent and culturally competent nursing care.

The following TCN scholars and leaders have enhanced, expanded, and advanced the specialty through their research, teaching, publications, conceptual models, frameworks, and/or theories: Josepha Campinha-Bacote (Campinha-Bacote, 2011), Geri-Ann Galanti (Gilanti, 2014), Joyce Newman Giger (Giger, 2013), Marianne Jeffreys (Jeffreys & Dogan, 2014), Larry Purnell (Purnell, 2014), Marilyn Ray (Davidson & Ray, 2011; Ray, 2010; Ray, Turkel, & Cohn, 2011), Priscilla Sagar (Sagar, 2012, 2014, 2015), Rachel Spector (Spector, 2013), and the late Ruth Davidhizar.

The Core Curriculum

In collaboration with a group of other TCN scholars and experts globally, the editor and associate editor of the JTN published the Core Curriculum in Transcultural Nursing and Health Care to "establish a core base of knowledge that supports TCN practice" (Douglas & Pacquiao, 2010, p. S5). The Core Curriculum marks the culmination of many years of research and theory development in TCN and draws on knowledge and research from the natural, social, and behavioral sciences; philosophy, theology, and religious studies; history; the fine arts; and applied or professional disciplines such as medicine, social work, education, and other fields. The Core Curriculum clearly identifies, delineates, and authoritatively establishes the core of knowledge that supports TCN practice.

The Core Curriculum includes the following:

- Contributions by many of the foremost experts in TCN from around the world who provide concrete and specific curricular outline for TCN.
- A comprehensive compendium that contains an overview of the key knowledge, research, evidence, and general content areas that collectively form the foundation for TCN practice.
- Content on subjects such as global health; comparative systems of health care delivery; cross-cultural communication; culturally based health and illness beliefs and practices across the lifespan; culturally based healing and care modalities; cultural health assessment; educational issues for students, organizational staff,

patients, and communities; organizational cultural competency; research methodologies for investigating cultural phenomena and evaluating interventions; and professional roles and attributes of the transcultural nurse.

- Content that will prepare nurses to take one or both of the examinations leading to transcultural nursing certification.
- Basic certification in transcultural nursing (CTN-B) and advanced certification in transcultural nursing (CTN-A). Both exams are offered by the TCNS's Certification Commission (Transcultural Nursing Certification Commission, 2007) and appear on the list of Magnet national certifications for inclusion on the Demographic Data Collection Tool. See Sagar (2015) for further information about certification in TCN.

The Core Curriculum also is used in schools of nursing, hospitals, health departments, and other health care organizations to determine the key content to be included in seminars, workshops, conferences, and credit-bearing and continuing professional development courses on TCN and cultural competency. Those interested in cultural competence, multiculturalism, diversity, and related topics from multiple disciplines will also find valuable information in the Core Curriculum. As scientific, technological, and discipline-specific advances are made in TCN, the Core Curriculum will be updated and refined.

The coauthors of this book contributed to the Core Curriculum, as did many of the chapter contributors; therefore, the key concepts contained in the Core Curriculum also are found in this book.

Andrews/Boyle Transcultural Interprofessional Practice (TIP) Model

Conceptual frameworks, theoretical models, and theories in nursing are structured ideas about human beings and their health. Models enable nurses and other health care team members to organize and understand what happens in

practice, critically analyze situations for clinical decision making, develop a plan of care, propose appropriate nursing interventions, predict the outcomes from the care, and evaluate the effectiveness of the care provided (Alligood, 2014).

Goals, Assumptions, and Components of the Model

The goals of the Andrews/Boyle TIP Model are to:

- Provide a systematic, logical, orderly, scientific process for delivering culturally congruent, culturally competent, safe, affordable, accessible, and quality care to people from diverse backgrounds across the lifespan
- Facilitate the delivery of nursing and health care that is beneficial, meaningful, relevant, culturally congruent, culturally competent, and consistent with the cultural beliefs and practices of clients from diverse backgrounds
- Provide a conceptual framework to guide nurses in the delivery of culturally congruent and competent care that is theoretically sound, evidence based, and utilizes best professional practices

Fundamental assumptions underlying the TIP Model include those related to TCN (Box 1-1), humans (Box 1-2), and cross-cultural communication between and among team members (Box 1-3). These assumptions are ideas that are formed or taken for granted as having veracity without proof or evidence. Assumptions are useful in providing a basis for action and in creating "what if..." scenarios to simulate possible situations until such time as there is proof or evidence available to corroborate or refute the assumption.

The TIP Model consists of the following interconnected and interrelated components: the **context** from which people's health-related values, attitudes, beliefs, and practices emerge; the **interprofessional health care team; communication**; and the **problem-solving process**.

Cultural Context

Derived from the Latin *contexere* (*con-* meaning together and *texere* meaning to weave or

Box 1-1 Assumptions about Transcultural Nursing

- Transcultural nursing is a theoretical and evidence-based formal area of study and practice within professional nursing that focuses on people's culturally based beliefs, attitudes, values, behaviors, and practices related to wellness, health, birth, illness, healing, dying, and death.
- Transcultural nursing requires that nurses engage in an ongoing process of constructively critical, reflective self-assessment that enables them to identify their own culturally based values, attitudes, beliefs, behaviors, biases, stereotypes, prejudices, and practices.
- Transcultural nursing knowledge is interconnected with the knowledge, research, and scholarship of other disciplines in the natural sciences (e.g., biology, chemistry, physics), social and behavioral sciences (e.g., anthropology, sociology, psychology, economics, political science), professional disciplines (e.g., medicine, pharmacy, social work, education), and the humanities (e.g., music, art, history, languages, philosophy, theater).
- Transcultural nursing practice encompasses autonomous and collaborative care of individuals of all ages across the lifespan whether they are sick or well, able or disabled.
- Transcultural nursing engages nurses the care of families, groups, populations, and communities globally.
- Transcultural nursing includes the promotion of health, prevention of disease, and the care of sick, ill, disabled, and dying people from diverse cultures across the lifespan from birth to old age.
- Transcultural nursing roles include advocacy, research, health policy development, health systems leadership, management, education, clinical practice, and consultation.
- Transcultural nursing practice requires that nurses establish and maintain a caring, empa-

thetic, therapeutic relationship with clients and a collaborative, collegial relationship with other members of the interprofessional health care team.
- Transcultural nursing assessment is facilitated when the nurse's communications are client-centered and focused on establishing and maintaining a therapeutic nurse–client relationship.
- Transcultural nursing practice requires that nurses be aware of changes in the world that influence and challenge their knowledge of the unfolding meaning of diversity and the need for the delivery of nursing and health care that is respectful and responsive to individual needs and differences of the people and communities served.
- Transcultural nursing practice encompasses autonomous and collaborative care of individuals of all ages, families, groups, and communities, sick or well and in all settings.
- Transcultural nursing practice requires that nurses establish and maintain a caring, empathetic, therapeutic relationship with clients; formally educated and/ or licensed credentialed healers, such as registered nurses, licensed physicians, and other health professionals; and folk, traditional, religious, spiritual, and other healers identified by clients as significant to their health and well-being.
- In transcultural nursing practice, the nurse's communications are other oriented and focused on what is best for the client's health well-being, recovery, or peaceful death.
- Transcultural nursing practice requires that nurses be respectful and responsive to individual needs and differences of the people and communities served.

braid), the term context refers to the conditions, circumstances, and/or situations that exist when and where something happens, thereby providing meaning to what transpired. In the TIP Model, the following factors contribute to

the cultural context of human experiences and need to be assessed, interpreted, examined, and evaluated when clients interact with nurses and other members of the interprofessional health care team: environmental, social, economic,

Box 1-2 Assumptions about Humans

- Humans are complex biological, cultural, psychosocial, spiritual beings who experience health and illness along a continuum throughout the span of their lives from birth to death.
- All humans have the right to safe, accessible, and affordable nursing and health care, regardless of national origin, race, ethnicity, gender, age, socioeconomic background, religion, sexual orientation, size, and related characteristics.
- Whether rich or poor; educated or illiterate; religious or nonbelieving; male or female; black, white, yellow, red, or brown, each person deserves to be respected by nurses and other health members of the health care team.
- As people from different racial, ethnic, and cultural backgrounds travel and comingle with those having backgrounds that differ from their own, the likelihood of intermarriage and offspring of mixed racial and ethnic heritage increases.
- Regardless of their national origin or current citizenship, humans around the world share culture-universal needs for food, shelter, safety, and love; seek well-being and health; and endeavor to avoid, alleviate, or eliminate the pain and suffering associated with disease, illness, dying, and death.
- Although humans have common culture-universal needs, they also have culture-specific needs that are interconnected with their health-related values, attitudes, beliefs, and practices.
- In times of health and illness, humans seek the therapeutic (beneficial) assistance of various types of healers to promote health and well-being, prevent disease, and recover from illness or injury.
- Humans seek therapeutic interventions from family and significant others; credentialed or licensed health care providers; folk, traditional, indigenous, religious, and/or spiritual healers; and companion or therapy animals and pets as they perceive appropriate for their condition, situation, or problem.
- Interventions are judged to have a therapeutic effect when they result in a desirable and beneficial outcome, whether the outcome was expected, unexpected, or even an unintended consequence of the intervention.

Box 1-3 Assumptions about Effective Communication

- Effective communication begins with an assessment of the client's ability to read, write, speak, and comprehend messages.
- Effective communication in contemporary society sometimes requires literacy in the use of computers, smartphones, and numerous technology-assisted medical or health devices.
- Effective communication includes the ability to convey sincere interest in others, patience, and willingness to intervene or begin again when misunderstandings occur.
- To provide safe, quality, affordable, accessible, efficacious, culturally congruent, and culturally competent nursing and health care, members of the interprofessional health care team must communicate effectively.
- Communication occurs verbally, nonverbally, in writing, and in combination with technology.
- Communication should be appropriate for the client's age, gender, health status, health literacy, and related factors.
- When nurses communicate with others from cultural and linguistic backgrounds different from their own, the probability of miscommunication increases significantly.
- In promoting effective cross-cultural communication with clients from diverse backgrounds, nurses should avoid technical jargon, slang, colloquial expressions, abbreviations, and excessive use of medical terminology.

religious, philosophical, moral, legal, political, educational, biological (genetic/inherited factors), and technological. In TCN, culture is the lens through which nurses see the world, their clients, and other members of the team. When culture is interwoven with the other factors (see Figure 1-4), it forms the health-related cultural values, attitudes, beliefs, and practices of humans worldwide, including clients and other members of the team.

Interprofessional Health Care Team

The transcultural interprofessional health care team has at its core the *client*, who is the team's *raison d'etre* (reason for being). In addition to the client, the team may have one or more of the following members:

- The *client's family*, and *others significant in his or her life*, including a legally appointed *guardian* who might not be genetically related
- *Credentialed health professionals* such as nurses; physicians; physical, occupational, respiratory, music, art, dance, recreational, and other therapists; social workers; health navigators; public and community health workers; and related professionals with formal academic preparation, licensure, and/or certification
- *Folk, indigenous, or traditional healers*—unlicensed individuals who learn healing arts and practices through study, observation, apprenticeship, imitation, and sometimes by inheriting healing powers, for example, herbalists, curanderos, medicine men/women, Amish brauchers, bonesetters, lay midwives, sabadors, and healers with related names

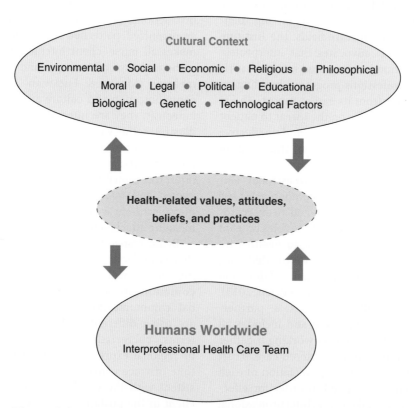

Figure 1-4. Influence of cultural context on health values, beliefs, and practices of the interprofessional health care team. (© Margaret M. Andrews.)

- *Religious or spiritual healers*—clergy or lay members of religious groups who heal through prayer, religious or spiritual rituals, faith healing practices, and related actions or interventions, for example, priests, priestesses, elders, rabbis, imams, monks, Christian Science practitioners, and others believed to have healing powers derived from faith, spiritual powers, or religion.
- *Others* identified by the client as significant to his or her health, well-being, or healing such as companion animals or pets as culturally appropriate.

The World Health Organization defines **interprofessional collaboration** as multiple health workers from different professional backgrounds working together with patients, families, caregivers, and communities to deliver the highest quality of care (World Health Organization, 2013). In collaboration with leaders in nursing, dentistry, and other health care fields, the Institute of Medicine (2011) advocates that interprofessional collaboration be integrated into the curricula of health professions programs, building on recommendations from its earlier report, *To Err is Human*, which focuses on the threat to patient safety caused by human error and ineffective interprofessional communication (Institute of Medicine, 1999).

To be successful in interprofessional collaboration, the following core competencies are required: values and ethics related to interprofessional practice, knowledge of the roles of team members, and a team approach to health care (Fulmer & Gaines, 2014; Institute of Medicine, 1999, 2011; Interprofessional Education Collaborative Expert Panel, 2011; O'Brien, 2013). Interprofessional collaboration is a partnership that starts with the client and includes all involved health care providers working together to deliver client and family-centered care. Trust must be established and an appreciation of each other's roles must be gained in order for effective collaboration to take place (Interprofessional Education Collaborative Expert Panel). Health

professionals must recognize their own individual scope of practice and skill set and have an awareness of and appreciation for other health professionals' capacity to contribute to the delivery of care to clients in order to achieve optimal health outcomes. Working as a member of an interprofessional team requires communication, cooperation, and collaboration (Fulmer & Gaines, 2014; Institute of Medicine, 2011; Interprofessional Education Collaborative Expert Panel, 2011).

Communication

Derived from the Latin verb *communicare*, meaning to share, **communication** refers to the meaningful exchange of information between one or more participants. The information exchanged may be conveyed through ideas, feelings, intentions, attitudes, expectations, perceptions, instructions, or commands. Communication is an organized, patterned system of behavior that makes all nurse–client interactions possible. It is the exchange of messages and the creation of meaning (Munoz & Luckman, 2008). Because communication and culture are acquired simultaneously, they are integrally linked. Figure 1-5 illustrates the ways in which communication, cultural context, and health-related values, attitudes, beliefs, and practices of members of the interprofessional health care team are interconnected and interrelated. In effective communication, there is mutual understanding of the meaning attached to the messages.

Being respectful and polite, using language that is understood by the other(s), and speaking clearly will facilitate **verbal** (or spoken) **communication**. Barriers to effective verbal communication occur when participants are using different languages; when technical terms, abbreviations, idioms, colloquialisms, or regional expressions are used; or when the tone of voice conveys a message that is inconsistent with the words spoken, for example, a client in the postanesthesia care unit following major surgery verbally denies having pain, but

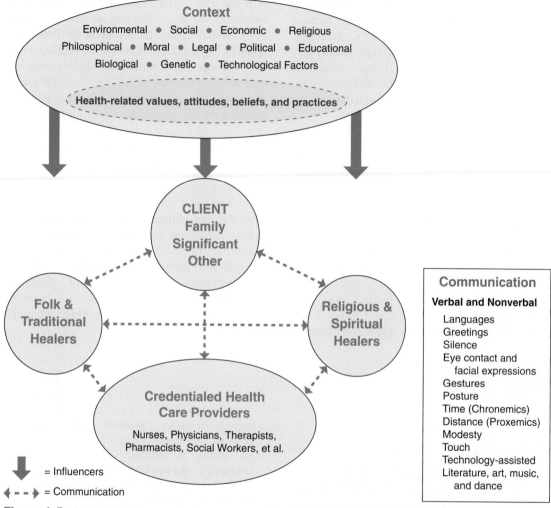

Figure 1-5. Cross-cultural communication among members of the interprofessional health care team—clients, family, significant others, credentialed health professionals, and folk, traditional, religious, and spiritual healers. (© Margaret M. Andrews.)

the nurse observes that the client has clenched teeth, taught muscles, pursed lips, and a wrinkled brow, all of which are nonverbal indicators of pain. Whereas **language** refers to what is said, **paralanguage** refers to *how* it is said and relates to all aspects of the voice that are not part of the verbal message. Paralanguage may modify or nuance meaning or convey emotion through rhythm, pitch, stress, volume, speed, hesitations, or intonation. For example, consider the sentence, "I would like to help you." By placing the emphasis on the words I, like, help, and you in four different sentences, the meaning of the sentence changes significantly. **Nonverbal communication** refers to how people convey meaning without words, for example, through the use of facial expressions, gestures, posture (body language), and the physical distance between the communicators (proxemics).

The many nuances of verbal and nonverbal communication are interconnected, interwoven, interrelated, and often embedded in one another.

Aspects of communication that are of particular importance for the transcultural nurse include language, the use of interpreters, greetings, silence, eye contact and facial expressions, gestures, posture, chronemics (time), proxemics, modesty, touch, technology-assisted communication, and literature, art, music, and dance.

Language

More than 6,000 languages are spoken throughout the world; 382 individual languages and language groups are spoken in the United States alone, where nearly 60 million people, ages 5 years or older, speak a language other than English at home (U.S. Census Bureau, 2013a). Fifty-six percent of the people who speak a language other than English at home report they speak English "very well" (U.S. Census Bureau, 2013b, p. 9). Spanish is the second most commonly spoken language in the United States, spoken by 37 million people age 5 and older; 9%

of those individuals indicated that they did not speak English at all (U.S. Census Bureau, 2013b, p. 3). After English (230.9 million speakers) and Spanish (37.5 million), Chinese (2.8 million) was the language most commonly spoken at home (U.S. Census Bureau, 2013b, pp. 5–6). Language is one of the primary ways that culture is transmitted from one generation to the next.

Interpreters

One of the greatest challenges in cross-cultural communication for nurses occurs when the nurse and client speak different languages. After assessing the language skills of the client who speaks a different language from the nurse, the nurse may be in one of two situations: either struggling to communicate effectively through an interpreter or communicating effectively when there is no interpreter. Box 1-4 provides recommendations for overcoming language barriers.

Box 1-4 Overcoming Language Barriers

Using an Interpreter

- Before locating an interpreter, determine the language the client speaks at home; it may be different from the language spoken publicly (e.g., French is sometimes spoken by well-educated and upper-class members of certain Asian or Middle Eastern cultures).
- After assessing client's health literacy, use electronic devices such as cell phones, tablets, and laptop computers to connect client with Web-based translation programs.
- Avoid interpreters from a rival tribe, state, region, or nation (e.g., a Palestinian who knows Hebrew may not be the best interpreter for a Jewish client).
- Be aware of gender differences between interpreter and client. In general, the same gender is preferred.
- Be aware of age differences between interpreter and client. In general, an older, more

mature interpreter is preferred to a younger, less experienced one.
- Be aware of socioeconomic differences between interpreter and client.
- Ask the interpreter to translate as closely to verbatim as possible.
- Expect an interpreter who is not a relative to seek compensation for services rendered.

Recommendations for Institutions

- Keep pace with assistive equipment and technology for people who are deaf, hard of hearing, blind, visually impaired, and/or disabled.
- Maintain a computerized list of interpreters, including those certified in sign language, who may be contacted as needed.
- Network with area hospitals, colleges, universities, and other organizations that may serve as resources.

What To Do When There Is No Interpreter

- Be polite and formal.
- Greet the person using the last or complete name. Gesture to yourself and say your name. Offer a handshake or nod. Smile.
- Proceed in an unhurried manner. Pay attention to any effort by the patient or family to communicate.
- Speak in a low, moderate voice. Avoid talking loudly. There is often a tendency to raise the volume and pitch of your voice when the listener appears not to understand, but this may lead the listener to perceive that the nurse is shouting and/or angry.
- Use any words known in the patient's language. This indicates that the nurse is aware of and respects the client's culture.
- Use simple words, such as *pain* instead of *discomfort*. Avoid medical jargon, idioms, and slang. Avoid using contractions. Use nouns repeatedly instead of pronouns. For example, do *not* say, "He has been taking his medicine, hasn't he?" Do say, "Does Juan take medicine?"
- Pantomime words and simple actions while verbalizing them.
- Give instructions in the proper sequence. For example, do *not* say, "Before you rinse the bottle, sterilize it." Do say, "First, wash the bottle. Second, rinse the bottle."
- Discuss one topic at a time. Avoid using conjunctions. For example, do *not* say, "Are you cold and in pain?" Do say, "Are you cold [while pantomiming]?" "Are you in pain?"
- Validate whether the client understands by having him or her repeat instructions, demonstrate the procedure, or act out the meaning.
- Write out several short sentences in English, and determine the person's ability to read them.
- Try a third language. Many Southeast Asians speak French. Europeans often know three or four languages. Or, try Latin words or phrases.
- Ask if any of the client's family and friends could serve as an interpreter.
- Obtain phrase books from a library or bookstore, make or purchase flash cards, contact hospitals for a list of interpreters, and use both formal and informal networking to locate a suitable interpreter.

Adapted from Andrews, M. (2000). Transcultural considerations in health assessment. In C. Jarvis (Ed.), *Physical examination and health assessment* (p. 69). Philadelphia, PA: W.B. Saunders.

Even a person from another culture or country who has a basic command of the language spoken by the majority of nurses and other health professionals may need an interpreter when faced with the anxiety-provoking situation of entering a hospital, encountering an unfamiliar symptom, or discussing a sensitive topic such as birth control or gynecologic or urologic concerns. A trained medical interpreter knows interpreting techniques, has knowledge of medical terminology, and understands patients' rights. The trained interpreter is also knowledgeable about cultural beliefs and health practices. This person can help bridge the cultural gap and can give advice concerning the cultural appropriateness of nursing and medical recommendations.

Although the nurse is in charge of the focus and flow of the interview, the interpreter should be viewed as an important member of the health care team. It can be tempting to ask a relative, a friend, or even another client to interpret because this person is readily available and likely is willing to help. However, this violates confidentiality for the client, who may not want personal information shared. Furthermore, the friend or relative, though fluent in ordinary language usage, is likely to be unfamiliar with medical terminology, hospital or clinic procedures, and health care ethics. In ideal circumstances, ask the interpreter to meet the client beforehand to establish rapport and obtain basic descriptive information about the client such as age, occupation, educational level, and attitude toward health care. This eases the interpreter and client into the relationship and allows the client to talk about aspects of his or her life that are relatively nonthreatening.

When using an interpreter, expect that the interaction with the client will require more time than is needed if the nurse and client speak the same language. It will be necessary to organize nursing care so that the most important interactions or procedures are accomplished first, before the client becomes fatigued. In the absence of an interpreter, try using electronic devices with translation software and other applications that may be helpful in effectively communicating and delivering care for people who speak a language different from the nurse.

Greetings

Some cultures value formal greetings at the start of the day or whenever the first encounter of the day occurs—a practice found even among close family members. When communicating with people from cultures that tend to be more formal, it is important to call a person by his or her title, such as Mr., Mrs., Ms., Dr., Reverend, and related greeting as a sign of respect, and until such time as the individual gives permission to address them less formally. The recommended best practice at the time the nurse initially meets a client or new member of the health care team is to state his or her name and then ask the client or team member by what name he or she prefers to be called.

Silence

Wide cultural variations exist in the interpretation of silence. Some individuals find silence extremely uncomfortable and make every effort to fill conversational lags with words. By contrast, many Native Americans consider silence essential to understanding and respecting the other person. A pause following a question signifies that what has been asked is important enough to be given thoughtful consideration. In traditional Chinese and Japanese cultures, silence may mean that the speaker wishes the listener to consider the content of what has been said before continuing. Other cultural meanings of silence may be found. Arabs may use silence out of respect for another's privacy, whereas people of French, Spanish, and Russian descent may interpret it as a sign of agreement. Asian cultures often use silence to demonstrate respect for elders. Among some African Americans, silence is used in response to a question perceived as inappropriate.

Eye Contact and Facial Expressions

Eye contact and facial expressions are the most prominent forms of nonverbal communication. Eye contact is a key factor in setting the tone of the communication between two people and differs greatly between cultures and countries. In the United States, Canada, Western Europe, and most parts of Australia, eye contact is interpreted similarly: conveying interest, active engagement with the other person, forthrightness, and honesty. People who avoid eye contact when speaking are viewed negatively and may be perceived as withholding information and/or lacking in confidence. In some parts of Asia, Africa, and the Middle East, and certain Native American nations, however, direct eye contact may be seen as disrespectful, a sign of aggression, or a sign that the other person's authority is being challenged. In some cultures, staring at someone for a prolonged period of time communicates that the person doing the staring has a sexual interest in the other person. People who make eye contact, but only briefly, are viewed as respectful and courteous. In some Native American cultures, the person might look at the floor while someone in a position of authority is speaking as a sign of respect and interest. Among some African American and White cultures, *occulistics* (eye rolling) takes place when someone speaks or behaves in a manner that is regarded as inappropriate.

Strongly influenced by a person's cultural background, facial expressions include *affective displays* that reveal emotions, such as happiness through a smile or sadness through crying, and various other nonverbal gestures that may be perceived as appropriate or inappropriate according to the person's age and gender. These nonverbal expressions are often unintentional and can conflict with what is being said verbally.

Gestures

Gestures that serve the same function as words are referred to as *emblems*. Examples of emblems include signals that mean okay, the "thumbs up" gesture, the "come here" hand movement, or the hand gesture used when hitchhiking. Gestures that accompany words to illustrate a verbal message are known as *illustrators*. Illustrators mimic the spoken word, such as pointing to the right or left while verbally saying the words right or left. *Regulators* convey meaning through gestures such as raising one's hand before verbally asking a question. Regulators also include head nodding and short sounds such as "uh huh" or "Hmmmm" and other expressions of interest or boredom. Without feedback, some people find it difficult to carry on a conversation. *Adaptors* are nonverbal behavior that either satisfy some physical need such as scratching or adjusting eyeglasses or represent a psychological need such as biting fingernails when nervous, yawning when bored, or clenching a fist when angry. Although normally subconscious, adaptors are more likely to be restrained in public places than in private gatherings of people. Adaptive behaviors often accompany feelings of anxiety or hostility (Galvin, Prescott & Huseman, 1988). All of the nonverbal communication previously described varies widely cross-culturally and cross-nationally.

Posture

Posture reflects people's emotions, attitudes, and intentions. Posture may be open or closed and is believed to convey an individual's degree of confidence, status, or receptivity to another person. An open posture is characterized by hands apart or comfortably placed on the arms of a chair while directly facing the person speaking. The person often leans forward, toward the speaker. Open posture communicates interest in someone and a readiness to listen. Someone seated in a closed posture might have his or her arms folded, legs crossed, or be positioned at a slight angle from the person with whom they are interacting. The person may also allow his or her eyes to dart quickly from one spot to another in an unfocused, distracted manner. Closed posture usually conveys disinterest or discomfort.

Chronemics

There are cultural variations in how people understand and use time. **Chronemics** is the study of the use of time in nonverbal communication. The manner in which a person perceives and values time, structures time, and reacts to time contributes to the context of communication. Social scientists have discovered that individuals are divided in two major groups in the ways they approach time: **monochronic** or **polychronic**. In monochronic cultures, such as many groups in the United States, Northern Europe, Israel, and much of Australia, time is seen as a commodity, and people tend to use expressions such as "waste time" or "lose time" or "time is money." Given that time is so highly valued, showing up late, especially for a meeting or a dinner, is usually perceived as very disrespectful to the individuals who are made to "waste their time" waiting (Lombardo, n.d.). A monochronic culture functions on clock time. People tend to focus on one thing at a time and usually prefer to complete objectives in a systematic way. In a meeting, for example, it's considered culturally appropriate to follow the predetermined agenda and avoid straying from the agenda by talking about unrelated topics (Rutledge, 2013).

People in polychronic cultures, such as some groups in Southern Europe, Latin America, Africa, and the Middle East, take a very different view of time. People from these cultures often believe that time cannot be controlled, and it is flexible. Days are planned based on events rather than the clock. For many people in these cultures, when one event is finished, it is time to start the next, regardless of what time it is. In a polychronic culture, following an agenda might not be very important. Instead, many tasks, such as building relationships, negotiating, and/or problem solving, can be accomplished at the same time. In many Asian cultures, such as Japanese,

Chinese, and Taiwanese groups, people tend to arrive a little early. In many parts of Europe, the United States, Canada, Israel, and Australia, people tend to arrive precisely on time and may perceive it as an inconvenience to others if they arrive too early. In many parts of Latin America, Arab areas in the Middle East, and Africa, people tend to be more flexible in their notion of arrival times and may show up significantly later than the mutually agreed-upon time. Among certain Native American groups, an appointment or event begins "when everyone arrives," and there is considerable tolerance for those who show up after the appointed time. These examples are stereotypes, and not all of members of a culture or subculture will perceive time in the same manner.

Proxemics

Another form of nonverbal communication is manifested in closeness and **personal space**. The study of space and how differences in that space can make people feel more relaxed or more anxious is referred to as **proxemics**, a term that was coined in the 1950s by the anthropologist and cross-cultural researcher Edward T. Hall. Distances have been identified based on the relationship between or among the people involved: (1) *Intimate space* (touching to 1 foot) is typically reserved for whispering and embracing; nurses and other health care providers, however, sometimes need to enter this intimate space when providing care for clients. (2) *Personal space* (ranges from 2 to 4 feet) is used among family and friends or to separate people waiting in line at the drug store or ATM machine. (3) *Social space* (4 to 10 feet) is used for communication among business or work associates and to separate strangers, such as those taking a course on natural child birth. (4) *Public space* (12 to 25 feet) is the distance maintained between a speaker and the audience (Hall, 1984, 1990).

Cultural and ethnic variations occur in proxemics. For example, when having a conversation, people from Arab parts of the Middle East, France, and Latin America generally prefer to stand closer to one another than those from Canadian, American, and British cultures, who also tend to feel more uncomfortable when they have to sit close to one another (Munoz & Luckmann, 2008). There are also important gender and age factors to consider in cross-cultural communication. In general, clients are likely to prefer a nurse or other health care provider of the *same gender*, particularly when care requires entering his or her personal space and/or touching the client. Similarly, the same gender may be preferred when the health history and/or physical examination includes the reproductive organs. In some ethnic and religious groups, it may be inappropriate or forbidden for health care providers of the opposite gender to shake hands, provide care, or otherwise touch the client. For example, observant Muslim women are not permitted to shake hands with male physicians, nurses, or other health professionals. As a sign of respect to the man, some Muslim women will place one or both arms over their chest and slightly bow their head. Whenever an observant Muslim is having a conversation with a person of the opposite gender, a third person needs to be present to avoid the appearance of impropriety. Among some people from Chinese, Japanese, or other Asian cultures, there may be both gender and age factors to be considered in cross-cultural communication.

Modesty

Modesty is a form of mixed nonverbal and verbal communication that refers to reserve or propriety in speech, dress, or behavior. It conveys a message that is intended to avoid encouraging sexual attention or attraction in others (aside from a person's spouse). In cultures that have been studied by anthropologists or transcultural nurses, men and women have cultural beliefs about modesty and rules concerning which behavior and dress are appropriate in various situations and circumstances. The following are examples of groups that have required rules or optional guidelines pertaining to modesty.

Traditional Muslim women beyond the age of puberty wear a headscarf to cover their head and hair as a sign of modesty and religious faith. The word **hijab** describes the act of covering up generally but is sometimes used to describe the headscarves worn by Muslim women (Figure 1-6). These scarves come in many styles and colors and have different names around the world, such as niqab, al mira, Shayla, khimar, chador, and burka. The type of hijab most commonly worn in the United States, Canada, Australia, and Western Europe covers the head and neck but leaves the face clear. In various parts of the Arab world, cultural expectations for women may include covering the head, face, neck, or the entire body in order to conform to certain standards of modesty established by various Islamic denominations and groups. The burka is the most concealing of all Islamic coverings. It is a one-piece veil that conceals the face and body, often leaving just a mesh screen to see through. There are differences between modesty at home and modesty in public. At home, Muslim women typically do not wear veils, scarves, or other coverings in the presence of male family members such as their fathers, husbands, sons, and other male or female relatives.

Women from observant Orthodox and Hasidic Judaism, Amish, Mennonite, and some conservative Catholics cover their heads, arms, and/or legs as a cultural and/or religious expression of modesty and often as a sign of their affiliation with a particular religious order within Catholicism. The Hebrew word *tznius* or *tzniut* means modesty. It is generally used in reference to women and also relates to humility and general conduct, especially between men and women. Hasidic, Sikh, and Amish men often cover their heads and/or wear clothing that conveys modesty. For Buddhists, modesty is the quality of being unpretentious about one's virtues or achievements. The most important thing is not what type of clothes an individual wears or their color, but the quality of his or her heart. Buddhist monks have modesty guidelines pertaining to the manner in which they wear their robes, never allowing skin to show on both sides of the body.

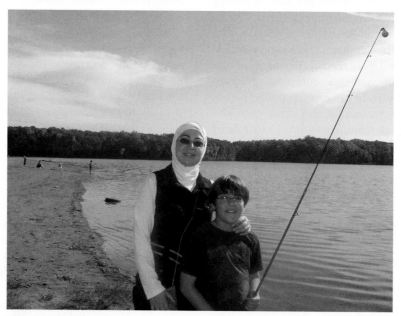

Figure 1-6. When in public places, some Muslim women wear a headscarf (hijab) to cover their hair, head, and neck, as a sign of modesty and religious faith.

The Church of Jesus Christ of Latter-day Saints (LDS), also known as the Mormon Church, has issued official statements on modesty and dress for its members. Modesty is an attitude of propriety and decency in dress, grooming, language, and behavior. Clothing such as "short shorts" and short skirts, shirts that do not cover the stomach, and clothing that does not cover the shoulders or is low cut in the front or the back are discouraged. Men and women are also encouraged to avoid extremes in clothing or hairstyles. Most LDS members do not wear sleeveless shirts or blouses or shorts that fail to reach the knee. Women do not wear pants or slacks to religious services, and members of both genders attend services well-groomed and well-dressed (Church of Jesus Christ of Latter Day Saints, 2014).

All cultures have rules, often unwritten, concerning who may touch whom, where, when, how, for what reason, and for how long. In general, it is best for nurses to refrain from touching clients or coworkers of either gender unless necessary for the accomplishment of a job-related task, such as the provision of safe client care. Typically, people from Asian cultures are not as overtly demonstrative of affection or as tactile as Whites, Hispanics, or African Americans. Generally, they refrain from public embraces, kissing, loud talking, laughter, and boisterous behavior in public. Affection is expressed in a more reserved manner, usually in private rather than public places. In some instances, nurses and other members of the health care team from cultures that differ from the client's may send unintended messages through their use of touch. Special attention to male–female relationships and to the age of the client is warranted in nurse–client interactions and especially when it is necessary to touch members of the opposite gender.

Technology-Assisted Communication

Communication sometimes uses a combination of verbal, nonverbal, and written signals. With innovations in health care devices and software, technological advances are changing how care is delivered and the nature of the nursing profession. One of the major challenges of technology from a transcultural perspective is the gap between the regions and nations that have greater resources than others. While some strides are being made, it will still be many years before technological capabilities are mobilized in ways that benefit people globally by enhancing safe, quality, accessible, affordable, evidence-based, culturally congruent, and culturally competent nursing and health care. This is a matter of social justice that needs to be addressed as an integral component of TCN.

Although linguists have known that language changes over time, the digital language is changing faster than any other language in recorded history. For example, the first chat room was invented at the University of Illinois in 1973. In 1992, the first mobile text message was sent. By 2012, people in the world were sending 200,000 texts per second (Eisinger, 2012).

Ninety percent of Whites, 90% of African Americans, and 92% of Hispanics own cell phones (Pew Internet Research Center, 2014). Seventy-two percent of all English-speaking adults send text messages (68% of Whites, 79% of Blacks, and 83% of Hispanics). As text messaging increases, the number of minutes spent on the phone decreases. The average person in the United States looks at his or her phone 150 times per day (My Cloud Media Company, 2014). In many health care agencies, nurses are given smartphones, pagers, tablets, and other technology-assisted devices for job-related activities to improve patient outcomes.

While the Internet, social media, and texting enable people to communicate more often, use of technology is primarily about saving time or taking digital shortcuts. It has become easy for nurses to use technology instead of interacting more directly with clients or other members of the health care team. While the digital shortcuts may be expedient and time-saving, the quality of the communication for this generation and the next is currently being studied to determine the ways in which technology is rewriting the

neuropathways in children's brains (Brackett et al., 2013). Between television, tablets, video games, and smartphones, the average child in the United States spends nearly 8 hours each day staring at a screen (Blue Cross/Blue Shield, 2014). When children—or adults—spend so much time communicating through technology, they're not developing their verbal or emotional skills; screen time needs to be balanced with face time. An emoji cannot truly convey emotion—☺ is not the same as a human smile—nor can a text message replace a warm embrace or hug when a client needs emotional support from family and friends during times of injury or illness. Nurses and other members of the health care team need to communicate in multiple ways, balancing face to face and digital interactions. It is important for the nurse to identify the client's preferred mode for communication as an integral component of the overall assessment of communication used by the client, his or her family, and significant others.

Literature, Art, Music, and Dance

The literature, art, music, and dance of various cultural groups communicate to the world the cherished values, beliefs, history, traditions, and contributions of people from nations, tribes, and population groups. The creative products, in the form of books, poems, artwork, music, and dance, describe the social climate of the day; portray religious, racial, gender, political, class, and other perspectives; and serve as unique historical documents and artifacts to help people better see, hear, know, understand, and appreciate the richness of the world's diverse cultures as they are communicated through the literary works, artistic and musical creations, and dance of people from cultures around the world.

Problem-Solving Process

The TIP Model is intended to guide members of the interprofessional health care team in determining what decisions, actions, and interventions the client needs to achieve an optimal state of

well-being and health. As indicated in Figure 1-7, the model helps nurses to conceptualize the care of people from diverse backgrounds in a logical, orderly, systematic, scientific five-step process:

1. A comprehensive cultural **assessment**. The cultural assessment includes a self-assessment and a holistic assessment of the client that includes a health history and physical examination (Chapter 3 provides an in-depth discussion of these topics).

2. **Mutual goal setting** that takes into account the perspectives of each member of the health care team—the client, the client's family and significant others, and all those who are co-participants with the client in the decision-making and goal-setting processes including credentialed health professionals and folk, traditional, indigenous, religious, and/or spiritual healers.

3. **Planning** care that includes input from and dialogue with members of the interprofessional health care team.

4. **Implementation** of the care plan through a wide range of actions and interventions.

5. **Evaluation** of the care plan from multiple, diverse perspectives to determine the degree to which the plan (a) is effective in achieving the intended goal(s); (b) provides care that is *culturally congruent* with and fits the client's culturally based beliefs and practices related to wellness, health, illness, disease, healing, dying, and death; (c) reflects the delivery of *culturally competent* care by nurses and other members of the interprofessional team; (d) provides *quality* care that is *safe, affordable,* and *accessible*; and (e) integrates *research, evidence-based, and best practices* (Melnyk, 2015) into the care.

Data from the formal evaluation of the plan guide the nurses and other team members in determining if modifications or changes to the plan are necessary to accomplish the mutual goal(s) in step two or if new goals need to be discussed, proposed, planned, and established. If changes are needed, return to assessment, the first step

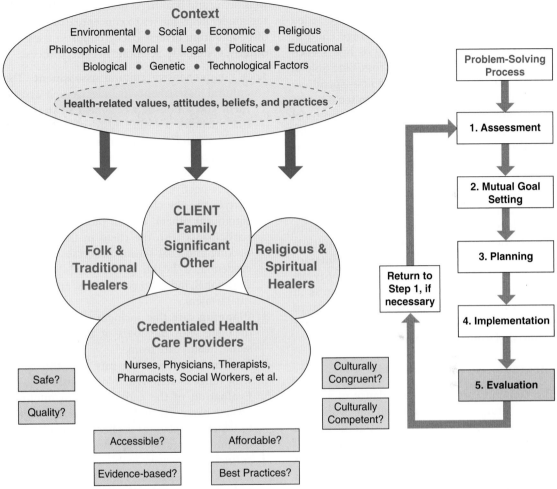

Figure 1-7. The five-step problem-solving process is a key part of the Transcultural Interprofessional Practice (TIP) Model. This client-centered model also includes the context from which people's health-related values, attitudes, beliefs, and practices emerge; the interprofessional health care team; and communication. (© Margaret M. Andrews.)

in the problem-solving process, and repeat the other steps as appropriate until each of the mutual goals is met.

As indicated in Benner's classic work titled, From Novice to Expert, in the acquisition and development of problem-solving skills, a nurse passes through levels of proficiency: novice, advanced beginner, competent, proficient, and expert (Benner, 1984). The development of proficiency in using the previously described problem-solving process requires time and repeated

simulated and/or in situ clinical experiences. As Benner aptly observes, the process leading to proficiency as an expert takes place gradually and seldom follows a direct pathway from novice to expert, rather a nurse passes through the intermediate stages, sometimes regressing to an earlier stage of competence, other times catapulting to a more advanced stage (Benner, 1984; Benner, Sutphen, Leonard, & Day, 2010). The process of developing competence in clinical problem solving is uneven and nonlinear, as is the process of

developing cultural competence, a topic that is discussed in the next chapter.

Summary

In this chapter, we examined the historical and theoretical foundations of TCN and its close ties with anthropology. In the mid-20th century, Madeleine Leininger, a visionary nurse–anthropologist, created the infrastructure to support, develop, and expand TCN by establishing the TCNS, the JTN, graduate programs in TCN at schools of nursing, and by creating the ethnonursing research method. We also explored the contributions of selected TCN leaders and scholars to the advancement of TCN practice, research, and theory. Lastly, we described the TIP Model that serves as a framework for nurses seeking to collaborate with clients and other members of the health care team in the delivery of quality nursing care that is beneficial, meaningful, relevant, culturally congruent, culturally competent, and consistent with the cultural beliefs and practices of clients from diverse backgrounds.

REVIEW QUESTIONS

1. When Dr. Madeleine Leininger established transcultural nursing in the middle of the 20th century, she identified eight reasons why this specialty was needed. Review the reasons and discuss the relevance of these reasons in contemporary nursing and health care.
2. In your own words, describe the meaning of culture and its relationship to nursing.
3. Identify at least five nonethnic cultures and describe the characteristics of each.
4. Describe the composition of the interprofessional health care team in the Transcultural Interprofessional Practice (TIP) Model and identify factors that facilitate effective communication between and among team members.
5. Identify six examples of nonverbal communication and briefly describe each one.

6. In the Transcultural Interprofessional Practice Model, what criteria are used to determine the effectiveness of the plan of care in meeting mutual goals established by the patient and other members of the interprofessional health care team?

CRITICAL THINKING ACTIVITIES

1. Visit the TCNS's official website (http://www.tcns.org).

   a. Briefly summarize the information you find at the website.
   b. Critically evaluate the strengths and limitations of this information source and the data available. What else would you like to know about transcultural nursing that isn't available on this website?
   c. Critically reflect on the information about transcultural nursing that you've learned and indicate how it will help you to provide nursing care for people from cultures that differ from your own.
   d. Search for other websites on transcultural nursing. What are the similarities and differences in the perspectives on transcultural nursing presented by the TCNS and other websites? How is it helpful or unhelpful to review different viewpoints on the same subject?

2. Read the following article: Andrews, M., & Friesen, L. (2011). Finding electronically available information on cultural competence in health care. *Online Journal of Cultural Competence in Nursing and Healthcare, 1*(4), 27–47. (available on the OJCCNH website). Using the key word *transcultural nursing*, search for online resources that were posted during the past year. How many references did you find? If you want information about a specific cultural, ethnic, or minority group, what key words will help you to narrow the search? Consult a reference librarian for assistance if you need help.

3. Conduct an electronic search for websites about modesty among observant Muslims and Orthodox and Hasidic Jews.

   a. Evaluate the credibility, accuracy, veracity, and currency of each website and the information available on the topic.
   b. Compare and contrast the beliefs and practices of each group for men and women.
   c. What are the clinical implications of this information?

4. Maria Rodriguez is a 61-year-old female who self-identifies as being Mexican American. She reads, writes, and speaks Spanish; it is her primary language. Although she speaks English well enough to manage activities of daily living, she has difficulty reading and comprehending medical documents in English. Maria is scheduled to be discharged from the hospital on her 3rd day postoperatively following a below-the-knee amputation of her right leg. She is diagnosed with peripheral vascular disease, diabetes mellitus, obesity, and hypertension. Maria lives alone in a two-story single dwelling. Her son, age 30, is on active duty in Iraq. Her 21-year-old daughter is 8 months pregnant and lives out-of-state. Unable to manage her care at home, Maria is unhappy that she will need to be discharged to a rehabilitation center for the next several weeks. She tells the nurse manager that she is severely depressed and threatens to commit suicide. Using the Transcultural Interprofessional Practice (TIP) Model as a guiding framework, analyze the case and develop a plan of care for Maria.

REFERENCES

Alligood, M. R. (2014). *Nursing theory: Utilization and application.* Maryland Heights, MO: Mosby-Elsevier.

American Anthropological Association. (n.d.). What is anthropology? Retrieved from http://aaanet.org/whatisanthropology.cfm

American Nurses Association. (2013). What is nursing? Retrieved from http://www.nursingworld.org/especially foryou/what-is-nursing

Benner, P. (1984). *From novice to expert: Excellence and power in clinical nursing practice.* Menlo Park, CA: Addison-Wesley.

Benner, P., Sutphen, M., Leonard, V., Day, L. (2010). *Educating nurses: A call for a radical transformation.* San Francisco, CA: Jossey-Bass.

Blue Cross/Blue Shield. (2014). Limit screen time for a happier family. *Living Healthy, Fall,* 2014, 16.

Brackett, M. A., Bertoli, M., Elbertson, N., Bausseron, E., Castillo, R., & Salovey, P. (2013). Emotional intelligence: Reconceptualizing the cognition-emotion link. In M. D. Robinson, E. Watkins, & E. Harmon-Jones (Eds.), *Handbook of cognition and emotion* (pp. 365–379). New York: Guilford Press.

Branch, M. F., & Paxton, P. P. (Eds.) (1976). *Providing safe nursing care for ethnic people of color.* New York: Appleton-Century-Crofts.

Brink, P. J. (1976). *Transcultural nursing care.* Englewood Cliffs, NJ: Prentice-Hall, Inc.

Campinha-Bacote, J. (2011). Delivering patient-centered care in the midst of cultural conflict: The role of cultural competence. *Online Journal of Issues in Nursing, 16*(2), doi: 10.3912/OJIN.Vol16No02Man05

Church of Jesus Christ of Latter Day Saints. (2014). Modesty. Retrieved at http://lds.org.topics/modesty?language=eng

Clark, L. (2013). Humanizing gaze for transcultural nursing research will tell the story of health disparities. *Journal of Transcultural Nursing 25*(2), 122–128.

Council on Nursing and Anthropology, n.d. Retrieved from. http://www.conaa.org/about/htm.

Courtney, R., & Wolgamott, S. (2015). Using Leininger's theory as the building block for cultural competence and cultural assessment for a collaborative care team in a primary care setting. In M. R. McFarland & H. B. Wehbe-Alamah (Eds.), *Leininger's culture care diversity and universality: A worldwide nursing theory* (pp. 345–368). Burlington, MA: Jones and Bartlett Learning.

Davidson, A., Ray, M., & Turkel, M. (Eds.) (2011). *Nursing, caring, and complexity science: For human-environment well-being.* New York: Springer Publishing Company.

deRuyter, L. M. (2015). Culture care education and experience of African American students in predominantly EuroAmerican associate degree nursing programs. In M. R. McFarland & H. B. Wehbe-Alamah (Eds.), *Leininger's culture care diversity and universality: A worldwide nursing theory* (pp. 389–442). Burlington, MA: Jones and Bartlett Learning.

Douglas, M. K., & Pacquiao, D. F. (Eds.). (2010). Core curriculum in transcultural nursing and health care [supplement]. *Journal of Transcultural Nursing, 2*(1)(Suppl. 1), 53S–136S.

Eipperle, M. (2015). Application of the three modes of culture care decisions and actions in advanced practice primary care. In M. R. McFarland & H. B. Wehbe-Alamah (Eds.), *Leininger's culture care diversity and universality: A worldwide nursing theory* (pp. 317–344). Burlington, MA: Jones and Bartlett Learning.

Eisinger, D. (2012). Short Message Service (SMS) birthday: 20 years after first text message, 200,000 now sent per second. Retrieved from http://www.newsmax.com/TheWire/text-sms-20-birthday/2012/12/03/id/466297/

Fulmer, T., & Gaines, M. (Eds.). (2014). Conference conclusions and recommendations. In G. E. Thibault, T. Fulmer, & M. Gaines. 2014 Conference conclusions and recommendations. *Partnering with patients, families, and communities to link interprofessional practice and education.* Proceedings of a conference sponsored by the Josiah Macy Foundation, Arlington, VA, 3-6 April (pp. 27–45). New York, NY: Josiah Macy Foundation.

Galvin, M., Prescott, D., & Huseman, R. C. (1988). *Business communication: Strategies and skills.* New York: Holt, Rinehart, & Winston.

Giger, J. N. (2013). *Transcultural nursing: Assessment and intervention* (6th ed.), Saint Louis, MO: Mosby/Elsevier.

Gilanti, J. (2014). *Cultural sensitivity: pocket guide for health care professionals.* Philadelphia, PA: University of Pennsylvania Press.

Hall, E. T. (1984). *The dance of life: The other dimension of time.* New York: Anchor Press Double Press/Doubleday.

Hall, E. T. (1990). *Distance: The hidden dimension.* New York: Anchor Press/Doubleday.

Hesmondhalgh, D., & Saha, A. (2013). Race, ethnicity, and cultural production. *Popular Communication, 11*(3), 179–193.

Hunt, L. M., Truesdell, N. D., & Kreiner, M. J. (2013). Genes, race, and culture in clinical care. *Medical Anthropology Quarterly, 27*(2), 253–271.

Institute of Medicine. (1999). *To err is human.* Washington, DC: The National Press.

Institute of Medicine. (2011). *The future of nursing: Leading change, advancing health.* Washington, DC: The National Academic Press.

International Council of Nurses. (2014). Definition of Nursing. Retrieved at http://www.icn.ch/about-icn/icn-definition-of-nursing/

Interprofessional Education Collaborative Expert Panel. (2011). Core competencies for interprofessional collaborative practice: Report of an expert panel. Washington, DC: Interprofessional Education Collaborative.

Jeffreys, M. R., & Dogan, E. (2014). Evaluating cultural competence in the clinical practicum. *Nursing education perspectives, 34*(2), 88–94.

Larson, M. (2015). The Greek connection: Discovering the cultural and social care dimensions of the Greek culture using Leininger's Theory of Culture Care: A model for a baccalaureate study- abroad experience. In M. R.

McFarland & H. B. Wehbe-Alamah (Eds.), *Leininger's culture care diversity and universality: A worldwide nursing theory* (pp. 503–520). Burlington, MA: Jones and Bartlett Learning.

Leininger, M. M. (1970). *Nursing and anthropology: Two worlds to blend.* New York: John Wiley & Sons.

Leininger, M. M. (1978). *Transcultural nursing: Concepts, theories and practices.* New York: John Wiley & Sons.

Leininger, M. M. (1991). *Culture care diversity and universality: A theory of nursing.* New York: National League for Nursing.

Leininger, M. M. (1995). *Transcultural nursing: Concepts, theories, research and practices.* New York: McGraw-Hill.

Leininger, M. M. (1997). Future directions in transcultural nursing in the 21st century. *International Nursing Review, 44*(1), 19–23.

Leininger, M. M. (1998). Twenty five years of knowledge and practice development transcultural nursing society annual research conferences. *Journal of Transcultural Nursing, 9*(2), 72–74.

Leininger, M. M. (1999). What is transcultural nursing and culturally competent care? *Journal of Transcultural Nursing, 10*(1), 9.

Leininger, M. M., & McFarland, M. R. (2002). *Transcultural nursing: Concepts, theories and practices.* New York: McGraw-Hill.

Leininger, M. M., & McFarland, M. R. (2006). *Culture care diversity and universality: A worldwide theory for nursing* (2nd ed.). Sudbury, MA: Jones & Bartlett, Publishers.

Lombardo, J. (n.d.). Monochronic and polychronic cultures: Definitions and communication styles. Retrieved at http://education-portal.com/academy/lesson/monochronic-vs-polychronic-cultures-definitions-communication-styles.html

McFarland, M. R., & Wehbe-Alamah, H. B. (2015a). *Leininger's culture care diversity and universality: A worldwide theory of nursing* (3rd ed.). Burlington, MA: Jones & Bartlett Learning.

McFarland, M. R., & Wehbe-Alamah, H. B. (2015b). The theory of culture care diversity and universality. In M. R. McFarland & H. B. Wehbe-Alamah (Eds.), *Leininger's culture care diversity and universality: A worldwide nursing theory* (pp. 1–34). Burlington, MA: Jones and Bartlett Learning.

McFarland, M. R., & Wehbe-Alamah, H. B. (2016). *Transcultural nursing: Concepts, theories, research, and practices* (4th ed.). New York: McGraw-Hill, Medical Publishing Division.

McFarland, M. R., Wehbe-Alamah, H., Wilson, M., & Vossos, H. (2011). Synopsis of findings discovered within a descriptive meta-synthesis of doctoral dissertations guided by the Culture Care Theory with use of the ethnonursing research method. *Online Journal of Cultural Competence in Nursing and Health Care, 1*(2), 24–39.

McFarland, M. R., Mixer, S. J., Webhe-Alamah, H., & Burk, R. (2012). Ethnonursing: A qualitative research method

for all disciplines. *International Journal of Qualitative Methods, 11*(3), 259–279. University of Alberta, Canada.

McFarland, M. R., Wehbe-Alamah, H. B., Vossos, H., & Wilson, M. (2015). Synopsis of findings discovered within a descriptive metasynthesis of doctoral dissertations guided by the culture care theory with use of the ethnonursing research method. In M. R. McFarland & H. B. Wehbe-Alamah (Eds.), *Leininger's culture care diversity and universality: A worldwide nursing theory* (pp. 287–315). Burlington, MA: Jones and Bartlett Learning.

McKenna, M. (1985). Anthropology and nursing: The interaction between two fields of inquiry. *Western Journal of Nursing Research, 6*(4), 423–431.

Mead, M. (1937). *Cooperation and collaboration among primitive peoples.* New York: McGraw-Hill.

Melnyk, B. (2014). Evidence-based practice in nursing and healthcare, 3rd edition. Philadelphia: Wolters Kluwer Health.

Mixer, S. J. (2015). Application of culture care theory in teaching cultural competence and culturally congruent care. In M. R. McFarland & H. B. Wehbe-Alamah (Eds.), *Leininger's culture care diversity and universality: A worldwide nursing theory* (pp. 369–388). Burlington, MA: Jones and Bartlett Learning.

Morris, E. (2015). An examination of subculture as a theoretical social construct through an ethnonursing study of urban African American adolescent gang members. In M. R. McFarland & H. B. Wehbe-Alamah (Eds.), *Leininger's culture care diversity and universality: A worldwide nursing theory* (pp. 255–286). Burlington, MA: Jones and Bartlett Learning.

Munoz, C., & Luckman, J. (2008). *Transcultural communication in nursing* (2nd ed.). Clifton Park, NJ: Delmar Learning.

My Cloud Media Company. (2014). Why SMS text messaging marketing is worth the effort. Retrieved at http://www.mycloudmedia.co.uk/blog/sms-text-message-marketing-worth-effort/

National Human Genome Institute (2014). Fact sheet on science, research, ethics, and the institute. National Institutes of Health, last updated August 7, 2014. Retrieved from http://www.genome.gov/10000202

O'Brien, J. (2013). Interprofessional Collaboration. RN.com. Retrieved at http://www.rn.com/getpdf.php/1892.pdf?Main_Session=0c7d338fb741e35dc663010a8e86bc8b

Omeri, A. (2015). Culture care diversity and universality: A pathway to culturally congruent practices in transcultural nursing education, research, and practice in Australia. In M. R. McFarland & H. B. Wehbe-Alamah (Eds.), *Leininger's culture care diversity and universality: A worldwide nursing theory* (pp. 443–474). Burlington, MA: Jones and Bartlett Learning.

Orque, M. S., Bloch, B., & Monrroy, L. S. (1983). *Ethnic nursing care.* St. Louis, MO: C.V. Mosby.

Osborne, O. (1969). Anthropology and nursing: Some common traditions and interests. *Nursing Research, 18*(3), 251–255.

Pew Internet Research Center. (2014). Mobile technology fact sheet. Retrieved from http://pewinternet.org/fact-sheets/mobile/technology-fact-sheet

Purnell, L. (2014). *Guide to culturally competent health care.* Philadelphia, PA: F.A. Davis Company.

Ray, M. (2010). *Transcultural caring dynamics in nursing and health care.* San Francisco, CA: Jossey Boss Wiley.

Ray, M., Turkel, M., & Cohn, J. (2011). Relational caring complexity: The study of caring and complexity in health care hospital organizations. In A. Davidson, M. Ray & M. Turkel (Eds.), *Nursing, caring and complexity science: For human-environment well-being* (pp. 95–117). New York: Springer Publishing Company.

Ray, M. & Turkel, M. (2014). Caring as emancipatory nursing praxis: The theory of Relational Caring Complexity. *Advances in Nursing science, 37*(2), 132–146.

Raymond, L. M., & Omeri, A. (2015). Transcultural midwifery: Culture care for Mauritian immigrant childbearing families living in New South Wales, Australia. In M. R. McFarland & H. B. Wehbe-Alamah (Eds.), *Leininger's culture care diversity and universality: A worldwide nursing theory* (pp. 183–254). Burlington, MA: Jones and Bartlett Learning.

Rutledge, B. (2013). Cultural differences—Monochronic vs polychronic. *The Articulate CEO*, February, 2013. Retrieved at http://hearticulateceo.typepad.com/my-blog/2011/08/cultural-differences-monochronic-versus-polychronic.html

Sagar, P. L. (2012). *Transcultural nursing theory and models: Application in nursing education, practice, and administration.* New York: Springer Publishing Company.

Sagar, P. L. (2014). *Transcultural nursing education strategies.* New York: Springer Publishing Company.

Sagar, P. L. (2015). Transcultural nursing certification: Its role in nursing education, practice, and administration. In M. R. McFarland & H. B. Wehbe-Alamah. *Leininger's Culture Care Diversity and Universality: A worldwide theory of nursing* (3rd ed., pp. 579–592). Burlington, MA: Jones & Bartlett Learning.

Schacter, D. L., Wegner, D., & Gilbert, D. (2007). *Psychology.* Worth Publishers, 26–27.

Spector, R. E. (2013). *Cultural diversity in health and illness* (8th ed.). Upper Saddle River, NJ: Pearson.

Stanford Center on Poverty and Inequality. (2014). *State of the union: Poverty and inequality report 2014.* Palo Alto, CA: Author.

Transcultural Nursing Certification Commission. (2007). *Transcultural Nursing Certification revision.* Conducted at Transcultural Nursing Certification Committee Meeting, Fenton, MI, March 23–25, 2007.

Transcultural Nursing Society. (2007). Transcultural Nursing Society: Historical moments. *Transcultural Nursing Society Newsletter, 16*(1), 9.

Tylor, E. B. (1871). *Primitive culture.* Volumes 1 and 2. London, UK: Murray.

U.S. Census Bureau. (2013a). Language use in the United States: 2011. Retrieved from http://www.census.gov/prod/2013pubs/acs-22.pdf

U.S. Census Bureau. (2013b). Language use. U.S. Department of Commerce. Retrieved September 12, 2014, from U.S. Census Bureau: https://www.census.gov/hhes/socdemo/language/about/faqs.html#Q3

Wehbe-Alamah, H. B. (2015). Folk care beliefs and practices of traditional Lebanese and Syrian Muslims in the Midwestern United States. In M. R. McFarland & H. B. Wehbe-Alamah (Eds.), *Leininger's culture care diversity and universality: A worldwide nursing theory* (pp. 137–181). Burlington, MA: Jones and Bartlett Learning.

Wehbe-Alamah, H. B., & McFarland, M. R. (2015a). The ethnonursing research method. In M. R. McFarland & H. B. Wehbe-Alamah (Eds.), *Leininger's culture care diversity and universality: A worldwide nursing theory* (pp. 35–71). Burlington, MA: Jones and Bartlett Learning.

Wehbe-Alamah, H. B., & McFarland, M. R. (2015b). Leininger's enablers for use with the ethnonursing research method. In M. R. McFarland & H. B. Wehbe-Alamah (Eds.), *Leininger's culture care diversity and universality: A worldwide nursing theory* (pp. 73–100). Burlington, MA: Jones and Bartlett Learning.

World Health Organization. (2013). Interprofessional collaborative practice in primary health care: Nursing and midwifery perspectives. Human Resources for Health Observor, No. 13. Retrieved from http://www.who.int/hrh/resources/observer13/en/

Zimitri, E. (2013). Throwing the genes: A renewed biological imaginary of 'race', place and identification. *Theoria: A Journal of Social and Political Theory*, 60(136), 38–53.

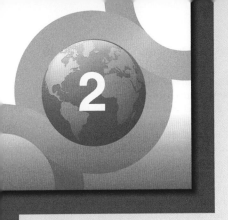

2

Culturally Competent Nursing Care

● Margaret M. Andrews

Key Terms

Cross-cultural communication
Cultural assessment
Cultural competence (individual and organizational)
Cultural self-assessment
Cultural stereotype
Cultural baggage
Culture of the deaf

Diversity
Disabling hearing loss
Discrimination
Emigrate
Folk healer
Hard of hearing
Health Disparity
Health Tourism
Healthy People 2020
Immigrate
Immigrant

Interprofessional collaborative practice
Language access services
Prejudice
Racism
Refugee
Self-location
Social determinants of health
Traditional healer
Vulnerable populations

Learning Objectives

1. Critically analyze the complex integration of knowledge, attitudes, and skills needed for the delivery of culturally competent nursing care.
2. Compare and contrast individual cultural competence and organizational cultural competence.
3. Evaluate guidelines for the practice of culturally competent nursing care.
4. Use a transcultural interprofessional framework for the delivery of culturally congruent and culturally competent nursing care for clients with special needs.

In this chapter, we provide an overview of the rationale for cultural competence in the delivery of nursing care and describe individual and organizational cultural competence, topics that will be discussed throughout the remainder of the book. We analyze cultural self-assessment, a valuable exercise that enables nurses to gain insights into their own unconscious cultural attitudes (biases, cultural stereotypes, prejudice, and tendencies

to discriminate against people who are different from themselves). We discuss the need for cultural knowledge about other ethnic and nonethnic groups and psychomotor skills that are required for the delivery of culturally congruent and competent nursing care. We examine the use of the problem-solving process—assessment, mutual goal setting, planning, implementation, and evaluation—in the delivery of culturally congruent and competent

care for clients from diverse backgrounds. We explore the roles and responsibilities of nurses and other members of the interprofessional health care team in the delivery of culturally competent care and the need for effective cross-cultural communication. We analyze the importance of assessing the cultural context and social determinants of health (World Health Organization, n.d.) that influence the delivery of culturally competent care for clients from diverse cultures, for example, environmental, social, economic, religious, philosophical, moral, legal, political, educational, biological, and technological factors. By introducing national and global guidelines for the delivery of culturally competent nursing care and identifying cultural assessment instruments, we provide nurses with tools to guide them in the delivery of care that is culturally acceptable and congruent with the client's beliefs and practices, culturally competent, affordable, accessible, and rooted in state of the science research, evidence-based, and best practices. Lastly, we examine clients with special needs including those at high risk for health disparities, those who are deaf, and those with communication and language needs.

Rationale for Culturally Competent Care

Multiple factors are converging at this time in history to heighten societal awareness of cultural similarities and differences among people. In many parts of the world, there is growing awareness of social injustice for people from diverse backgrounds and the moral imperative to safeguard the civil and health care rights of vulnerable populations. **Vulnerable populations** are groups that are poorly integrated into the health care system because of ethnic, cultural, economic, geographic (rural and urban settings), or health characteristics, such as disabilities or multiple chronic conditions (Office of Minority Health & Equity, 2013).

Immigration and migration result in growing numbers of **immigrants**, people who move from one country or region to another for economic, political, religious, social, and personal reasons. The verb **emigrate** means to leave one country or region to settle in another; **immigrate** means to enter another country or region for the purpose of living there. People *emigrate from* one country or region and *immigrate to* a different nation or region.

In the United States, for example, 41 million people (13% of the population) are foreign-born, a term used by the Census Bureau in reference to anyone who is not a US citizen at birth, including those who eventually become citizens through naturalization (U.S. Census Bureau, 2012). Additionally, an estimated 8 to 10 million people from other countries are living in the United States without documentation. In many countries, national borders have become increasingly porous and fluid, enabling people to move more freely from one country or region to another.

Nurses respond to global health care needs such as infectious disease epidemics and the growing trends in **health tourism,** in which patients travel to other countries for medical and surgical health care needs. By traveling to another nation, clients often obtain more affordable care services or receive specialized care that is unavailable in their own country. Nurses also respond to natural and human-made disasters around the world and provide care for **refugees** (people who flee their country of origin for fear of persecution based on ethnicity, race, religion, political opinion, or related reasons) and other casualties of civil unrest or war in politically unstable parts of the world. In all of these situations, nurses are expected to demonstrate effective cross-cultural communication and deliver culturally congruent and culturally competent nursing care to people from diverse countries and cultures.

Technological advances in science, engineering, transportation, communication, information and computer sciences, health care, and health professions education result in increased electronic and face-to-face communications

between nurses and people from diverse backgrounds. Population demographics, health care standards, laws, and regulations make cultural competence integral to nursing practice, education, research, administration, and interprofessional collaborations.

Interprofessional collaborative practice refers to multiple health providers from different professional backgrounds working together with patients, families, caregivers, and communities to deliver the highest quality care (World Health Organization [WHO], 2010). Interprofessional teams have a collective identity and shared responsibility for a client or group of clients. Culturally competent care is an extension of interprofessional collaborative practice (Institute of Medicine, 2011; Interprofessional Education Collaborative Expert Panel, 2011; Oelke, Thurston, & Arthur, 2013), involving clients and their families; credentialed or licensed health professionals; folk or traditional healers from various philosophical perspectives, such as herbalists, medicine men or women, and others; and religious and spiritual leaders, such as rabbis, imams, priests, elders, monks, and other religious representatives or clergy, all of whom are integral members of the interprofessional team. The religious and spiritual healers are especially helpful when the client is discerning which decision or action in health-related matters is best, especially when there are moral, ethical, or spiritual considerations involved (see Chapter 13, Religion, Culture, and Nursing and Chapter 14, Cultural Competence in Ethical Decision Making).

Guidelines for the Practice of Culturally Competent Nursing Care

A set of guidelines for implementing culturally competent nursing care was recently developed by a task force consisting of members of the American Academy of Nursing (AAN) Expert Panel on Global Nursing and Health and the Transcultural Nursing Society (TCNS). In addition to endorsement by the membership of the AAN and TCNS, these guidelines have been endorsed by the International Council of Nurses. Intended to present universally accepted guidelines that can be embraced by nurses around the world, the ten items listed in Table 2-1 provide a useful framework for implementing culturally competent care. The guidelines include knowledge of culture; education and training in culturally competent care; critical reflection; cross-cultural communication; culturally competent practice; cultural competence in systems and organizations; patient advocacy and empowerment; multicultural workforce (see Chapter 12, Cultural Diversity in the Health Care Workforce); cross-cultural leadership; and evidence-based practice and research. The guidelines have their foundation in principles of social justice, such as the belief that everyone is entitled to fair and equal opportunities for health care and to have their dignity protected. The guidelines and accompanying descriptions are intended to serve as a resource for nurses in clinical practice, administration, research, and education (Douglas et al., 2014).

Definitions and Categories of Cultural Competence

There is no universally accepted definition of cultural competence. Rather, there are hundreds of definitions that have "evolved from diverse perspectives, interests, and needs and are incorporated in state legislation, Federal statutes and programs, private sector organizations, and academic settings" (National Center for Cultural Competence, n.d.a). Although definitions vary, there is general consensus that cultural competence conceptually can be divided into two major

Table 2-1: Guidelines for the Practice of Culturally Competent Nursing Care

Guideline	Description
1. Knowledge of Cultures	Nurses shall gain an understanding of the perspectives, traditions, values, practices, and family systems of culturally diverse individuals, families, communities, and populations they care for, as well as knowledge of the complex variables that affect the achievement of health and well-being.
2. Education and Training in Culturally Competent Care	Nurses shall be educationally prepared to provide culturally congruent health care. Knowledge and skills necessary for assuring that nursing care is culturally congruent shall be included in global health care agendas that mandate formal education and clinical training as well as required ongoing, continuing education for all practicing nurses.
3. Critical Reflection	Nurses shall engage in critical reflection of their own values, beliefs, and cultural heritage in order to have an awareness of how these qualities and issues can impact culturally congruent nursing care.
4. Cross-Cultural Communication	Nurses shall use culturally competent verbal and nonverbal communication skills to identify client's values, beliefs, practices, perceptions, and unique health care needs.
5. Culturally Competent Practice	Nurses shall utilize cross-cultural knowledge and culturally sensitive skills in implementing culturally congruent nursing care.
6. Cultural Competence in Health Care Systems and Organizations	Health care organizations should provide the structure and resources necessary to evaluate and meet the cultural and language needs of their diverse clients.
7. Patient Advocacy and Empowerment	Nurses shall recognize the effect of health care policies, delivery systems, and resources on their patient populations and shall empower and advocate for their patients as indicated. Nurses shall advocate for the inclusion of their patient's cultural beliefs and practices in all dimensions of their health care.
8. Multicultural Workforce	Nurses shall actively engage in the effort to ensure a multicultural workforce in health care settings. One measure to achieve a multicultural workforce is through strengthening of recruitment and retention efforts in the hospitals, clinics, and academic settings.
9. Cross-Cultural Leadership	Nurses shall have the ability to influence individuals, groups, and systems to achieve outcomes of culturally competent care for diverse populations. Nurses shall have the knowledge and skills to work with public and private organizations, professional associations, and communities to establish policies and guidelines for comprehensive implementation and evaluation of culturally competent care.
10. Evidence-Based Practice and Research	Nurses shall base their practice on interventions that have been systematically tested and shown to be the most effective for the culturally diverse populations that they serve. In areas where there is a lack of evidence of efficacy, nurse researchers shall investigate and test interventions that may be the most effective in reducing the disparities in health outcomes.

Reprinted by permission of the Journal of Transcultural Nursing.

categories: (1) **individual cultural competence,** which refers to the care provided for an individual client by one or more nurses, physicians, social workers, and/or other health care, education, or social services professionals, and (2) **organizational cultural competence,** which focuses on the collective competencies of the members of an organization and their effectiveness in meeting the diverse needs of their clients, patients, staff, and community.

Before nurses can provide culturally competent care for individual clients or contribute to organizational cultural competence, they need to engage in a cultural self-assessment to identify their cultural baggage. **Cultural baggage** refers to the tendency for a person's own culture to be foremost in his/her assumptions, thoughts, words, and behavior. People are seldom consciously aware that culture influences their world view and interactions with others.

Cultural Self-Assessment

The purpose of the **cultural self-assessment** is for nurses to critically reflect on their own culturally based attitudes, values, beliefs, and practices and gain insight into, and awareness of, the ways in which their background and lived experiences have shaped and informed the person the nurse has become today. The nurse's cultural self-assessment is a personal and professional journey that emphasizes strengths as well as areas for continued growth, thereby enabling nurses to set goals for overcoming barriers to the delivery of culturally congruent and competent nursing care (Chettih, 2012; Douglas et al., 2014; McClimens, Brewster, & Lewis, 2014; National Center for Cultural Competence, n.d.a, National Center for Cultural Competence [NCCC], n.d.b; Timmins, 2006).

Part of the cultural self-assessment process includes nurses' awareness of their human tendencies toward bias, ethnocentrism, cultural imposition, cultural stereotyping, prejudice, and discrimination. **Bias** refers to the tendency, outlook, or inclination that results in an unreasoned judgment, positive or negative, about a person, place, or object.

"If anyone, no matter who, were given the opportunity of choosing from amongst all the nations in the world the set of beliefs which he thought best, he would inevitably—after careful considerations of their relative merits—choose that of his own country."

Herodotus, ancient Greek historian,
Histories, circum. 450 to 420 B.C.

The term **ethnocentrism** refers to the human tendency to view one's own group as the center of and superior to all other groups. People born into a particular culture grow up absorbing and learning the values and behaviors of the culture, and they develop a worldview that considers their culture to be the norm. Other cultures that differ from that norm are viewed as inferior. Ethnocentrism may lead to pride, vanity, belief in the superiority of one's own group over all others, contempt for outsiders, and cultural imposition. Box 2-1 identifies other examples of —"-isms," preconceived, unfavorable, judgments about people based on personal characteristics of another. "-Isms" are derived from cultural baggage, biases, stereotypes, prejudice, and/or discrimination related to someone with a background that differs from one's own. As indicated in Evidence-Based Practice 2-1, **racism,** the belief that one's own race is superior and has the right to dominate others, has a profound impact on the body's stress management system. Exposure to racism over prolonged periods of time may result in severe cardiovascular disease.

Cultural imposition is the tendency of a person or group to impose their values, beliefs, and practices onto others. **Cultural stereotype** refers to a preconceived, fixed perception or impression of someone from a particular cultural group without meeting the person. The perception generally has little or no basis in fact, but nonetheless is perpetuated by individuals who are unwilling to re-examine or change their perceptions even when faced with new evidence that disproves the incorrect perception. Cultural stereotypes fail to recognize individual differences, group changes that occur over

Box 2-1 Selected Examples of "-isms" Based on Preconceptions about Others

Characteristic	Type of -ism
Race	Racism
Ethnicity	Ethnocentrism
National origin	Nationalism
Socioeconomic class	Classism
Gender	Sexism, feminism
Sexual orientation	Homophobism*
Disability	Ableism*
Religion	Islamism* (political ideology associated with some denominations of Islam) Anti-Semitism (anti-Jewish) Anti- (name of religion), e.g., anti-Mormonism
Political opinion	Anti- (name of ideology), e.g., anti-capitalism, anti-communism
Size	Sizeism*

*Neologism—a newly coined term or phrase that is in the process of entering common or mainstream use, but isn't yet found in dictionaries.

time, and personal preferences. Ethnocentrism, cultural imposition, and cultural stereotypes are barriers to effective cross-cultural communication and the provision of culturally competent care, as are prejudice and discrimination.

Prejudice refers to inaccurate perceptions of others or preconceived judgments about people based on ethnicity, race, national origin, gender, sexual orientation, social class, size, disability, religion, language, political opinion, or related personal characteristics (Dunagan, Kimble, Gunby, & Andrews, 2014). Whereas prejudice concerns perceptions and attitudes, **discrimination** refers to the *act* or behavior of setting one individual or group apart from another, thereby treating one person or group differently from other people or groups. In the context of civil rights law, *unlawful* discrimination refers to unfair or unequal treatment of an individual or group based on age, disability, ethnicity, gender, marital status, national origin, race religion, and sexual orientation (Goico, 2014; Titles I and V of the Americans with Disabilities Act of 1990; Title VII of the Civil Rights Act of 1964, Public Law 88–352).

By engaging in cultural self-assessments and demonstrating genuine interest in and curiosity about the client's cultural beliefs and practices, nurses learn to develop their cultural competency and learn to put aside their own ethnocentric tendencies. Box 2-2 contains a cultural self-assessment tool that enables nurses to gain insights into how they relate to people from five different categories: racial/ethnic groups, social issues/problems, religious differences, physical and emotional handicaps, and different political perspectives. After completing and scoring the cultural self-assessment contained in Box 2-2, continue to the next section, which focuses on the cultural assessment of clients.

Cultural Assessment of Clients

The foundation for culturally competent and culturally congruent nursing care is the **cultural assessment**, a term that refers to the collection of data about the client's health state. There are two major categories of data: *subjective data* (i.e., what clients say about themselves during the

Box 2-2 How Do You Relate to Various Groups of People in the Society?

Described below are different levels of response you might have toward a person.

Levels of Response

1. *Greet*: I feel I can *greet* this person warmly and welcome him or her sincerely.
2. *Accept*: I feel I can honestly *accept* this person as he or she is and be comfortable enough to listen to his or her problems.
3. *Help*: I feel I would genuinely try to *help* this person with his or her problems as they might relate to or arise from the label–stereotype given to him or her.
4. *Background*: I feel I have the *background* of knowledge and/or experience to be able to help this person.
5. *Advocate*: I feel I could honestly be an *advocate* for this person.

The following is a list of individuals. Read down the list and place a checkmark next to anyone you would *not* "greet" or would hesitate to "greet." Then, move to response level 2, "accept," and follow the same procedure. Try to respond honestly, not as you think might be socially or professionally desirable. Your answers are only for your personal use in clarifying your initial reactions to different people.

Level of Response

	1	2	3	4	5
Individual	Greet	Accept	Help	Background	Advocate
1. Haitian	☐	☐	☐	☐	☐
2. Child abuser	☐	☐	☐	☐	☐
3. Jew	☐	☐	☐	☐	☐
4. Person with hemophilia	☐	☐	☐	☐	☐
5. Neo-Nazi	☐	☐	☐	☐	☐
6. Mexican American	☐	☐	☐	☐	☐
7. IV drug user	☐	☐	☐	☐	☐
8. Catholic	☐	☐	☐	☐	☐
9. Senile, elderly person	☐	☐	☐	☐	☐
10. Teamster Union member	☐	☐	☐	☐	☐
11. Native American	☐	☐	☐	☐	☐
12. Prostitute	☐	☐	☐	☐	☐
13. Jehovah's Witnesses	☐	☐	☐	☐	☐
14. Cerebral palsied person	☐	☐	☐	☐	☐
15. Equal Rights Amendment (ERA) proponent	☐	☐	☐	☐	☐
16. Vietnamese American	☐	☐	☐	☐	☐
17. Gay/lesbian	☐	☐	☐	☐	☐
18. Atheist	☐	☐	☐	☐	☐
19. Person with AIDS	☐	☐	☐	☐	☐

How Do You Relate to Various Groups of People in the Society?

Level of Response

Individual	1 Greet	2 Accept	3 Help	4 Background	5 Advocate
20. Communist	☐	☐	☐	☐	☐
21. Black American	☐	☐	☐	☐	☐
22. Unmarried pregnant teenager	☐	☐	☐	☐	☐
23. Protestant	☐	☐	☐	☐	☐
24. Amputee	☐	☐	☐	☐	☐
25. Ku Klux Klansman	☐	☐	☐	☐	☐
26. White Anglo-Saxon	☐	☐	☐	☐	☐
27. Alcoholic	☐	☐	☐	☐	☐
28. Amish person	☐	☐	☐	☐	☐
29. Person with cancer	☐	☐	☐	☐	☐
30. Nuclear armament proponent	☐	☐	☐	☐	☐

Scoring Guide: The previous activity may help you anticipate difficulty in working with some clients at various levels. The 30 types of individuals can be grouped into five categories: ethnic/racial, social issues/problems, religious, physically/mentally handicapped, and political. Transfer your checkmarks to the following form. If you have a concentration of checks within a specific category of individuals or at specific levels, this may indicate a conflict that could hinder you from rendering effective professional help.

Level of Response

Individual	1 Greet	2 Accept	3 Help	4 Background	5 Advocate
Ethnic/racial					
1. Haitian American	☐	☐	☐	☐	☐
6. Mexican American	☐	☐	☐	☐	☐
11. Native American	☐	☐	☐	☐	☐
16. Vietnamese American	☐	☐	☐	☐	☐
21. Black American	☐	☐	☐	☐	☐
26. White Anglo-Saxon	☐	☐	☐	☐	☐
Social issues/problems					
2. Child abuser	☐	☐	☐	☐	☐
7. IV drug user	☐	☐	☐	☐	☐
12. Prostitute	☐	☐	☐	☐	☐
17. Gay/lesbian	☐	☐	☐	☐	☐
22. Unmarried pregnant teenager	☐	☐	☐	☐	☐
27. Alcoholic	☐	☐	☐	☐	☐

(continued)

Religious

	1	2	3	4	5
3. Jew	☐	☐	☐	☐	☐
8. Catholic	☐	☐	☐	☐	☐
13. Jehovah's Witnesses	☐	☐	☐	☐	☐
18. Atheist	☐	☐	☐	☐	☐
23. Protestant	☐	☐	☐	☐	☐
28. Amish person	☐	☐	☐	☐	☐

How Do You Relate to Various Groups of People in the Society?

Level of Response

Individual	1 Greet	2 Accept	3 Help	4 Background	5 Advocate
Physically/mentally handicapped					
4. Person with hemophilia	☐	☐	☐	☐	☐
9. Senile elderly person	☐	☐	☐	☐	☐
14. Cerebral palsied person	☐	☐	☐	☐	☐
19. Person with AIDS	☐	☐	☐	☐	☐
24. Amputee	☐	☐	☐	☐	☐
29. Person with cancer	☐	☐	☐	☐	☐
Political					
5. Neo-Nazi	☐	☐	☐	☐	☐
10. Teamster Union member	☐	☐	☐	☐	☐
15. ERA proponent	☐	☐	☐	☐	☐
20. Communist	☐	☐	☐	☐	☐
25. Ku Klux Klansman	☐	☐	☐	☐	☐
30. Nuclear armament proponent	☐	☐	☐	☐	☐

Reproduced with permission of the author Randall-David, E. (1989). *Strategies for working with culturally diverse communities and clients* (pp. 7–9). U.S. Department of Health and Human Services, Health Resources and Services Administration, Maternal and Child Health Bureau, National Hemophilia Program.

admission or intake interview) and *objective data* (i.e., what health professionals observe about clients during the physical examination through observation, percussion, palpation, and auscultation). See Chapter 3, Cultural Competence in the Health History and Physical Examination, for an in-depth discussion of cultural competence in the health history and physical examination (cf., Jarvis, 2014).

When conducting a comprehensive cultural assessment of clients, nurses need to be able to successfully form, foster, and sustain relationships with people who may frequently come from a cultural background that is different from the nurse's, thus making it necessary to quickly establish rapport with the client. The ability to see the situation from the client's point of view is known as an **emic** or insider's perspective; looking at the situation from an outsider's vantage point is known as an **etic** perspective. The ability to successfully form, foster, and sustain relationships with members of a culture that differs from one's own requires effective cross-cultural communication. **Cross-cultural communication** is based on knowledge of many factors, such as the other person's values, perceptions, attitudes, manners,

Racism and Cardiovascular Disease

Risk factors for premature death and increased susceptibility to cardiovascular disease include **social determinants of health** (SDH), which are the conditions in which people are born, grow, live, work, and age. These circumstances are shaped by the distribution of money, power, and resources at global, national, and local levels (World Health Organization, n.d.). The SDH also include socio-economic factors such as employment, income, working conditions, education, and health literacy; environmental factors such as housing and food security; and biological factors such as age, gender, health, and race. Racism is an influential SDH because it shapes a person's health and well-being and is interwoven with life opportunities across the lifespan, even when there is no socioeconomic hardship (Etowa & McGibbon, 2012; Galabuzi, 2006). These opportunities may include equitable access to jobs, housing, education, and health. Racism stems from discrimination, bias, and cultural stereotyping. The experience of discrimination is a key factor in producing health disparities and poor health outcomes. Discrimination frequently produces the stressors that lead to health problems and is a barrier to accessing and using health services. Discrimination also limits the person's right to a wide array of opportunities and resources due to characteristics such as race, gender, and culture. Although a person's race may predetermine genetic differences in health outcomes, such as sickle cell anemia in African Americans and/or Tay–Sachs disease in Jews, racism is a key SDH. When discriminatory practices become embedded in societal systems, such as the health and education systems, they are referred to as "systemic" and become interwoven with racist health policies and practices within the health care delivery system.

Racism impacts the ability of individuals, families, and communities to access health care. The results of research indicate that, when seeking health care, the experience of discrimination can range from 50% (Thomas, 2008) to 68% (Peters, 2006). The results of one study, in which the investigators shadowed black patients as they navigated the health care

system, reveal that 20% to 30% did not receive any follow-up or referral appointments for community services after discharge (Woodger & Cowan, 2010). Female immigrants in Canada identified language and culture as barriers to accessing care.

Black patients with cardiovascular disease in the United States were likely to receive lower quality care, for example, fewer cardiac catheterizations, and receive fewer diagnostic and treatment options than white counterparts, even when controlling for insurance and socioeconomic background (Redburg, 2005). Black men with cardiovascular disease were more likely to die from the illness than white men, after controlling for age and income (Thomas, Eberly, Smith, Neaton, & Stamler, 2005).

Racism has a profound impact on the body's stress management system, the sympathetic adrenal medulla (SAM) and the hypothalamus–pituitary–adrenal cortex (HYPAC) (McGibbon, 2012). In the presence of chronic racism-related stresses, the SAM-HYPAC system becomes overwhelmed, leading to a release of catecholamines such as epinephrine. Due to the presence of epinephrine, both blood pressure and heart rate are raised significantly; therefore, racism influences the prevalence of hypertension through stress exposure and reactivity. The prolonged elevation of blood pressure, in turn, causes strain on the myocardium and left ventricular hypertrophy as a compensatory mechanism to offset the increased vascular resistance produced by hypertension. The process of sustained sympathetic activation eventually causes heart failure.

Other body systems also react with the kidneys responding to hypertension through activation of the renin–angiotensin system (Swann, 2011). When a person experiences racism on a daily basis, the stress response becomes overwhelmed, and the adrenal system is no longer able to maintain homeostasis. Chronic adrenal fatigue can cause depression, obesity, hypertension, diabetes, cancer, ulcers, allergies, eczema, autoimmune diseases, headaches, and liver disease (Varcorolis & Halter, 2010).

(continued)

Racism and Cardiovascular Disease (continued)

In summary, chronic, persistent racism can lead to hypertension, heart failure, myocardial infarction, and stroke. Black clients may also respond differently to some cardiac medications. People experiencing racism appear to be more likely to develop cardiovascular disease due to the physiological impact of racism because no significant genetic variants are linked to cardiovascular disease among African Americans or African Canadians (Peters, 2006).

Clinical Implications

Nurses need to position themselves strategically to bring about change in the Canadian and US health care systems by acting as patient advocates, addressing racism for individual clients, and acting collectively as members of the nursing profession to rid the system of racism through systemic changes. Strategies for action include the following:

- Engaging in self-reflexive practice through which nurses examine the ways that their own social and cultural backgrounds, experiences, beliefs, and attitudes affect practice
- Acknowledging the nurse's own **self-location** (e.g., race, culture, class, gender, socioeconomic status, disability, and other social identities) influences one's own beliefs, attitudes, and the therapeutic nurse–client relationship
- Revitalizing the undergraduate and graduate nursing curricula through transformative education about racism and antiracist practices, thereby openly addressing how inequities in the SDH can intersect and overlap to deepen disadvantage and how advocacy by nurses can bring about change
- Providing leadership in analyzing organizational approaches to racial diversity and workplace policies to foster inclusiveness, equity, and justice in the Canadian and US health systems, for example, establish an Aboriginal Health Worker role on an inpatient cardiac unit
- Conducting research on Canadian and US populations experiencing racism in their daily lives and within the health system with goal of strengthening cardiovascular care for African Canadian and African American clients and ensuring that people from a variety of racial backgrounds are represented in investigations and on research councils that review proposals and allocate funds for cardiovascular research

Reference: Jackson, J., McGibbon, E., & Waldron, I. (2013). Racism and cardiovascular disease: Implications for nursing. *Canadian Journal of Cardiovascular Nursing, 23*(4), 12–18.

Additional References

Etowa, J., & McGibbon, E. (2012). Racism as a determinant of health. In E. McGibbon (Ed.). *Oppression: A social determinant of health* (pp. 120–138). Toronto, ON: Brunswick Books.

Galabuzi, G.-E. (2006). *Canada's economic apartheid.* Toronto, ON: Canadian Scholar's Press.

Peters, R. (2006). The relationship of racism, chronic stress emotions, and blood pressure. *Journal of the National Medical Association, 98,* 1532–1540.

Redburg, R. F. (2005). Gender, race and cardiac care: Why the differences? *Journal of the American College of Cardiology, 46,* 1852–1854.

Swann, J. I. (2011). Understanding the common triggers and effects of stress. *British Journal of Healthcare Assistants, 5,* 483–486.

Thomas, K. L. (2008). Discrimination: A new cardiovascular risk factor? *American Heart Journal, 156,* 1023–1025.

Thomas, A. J., Eberly, L. E., Smith, G. D., Neaton, J. D., Stamler, J. (2005). Race/ethnicity, income, major risk factors, and cardiovascular disease mortality. *American Journal of Public Health, 95,* 1417–1423.

Varcarolis, E. M., & Halter, M. (2010). *Foundations of psychiatric mental health nursing.* St. Louis, MO: Saunders

Woodger, D., & Cowan, J. (2010). Institutional racism in healthcare services: Using mainstream methods to develop a practical approach. *Ethnicity and Inequalities in Health and Social Care, 3,* 36–44.

World Health Organization (n.d.). What are the social determinants of health? Retrieved at *http://www.int/social_determinants/en/*

social structure, decision-making practices, and an understanding of how members of groups communicate both verbally and nonverbally.

Knowledge about a client's family and kinship structure helps nurses to ascertain the values, decision-making patterns, and overall communication within the household. It is necessary to identify the significant others whom clients perceive to be important in their care and who may be responsible for decision making that affects their health care. For example, for many clients, familism—which emphasizes interdependence over independence, affiliation over confrontation, and cooperation over competition—may dictate that important decisions affecting the client be made by the family, not the individual alone. When working with clients from cultural groups that value cohesion, interdependence, and collectivism, nurses may perceive the family as being overly involved and usurping the autonomy of both the client and the nurse. At the same time, clients are likely to perceive the involvement with family as a source of mutual support, security, comfort, and fulfillment.

The family is the basic social unit in which children are raised and where they learn culturally based values, beliefs, and practices about health and illnesses. The essence of family consists of living together as a unit. Relationships that may seem obvious sometimes warrant further exploration when the nurse interacts with clients from culturally diverse backgrounds. For example, most European Americans define siblings as two persons with the same mother, the same father, the same mother and father, or the same adoptive parents. In some Asian cultures, a sibling relationship is defined as any infant breast-fed by the same woman. In other cultures, certain kinship patterns, such as maternal first cousins, are defined as sibling relationships. In some African cultures, anyone from the same village or town may be called brother or sister.

Among some Hispanic groups, for example, female members of the nuclear or extended family such as sisters and aunts are primary providers of care for infants and children. In some African American families, the grandmother may be the decision maker and primary caretaker of children. To provide culturally congruent and competent care, nurses must effectively communicate with the appropriate decision maker(s).

When making health-related decisions, some clients may seek assistance from other members of the family. It is sometimes culturally expected that a relative (e.g., parent, grandparent, eldest son, or eldest brother) will make decisions about important health-related matters. For example, in Japan, it is the obligation and duty of the eldest son and his spouse to assume primary responsibility for aging parents and to make health care decisions for them. Among the Amish, the entire community is affected by the illness of a member and pays for health care from a common fund. The Amish join together to meet the needs of both the sick person and his or her family throughout the illness, and the roles of dozens of people in the community are likely to be affected by the illness of a single member. The individual value orientation concerning relationships is predominant among the dominant cultural majority in North America. Although members of the nuclear family may participate to varying degrees, decision making about health and illness is often an individual matter. Nurses should ascertain the identity of all key participants in the decision-making process; sometimes, decisions are made after consultation with family members, but the individual is the primary decision maker.

Individual Cultural Competence

Individual cultural competence is a complex integration of knowledge, attitudes, values, beliefs, behaviors, skills, practices, and cross-cultural nurse–client interactions that include effective communication and the provision of safe, affordable, accessible, research, evidence-based, and best practices, acceptable, quality, and efficacious nursing care for clients from diverse backgrounds. The term diverse or **diversity** refers to the client's uniqueness in the dimensions of race; ethnicity; national origin; socioeconomic background; age;

gender; sexual orientation; philosophical and religious ideology; lifestyle; level of education; literacy; marital status; physical, emotional, and psychological ability; political ideology; size; and other characteristics used to compare or categorize people.

Although the connotation of diversity is generally positive, Talabere (1996) argues that it is itself an ethnocentric term because it focuses on "how different the other person is from me" rather than "how different I am from the other." In using the term *cultural diversity*, the white panethnic group is frequently viewed as the norm against which the differences in everyone else (ethnocentrically referred to as nonwhites) are measured or compared.

Cultural competence is not an end point, but a dynamic, ongoing, lifelong, developmental process that requires self-reflection, intrinsic motivation, and commitment by the nurse to value, respect, and refrain from judging the beliefs, language, interpersonal styles, behaviors, and culturally based, health-related practices of individuals and families receiving services as well as the professional and auxiliary staff who are providing such services. Culturally competent nursing care requires effective cross-cultural communication, a diverse workforce, and is provided in a variety of social, cultural, economic, environmental, and other contexts across the life span (Roberts, Warda, Garbutt, & Curry, 2014). Scholars from nursing, medicine, psychology, and many disciplines have written about cultural competence (American Medical Association, 2013; Andrews, 2013; Andrews & Collins, 2015; Andrews et al., 2011; Basuray, 2014; Betancourt, Green, & Carrillo, 2002; Campinha-Bacote, 2003, 2011; Cross, Bazron, Dennis, & Isaacs, 1989; Douglas & Pacquiao, 2010; Douglas et al., 2014; Institute of Medicine, 2011; Leininger, 1970, 1978, 1991, 1995, 1999; Leininger & McFarland, 2002, 2006; McFarland & Wehbe-Alamah, 2015; Purnell, 2014; Purnell & Paulanka, 2013; Spector, 2013).

Given the large number of cultures and subcultures in the world, it's impossible for nurses to know everything about them all; however, it is possible for nurses to develop excellent cultural assessment and cross-cultural communication skills and to follow a systematic, orderly process for the delivery of culturally competent care. Nurses are encouraged to study in-depth the top two or three cultural groups that they encounter most frequently in their clinical practice and develop the affective (feelings or emotions), cognitive (conscious mental activities such as thinking), and psychomotor (combined thinking and motor) skills necessary to deliver culturally competent nursing care. As new groups move into a geographic area, nurses need to update their knowledge and skills in order to be responsive to the changing demographics. For nurses in large multicultural urban centers, the challenge of keeping pace with client diversity is complex and needs to become an integral component of the nurse's continuing professional development. Professional organizations, employer-sponsored in-service programs, and Web-based resources provide nurses with valuable sources of information on culturally based health beliefs and practices of clients from diverse backgrounds.

Figure 2-1 provides a more detailed view of the five-step problem-solving process for delivering culturally congruent and competent nursing care for individual clients introduced in Chapter 1. Clients (the individual, their family, and significant others) are at the center and are the focus of the interprofessional health care team (which includes credentialed and/or licensed health professionals, folk, traditional, religious, and spiritual healers).

Step one of the process is assessment—of both the nurse and the client. This begins with nurses' *self-assessment* of their attitudes, values, and beliefs about people from backgrounds that differ from their own; their *knowledge* of their own self-location (cultural, gender, class, and other social self-identities) compared to those of clients and other team members; and the *psychomotor skills* needed for the delivery of culturally

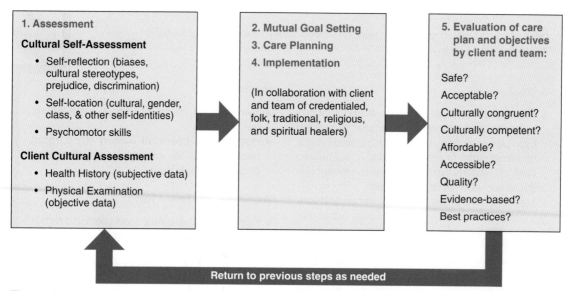

Figure 2-1. The five-step problem-solving process for delivering culturally congruent and competent nursing care for individual clients (Copyright Margaret M. Andrews).

congruent and competent care (see Box 2-3). The self-assessment includes self-reflection and reflexivity (analysis of cause–effect relationships) for the purpose of uncovering the nurse's unconscious biases, cultural stereotypes, prejudices, and discriminatory behaviors. Nurses then have the opportunity to change, or rectify, affective, cognitive, or psychomotor deficits by reframing their attitude toward certain individuals and groups from diverse backgrounds, learning more about the cultures and subcultures most frequently encountered in their clinical practice, and developing psychomotor skills that enhance their ability to use and their clinical skills to deliver culturally congruent and competent nursing care.

The comprehensive cultural assessment of the client and his/her family and significant others (people, companion animals, and pets) requires nurses to gather subjective and objective data through the health history and the physical examination (see Chapter 3). The nurse should consider the influence of the following factors: environmental, social, economic, religious, philosophical, moral, legal, political, educational, biological (genetic and acquired diseases, conditions,

disorders, injuries, and illnesses), and technological. In addition, the nurse may have professional and organizational cultures that influence the nurse–patient interaction, such as hospital or agency policies that determine visiting hours, or laws governing the nurse's scope of practice and professional responsibilities within a particular jurisdiction or setting. The influence of cultural and health belief systems (on the nurse and the client) must also be considered in relation to disease causation, healing modalities, and choice of healer(s). See Chapter 4, The Influence of Cultural Belief Systems on Health Care Practices, for detailed information.

In steps two through four, the nurse collaborates with the client, the client's family and significant others, and members of the health care team (credentialed, folk, traditional, religious, and spiritual healers). The terms folk healer and traditional healer sometimes are used interchangeably. Folk healers typically learn healing practices through an apprenticeship with someone experienced in folk healing. Folk healers primarily use herbal remedies, foods, and inanimate objects in a therapeutic manner. Traditional

Box 2-3 Selected Examples of Psychomotor Skills Useful in Transcultural Nursing

Assessment

- Techniques for assessing biocultural variations in health and illness, for example, assessing cyanosis, jaundice, anemia, and related clinical manifestations of disease in darkly pigmented clients; differentiating between mongolian spots and ecchymoses (bruises)
- Measurement of head circumference and fontanelles in infants using techniques not in violation of taboos for selected cultural groups
- Growth and development monitoring for children of Asian heritage using culturally appropriate growth grids
- Cultural modification of the Denver II and other developmental tests used for children
- Conducting culturally appropriate obstetric and gynecologic examinations of women from various cultural backgrounds

Communication

- Speaking and writing the language(s) used by clients
- Using alternative methods of communicating with non–English-speaking clients and families when no interpreter is available (e.g., pantomime)

Hygiene

- Skin care for clients of various racial/ethnic backgrounds
- Hair care for clients of various ethnic/racial backgrounds, for example, care of African American clients' hair

Activities of Daily Living

- Assisting Chinese American clients to regain the use of chopsticks as part of rehabilitation regimen after a stroke
- Assisting paralyzed Amish client with dressing when buttons and pins are used
- Assisting West African client who uses "chewing stick" with oral hygiene

Religion

- Emergency baptism and anointing of the sick for Roman Catholics
- Care before and after ritual circumcision by *mohel* (performed 8 days after the birth of a male Jewish infant)

or indigenous healers often are divinely chosen and/or learn the art of healing by applying knowledge, skills, and practices based on experiences indigenous to their culture, for example, Native American medicine men/women and shamans. The focus of most traditional and indigenous healers is on establishing and restoring balance and harmony in the body–mind–spirit through the use of spiritual healing interventions, such as praying, chanting, drumming, dancing, participating in sweat lodge rituals, and storytelling. The definition and scope of practice of religious and spiritual healers varies widely, but these healers often help clients analyze complex health-related decisions involving moral and/or ethical issues

(see Chapter 13, Religion, Culture and Nursing, and Chapter 14, Cultural Competence in Ethical Decision Making). All healers whom the client wants to be involved in care should be included in steps two to five to the extent this is feasible.

In *step two*, mutual goals are set, and objectives are established to meet the goals and desired health outcomes.

In *step three*, the plan of care is developed using approaches that are client centered and culturally congruent with the client's socioeconomic, philosophical, and religious beliefs, resources, and practices. Members of the health care team assume roles and responsibilities according to their educational background, clinical knowledge,

and skills. For credentialed or licensed members of the team such as nurses, physicians, physical, occupational and respiratory therapists, social workers, and similar health professions, roles, responsibilities, and scope of practice are delineated by ministries of health, provincial or state health professions licensing, and/or registration boards. In most instances, the credentialed or licensed healer has formal academic preparation and has passed an examination that tested knowledge and skills deemed necessary for clinical practice.

In *step four*, decisions, actions, treatments, and interventions that are congruent with the patient's health-related cultural beliefs and practices are implemented by those team members who are best prepared to assist the client. In some instances, there is overlapping of scope of practice, roles, and responsibilities between and among team members (Figure 2-2). Client-centered interprofessional team conferences are usually helpful in sorting out roles and responsibilities of team members when there is lack of clarity about who will deliver a particular service.

Lastly, in *step five*, the client and members of the health care team collaboratively evaluate the care plan and its objectives to determine if the care is safe; culturally acceptable, congruent, and competent; affordable; accessible; of high quality; and based on research, scientific evidence, and/or best practices. If modifications or changes are needed, the nurse should return to previous steps and repeat the process. Throughout the five steps of the process for the delivery of culturally congruent and competent nursing care, the nurse behaves in an empathetic, compassionate, caring manner that matches, "fits," and is consistent with the client's cultural beliefs and practices.

Organizational Cultural Competence

According to the National Center for Cultural Competence (National Center for Cultural Competence, n.d.), cultural competence requires that *organizations* have the following characteristics:

- A defined set of values and principles and demonstration of behaviors, attitudes, policies, and

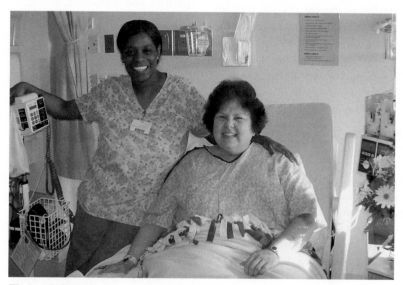

Figure 2-2. Effective cross-cultural communication is vital to the establishment of a strong nurse–client relationship. It is important to understand both verbal and nonverbal cues when communicating with people from different cultural backgrounds (Margaret M. Andrews).

structures that enable them to work effectively cross-culturally

- The capacity to (1) value diversity, (2) conduct self-assessments, (3) manage the dynamics of difference, (4) acquire and institutionalize cultural knowledge, and (5) adapt to diversity and the cultural contexts of the communities they serve
- Incorporation of the previously mentioned items in all aspects of policy making, administration, practice, and service delivery and systematic involvement of consumers, key stakeholders, and communities (National Center for Cultural Competence, n.d.c; Marrone, 2014; Ray, 2010a, 2010b)

Organizational cultural competence is discussed in detail in Chapter 9, Creating Culturally Competent Organizations. Appendix C contains the Andrews/Boyle Transcultural Nursing Assessment Guide for Health Care Organizations and Facilities.

Clients with Special Needs

In the remainder of this chapter, we discuss the delivery of culturally competent nursing care for three groups of clients with special needs: those at high risk for health inequities and health disparities, those who are deaf, and those with communication and special language needs.

Health Disparities

The Health Resources and Services Administration defines health disparities as population-specific differences in the presence of disease, health outcomes, or access to health care. These differences can affect how frequently a disease affects a group, how many people get sick, or how often the disease causes death (U.S. Department of Health and Human Services, 2012). Many different populations are affected by disparities. These include the following:

- Racial and ethnic minorities
- Residents of rural areas
- Women, children, and the elderly

- Persons with disabilities
- Other special populations such as the deaf

In the United States, health disparities are a well-known problem among panethnic minority groups, particularly African Americans, Asian Americans, Native Americans, and Latinos. When examining health disparities globally, the World Health Organization uses the term health inequities (American Medical Association, n.d.).

Recent studies indicate that despite the steady improvements in the overall health of the United States, clients from racial and ethnic minority backgrounds experience a lower quality of health services, are less likely to receive routine medical procedures, and have higher rates of morbidity and mortality than nonminorities. Disparities in health care exist even when controlling for gender, condition, age, and socioeconomic status (American Medical Association, 2013; Clark, 2014; Frieden, 2013; Mandal, 2014; Purnell et al., 2011). The U.S. Department of Health, Health Resources and Services Administration, identifies culturally competent nursing care as an effective approach in reducing and eliminating health disparities and inequities in high-risk populations such as Blacks, Latinos, and American Indians. Studies demonstrate that these groups have a higher prevalence of chronic conditions, along with higher rates of mortality and poorer health outcomes, when compared with counterparts in the general population. For example, the incidence of cancer among African Americans is 10% higher than it is for Whites. African Americans and Latinos are also approximately twice as likely to develop diabetes as counterparts in the general population. Throughout the remaining chapters of the book, there will be discussion of the delivery of culturally congruent and culturally competent nursing care for clients from diverse backgrounds across the lifespan (Frieden, 2013).

Culture of the Deaf

Although nurses tend to think about clients from racially and ethnically diverse backgrounds, when discussing culturally competent nursing

care, there are many people who self-identify with *nonethnic cultures* and/or with more than one culture or subculture. For example, more than 5% of the world's population (360 million adults and 32 million children) experience disabling hearing loss (World Health Organization, 2014). Additionally, nurses will encounter clients who are both Black and deaf, gay and deaf, Native American and deaf, and many other combinations of two or more cultures (Holcomb, 2013). **Disabling hearing loss** is defined as the loss of greater than 40 decibels in the better ear in adults and the loss of greater than 30 decibels in the better ear in children. Disabling hearing loss means that a client has very little or no hearing, which has consequences for interpersonal communication, psychosocial well-being, quality of life, and economic independence. Hearing loss may affect one or both ears, can be congenital or acquired, and occurs on a continuum from mild to severe. Hearing loss leads to difficulty in hearing conversational speech or loud sounds. Clients who are **hard of hearing** usually communicate through spoken language and can benefit from hearing aids, captioning, and assistive listening devices (National Institute on Deafness and Other Communication Disorders, 2014; World Health Organization, 2014).

If hearing loss develops in childhood, it impedes speech and language development and, in severe cases, requires special education. In adulthood, disabling hearing loss can lead to embarrassment, loneliness, social isolation, stigmatization, prejudice, abuse, mental health problems such as depression, difficulties in interpersonal relationships with partners and children, restricted career choices, occupational stress, and lower earnings when compared with counterparts who do not have disabling hearing loss. Approximately one-third of people over 65 years of age are affected by disabling hearing loss. The prevalence in this age group is greatest in South Asia, Asia Pacific, and sub-Saharan Africa (World Health Organization, 2014).

Some clients with congenital deafness or others with significant hearing losses may benefit from cochlear implants, but the decision to have a cochlear implant is interconnected with an animated debate within and between members of the deaf culture and members of the culture of medicine concerning the appropriateness of cochlear implants. The fundamental issues underlying the debate concern the philosophical belief about deafness and the concept of deaf culture.

From an emic perspective, many deaf people see their bodies as well, whole, and nonimpaired, and they self-identify as members of a linguistic minority, not with the culture of disability (Harris, 2014; Holcomb, 2013; Humphries, 2014). As members of a cultural minority, some deaf people perceive themselves as being on a journey of cultural awareness, one of several stages on the way to achieving a positive sense of self and deaf identity. On the other hand, others who are deaf advocate reframing the concept of a deaf culture and conceptualizing it as the deaf experience based on values stemming from a visual orientation. Recognizing that literature and the arts provide forums for cultural awareness, appreciation, and expression of ideas and feelings, there are a growing number of deaf people using these media to communicate their experiences with one another and with hearing members of society (Harris, 2014; Holcomb, 2013).

From an etic (outsider's) perspective, some physicians and other members of the hearing society embrace concepts about deaf peoples' bodies that emphasize their differences from the bodies of people in the hearing society, thereby placing unwanted, unwarranted, and unnecessary limitations on deaf people's lives and capabilities. In the biological sciences, for example, the bodies of hearing people historically have been constructed with a normative bias. In other words, the body that hears is the normative prototype (Humphries, 2014). Some physicians engage in the cultural imposition of medical and surgical interventions on members of the deaf culture through eugenics (a science that tries to improve the human race by controlling which people become parents), genetic engineering, and insistence that deaf people should use hearing aids,

agree to cochlear implant surgery, and embrace other technologies that profoundly change their lives and their culture (Harris, 2014; Holcomb, 2013; Humphries, 2014).

Box 2-4 uses the framework of the five-step process for delivering culturally congruent and competent nursing care for people who self-identify as members of the deaf culture, beginning with a cultural assessment of self and the client, mutual goal setting, planning, implementation, and evaluation. Box 2-5 identifies measures that nurses can take to prevent deafness.

There are hundreds of sign language dialects in use around the world. Each culture has developed its own form of sign language to be compatible with the language spoken in that country. In the United States, an estimated 500,000 people communicate by using American Sign Language (ASL), including many who are deaf and hearing impaired, and family members, friends, or teachers of people with hearing impairments (Harrington, 2010). An ASL interpreter is often helpful in avoiding communication difficulty when caring for someone who is deaf or hearing impaired. Signaling and assistive listening devices, alerting devices, telecommunication devices for the deaf (TDD), and telephone amplifiers might also help promote effective communication and

---

Box 2-4 Culturally Congruent and Competent Care for Deaf Clients

1. Cultural Assessment
Self-Assessment:

What is your attitude toward people who are deaf? Do you think of people who are deaf as able-bodied or disabled? How do you feel about those who use hearing aids and other assistive devices for hearing?

How do you assess your self-location with regard to culture, gender, class, age, and other self-identities compared to the client's background?

What do you know about deafness, for example, causes, categories or types, and assistive devices?

Do you know anyone who is deaf? If so, how do you feel about the interactions you had with this person(s)?

Client Assessment:

Health History (Subjective Data) *See Appendix A, Transcultural Nursing Assessment Guide for Individuals and Families, for questions you might want to pose in the following categories:*

Cultural affiliations or self-identities associated with deafness?

Client's preferred method for communication? Sign language? Written communication? Verbal communication? Are any assistive devices needed for effective communication? Has exclusion from communication significantly impacted everyday life? Is there any evidence of feelings

of loneliness, isolation, and frustration, particularly for older adults with hearing loss?

Cultural sanctions and restrictions?

Economic or financial concerns?

Adults with hearing loss have a much higher unemployment rate and earn less than counterparts who have hearing. Is the client employed?

Education and health literacy levels?

In developing countries, children with hearing loss and deafness rarely receive any schooling. What is the educational and health literacy level of the client? Improving access to education and vocational rehabilitation services, and raising awareness, especially among employers, would decrease unemployment rates among adults with hearing loss.

Health-related beliefs and practices?

Kinship and social support network?

Nutrition and diet?

Religion and spirituality?

Values orientation of the client, including his/her perspective on culturally acceptable interventions to improve hearing?

Physical Examination (Objective Data) *See Chapter 3, Cultural Competence in the Health History and Physical Examination.*

2. **Mutual Goal Setting**
3. **Care Planning**
4. **Implementation of Care Plan**
5. **Evaluation of Care**

    Culturally acceptable, congruent, and competent?
    Affordable?
    Accessible?
    Quality?
    Evidence based?
    Best practices?

> In collaboration with client's family, significant others, credentialed, licensed members of the health care team (e.g., audiologist, speech–language pathologist), folk, traditional, religious, and/or spiritual healers

facilitate the provision of culturally competent care in home, community, hospital, and other settings.

Communication and Language Assistance

With growing concerns about racial, ethnic, and language disparities in health and health care and the need for health care systems to accommodate increasingly diverse patient populations, **language access services** (LAS) have become a matter of increasing national importance. Currently, about 20% of the US population speaks a language other than English at home, and 9% has limited English proficiency. By 2050, more than half the population will come from racial or ethnic minority backgrounds. Diversity is even greater when dimensions such as geography, socioeconomic status, disability status, sexual orientation, and gender identity are considered. Attention to these trends is critical for ensuring that health disparities narrow, rather than widen, in the future. In 2013, the Office of Minority Health released an

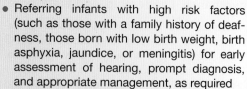

Box 2-5 Prevention of Deafness

50% of all cases of hearing loss can be prevented through primary prevention. Strategies for prevention include:

- Immunizing children against childhood diseases, including measles, meningitis, rubella, and mumps
- Immunizing adolescent girls and women of reproductive age against rubella before pregnancy
- Screening for and treating syphilis and other infections in pregnant women
- Improving antenatal and perinatal care, including promotion of safe childbirth
- Avoiding the use of ototoxic drugs, unless prescribed and monitored by a qualified physician,

nurse practitioner, or other health care provider
- Referring infants with high risk factors (such as those with a family history of deafness, those born with low birth weight, birth asphyxia, jaundice, or meningitis) for early assessment of hearing, prompt diagnosis, and appropriate management, as required
- Reducing exposure (both occupational and recreational) to loud noises by creating awareness, using personal protective devices, and developing and implementing suitable legislation

Data from World Health Organization (2014).

update of the National Standards for Culturally and Linguistically Appropriate Services in Health and Health Care (the National CLAS Standards, see Box 2-6).

Standards under the theme "Communication and Language Assistance" include the recommendation that language assistance should be provided as needed, in a manner appropriate to the organization's size, scope, and mission (U.S. Census Bureau, 2013a, 2013b). Clients are informed about the availability of assistance in their preferred language after being asked to indicate their language needs (Jones & Boyle, 2011; Office of Minority Health, 2013, n.d.; Siaki, 2011). Health care organizations and providers that receive federal financial assistance without providing free language assistance services could be in violation of Title VI of the Civil Rights Act of 1964 and its implementing regulations. The director of the U.S. Department of Health and Human Services Office for Civil Rights encourages requests for information and technical assistance concerning the law (Hoh, Garcia, & Alvarez, 2014).

Box 2-6 National Standards for Culturally and Linguistically Appropriate Services in Health and Health Care

The National Standards for Culturally and Linguistically Appropriate Services in Health and Health Care (the National CLAS Standards) aim to improve health care quality and advance health equity by establishing a framework for organizations to serve the nation's increasingly diverse communities.

Principal Standard

1. Provide effective, equitable, understandable, and respectful quality care and services that are responsive to diverse cultural health beliefs and practices, preferred languages, health literacy, and other communication needs.

Governance, Leadership, and Workforce

2. Advance and sustain organizational governance and leadership that promotes CLAS and health equity through policy, practices, and allocated resources.
3. Recruit, promote, and support a culturally and linguistically diverse governance, leadership, and workforce that are responsive to the population in the service area.
4. Educate and train governance, leadership, and workforce in culturally and linguistically appropriate policies and practices on an ongoing basis.

Communication and Language Assistance

5. Offer language assistance to individuals who have limited English proficiency and/or other communication needs, at no cost to them, to facilitate timely access to all health care and services.
6. Inform all individuals of the availability of language assistance services clearly and in their preferred language, verbally and in writing.
7. Ensure the competence of individuals providing language assistance, recognizing that the use of untrained individuals and/or minors as interpreters should be avoided.
8. Provide easy-to-understand print and multimedia materials and signage in the languages commonly used by the populations in the service area.

Engagement, Continuous Improvement, and Accountability

9. Establish culturally and linguistically appropriate goals, policies, and management accountability, and infuse them throughout the organizations' planning and operations.

10. Conduct ongoing assessments of the organization's CLAS-related activities and integrate CLAS-related measures into assessment measurement and continuous quality improvement activities.
11. Collect and maintain accurate and reliable demographic data to monitor and evaluate the impact of CLAS on health equity and outcomes and to inform service delivery.
12. Conduct regular assessments of community health assets and needs and use the results to plan and implement services that respond to the cultural and linguistic diversity of populations in the service area.
13. Partner with the community to design, implement, and evaluate policies, practices, and services to ensure cultural and linguistic appropriateness.
14. Create conflict and grievance resolution processes that are culturally and linguistically appropriate to identify, prevent, and resolve conflicts or complaints.
15. Communicate the organization's progress in implementing and sustaining CLAS to all stakeholders, constituents, and the general public.

Source: Office of Minority Health (2014).

Summary

In this chapter, the reader was introduced to individual and organizational cultural competence and provided with the knowledge and skills needed to deliver culturally congruent and competent nursing care to individual clients from diverse cultures. Nurses are encouraged to think about out the delivery of care as a five-step process consisting of (1) a constructively critical self-assessment of the nurse's own attitudes, knowledge, and skills and a cultural assessment of clients from diverse backgrounds by gathering subjective and objective data using the health history and physical examination; (2) mutual goal setting in collaboration with the client and other members of the interprofessional health care team (family, significant others, credentialed, licensed, folk, traditional, religious, and/or spiritual healers); (3) development of the plan of care; (4) implementation of the care plan; and (5) evaluation of the plan for client acceptance, cultural congruence, cultural competence, affordability, accessibility, and use of research, evidence, and best practices. If necessary, the steps in the process may be repeated. Interprofessional collaboration with the client and members of the health care team is integral to the provision of culturally congruent and competent nursing care. Lastly, we examined clients with special needs including those at high risk for health disparities, those who are deaf, and those with communication and language needs.

REVIEW QUESTIONS

1. Compare and contrast individual and organizational cultural competence.
2. Describe the five steps in the process for delivering culturally congruent and competent care for clients from diverse backgrounds.
3. In your own words, define the following terms: cultural baggage, ethnocentrism, cultural imposition, prejudice, and discrimination.
4. Identify key strategies to assist clients with communication and language needs.

CRITICAL THINKING ACTIVITIES

1. After critically analyzing the definitions of cultural competence presented in the chapter, craft a definition of the term in your own words.

2. In discussions of culturally competent nursing care, the culture of the deaf and hearing impaired is sometimes overlooked because it is categorized as a nonethnic culture. Search the Internet for information on the culture

of the deaf. What cultural characteristics do deaf people have in common with members of other cultural groups? If a client is both deaf and self-identifies as a member of another ethnic or nonethnic culture, how does this influence your ability to deliver culturally congruent and culturally competent nursing care?

3. To provide culturally competent nursing care, you should engage in a cultural self-assessment. Answer the questions in Box 2-2, How Do You Relate to Various Groups of People in the Society? Score your answers using the guide provided. What did you learn about yourself? How would you approach learning more about the health-related beliefs and practices of groups for which you need more background knowledge? What resources might you use in your search for information?

4. At the request of the Bureau of Primary Health Care, Health Resources and Services Administration, U.S. Department of Health and Human Services, staff at the National Center for Cultural Competence (NCCC) developed the *Cultural Competence Health Practitioner Assessment,* which is available online. Visit the NCCC website and complete this assessment.

5. Mary Johnson is an African American nurse working in the Post-Anesthesia Care Unit (PACU). When Mrs. Li, a recent immigrant from China, arrives in the PACU following a major bowel resection for cancer, Mary assesses Mrs. Li for pain. Mary notes that Mrs. Li is not complaining about pain, is lying quietly in her bed, and has a stoic facial expression. Mary comments to another nurse that "all Chinese patients seem to do just fine without post-operative pain medications. I'm not going to administer any analgesics unless she asks me for something." Do you agree with Nurse Johnson's assessment of Mrs. Li's pain? What nonverbal manifestations of pain would you assess? How would you reply to Nurse Johnson's statement that she doesn't intend to administer any pain medication?

REFERENCES

American Medical Association. (2013). *Health literacy and patient safety: Helping patients understand.* Chicago, MA: Author.

American Medical Association. (n.d.). Eliminating health disparities. Retrieved from http://www.ama-assn.org/ama/pub/physician-resources/public-health/eliminating-health-disparities.page

Andrews, J. D. (2013). *Cultural, ethnic, and religious reference manual for healthcare providers* (4th ed.). Kernersville, NC: JAMARDA Resources.

Andrews, M. M., & Collins, J. W. (2015). Using Leininger's theory as the organizing framework for a federal project on cultural competence. In M. R. McFarland & H. B. Wehbe-Alamah (Eds.), *Leininger's culture care diversity and universality: A worldwide nursing theory* (pp. 537–582). Burlington, MA: Jones and Bartlett Learning.

Andrews, M., Thompson, T., Wehbe-Alamah, H., McFarland, M. R., Hasenau, S., Horn, B., ..., Vint, P. (2011). Developing a culturally competent workforce through collaborative partnerships. *Journal of Transcultural Nursing, 22*(3), 300–306.

Basuray, J. (2014). *Culture & health: Concept and practice* (2nd ed.). Ronkonkoma, NY: Linus Publications, Inc.

Betancourt, J., Green, A., & Carrillo, E. (2002). *Cultural competence in health care: Emerging frameworks and practical approaches.* The Commonwealth Fund. Retrieved from http://www.commonwealthfund.org/usr_doc/betancourt_culturalcompetence_576.pdf

Campinha-Bacote, J. (2003). *The process of cultural competence in the delivery of healthcare services* (4th ed.). Cincinnati, OH: Transcultural C.A.R.E. Associates.

Campinha-Bacote, J. (May 31, 2011). Delivering patient-centered care in the midst of a cultural conflict: The role of cultural competence. *Online Journal of Issues in Nursing, 16*(2), Manuscript 5.

Chettih, M. (2012). Turning the lens inward: Cultural competence and providers' values in health care decision making. *Gerontologist, 52*(6), 739–747.

Clark, L. (2014). A humanizing gaze for transcultural nursing research will tell the story of health disparities. *Journal of Transcultural Nursing, 25*(2), 122–128.

Cross, T., Bazron, B., Dennis, K., & Isaacs, M. (1989). *Towards a culturally competent system of care, Vol. I.* Washington, DC: Georgetown University Child Development Center, CASSP Technical Assistance Center.

Douglas, M. K., & Pacquiao, D. F. (2010). Core curriculum for transcultural nursing and health care. *Journal of Transcultural Nursing, 21*(4 Suppl), 5S–417S.

Douglas, M. K., Rosenkoetter, M., Pacquiao, D. F., Callister, L. C., Hattar-Pollara, M., Lauderdale, J., ... Purnell, L.

(2014). Guidelines for implementing culturally competent nursing care. *Journal of Transcultural Nursing, 25*(20), 109–121.

Dunagan, P. B., Kimble, L. P., Gunby, S.S., & Andrews, M. M. (2014). Attitudes of prejudice as a predictor of cultural competence among baccalaureate nursing students. *Journal of Nursing Education, 53*, 320–328. doi: 10.3928/01484834-20140521-13

Frieden, T. R. (2013). CDC Health disparities and inequalities report—United States, 2013. Forward. *Morbidity and mortality weekly report. Surveillance summaries (Washington, D.C.: 2002), 62*(Suppl 3), 1–2.

Goico, A. L. (2014). EEOC expands pregnancy discrimination definitions and offers new guidance that increases employer obligations to pregnant employees. *Employee Relations Law Journal, Winter 2014*, 39–43.

Harrington, T. (2010). Sign language: Ranking and number of users. Retrieved from http://libguides.gallaudet.edu/content.php?pid=114804&sid=991835

Harris, R. (2014). Introduction to American deaf culture. *Sign Language Studies, 14*(3), 406–410.

Hoh, H. K., Garcia, J. N., Alvarez, M. H. (2014). Culturally and linguistically appropriate services—Advancing health with CLAS. *New England Journal of Medicine, 371*, 198–201.

Holcomb, T. K. (2013). *Introduction to American deaf culture.* New York: Oxford University Press.

Humphries, T. (2014). Our time: The legacy of the twentieth century. *Sign Language Studies, 15*(1), 57–73.

Institute of Medicine. (2011). *Future of nursing: Leading change, advancing health.* Washington, DC: National Academies Press.

Interprofessional Education Collaborative Expert Panel. (2011). *Core competencies for interprofessional collaborative practice: Report of an expert panel.* Washington, DC: Interprofessional Education Collaborative.

Jarvis, C. (2014). *Physical examination and assessment,* Saint Louis, MO: Elsevier.

Jones, E. G. & Boyle, J. S. (2011). Working with translators and interpreters in research: Lessons learned. *Journal of Transcultural Nursing, 22*(2), 109–115.

Leininger, M. M. (1970). *Nursing and anthropology: Two worlds to blend.* New York: John Wiley & Sons.

Leininger, M. M. (1978). *Transcultural nursing: Concepts, theories and practices.* New York: John Wiley & Sons.

Leininger, M. M. (1991). *Culture care diversity and universality: A theory of nursing.* New York: National League for Nursing.

Leininger, M. M. (1995). *Transcultural nursing: Concepts, theories, research and practices.* New York: McGraw-Hill.

Leininger, M. M. (1999). What is transcultural nursing and culturally competent care? *Journal of Transcultural Nursing, 10*(1), 9.

Leininger, M. M., & McFarland, M. R. (2002). *Transcultural nursing: Concepts, theories, research and practices.* New York: McGraw-Hill.

Leininger, M. M., & McFarland, M. R. (2006). *Culture care diversity and universality: A worldwide theory for nursing* (2nd ed.). Sudbury, MA: Jones & Bartlett, Publishers.

Mandal, A. (2014). What are health disparities? Retrieved from http://www.news-medical.net/health/Health-Disparities-What-are-Health-Disparities.aspx

Marrone, S. (2014). Organizational cultural competence. Transcultural Nursing Society Annual Conference, October, 2014, Charleston, SC.

McClimens, A., Brewster, J., & Lewis, R. (2014). Recognising and respecting patients' cultural diversity. *Nursing Standard, 12*(28), 45–52.

McFarland, M. R., & Wehbe-Alamah, H. B. (2015). The theory of culture care diversity and universality. In M. R. McFarland & H. B. Wehbe-Alamah (Eds.), *Leininger's culture care diversity and universality: A worldwide nursing theory* (pp. 1–34). Burlington, MA: Jones and Bartlett Learning.

National Center for Cultural Competence. (n.d.a). Definitions of cultural competence. (Georgetown University Center for Child and Human Development). Retrieved September 12, 2014, from Curricula Enhancement Module Series: http://www.ncccurricula.info/culturalcompetence.html

National Center for Cultural Competence. (n.d.c). Organizational cultural competence. Retrieved from http://www.ncccurricula.info/culturalcompetence.html

National Center for Cultural Competence (NCCC). (n.d.b). Foundations of cultural and linguistic competence. Retrieved September 10, 2014 from http://nccc.georgetown.edu/foundations/index.html

National Institute on Deafness and Other Communication Disorders. (2014, August 12). National Institute on Deafness and Other Communication Disorders (NIDCD). U.S. Department of Health and Human Services. Retrieved September 12, 2014, from National Institutes of Health: http://www.nidcd.nih.gov/Pages/default.aspx

Oelke, N. D., Thurston, W. E., & Arthur, N. (2013). Intersections between interprofessional practice, cultural competence, and primary healthcare. *Journal of Interprofessional Care, 27*(5), 267–272. doi: 10.3109/13561820.2013.785502

Office of Minority Health. (2013). The national CLAS standards. Retrieved from http://minorityhealth.hhs.gov/templates/browse.aspx?lvl=2&lvlid=15

Office of Minority Health. (2014, June 19). The Center for Linguistic and Cultural Competency in Health Care. U.S. Department of Health and Human Services. Retrieved September 12, 2014, from Office of Minority Health website: http://minorityhealth.hhs.gov/omh/browse.aspx?lvl=2&lvlid=34

Office of Minority Health. (n.d.). National standards for culturally and linguistically appropriate services in health and health care. Retrieved from https://www.thinkculturalhealth.hhs.gov/pdfs/NationalCLASStandardsFactSheet.pdf

Office of Minority Health & Equity (OMHHE). (2013, March 22). Minority health. Centers for Disease Control and Prevention. Retrieved September 13, 2014, from Centers

for Disease Control and Prevention website: http://www.
cdc.gov/minorityhealth/omhhe.html

Purnell, L. (2014). *Guide to culturally competent health care.*
Philadelphia, PA: F.A. Davis Company.

Purnell, L., & Paulanka, B. J. (Eds.). (2013). *Transcultural health
care: A culturally competent approach.* Philadelphia, PA: F.
A. Davis.

Purnell, L., Davidhizar, R., Giger, J., Fishman, D., Strickland, O., &
Allison, D. (2011). Guide to developing a culturally competent
organization. *Journal of Transcultural Nursing, 22*(1), 5–14.

Ray, M. (2010a). Creating caring organizations and cultures
through communitarian ethics. *Journal of the World
Universities Forum, 3*(5), 41–52.

Ray, M. (2010b). *Transcultural caring dynamics in nursing
and health care.* Philadelphia, PA: F.A. Davis Company.

Roberts, S., Warda, M., Garbutt, S., & Curry, K. (2014). Use
of high-fidelity simulation to teach cultural competence in
the nursing curriculum." *Journal of Professional Nursing,
30*(3), 259–265.

Siaki, L. (2011). Translating a questionnaire for use with
Samoan adults: Lessons learned. *Journal of Transcultural
Nursing, 22*(2), 122–128.

Spector, R.E. (2013). *Cultural diversity in health and illness.*
(8th ed.). Upper Saddle River, NJ: Pearson.

Talabere, L. R. (1996). Meeting the challenge of culture care in
nursing: Diversity, sensitivity, and congruence. *Journal of
Cultural Diversity, 3*(2), 53–61.

Timmins, F. (2006). Critical practice in nursing care: Analysis,
action and reflexivity. *Nursing Standard, 20*, 49–54.

Title VII of the Civil Rights Act of 1964 (Public Law 88–352)
retrieved at http://www.eeoc.gov/laws/statutes/ada.cfm-
www.eeoc.gov/laws/statutes/titlevii.cfm

Titles I and V of the Americans with Disabilities Act of 1990
(Pub. L. 101–336) (ADA) retrieved at http://www.eeoc.
gov/laws/statutes/ada.cfm

U.S. Census Bureau. (2012). Selected social characteristics
in the United States. http://factfinder2.census.gov/faces/
tableservices/jsf/pages/productview.xhtml?pid=ACS_12_
1YR_DP02&prodType=table

U.S. Census Bureau. (2013a). Language use. (U.S. Department
of Commerce) Retrieved September 12, 2014, from U.S.
Census Bureau https://www.census.gov/hhes/socdemo/
language/about/faqs.html#Q3

U.S. Census Bureau. (2013b). Language Use in the United
States: 2011. Retrieved from http://www.census.gov/
prod/2013pubs/acs-22.pdf

U.S. Department of Health and Human Services (2012). *HHS
Action Plan to reduce racial and ethnic health disparities.*
Washington, DC: U.S. Department of Human Services.

World Health Organization. (2014, February). Deafness
and hearing loss. Retrieved from http:// www.who.int/
mediacentre/factsheets/fs300/en/

World Health Organization. (n.d.). What are the social determinants of health? Retrieved at http://www.int/social_
determinants/en/

World Health Organization (WHO). (2010). Framework for
action on interprofessional education and collaborative
practice. Geneva, Switzerland: World Health Organization.

Cultural Competence in the Health History and Physical Examination

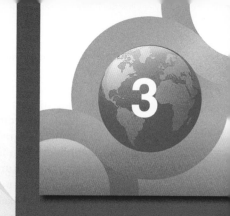

Margaret M. Andrews and Margaret Murray-Wright

Key Terms

Albinism
Addison's disease
Biocultural variations
Cafe' au lait spots
Clinical decision making
Copy-number variants
Cultural assessment
Cultural care accommodation
   or negotiation
Cultural care repatterning or
   restructuring
Cultural care preservation or
   maintenance

Cultural norms
Culture-bound syndromes
Cyanosis
Ecchymoses
Epigenetics
Erythema
Ethnohistory
Evaluation
Genetics
Genome
Genomics
Genotyping
Jaundice
Leukoedema
Lactose intolerance

Mongolian spots
Oral hyperpigmentation
Pain
Pallor
Petechiae
Pharmacogenomics
Presbycusis
Single-nucleotide
   polymorphisms
Steatorrhea
Uremia
Vitiligo

Learning Objectives

1. Explore the process and content needed for a comprehensive cultural assessment of clients from diverse cultures.
2. Identify biocultural variations in health and illness for individuals from diverse cultures.
3. Integrate concepts from the fields of genetics and genomics into the cultural assessment of clients from diverse cultural backgrounds.
4. Discuss biocultural variations in common laboratory tests.
5. Critically review transcultural perspectives in the health history and physical examination.

In this chapter, we provide cultural prompts or cues that enable nurses to customize or tailor their cultural assessment according to the client's genetic background, biographic makeup, and his/her self-identified cultural affiliation(s). We define and describe the cultural assessment and then discuss transcultural perspectives on the health history, the physical examination, and **clinical decision making** and actions.

In many instances, the health history and physical examination are interconnected and interrelated. For example, the client might complain about shortness of breath during the history, and the nurse might hear the client wheezing during the interview. After the interview is finished, the nurse gathers additional data during the physical examination by observing the client for clinical manifestations of cyanosis, nasal flaring, intercostal retraction, and by auscultating the lungs. Based on the findings in the physical examination, the nurse might ask additional questions, such as the length of time the client has experienced the symptoms, check for family history of respiratory disease, and pursue additional assessment related to the respiratory and cardiovascular systems.

The health history includes cultural perspectives on biographic and genetic data, medications, reasons for seeking care, present health and history of the present illness, past health, family and social history, and the review of systems. In the physical examination, the nurse compares and contrasts normal and abnormal cultural variations in measurements, general appearance, skin, sweat glands, head (hair, eyes, ears, mouth), mammary plexus, and the musculoskeletal system. We also discuss biocultural variations in pain and illness and cultural considerations in selected laboratory tests for which there is evidence of racial and/or ethnic differences. Lastly, we explore transcultural perspectives in clinical decision making and actions. After completing a comprehensive cultural assessment through the health history, physical examination, and analysis of laboratory test results, the next steps are to analyze the subjective and objective data, set mutual goals with the client, develop a plan of care, confer with and make referrals to other members of the interprofessional health care team as needed, and implement a plan of care, either alone or with others.

Cultural Assessment

With 318 million people, the United States is the third most populous nation in the world (behind China and India). By the year 2050, nearly 50% of the U.S. population will be comprised of people from diverse racial and ethnic backgrounds, that is, non-white groups. Hispanic and Asian populations are expected to double between now and 2050 and are followed in growth by Blacks, Native Americans, Native Hawaiians, and other Pacific Islanders (U.S. Census Bureau, 2014a). With growing diversity comes the need for nurses to develop their knowledge and skills in cultural assessment. In the course of their professional careers, nurses might need to assess people from many different racial and ethnic groups and from numerous nonethnic cultures.

Cultural assessment, or *culturologic assessment*, refers to a systematic, comprehensive examination of individuals, families, groups, and communities regarding their health-related cultural beliefs, values, and practices. Although the focus in this chapter is on the individual client, there are some instances in which clients' families and others in close contact might need to be involved, for example, when the cultural assessment reveals the presence of a genetic, infectious, or communicable disorder. Cultural assessments form the foundation for the clients' plan of care, providing valuable data for setting mutual goals, planning care, intervening, and evaluating the care. The goal of the cultural assessment is to determine the nursing and health care needs of people from diverse cultures and intervene in ways that are culturally acceptable, congruent, competent, safe, affordable, accessible, high quality, and based on current research, evidence, and best practices (Leininger & McFarland, 2002; McFarland & Wehbe-Alamah, 2015).

Given that they deal with cultural values, belief systems, and lifeways, cultural assessments tend to be broad and comprehensive. It is sometimes necessary to conduct an abbreviated assessment when time is limited, the client's reason for seeking care is urgent or time sensitive, the client is unable to provide all of the necessary data, or other circumstances require a shorter, more focused assessment. The cultural assessment consists of both *process* and *content*. *Process* refers to how to approach to the client, consideration of verbal and nonverbal communication, and the sequence and order in which data are gathered. The *content* of the cultural assessment consists of the actual data categories in which information about clients is gathered. Nurses are required to complete assessments before and/or at the time of admission to health care facilities, when opening home health care cases, and prior to many types of medical and surgical procedures. Depending on the circumstances, assessments may be very brief, or they may be detailed and in-depth. Ideally, the cultural assessment is integrated into the overall assessment of the client, family, and significant others. It is usually impractical to expect that nurses will have the time to conduct a separate cultural assessment, so questions aimed at gathering cultural data should be integrated into the overall assessment using the format provided by health care facilities, agencies, or organization for their admissions or intake assessment.

Appendix A is the Andrews and Boyle Transcultural Nursing Assessment Guide for Individuals and Families for use when initially assessing clients from diverse backgrounds, for example, when conducting an admission assessment or opening a case in home health care or ambulatory settings. The major categories in this guide include cultural affiliations, values orientation, communication, health-related beliefs and practices, nutrition, socioeconomic considerations, organizations providing cultural support, education, religion, cultural aspects of disease incidence, biocultural variations, and developmental considerations across the lifespan. Appendix B is the Andrews and Boyle

Transcultural Nursing Assessment Guide for Groups and Communities. The major categories in this guide include family and kinship systems, social life and networks, political or government systems, language and traditions, worldview, values, norms, religious beliefs and practices, health beliefs and practices, and health care systems.

Transcultural Perspectives on the Health History

The purpose of the health history is to gather *subjective data*—a term that refers to things that people say or relate about themselves. The health history provides a comprehensive overview of a client's past and present health, and it examines the manner in which the person interacts with the environment. The health history enables the nurse to assess health strengths, including cultural beliefs and practices that might influence the nurse's ability to provide culturally competent nursing care. The history is combined with the *objective data* from the physical examination and the laboratory results to form a diagnosis about the health status of a person.

For the well client, the history is used to assess lifestyle, which includes activity, exercise, diet, and related personal behaviors and choices that nurses may gather to identify potential risk factors for disease. For the ill client, the health history includes a chronologic record of the health problem(s). For both well and ill clients, the health history is a screening tool for abnormal symptoms, health problems, and concerns. The health history also provides valuable information about the coping strategies and health-related behaviors and responses used previously by clients and family members.

In many health care settings, the client is expected to fill out a printed history form or checklist. From a transcultural perspective, this approach has both positive and negative aspects. On the positive side, this approach provides the client with ample time to recall details such as relevant family history and the dates of health-related

events such as surgical procedures and illnesses. It is expedient for nurses because it takes less time to review a form or a checklist than to elicit the information in a face-to-face or telephone interview.

However, this approach has limitations. First, the form is likely to be in English. Those whose primary language is not English might find the form difficult or impossible to complete accurately. Although some health care facilities provide forms translated into Spanish, French, or other languages, translating forms can be costly and is not always effective. In some instances, the literal translation of medical terms is not possible. In other instances, the symptom or disease is not recognized in the culture with which the client identifies. For example, in asking about symptoms of depression, there might be many cultural factors that influence the client's interpretation of the question. In Chinese languages, there is no literal translation for the word *depression*. In Chinese culture, it is more acceptable to somaticize emotional pain with expressions of physical discomfort such as chest pain or "heaviness of the heart" (Ryder & Chentsova-Dutton, 2012; Yu & Lee, 2012). In rural Guatemala, Mayans might refer to "*dolor de corazón*" or pain in the heart (Godoy-Paiz, Toner, & Vidal, 2011; Pedersen et al., 2012). "*Nervios*" may be cited by Guatemalan Mayan women as the cause of somatic disorders such as ulcers, diabetes, and dizziness (Godoy-Paiz et al., 2011). If health care providers fail to understand the cultural meaning of the symptom "heaviness of the heart," or "pain in the heart," unnecessary, invasive, and costly tests might be performed to rule out cardiovascular disease. In some instances, clients might be unable to read or write in any language; thus, an assessment of the client's literacy level should precede the use of printed history forms or checklists.

Although there is wide variation in health history formats, most contain the following categories: *biographic data, reason for seeking care, review of medications and allergies, present health or history of present illness, past history, family and social history,* and *review of systems. Genetic data* are also an important area for the transcultural nurse to consider as part of the health history. This chapter will not provide a comprehensive overview of these categories, but will present them as they relate to providing culturally congruent and culturally competent nursing care.

Biographic Data

Although the biographic information (name, address, phone, age, gender, preferred language, and so forth) might seem straightforward, several cultural variations in recording age are important to note. In some Asian cultures, an infant is considered 1 year old at birth. Having an accurate age has many clinical implications, including assessing developmental milestones and determining appropriate medication dosages, and certain legal implications as well. For many reasons, age may not be reported correctly. Some clients may not wish to report their correct age; other clients may not know or be able to provide a specific age in the way health care providers may expect it.

One of the first areas that nurses should assess is the client's self-reported cultural affiliation. With what cultural group(s) does the client report affiliation? Where was the client born? What is the ancestry or **ethnohistory** of the client? When the client self-identifies with multiple races or ethnicities, it is often useful to determine with which group the client *primarily* identifies. Knowledge of the client's ethnohistory is important in determining risk factors for genetic and acquired diseases and in understanding the client's cultural heritage. In addition to the standard descriptive information about clients, it is necessary to record who has furnished the data. Whereas this is usually the client, the source might be a relative, guardian, or friend. Note whether an interpreter is used and indicate the relationship to the client.

Genetic Data

Genetics is a branch of biology that studies heredity and the variations of inherited characteristics. A rapidly evolving science, genetics

exerts a significant influence on the health of people from cultures around the world. Whereas genetics scrutinizes the functioning and composition of a specific gene, **genomics** addresses all genes and their interrelationship to identify their combined influence on the growth and development of the organism. To date, the locations of more than 25,000 genes have been mapped to a specific human chromosome and most to a specific region on the chromosome. A **genome** is an organism's complete set of DNA, including all of its genes. Each genome contains all of the information needed to build and maintain that organism. In humans, a copy of the entire genome—more than 3 billion DNA base pairs—is contained in all cells that have a nucleus. Genetic mapping is continuing at a rapid rate, and these numbers and discoveries are constantly being updated. **Epigenetics** is the study of how genes are influenced by forces such as the environment, obesity, or medication. Although the children in Figure 3-1 are twins, epigenetic modifications can cause individuals with the same DNA sequences to have different disease profiles (McCance & Huether, 2014). As a result of epigenetic research,

the critical role played by external forces is better understood and can now be integrated into client assessment and care.

While each person has approximately 30,000 genes, any two individuals share 99.9% of their DNA sequence, reflecting that the diversity among individuals accounts for approximately 0.1% of the DNA (Porth, 2015). Although humans are more alike than different, the growing inventory of human genetic variation facilitates an understanding of why susceptibility to common diseases differs among individual clients and populations. These genetic variations provide the knowledge needed to safely administer medications and counsel clients regarding the prevention and risk of disease. This discussion provides a foundation in genetic and genomic science to ensure that the nursing assessment is customized according to each client's unique background and current care needs.

Human genetic variation contributes significantly to the physical variation occurring among individuals. The two most important components of human genetic variation are **single-nucleotide polymorphisms** (SNPs) and **copy-number**

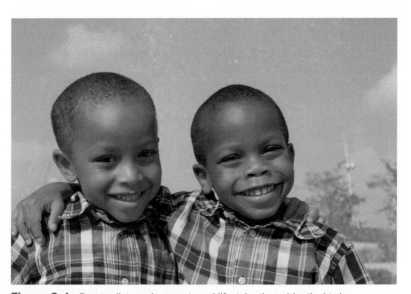

Figure 3-1. Due to diet, environment, and lifestyle, these identical twins may have entirely different disease profiles as they mature into adulthood (Felix Mizioznikov/Shutterstock.com).

variants. SNPs are single DNA base pairs that differ among individual DNA sequences; copy-number variants are larger blocks of DNA sequence that vary. Most common SNPs are shared among populations from different continents, which reflect continued migration and gene flow among humans through history. Many studies have shown that 85% to 90% of genetic variation can be found within any human population. Samples of persons from Great Brain and Ghana have genetic similarity. Only an additional 10% to 15% of variation is gained when the entire human population is considered. A genetic variation may be relatively common in one population, but absent in another due to a recent emergence of a variant that has not yet had time to spread. Hereditary hemochromatosis, a disorder that causes the body to absorb too much iron from food, is common in Europe, but very rare elsewhere. Hereditary lactase is prevalent among European and African pastoral populations where milk consumption beyond childhood has had a selective advantage (Rotimi & Jorde, 2010).

Genetic research studies are now readily available regarding the safety and efficacy of medications for a variety of conditions. This information extends far beyond traditional inherited disease such as sickle cell anemia or cystic fibrosis. This growing inventory of human variation facilitates an understanding of why susceptibility to common disease varies among individuals and populations. Analyses of two key heart failure (HF) trials comparing African Americans to Whites reveal significant ethnic differences in response to treatment.

The African-American Heart Failure Trial (A-HeFT) demonstrates that therapy with fixed-dose combined isosorbide dinitrate/hydralazine (BiDil) added to customary therapy significantly improved survival in self-identified African American men and women with advanced heart failure (Bress et al., 2013).

The 2013 American College of Cardiology Foundation/American Heart Association guidelines recommend combined isosorbide dinitrate (ISDN) and hydralazine to reduce mortality and morbidity for African Americans with symptomatic heart failure as earlier studies reflected a significant reduction in death and improvement in outcomes. Hypertension contributes to HF, especially in African Americans. The A-HeFT and its substudies demonstrated improvements in ventricular performance based on echocardiogram, morbidity, and mortality as well as a decrease in hospitalizations, potentially affecting burgeoning HF health care costs. The importance of genetic characteristics in determining response to ISDN–hydralazine was reinforced a decade after the original study. The Genetic Risk Assessment in Heart Failure substudy confirmed an important hypothesis and generated relevant pharmacogenomic data (Ferdinand et al., 2014).

Investigators have focused on genetic variations in populations, which may yield a more complete characterization of risk, and thereby permit more specifically targeted treatment of heart failure clients. In the future, more precise selection of β-blocker therapy for heart failure and hypertension based on genotype may be superior to selecting therapy based on a client's race/ethnicity.

Recent attention has been drawn to the association of chronic traumatic encephalopathy (CTE) with contact sports such as boxing, American football, soccer, hockey, and wrestling. Chronic CTE is a progressive neurodegenerative disease that is a long-term consequence of single or repetitive closed head injuries for which there is no treatment and no definitive premortem diagnosis. Researchers from Boston University discovered significant cases of CTE in college and professional football players. Subsequently, it was discovered that a significant number of these athletes had two copies of the ApoE4 gene variant; this version of the ApoE gene has been shown to substantially increase the risk of Alzheimer's disease. This raises questions about offering genetic screening for the ApoEv4 to linebackers, boxers, and parents whose children play sports that put players at risk for CTE. Sports transcend all cultures, yet may be more prevalent in certain racial and ethnic groups, for example, 68% of all NFL football players are African American (National

Football League, 2014). Juvenile traumatic brain injury leaves survivors facing a potential lifetime of cognitive, somatic, and emotional symptoms; therefore, prevention and education are currently the most compelling ways to combat CTE and are emphasized by nurses with parents, athletic trainers, and coaches (Hwang et al., 2011).

Apolipoprotein genotype also has a potential role in cognitive function of postmenopausal women with early-stage breast cancer (American Cancer Society, n.d.; Domchek, 2014). Koleck et al. (2014) examine the role of apolipoprotein E (APOE) in the cognitive function of postmenopausal women with early-stage breast cancer prior to the initiation of adjuvant therapy, that is, assisting in the prevention, amelioration, or cure of the disease. Performance or changes in performance on tasks of executive function, attention, verbal/visual learning, and memory were influenced. APOE genotype along with other biomarkers may be used in the future to assist nurses in identifying women with breast cancer most at risk for cognitive decline.

Nurses should consider how the client will use genetic and genomic information and be prepared to provide support if clients experience moral or ethical issues. Most hospitals have ethics committees, chaplains, pastoral teams, and other resources to assist clients facing moral and ethical dilemmas.

The addition of genetics and genomics to the traditional nursing assessment will inform and engage clients to make key decisions in their personal health care plan. By virtue of their race or ethnicity, clients are sometimes said to be "at risk" for certain diseases. Examples include diabetes mellitus among Native Americans, breast cancer among Ashkenazi Jews, and prostate cancer among African Americans. Particular forms of treatment are also believed to be more (or less) effective among certain racial/ethnic groups compared with others.

Among African Americans (compared with Whites), angiotensin-converting enzyme (ACE) inhibitors are less effective for essential hypertension and a therapeutic response to selective serotonin reuptake inhibitor (SSRI) antidepressants occurs at lower doses. Considerations

about health by racial and ethnic groups require the context that environmental factors and health disparities as well as genetic factors are operative in determining health risk. The nurse should avoid oversimplifying the relationship between race/ethnicity and genetics when communicating to clients and their families. Knowledge of race or ethnicity might prompt genetic testing or detailed family history taking in particular instances; however, the issues are often too complex for the nurse to make unqualified assertions to clients that they are "at risk" for a particular illness or unlikely to respond to therapies solely on the basis of their racial/ethnic background. In most instances, the full interprofessional health care team will be the best catalyst for client information and interventions. Table 3-1 provides an overview of the distribution of selected genetic traits and disorders by population or ethnic group. Knowledge of the client's race or ethnicity might prompt the nurse to gather a detailed family history and/or collaborate with physicians and nurse practitioners to order genetic testing.

Human genetic information is accumulating at a rapid pace, and more than 2,700 diseases can now be diagnosed by testing for specific mutations (National Center for Biotechnology, 2014). The following genetic screenings may be useful to clients, nurses, and other members of the health care team:

- *Drug efficacy or sensitivity*: **Pharmacogenomics**, the study of the role of inherited and acquired genetic variation in drug response, is an evolving field that facilitates the identification of biomarkers that can help health providers optimize drug selection, dose, and treatment duration as well as eliminate adverse drug reactions. For example, researchers have identified an HLA allele that is associated with hypersensitivity reactions to the anticonvulsant and mood-stabilizing drug carbamazepine (Tegretol) in persons of European descent (McCormack et al., 2011). For other drugs such as warfarin (Coumadin) and clopidogrel (Plavix), genetic testing for variants in specific genes may be warranted to help guide the drug dosage.

Table 3-1: Selected Genetic Diseases and Clinical Implications

Disease or Condition	Group Impacted	Clinical Implications
Alpha-1 antitrypsin deficiency (AAT) Autosomal recessive disorder resulting in early-onset emphysema and liver disease	Northern European, Scandinavian, and Iberian ancestry. Rare in Jewish, Black, and Japanese populations. AAT deficiency affects 1%–2% of patients with chronic obstructive pulmonary disease.	**Consider diagnosis in** adults with emphysema with onset at ≤40 years old and without risk factors (no history of smoking or occupational dust exposure) **Diagnosis made by** serum alpha-1 antitrypsin levels and confirmed with genetic testing.
Breast cancer **BRCA1 and BRCA2** Autosomal dominant; accounting for ~5% US cases	Ashkenazi Jewish women Estimated that 0.2%–0.33% of general population have gene mutations	**Counseling:** U.S. Preventive Services Task Force recommends genetic counseling and evaluation for BRCA testing for Ashkenazi Jewish women with any first-degree relative with breast or ovarian cancer or second-degree relatives on same side of family with breast or ovarian cancer.
G6PD deficiency (glucose-6-phosphate dehydrogenase deficiency) X-linked genetic defect with clinical manifestations of neonatal jaundice and/or acute or chronic hemolytic anemia triggered by medications, infections, and fava beans	Highest frequency found in: Africa, southern Europe (Mediterranean region), Middle East, Southeast Asia, central and southern Pacific islands Deficiency is found in 10% of Blacks and can occur in Sephardic Jews, Greeks, Iranians, Chinese, Filipinos, and Indonesians with a frequency ranging from 5% to 40% Kurdish Jews 50% of males reported to be affected Most common human enzyme defect worldwide	**Relevant history:** Ask about family history of G6PD deficiency and hemolytic factors that can be transmitted to infants via mother's milk (such as fava bean ingestion, drugs, or herbal remedies). Hemolytic anemia occurs about 24 hours after ingestion of fava beans. **Medication history:** Ask about recent history of medications that may have precipitated hemolytic anemia, such as antimalarials, nitrofurantoin (urinary tract infections), phenazopyridine (for dysuria), and topical application of henna.
Leiden V The most common hereditary abnormality of hemostasis predisposing to thrombosis Autosomal dominant inheritance single mutation causes mild hypercoagulable state	Highest in US and European white populations. Prevalence may be higher in some Middle Eastern countries including Jordan (12.3%) and Lebanon (14.4%).	**Relevant assessment:** May have no clinical symptoms Mutation is present in about 15%–20% patients with first deep vein thrombosis and up to 50% of patients with recurrent venous thromboembolism. **Medication history:** Risk for thromboembolism increased with oral contraceptives, hormonal replacement therapy (HRT), and selective estrogen receptor modulators (SERMs)

Table 3-1: Selected Genetic Diseases and Clinical Implications (continued)

Disease or Condition	Group Impacted	Clinical Implications
Sickle cell disease Autosomal recessive genetic disorder; patients with same genotype may have highly variable phenotypes, ranging from asymptomatic to life-threatening complications; interaction of environmental factors with genetic polymorphisms may explain disease variation Chronic inflammation, ischemia, and vasoocclusion contribute to chronic organ damage	African, Mediterranean, Middle Eastern, Indian ancestry, Caribbean, and parts of Central and South America Most prevalent disease detected by neonatal blood screening Alpha-thalassemia and beta-thalassemia may be coinherited Sickle cell trait occurs in 1 out of every 12 blacks Sickle cell disease affects 90,000 to 100,000 Americans; occurs in 1 out of every 500 Blacks; occurs in 1 out of every 36,000 Hispanic American births	**Relevant assessment**: Affected infants not identified through neonatal screening usually present clinically during infancy/early childhood with painful swelling of the hands and feet (dactylitis), pneumococcal sepsis or meningitis, severe anemia and acute splenic enlargement (splenic sequestration), acute chest syndrome, jaundice, pallor. **Counseling**: Many adolescents and young adults are unaware of their sickle cell trait status—higher risk for rhabdomyolysis during rigorous sports. Prenatal diagnosis may be made in first and second trimester. Preimplantation genetic diagnosis is available during in vitro fertilization. Embryos not affected with sickle cell disease may be selected.
Tay–Sachs disease Neurodegenerative disorder caused by inborn error of metabolism Genetic mutation results in central nervous system degeneration and loss of organ function	Ashkenazi Jews Incidence of 1/3,600 among Ashkenazi Jewish births Carrier rate of 1/30 among Jewish Americans of Ashkenazi descent Additional at-risk groups include French Canadians living in Eastern Quebec or New England; select Cajun communities in Louisiana; and Pennsylvania Dutch semi-isolates	**Relevant assessment** Classic or acute infantile is the most common type. Infants appear normal at birth. Rapidly progressive neurodegenerative disorder characterized by progressive motor weakness beginning at 3–6 months old; loss of developmental milestones and death within first few years of life.
Alpha-thalassemia Hereditary anemia caused by defect during hemoglobin production; various clinical phenotypes—from silent carrier to more severe	Inhabitants or descendants of Southeast Asia, Middle East, and Mediterranean countries 80%–90% may be carriers of alpha-thalassemia in tropical and subtropical regions. About 30% of African Americans	**Relevant assessment**: Patients can be asymptomatic or have mild symptoms of anemia including fatigue and dyspnea, poor growth in children, and jaundice Abnormal physical findings occur with more severe phenotypes.
Beta-thalassemia An autosomal recessive inherited anemia caused by absent or decreased beta-globin chain synthesis during hemoglobin production. Also referred to as Cooley's or Mediterranean anemia	Inhabitants or descendants of Mediterranean countries, Middle East, Central Asia, India, Southern China, Far East, South America, and north coast of Africa Estimated annual incidence of symptomatic individuals: 1 in 100,000 people globally; 1 in 10,000 people in European community	**Relevant assessment**: Symptoms emerge at 6–12 months: failure to thrive, feeding problems, diarrhea, fever, and progressive enlargement of abdomen due to hepatosplenomegaly Symptoms in patients who have not been treated or who have received inadequate transfusion treatments may include growth retardation, jaundice, and craniofacial changes.

continued

Table 3-1: Selected Genetic Diseases and Clinical Implications (continued)

Disease or Condition	Group Impacted	Clinical Implications
von Willebrand disease Bleeding disorder resulting in platelet and clotting defect Vary from mild to more severe forms Three types exist, most commonly autosomal dominant	Type three may be more prevalent in Swedish communities 7:3 female-to-male ratio Racial characteristics of all patients: 75.1% White 10.9% Hispanic 7.5% Black 2.6% Asian/Pacific Islander 0.4% American Indian/Alaska native	**Preoperative assessment**: May be asymptomatic All patients having major surgery should be screened. Symptoms typical of bleeding disorder, most commonly mucosal bleeding such as nosebleed, gingival bleeding, easy bruising, or menorrhagia (most common bleeding disorder in women who present with menorrhagia, 12%–20%).

Data from Centers for Disease Control and Prevention. (2014). Sickle cell disease: Data and statistics. Retrieved from www. CDC.gov/NCBDD/sicklecell/data.html; deSerres, F. J., & Blanco, L. (2012). Prevalence of α1-antitrypsin deficiency alleles PI*S and PI*Z worldwide and effective screening for each of the five phenotypic classes PI*MS, PI*MZ, PI*SS, PI*SZ, and PI*ZZ: A comprehensive review. *Therapeutic Advances in Respiratory Disease*, 6(5), 277–295; Galanello, R., & Origa, R. (2010). Beta-thalassemia. *Orphanet Journal of Rare Diseases*, 5, 11; Harteveld, C. L., & Higgs, D. R. (2010). Alpha-thalassaemia. *Orphanet Journal of Rare Diseases*, 5, 13; Kaback, M., & Desnick, R. J. (2011). Hexosaminidase A deficiency. *Gene Reviews*, 8(11); McCance, K. L., & Huether, S. E. (2014). *Pathophysiology: The biologic basis for disease in adults and children* (7th ed.). St. Louis, MO: Elsevier, Inc.; Mohr, H. (2006). Acquired von Willebrand syndrome: Features and management. *American Journal of Hematology*, 81(8), 616–623; Porth, C. M. (2015). *Essentials of pathophysiology: Concepts of altered health states* (4th ed.). Philadelphia, PA: Lippincott; Rotimi, C. N., & Jorde, L. B. (2010). Ancestry and disease in the age of genomic medicine. *New England Journal of Medicine*, 36, 1551–1558; Taylor, C., Kavanagh, P., & Zuckerman, B. (2014). Sickle cell train-neglected opportunities in the era of genomic medicine. *JAMA*, 311(15), 1495–1496.

- *Carrier screening*: Genetic tests can identify heterozygous carriers for many recessive diseases such as cystic fibrosis, sickle cell disease, and Tay–Sachs disease. A couple may wish to undergo carrier screening to help make reproductive decisions, especially in populations where specific diseases are relatively common, for example, Tay–Sachs disease in Ashkenazi Jewish populations and β-thalassemia in Mediterranean populations.
- *Prenatal diagnosis*: Amniocentesis is usually performed at 16 weeks' gestation; chorionic villus sampling (CVS) is carried out at 10 to 12 weeks' gestation; preimplantation genetic diagnosis (PGD) is carried out on early embryos (8 to 12 cells) prior to implantation; and fetal DNA analysis in maternal circulation is done at 6 to 8 weeks' gestation (Center for Disease Control and Prevention, 2013; Dotson et al., 2014; National Center for Biotechnology, 2014).

Review of Medications and Allergies

The review of medications includes all current prescription, over the counter, and home remedies, including herbs that a client might purchase or grow in a home garden. During the health history, note the name, dose, route of administration, schedule, frequency, purpose, and length of time that each medicine that has been taken. Because of cultural differences in clients' perceptions of what substances are considered medicines, it is important to ask about specific items by name. Inquire about vitamins, birth control pills, aspirin, antacids, herbs, teas, inhalants, poultices, vaginal and rectal suppositories, ointments, and any other items taken by the client for therapeutic purposes. The nurse also gathers data on the client's allergies to medicines and foods.

Table 3-2 provides an overview of commonly used herbs, their sources, uses, dosage, and

Table 3-2: Herbal Remedies

Aloe Vera

Source	Leaf of *Aloe barbadensis*
Action	Topical analgesic, anti-inflammatory, antioxidant, and antifungal agent
Traditional uses	Applied as topical ointment for treatment of inflammation, minor burns, sunburn, cuts, bruises, and abrasions; administered orally as a laxative
Current uses	Promotes wound healing in soft tissue injuries and is used as a folk or traditional remedy for diabetes, asthma, epilepsy, and osteoarthritis
	Aloe vera gel, contained in the leaves of the plant, is found in skin products such as lotions and sunblocks
	Prevents wound pain by inhibiting the action of the pain-producing agent bradykinin
Dosage	Apply topically as needed; the FDA ruled that aloe is not safe as a stimulant laxative
Warnings	Rarely, skin rash follows topical application
	Can cause diarrhea and abdominal cramps when taken orally and can decrease the absorption of many drugs

Dong-Quai (Chinese angelica, *Angelica sinensis*)

Source	Dried root of a member of the parsley family
Action	Smooth muscle relaxant; antispasmodic
Traditional uses	A highly regarded herb in Chinese medicine, also used in traditional Korean and Japanese medicine
	Has been called "female ginseng" because it is used for health conditions in women
	Used for both men and women to treat heart conditions, high blood pressure, inflammation, headache, infections, and nerve pain
	Believed to help nourish the blood and balance energy
Current uses	Used for menstrual cramps, anemia during menstruation, pregnancy, premenstrual syndrome (PMS), pelvic pain, recovery from childbirth or illness, muscle spasms, and fatigue or low energy
	Used in combination with other herbs for liver and spleen problems
Dosage	Varies by condition: Available in capsule, liquid extract, or in tea form
Warnings	Contraindicated for pregnant and breast-feeding women and persons with abdominal distention or diarrhea
	Not recommended for use with aspirin, ibuprofen, anticoagulants, antiplatelet drugs, diabetic clients taking insulin, or other herbs, such as Ginkgo biloba
	Large doses may cause contact dermatitis and photosensitivity.

Echinacea (*Echinacea angustifolia, E. pallida, E. purpurea*)

Source	Member of the daisy family; also known as purple coneflower
Action	Reduces cold symptoms
Traditional uses	Used to treat wounds and skin problems, such as acne or boils
Current uses	Enhances the immune system to fight infection and to treat colds, flu, and other illnesses. The parts of the plant above ground are used to make teas, juice, or extracts.

continued

Table 3-2: Herbal Remedies (continued)

Dosage	Follow directions on label; needed at onset of symptoms; usually taken for no longer than 2 weeks
Warnings	Contraindicated for pregnant or breast-feeding women, children, and those who are allergic to plants in the daisy family, including ragweed, chrysanthemums, marigolds, and daisies. Not recommended for people with severely compromised immune systems such as those with HIV/AIDS, tuberculosis, or multiple sclerosis

Evening Primrose Oil (*Oenothera biennis*)

Source	Seeds of the wildflower evening primrose
Action	Antihypertensive, immunostimulant, weight reduction
Traditional uses	Used as a folk remedy to treat eczema since the 1930s
Current uses	Believed to help inflammation, PMS, diabetes mellitus, eczema, fatigue, diabetic neuropathy, and rheumatoid arthritis
Dosage	Follow directions on label; will take at least 1 month to experience benefits
Warnings	Side effects include occasional reports of headache, nausea, and abdominal discomfort; not recommended for children.
	Some capsules may be altered with other types of oil such as soy or safflower.

Ginger

Current uses	Currently is used to treat postsurgery nausea; nausea caused by motion, chemotherapy, and pregnancy; rheumatoid arthritis; osteoarthritis, and joint and muscle pain
Dosage	Boil 1-oz dried ginger root in 1 cup water for 15–20 minutes.
	Follow label directions on ginger supplements.

Ginkgo (*Ginkgo biloba*)

Source	Extract from leaves of the ginkgo tree, one of the oldest types of trees in the world; is cultivated worldwide for its medicinal properties
Action	Antioxidant; improves blood circulation
Traditional uses	Used in traditional Chinese medicine for asthma, bronchitis, fatigue, circulatory disorders, sexual dysfunctions, and tinnitus
Current uses	Promotes vasodilation and improves memory, attention span, and mood in early stages of Alzheimer's disease or dementia by improving oxygen metabolism in the brain; used to treat intermittent claudication, sexual dysfunction, multiple sclerosis, tinnitus, and other health conditions
Dosage	Available in tablets, capsules, teas, and occasionally skin products
	Follow labels on supplements.
Warnings	Side effects may include headaches, diarrhea, nausea and vomiting, and dizziness.
	Some people have reported allergic skin reactions.
	Fresh ginkgo seeds can cause serious adverse reactions—including seizures and death.
	Contraindicated for women who are pregnant or breast-feeding
	Contraindicated for persons with clotting disorders or those who are about to have surgery
	Not recommended for children

Table 3-2: Herbal Remedies (continued)

Ginseng (*Panax quinquefolius* [American], *Panax ginseng* [Asian])

Source	Dried root of several species of the genus *Panax* of the family Araliaceae
Action	Tonic
Traditional uses	Treatment of anemia, atherosclerosis, edema, ulcers, hypertension, influenza, colds, inflammation, and disorders of the immune system (American)
	Treatment of shock, diaphoresis, dyspnea, fever, thirst, irritability, diarrhea, vomiting, abdominal distention, anorexia, and impotence; considered a "heat-raising" tonic for the blood and circulatory system (Asian)
Current uses	Used to enhance sexual experience and treat impotence, though there is no current research to support this claim
	Also used to improve athletic performance, strength, and stamina, as well as to treat diabetes and cancer (American)
	Used to treat diabetes, cancer, HIV/AIDS, and as an immunostimulant or to improve athletic performance (Asian)
	Improved sense of well-being (Asian)
Dosage	American: Follow directions on label.
	Asian: 100 mg BID
Warnings	American: May cause headaches, insomnia, anxiety, breast tenderness, rashes, asthma attacks, hypertension, cardiac arrhythmias, and postmenopausal uterine hemorrhage
	Should be used with caution for the following conditions: pregnancy, insomnia, hay fever, fibrocystic breasts, asthma, emphysema, hypertension, clotting disorders, and diabetes mellitus
	Asian: Same as American

Gotu Kola (*Centella asiatica*)

Source	Dried and powdered leaves of a member of the parsley family
Action	Improves memory
Traditional uses	In ancient India, considered a rejuvenating herb that increases intelligence, longevity, and memory while slowing the aging process
	In China, used as a tea for colds and for lung and urinary tract infections; used topically for snakebite, wounds, and shingles
Current uses	Acceleration of wound healing, diuretic, treatment of phlebitis, varicose veins, and scleroderma
Dosage	Follow directions on label; lower dose needed for children and older adults
Warnings	Sides effects include headaches and skin rash.
	Contraindicated for pregnant or breast-feeding women and children younger than 18 years
	Contraindicated for those diagnosed with liver disease

Saint John's wort (*Hypericum perforatum*)

Source	Tea made from the leaves and flowering tops of the perennial *H. perforatum*, which is particularly abundant in late June, the feast of St. John the Baptist

continued

Table 3-2: Herbal Remedies (continued)

Action	Antidepressant
Traditional uses	Used first in ancient Greece and historically to treat mental disorders and nerve pain. Also used to treat malaria, as a sedative, and topically for wounds, burns, and insect bites
	Also used by Native Americans to treat wounds, snake bites, and diarrhea
Current uses	Treatment of mild to moderate depression, anxiety, seasonal affective disorder, and sleep disorders
Dosage	300 mg daily
Warnings	Fair-skinned people may experience photosensitivity.
	Reduces effectiveness of some anticancer agents
	Can interact with antidepressants, birth control pills, cyclosporine, heart medications, HIV medications, anticoagulants, and seizure control medications
	Clinical manifestations of depression should be considered seriously.
	Encourage client to see a mental health care provider.

Valerian (*Valeriana officinalis*)

Source	Dried rhizome and roots of the tall perennial *V. officinalis*
Action	Mild tranquilizer and sedative
Traditional uses	Used as medicinal herb since Ancient Greece and Rome for insomnia
Current uses	Used as a mild tranquilizer and sedative; relieves muscle spasms, anxiety, headaches, depression, irregular heartbeat and trembling
	Especially effective for insomniac persons and older adults
Dosage	Available in capsules, tablets, liquid extracts, and teas
Warnings	Reported side effects include headache, gastrointestinal upset, and dizziness.
	Must not be taken in combination with other tranquilizers or sedatives
	Client should be cautioned against operating a motor vehicle after ingesting.
	Should discontinue use at least 1 week before surgery because it may interact with anesthesia

Table based on data from Bongki, P., Jun, J. H., Jung, J., You, S., & Lee, M. S. (2014). Herbal medicines for cancer cachexia: Protocol for a systematic review. *British Medical Journal Open, 4*, e005016. doi: 10.1136/bmjopne-2014-005016; Retrieved from Mayo Clinic (http://www.mayoclinic.org); Memorial Sloan-Kettering Cancer Center: About Herbs, Botanicals and Other Products (http://www.mskcc.org/cancer-care/integrative-medicine/about-herbs-botanicals-other-products), National Center for Complementary and Integrative Health. (2015). Herbs at a glance. Retrieved from https://nccih.nih.gov/health/herbsataglance.htm; University of Maryland Medical Center (https://umm.edu/health/medical/altmed/herb); Luca, A., Jimenez-Fonseca, P., & Gascon, P. (2013). Clinical evaluation and optimal management of cancer cachexia. *Critical Reviews in Oncology/Hematology, 88*(4), 625–636.

warnings, such as contraindications (e.g., pregnancy, childhood, people with compromised immune systems) and interactions with prescription drugs. Many of the active ingredients in herbs or plant-derived drugs are unknown and remain largely unregulated by government agencies, except for customs officials who make efforts to control the flow of illegal drugs. Fresh or dried herbs are usually brewed into a tea, with the dosage adjusted according to the chronicity or acuteness of the illness, age, and size of the client. Traditional Chinese medicine usually is used only as long as symptoms persist. Some clients extend the same logic to prescription

medicines. For example, they might stop taking an antibiotic as soon as the symptoms subside instead of completing the course of treatment for the prescribed length of time. Be sure to consider the potential interaction of herbs with prescription medicines. The root of the shrub *ginseng*, for example, is widely used for the treatment of arthritis, back and leg pains, and sores. Because ginseng is known to potentiate the action of some antihypertensive drugs, nurses need to ask clients whether they are experiencing side effects or toxicity and should frequently monitor the client's blood pressure. It might be necessary to withhold doses of the prescribed antihypertensive medicine if the blood pressure is low or to ask the client to discontinue or reduce the strength of the ginseng. When assessing the client's use of traditional Chinese medicine, nurses should be aware that some Chinese Americans who use herbs topically do not consider them drugs; therefore, nurses might not know that the person is taking these medicines. For further information about herbs, ask the client and family, consult an herbalist, search for reputable sources on the Internet, or check reference books on herbal remedies. People sometimes fail to disclose that they are taking herbs or plant-based medicines because they're concerned that their health care provider will disapprove. The National Center for Complementary and Integrative Health (2012) provides fact sheets with basic information about specific herbs or botanicals—common names, what the science says, potential side effects and cautions, and resources for more information.

For many years, people have attempted to identify plants, marine organisms, arthropods, animals, and minerals with healing properties. According to the World Health Organization (2013), 80% of people residing in less developed countries use indigenous medicinal plants for many of their primary health care needs. The estimated global market for botanical and plant-derived drugs is valued at $22.1 billion and is projected to grow to $26.6 billion by 2017 (BCC Research, 2013). Currently, respiratory problems such as asthma represent the largest medical application of plant-derived drugs, accounting for 24% of total sales of plant-derived medicines. Cancer treatment is expected to become the largest application of plant-derived drugs, capturing 30% of the market by 2017 (BCC Research, 2013). In particular, nurses should be aware of the widespread use of plant-derived medications among various cultures (see Table 3-2).

The client's genetic makeup results in distinctive patterns of drug absorption, metabolism, excretion, and effectiveness. Knowledge of clients' individual genotypes guides pharmacologic treatment and allows customization of choice of drug and dosage to ensure a therapeutic response and avoid toxicity (Casorbi, Bruhn, & Werk, 2013). For example, Evidence-Based Practice 3-1 describes genetically linked racial and ethnic differences in the conversion of codeine to morphine for analgesia. Another example concerns the possibility of reduced effectiveness of the widely prescribed platelet aggregation inhibitor clopidogrel (Plavix), which is used in the prevention of myocardial infarction and stroke. The cause of the reduced effectiveness is related to genetic variations in cytochrome P-450 and polypeptide 19 (CYP2C19). A black box warning from the U.S. Food and Drug Administration recommends that all clopidogrel users be tested. It is estimated that between 2% and 14% of the U.S. population are poor metabolizers. While previous studies have explored the impact of this variation in metabolism on heart disease, researchers found that a proportion of the poor/intermediate clopidogrel metabolizers have an increased risk of recurrent cerebrovascular events, including stroke. Only 26% of whites are intermediate or poor metabolizers, compared with 47% nonwhites. This finding is comparable to cardiovascular studies and warrants routine CYP2C19 testing and monitoring of people taking clopidogrel (Spokoyny et al., 2014). Table 3-3 identifies drug categories for which clients from certain racial or ethnic backgrounds respond differently from the general population.

Racial and Ethnic Variations in the Conversion of Codeine to Morphine for Analgesia

CYP2D6 is one of the most important enzymes involved in the metabolism of xenobiotics in the body. In particular, CYP2D6 is responsible for the metabolism and elimination of approximately 25% of clinically used drugs. Xenobiotics are foreign chemical substances found within an organism that are not normally naturally produced by or expected to be present within it. In humans, antibiotics are xenobiotics because the human body doesn't produce them itself nor are they typically part of normal food.

There is considerable variation in the efficiency and amount of CYP2D6 enzyme produced by individuals from different racial and ethnic backgrounds. For drugs that are metabolized by CYP2D6, certain individuals eliminate the drugs quickly (ultrarapid metabolizers) while others eliminate them slowly (poor metabolizers). If a drug is metabolized too quickly, it may decrease the drug's efficacy. If the drug is metabolized too slowly, toxicity may result. CYP2D6 catalyzes the conversion of codeine to morphine.

In 7% to 10% of US whites, an active form of the CYP2D6 enzyme, which is necessary to convert codeine into its active metabolite, morphine, is missing. These individuals experience the side effects of morphine without pain relief. Other variations in metabolic efficiency among ethnic groups are apparent. For example, Chinese produce less morphine from codeine than do Whites and also are less sensitive to morphine's effects. The reduced sensitivity to morphine may be due to decreased production of morphine-6-glucuronide.

Clinical Implications:

In approximately 10% of US Whites, codeine is ineffective as an analgesic, and 4% to 5% of the US population and 16% to 28% of North Africans, Ethiopians, and Arabs are ultrarapid metabolizers with increased sensitivity to codeine's effects, and therefore, nurses need to observe for the following signs of toxicity:

- Bluish-colored fingernails and lips
- Slow and labored breathing, shallow breathing, and no breathing

- Cold, clammy skin
- Coma (decreased level of consciousness and lack of responsiveness)
- Confusion
- Dizziness
- Drowsiness
- Fatigue
- Lightheadedness
- Low blood pressure
- Muscle twitches
- Pinpoint pupils
- Spasms of the stomach and intestines
- Weakness
- Weak pulse

Consider the possibility of metabolic genetic variations in any client who experiences toxicity or does not receive adequate analgesia from codeine or other opioid drugs (e.g., hydrocodone and oxycodone). Red heads also have variations. Dysfunctional melanocortin 1 receptor on certain cells that gives people their red hair also increases production of a hormone that causes heightened pain sensitivity.

References

Binkley, C. J., Beacham, A., Neace, W., Gregg, R. G., Liem, E. B., & Sessler, D. I. (2010). Genetic variations associated with red hair color and fear of dental pain, anxiety regarding dental care and avoidance of dental care. Journal of the American Dental Association, 140(7), 896–905

Liu, F., Struchalin, M. V., van Duijn, K., Hofman, A., Uitterlinden, A. G., van Duijn, C., …, Kayser, M. (2011). Detecting low frequent loss-of-function alleles in genome wide association studies with red hair color as example. PLoS One, 6(11), e28145

Sammer, C. F., Daali, Y., Wagner, M., Hopfgartner, G., Eap, C. B., Rebsamen, M. C., …, Desmueles, J. A. (2010). The effects of CYP2D6 and CYP3A activities on the pharmacokinetics of immediate release oxycodone. British Journal of Pharmacology, 160(4), 907–918

Teh, L. K., & Bertilsson, L. (2012). Pharmacogenomics of CYP2D6: Molecular genetics, interethnic differences and clinical importance. Drug Metabolism and Pharmacokinetic, 27(1), 55–67

Walko, C. M., & McLeod, H. (2012). Use of CYP2D6 genotyping in practice: Tamoxifen dose adjustment. Pharmacogenomics, 13(6), 691–707.

Table 3-3: Cultural Differences in Response to Drugs

Drug Category	Group	Remarks
Analgesics	Blacks	Despite decreased sensitivity to pain-relieving therapeutic action of drugs, there are increased gastrointestinal side effects, especially with acetaminophen.
Narcotic analgesics	Chinese	May be less sensitive to the respiratory depressant and hypotensive effects of morphine but more likely to experience nausea; have a significantly higher clearance of morphine
Antiarrhythmics	Arab Americans	Some may need lower dosage
Anticoagulants	Asian	Require lower doses of warfarin (Coumadin) than White counterparts
	Blacks	Require higher doses of warfarin (Coumadin) than White or Asian counterparts
Anticonvulsants	Chinese, Filipinos, Malaysians, Thai, Singaporeans, Taiwanese, East Indians, and Japanese	Higher toxicity observed with use of carbamazepine (Tegretol) including incidence of drug-induced Stevens–Johnson syndrome
Antihypertensives	Arab Americans	Some may need lower dosage
	Asian/Pacific Islanders	Respond best to calcium antagonists
	Blacks	Respond best to treatment with a single drug (vs. combined antihypertensive therapy)
		Research suggests favorable response to diuretics, calcium antagonists, and alpha-blockers
		Less responsive to beta-blockers (e.g., propranolol) and ACE inhibitors (e.g., enalapril, imidapril)
		Increased side effects such as mood response (e.g., depression) to thiazides (e.g., hydrochlorothiazide), which may explain reluctance to take drug as prescribed
Fat-soluble drugs	Asian Americans	Due to average lower percentage of body fat, dosage adjustments must be made for fat-soluble vitamins and other drugs, for example, vitamin K used to reverse the anticoagulant effect of Coumadin (warfarin); consider dietary intake of vitamins when calculating doses.
Immunosuppressants	Blacks	Black clients with kidney failure require higher doses of tacrolimus (Prograf, Advagraf, Protopic) to reach trough concentrations similar to those observed in White counterparts
Muscle relaxants	Native Alaskans	May experience prolonged muscle paralysis and an inability to breathe without mechanical ventilation for several hours postoperatively when succinylcholine has been administered in surgery

continued

Table 3-3: Cultural Differences in Response to Drugs (continued)

Drug Category	Group	Remarks
Mydriatics	Blacks	Higher dose required; less dilation occurs with dark-colored eyes.
Neuroleptics	Arab Americans	Some may need lower dosage.
	Asian/Pacific Islanders	Require lower dose than Whites or Blacks
Oxidizing drugs	Greeks, Italians, and others of Mediterranean descent with G6PD deficiency	The following drugs may precipitate a hemolytic crisis: primaquine, quinidine, thiazolsulfone, furazolidone, haloperidol, nitrofural, naphthalene, toluidine blue, phenylhydrazine, chloramphenicol, aspirin
Psychotropics	Asian/Pacific Islanders	Require lower dose, sometimes as little as half the normal dose for lithium and tricyclic antidepressants (TCAs) such as desipramine and trimipramine
	Blacks	Increased extrapyramidal side effects with TCAs such as haloperidol; relatively prolonged clearance and half-life of carbamazepine
	Hispanics	May require lower dosage and experience higher incidence of side effects with TCAs
	Jewish North Americans (Ashkenazi)	Agranulocytosis develops in 20% when clozapine (Clozaril or ODT) is used to treat schizophrenia; thus, the granulocyte count should be checked before the drug is administered.
Steroids	Blacks	When methylprednisolone is used for immunosuppression in renal transplant clients, there is increased toxicity such as steroid-associated diabetes; although Blacks are four times as likely to develop end-stage renal disease as Whites, they have the poorest long-term graft survival of any ethnic group.
Tranquilizers	Blacks	15%–20% are poor metabolizers of Valium (diazepam).

Table based partially on data from Bress, A., Han, J., Patel, S. R., Desai, A. A., Mansour, I., Groo, V., …, Cavallari, R. L. (2013). Association of Aldosterone Synthase Polymorphism (*CYP11B2* -344 T>C) and genetic ancestry with atrial fibrillation and serum aldosterone in African Americans with heart failure. *PLoS One, 8*(7), e71268; Buttaro, T. M., Trybulski, J., Polgar Bailey, P., & Sandberg-Cook, J. (2013). *Primary care: A collaborative practice*. St. Louis, MO: Elsevier; Casorbi, I., Bruhn, O., & Werk, A. N. (2013). Challenges in pharmacogenetics, *European Journal of Pharmacology, 69* (Suppl. 1), S17–S23; Center for Disease Control and Prevention. (2013). Genetic testing. Retrieved from http://www.cdc.gov/genomics/gtesting/index.htm; Marino, S. E., Birnbaum, A. K., Leppik, I. E., Conway, J. M., Musib, L. C., Brundage, R. C., … ,Cloyd, J. C. (2012). Steady-state carbamazepine pharmacokinetics following oral and stable-labeled intravenous administration in epilepsy clients: Effects of race and sex. *Clinical Pharmacology & Therapeutics, 91*(3), 483–488.

Reason for Seeking Care

The *reason* or *reasons for seeking care* refers to a brief statement in the client's own words describing why he/she is visiting a health care provider. This part of the health history previously was called the *chief complaint,* a term that is now avoided because it focuses on illness rather than wellness and tends to label the person as a complainer.

Symptoms are defined as phenomena experienced by individuals that signify a departure from normal function, sensation, or appearance and that might include physical aberrations. By

comparison, *signs* are objective abnormalities that the examiner can detect on physical examination or through laboratory testing. As individuals experience symptoms, they interpret them and react in ways that are congruent with their **cultural norms**, unconscious behavior patterns that are typical of specific groups. Such behaviors are learned from parents, teachers, peers, and others whose values, attitudes, beliefs, and behaviors take place in the context of their own culture. Some cultural norms are healthy; others are not.

Symptoms cannot be attributed to another person; rather, individual clients experience symptoms from their knowledge of bodily function and sociocultural interactions. Symptoms are perceived, recognized, labeled, reacted to, ritualized, and articulated in ways that make sense within the cultural worldview of the person experiencing them. Symptoms are defined according to the client's perception of the meaning attributed to the event. This perception must be considered in relation to other sociocultural factors and biologic knowledge. People develop culturally based explanatory models to explain how their illnesses work and what their symptoms mean. The search for cultural meaning in understanding symptoms involves a translation process that includes both the nurse's worldview and the client's. Assess the symptoms within the client's sociocultural and ethnohistorical context. It is important to use the same terms for symptoms that the client uses. For example, if the client refers to "swelling" of the leg, nurses should refrain from medicalizing that to "edema." Knowledge of the cultural expression of symptoms influences the decisions nurses make and will facilitate their ability to provide culturally congruent and culturally competent nursing care (Leininger & McFarland, 2002, 2006; McFarland & Wehbe-Alamah, 2015).

Present Health and History of Present Illness

Although all illnesses are defined and conceptualized through the lens of culture, the term **culture-bound syndromes** refers to more than 200 disorders created by personal, social, and cultural reactions to malfunctioning biological or psychological processes and can be understood only within defined contexts of meaning and social relationships (American Psychiatric Association, 2013; Kleinman, 1980; Simons & Hughes, 1985). When assessing clients with a culture-bound syndrome, it is important for the nurse to find out what the client, family, and other concerned individuals believe is happening; what prior efforts for help or cure have been tried; and what the results or outcomes from the treatment were.

Past Health

Past illnesses are important for multiple reasons. First, past illnesses may have residual effects on the current state of health or have sequelae that appear many months or years later. For example, the varicella-zoster virus responsible for chicken pox may remain latent until a person notices the characteristic rash or blisters of shingles; chicken pox and shingles are caused by the same herpes zoster virus. Although there has been a varicella vaccine available in the United States since 1995, protection from one dose is not lifelong, and a second dose is necessary 5 years after the initial immunization. Further, those born prior to 1995 and those born outside the United States may not be immunized. Second, the assessment of past illnesses includes other childhood conditions with known sequelae such as rheumatic fever, scarlet fever, and poliomyelitis. The nurse also gathers information about the date and nature of accidents, serious and chronic illnesses, hospitalizations, surgeries, obstetric history, and the last examination (Jarvis, 2015).

Family and Social History

In this era of genetics and genomics, a comprehensive and accurate family history highlights those diseases and disorders for which a client may be at increased risk. Table 3-4 provides an alphabetical listing of common diseases and identifies racial and ethnic groups for which the conditions are more prevalent. When conducting the

Table 3-4: Biocultural Aspects of Disease

Disease	Remarks
Alcoholism	American Indians have double the rate of Whites and 12% of all Native American deaths linked to alcohol; lower tolerance to alcohol among Chinese and Japanese Americans.
Anemia	High incidence among Vietnamese because of the presence of infestations among immigrants and low-iron diets; low hemoglobin and malnutrition found among 18.2% of Native Americans, 32.7% of Blacks, 14.6% of Hispanics, and 10.4% of White children under 5 years of age
Arthritis	*Increased incidence among Native Americans*
	Blackfoot 1.4%
	Pima 1.8%
	Chippewa 6.8%
Asthma	Six times greater for Native American infants <1 year; same as the general population for Native Americans aged 1–44 years
Bronchitis	Six times greater for Native American infants <1 year; same as the general population for Native Americans aged 1–44 years. Main cause of death for Aboriginal Canadian infants in the postnatal period
Cancer	*Nasopharyngeal*: high among Chinese Americans and Native Americans
	Breast: Black women 1½ times more likely than White
	Higher prevalence of BRCA1 and BRCA2 mutations (linked to breast and ovarian cancers) in Ashkenazi Jews, Norwegians, Dutch, and Icelandic peoples; also higher in African Americans, Hispanics, Asian Americans, and non-Hispanic Whites (National Cancer Institute, 2014)
	Colorectal: Blacks 40% higher than Whites
	Esophageal: No. 2 cause of death for Black men aged 35–54 years
	Incidence:
	White men 3.5/100,000
	Black men 13.3/100,000
	Liver: Highest among all ethnic groups are Filipino Hawaiians Latinos have twice the rate of Whites
	Stomach: Black men twice as likely as White men; low among Filipinos
	Cervical: 120% higher in Black women than in White women
	Mexican American and Puerto Rican women 2–3 times higher than Whites
	Uterine: 53% lower in Black women than White women
	Prostate: Black men have highest incidence of all groups
	Most prevalent cancer among Native Americans: biliary, nasopharyngeal, testicular, cervical, renal, and thyroid (females) cancer
	Lung cancer among Navajo uranium miners 85 times higher than among White miners
	Most prevalent cancer among Japanese Americans: esophageal, stomach, liver, and biliary cancer
	Among Chinese Americans, there is a higher incidence of nasopharyngeal and liver cancer than among the general population.

Table 3-4: Biocultural Aspects of Disease (continued)

Disease	Remarks
Cholecystitis	*Incidence*:
	Whites 0.3%
	Puerto Ricans 2.1%
	Native Americans 2.2%
	Chinese 2.6%
Colitis	High incidence among Japanese Americans
Diabetes mellitus	Three times as prevalent among Filipino Americans as Whites; higher among Hispanics than Blacks or Whites
	Death rate is 3–4 times as high among Native Americans aged 25–34 years, especially those in the West such as Utes and Tohono O'odham (Pimas and Papagos)
	Complications:
	Amputations: Twice as high among Native Americans vs. general US population
	Renal failure: 20 times as high as general US population, with tribal variation, for example, Utes have 43 times higher incidence
G6PD deficiency	Present among 30% of Black males
Influenza	Increased death rate among Native Americans aged 45+
Ischemic heart disease	Responsible for 32% of heart-related causes of death among Native Americans; Blacks have higher mortality rates than all other groups.
Lactose intolerance	Present among 66% of Hispanic women; increased incidence among Blacks and Chinese
Myocardial infarction	Leading cause of heart disease in Native Americans, accounting for 43% of death resulting from heart disease; low incidence among Japanese Americans
Otitis media	7.9% incidence among school-aged Navajo children vs. 0.5% in Whites
	Up to 1/3 of Eskimo children <2 years have chronic otitis media.
	Increased incidence among bottle-fed Native Americans and Eskimo infants
Pneumonia	Increased death rate among Native North Americans aged 45+
Psoriasis	Affects 2%–5% of Whites but <1% of Blacks; high among Japanese Americans
Renal disease	Lower incidence among Japanese Americans
Sickle cell anemia	Increased incidence among blacks
Trachoma	Increased incidence among Native Americans and Eskimo children (3–8 times greater than general population)
Tuberculosis	Highest among Asian Americans and Pacific Islanders
	Increased incidence among Native Americans
	Apache 2.0%
	Sioux 3.2%
	Navajo 4.6%

continued

Table 3-4: Biocultural Aspects of Disease (continued)

Disease	Remarks
	Aboriginals living on Canadian reserves are 10 times more likely to have TB than non-Aboriginal Canadians.
	Non-Whites 5.2 times more than Whites
Ulcers	Decreased incidence among Japanese Americans

Table based on data accessed on September 20, 2014 at American Cancer Society (http://www.cancer.org); American Diabetes Association (http://www.diabetes.org); American Heart Association (http://www.americanheart.org); Centers for Disease Control and Prevention (http://www.cdc.gov/DiseasesConditions/); Office of Minority Health (http://www.omhrc.gov/omh/whatsnew/2pgwhatsnew/special128a.htm); National Center for Health Statistics (http://www.cdc.gov/nchs); National Center on Minority Health & Health Disparities, National Institutes of Health (ncmhd.nih.gov); National Institute on Alcohol Abuse and Alcoholism (2014) Spotlight on Minority Health (http://www.cdc.gov/omh/populations/populations.htm).

family history, the nurse can refer to the table for conditions that tend to be more prevalent among certain groups. If clients are aware that they are at increased risk for a certain condition, they may seek early screening and periodic surveillance and may choose to adopt a healthier life style, for example, stop smoking, exercise regularly, and/or lose weight.

In addition to diagramming a family tree to identify familial relationships and the presence of disease conditions among those related to the client, the nurse should assess the broader socioeconomic factors influencing the client. The health history should include in-depth data pertaining to the client's family and/or close social friends, including identification of *key decision makers*. Although personal financial information is often a sensitive topic, it is important to determine the overall economic factors that influence a client. For example, regardless of race or ethnicity, people from lower socioeconomic categories have poorer health and shorter lives. There is a disproportionately high level of poverty among Blacks, Latinos/Latinas, American Indians/Alaska Natives (U.S. Census Bureau, 2014b), and First Nation People of Canada (Nicholls, 2014; Wells, 2014). Economic factors have been identified as causes of less favorable outcomes among clients with cancer (CDC, n.d., 2015). Research suggests that this is caused by a lack of health insurance and/or diminished access to health care services, both of which contribute to a situation

in which less affluent clients receive diagnosis and treatment later in the course of the disease (Becares et al., 2012; Dubay & Lebrun, 2012; Haeok, Fitzpatrick, & Baik, 2013; Kaiser Family Foundation, 2014; Obeig-Odoom, 2012; Pardasani & Bandyopadhylis, 2014).

See Appendix A for suggested interview topics aimed at eliciting information about family and social history.

Review of Systems

The purpose of the review of systems is threefold: (1) to evaluate the past and present health state of each body system, (2) to provide an opportunity for the client to report symptoms not previously stated, and (3) to evaluate health promotion practices. For example, when reviewing the gastrointestinal system with clients from Native American, Asian, African, and South American descent, the nurse should inquire about symptoms of lactose intolerance, such diarrhea, nausea, vomiting, abdominal cramps, bloating, and flatus, usually beginning 30 minutes to 2 hours after eating or drinking foods that contain lactose (e.g., milk, cheese, and ice cream). **Lactose intolerance** means that the body cannot easily digest lactose, a type of natural sugar found in milk and dairy products. Some people who have lactose intolerance cannot digest any milk products. Others can eat or drink small amounts of milk products or certain types of milk products without problems (Mayo Clinic, n.d.c, 2015).

Knowledge of current research on diseases prevalent in specific ethnic and racial groups might be useful in asking appropriate questions in the review of systems. For example, if the nurse is gathering review of systems information from a middle-aged African American man, it is useful to know that there is a statistically higher incidence of hypertension, sickle cell anemia, and type 2 diabetes in this group than in counterparts from other racial and ethnic groups. This will assist in customizing the review of systems questions and ensuring that symptoms of disease specific to the client's ethnic or racial heritage are included.

Transcultural Perspectives on the Physical Examination

There are a number of **biocultural variations** that nurses may encounter when conducting the physical examination of clients from different cultural backgrounds. Accurate assessment and **evaluation** of clients requires knowledge of normal biocultural variations among healthy members of selected populations, as well as variations that occur in illness. The data about biocultural variations presented here are evidence based and reflect the findings of classic studies that have been conducted over a period of years. The classic work of Dr. Theresa Overfield (1995), a renowned nurse–anthropologist who published extensively on biological variations in health and illness, is cited frequently in the discussion that follows. As more research on biocultural variations is conducted, there will be additions and modifications to the current body of knowledge.

The information provided here is intended to be helpful and illustrative, not exhaustive.

Biocultural Variations in Measurements

Racial and ethnic differences are found in measurements such as height (or length in infants and young children), body proportions, weight, and vital signs.

Height

Average heights for men and women from selected cultural groups are summarized in Table 3-5. In all groups, height increases up to 1.5 inches as socioeconomic status improves. First-generation immigrants might be up to 1.5 inches taller than their counterparts in the country of origin, due to better nutrition and decreased interference with growth by infectious diseases. During the past decade, the overall height of men from the United States increased by 0.7 inches; women from the United States grew an average of 0.5 inches taller. On average, white men are 0.5 inches (1.27 cm) taller than black males. White and black women, on the other hand, have approximately the same height (Jarvis, 2015; Overfield, 1995).

Body Proportions

Biocultural variations are found in the body proportions of individuals, largely because of differences in bone length. In comparing sitting/standing height ratios, Blacks of both genders have longer arms and legs and shorter trunks than Whites, Native Americans, or Asians. Because proportionately most of the body's weight is in the trunk, white men appear more obese than

Table 3-5: Biocultural Variations in Height for Selected Groups

Average Height (In Inches)				
All groups of men (*n*)	**White American**	**African American**	**Mexican America**	**Asian**
69.1	69.1	69.2	67.2	65.7
All groups of women (*n*)				
63.7	63.8	63.8	61.8	60.3

Table developed using data from Overfield, T. (1995). *Biologic variation in health and illness*. New York, NY: CRC Press.

their black counterparts. The reverse is true of women. Clients of Asian heritage are markedly shorter, weigh less, and have smaller body frames than their White counterparts and/or the overall population (Jarvis, 2015; Overfield, 1995).

Weight

Biocultural differences exist in the amount of body fat and the distribution of fat throughout the body. Generally, people from the lower socioeconomic class are more obese than those from the middle class, who are more obese than members of the upper class. On average, black men weigh less than their white counterparts throughout adulthood (166.1 pounds vs. 170.6 pounds). The opposite is true of women. Black women are consistently heavier than white women of every age (149.6 pounds vs. 137 pounds). Between the ages of 35 and 64 years, black women weigh on average 20 pounds more than white women. Mexican Americans weigh more in relation to height than non-Hispanic Whites because of differences in truncal fat patterns (Dixon, Pena, & Albright, 2012).

Some differences in the amount of body fat are related to socioeconomic factors, which in turn influence nutrition and exposure to communicable diseases. In a study of college age women in Hawaii, researchers found that current weight (body mass index [BMI]) appears to play a larger role in the desire for a lower body weight than does race/ethnicity, suggesting a desired BMI may be more personal than cultural. All of the young women were found to desire a body weight consistent with a normal BMI, including the Hawaiians/Pacific Islanders, who traditionally have been reported to value a larger body size. This possible shift in preference could potentially lead to an increase in the prevalence of eating disorders in this population (Schembre, Nigg, & Albright, 2011).

Around the world, people in cold climates tend to have more body fat, whereas those residing in warmer areas have less. Blacks have smaller skinfold thicknesses on their trunks and arms than

do their white counterparts (Overfield, 1995). Bottle-fed infants are heavier on average than those who are breast-fed, although their lengths are similar (Kliegman, Stanton, Saint Geme, Schor, & Behrman, 2011; Overfield, 1995).

Vital Signs

Although the average pulse rate is comparable across cultures, there are racial and gender differences in *blood pressure*. Black men have lower systolic blood pressures than their white counterparts from ages 18 to 34, but between the ages of 35 and 64, it reverses: Blacks have an average systolic blood pressure 5 mm Hg higher between 35 and 64 years of age. After age 65, there is no difference between the two races. Black women have a higher average systolic blood pressure than their white counterparts at every age. After age 45, the average blood pressure of black women might be as much as 16 mm Hg higher than that of white women in the same age group.

The incidence of hypertension is twice as high in African Americans as it is in Whites, and African Americans have the highest incidence of hypertension of anywhere in the world (American Heart Association, 2014). Studies have consistently reported a higher prevalence of hypertension in blacks than in whites, a main reason for the higher incidence of cardiovascular disease in blacks. The long list of causes for this higher prevalence suggests that the real reasons are still unknown. Biological differences in the mechanisms of blood pressure control or in the differences in the environment and habits of whites and blacks are among the potential causes. The higher prevalence of hypertension in blacks living in the United States as compared to those living in Africa demonstrates that environmental and behavioral characteristics are the more likely reasons for the higher prevalence in blacks living in the United States. These factors could act directly or by triggering mechanisms of blood pressure increase that are dormant in blacks living in Africa (American Heart Association, 2014; Fuchs, 2011; Jarvis, 2015). In Figure 3-2, a nurse

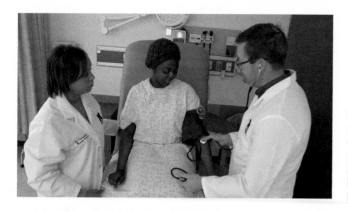

Figure 3-2. A nurse practitioner gathers subjective data during the health history and objective data (such as the blood pressure measurement) during the physical exam as part of the cultural assessment of a client being seen at an urban nurse-managed primary health care clinic.

practitioner checks the blood pressure of a client who is being seen for primary care services at an urban multicultural nurse-managed clinic.

Biocultural Variations in the Assessment of Pain

Pain is the most frequent and compelling reason that people seek health care and is sometimes referred to as the fifth vital sign. A universally recognized phenomenon, the term **pain** is defined as an unpleasant sensory and emotional experience conveyed by the brain through sensory neurons arising from actual or potential tissue damage to the body. Derived from the Greek word for penalty, pain is often associated with punishment in Judeo–Christian thought. Pain is a culture universal that is experienced by people in all parts of the world. Pain and ethnicity are multidimensional, subjective, and shaped by culture. The American Academy of Pain Medicine classifies pain as **acute** or **chronic**. In *acute pain*, a direct, one-to-one relationship exists between an injury and pain, and the pain is frequently short-lived and self-limiting. Acute pain, however, can become persistent and intractable if the underlying cause continues for a prolonged period. *Chronic pain* is described as pain that persists greater than 3 months. Chronic pain is now considered the most frequent cause of disability in industrialized nations globally. In the United States, an estimated 116 million people experience chronic pain, at a cost of $560 to $625 billion in health

care treatment and lost productivity (Institute of Medicine, 2011; Meghani et al., 2012).

In terms of pain measurement, it is generally believed that humans experience similar sensation thresholds. However, pain perception thresholds, pain tolerance, and encouraged pain threshold vary considerably among individuals from different racial and ethnic backgrounds. *Sensation threshold* refers to the lowest stimulus that results in tingling or warmth. *Pain threshold* refers to the point at which the individual reports that a stimulus is painful. Cultural background has an effect on this measure of pain as well as on pain threshold, the point at which the individual reports that a stimulus is painful, and pain tolerance, the point at which the individual withdraws or asks to have the stimulus stopped.

In a meta-analysis of 26 studies on racial and ethnic pain threshold and tolerance, Rahim-Williams, Riley, Williams, and Fillingim (2012) found that African Americans and non-Hispanic Whites are the most frequently studied groups. Both groups have the same pain threshold, but African Americans have lower pain tolerance. In a study of pain among African Americans and Whites, Mossey (2011) reported similar finding with African Americans having lower pain thresholds than Whites for cold, heat, pressure, and ischemia. Research on racial and ethnic group differences has translational merit for culturally competent clinical care and addressing and reducing pain treatment disparities among racially and ethnically diverse groups.

Research reveals that chronic disease, psychological distress, Medicaid insurance, and lower education levels are associated with higher incidences of severe pain (Meghani et al., 2012). Failure to adequately treat pain can lead to adverse outcomes, such as elevated heart rates postoperatively and increased risk of myocardial infarction, ischemic stroke, and hemorrhage resulting from elevated systemic vascular resistance and elevated levels of catecholamines. Other consequences of uncontrolled pain include reduced mobility, loss of strength, sleep disturbances, immune system impairment, increased susceptibility to disease, and medication dependence (Wang, Kennedy, Caggana, 2013; Wyatt, 2013).

The assessment of pain is complicated primarily because pain is an inherently subjective experience that necessitates the reliance on self-reporting, rather than objective measurements. Rating scales do not resolve uncertainties inherent in self-reporting methods. For example, self-report measures can be difficult to understand for people with limited English proficiency as well as for children and people with cognitive impairments. Pain assessment is influenced by three factors: (1) characteristics of the client, such as race and ethnicity; (2) the environmental context; and (3) the nurse's background and experience. Nurses and other health care providers sometimes project their own attitudes, beliefs, and opinions about pain onto their clients, a situation that encourages cultural stereotyping when assessing the client's self-reported level of pain (Tait & Chibnall, 2014).

Nurses and other health care providers are challenged to avoid bias when assessing pain and to take appropriate action commensurate with the level of self-reported pain. Research indicates that minority clients are likely to be more active in their communications when the clinical encounter is race concordant, that is, when the health care provider is from the same racial group, and to be less active in their communications when the encounter is race discordant, that is, the health care provider is from a different racial group than the client (Hsieh, Trip, & Li-Jun,

2011). Studies of primary care physicians reveal that provider race bias exists, especially between White providers and Black or Hispanic clients (Ezenwa & Fleming, 2012).

Negative stereotypes have been documented for members of racial and ethnic groups who experience pain. For example, some primary care physicians underestimate pain intensity in Black clients compared to other sociodemographic groups, and African Americans and Hispanics are sometimes perceived as requiring more scrutiny for potential drug abuse and misuse, despite evidence to the contrary (Becker et al., 2011; Kwok & Bhuvanakrishna, 2014; Tait & Chibnall, 2014). Blacks are more likely than non-Hispanic Whites to underreport pain unpleasantness in the clinical setting, especially in the presence of physicians who are perceived as having higher social status (Mossey, 2011) or are from a different racial background (Tait & Chibnall, 2014). Blacks demonstrate higher levels of posttreatment disability than whites for conditions such as low back pain, osteoarthritis, and other chronic pain conditions. Blacks also demonstrate more affective distress in response to chronic pain, with the distress contributing to levels of pain-related disability (Allen et al., 2010). Compared to non-Hispanic Whites, Native Americans have higher ischemic pain tolerance, higher electric pain threshold tolerance, lower ratings of electrical stimuli, and delay in withdrawing the hand from a noxious stimulus (nociceptive flexion reflex) (Palit et al., 2013). There is evidence that blacks and other minorities lack trust in the health care system and in their physicians (Hsieh et al., 2011; Palit et al., 2013; Tait & Chibnall, 2014; Wyatt, 2013); therefore, the client may fail to accurately report symptoms of pain, withhold information about the type and amount of medications he/she is using to control pain, and seek treatment for folk, traditional, religious, and/or spiritual healers when credentialed or licensed healers are unsuccessful in providing treatments that control pain to the client's satisfaction.

Factors contributing to racial and ethnic disparities in pain assessment include stereotypes

and biases of nurses conducting the client assessment, nurse–client communication, the nurse's ability to empathize with clients from racial/ethnic groups different from his/her own, the client's educational and socioeconomic background, and the client's pain reporting skills, pain coping ability, and level of trust of health care providers (Tait & Chibnall, 2014). The client's perception of the seriousness of the cause of pain (e.g., pain caused by cancer) may also influence the client's experience of pain (Kwok & Bhuvanakrishna, 2014).

Evidence-Based Practice 3-2 summarizes the results of a study of African American, Latino/Latina, and White clients with chronic pain who participated in a 4-week interdisciplinary team intervention that supported the notion that ethnic differences in pain assessment, perception, and treatment can be effectively managed using an interdisciplinary team approach, with nurses either leading or being key members of the team.

Biocultural Variations in General Appearance

In assessing general appearance, survey the person's entire body. Note the general health state and any obvious physical characteristics and readily apparent biologic features unique to the individual. In assessing the client's general appearance, consider four areas: physical appearance, body structure, mobility, and behavior. *Physical appearance* includes age, gender, level of consciousness, facial features, and skin color (evenness of color tone, pigmentation, intactness, and presence of lesions or other abnormalities). *Body structure* includes stature, nutrition, symmetry, posture, position, and overall body build or contour. *Mobility* includes gait and range of motion. *Behavior* includes such variables as facial expression, mood and affect, fluency of speech, ability to communicate ideas, appropriateness of word choice, grooming, and attire or dress. For example, observant members of the following groups often wear culture-specific attire: Amish, Mennonites, Hasidic and Orthodox Jews, and Muslims. Members of the Church of Jesus Christ

of Latter-day Saints (LDS), or Mormons, wear undergarments that symbolize their temple covenants. Many clients will want to leave the garments on during physical examinations. Nurses should respect the attire or clothing of people from diverse cultures and religions and those who ask to leave their garments on during the physical examination. In some instances, the client will not want nurses to handle their clothing.

In assessing a client's hygiene, it is useful to ask about typical bathing habits and customary use of various hygiene-related products. The level of self-care may suggest poor hygiene if unkempt and dirty. Recent immigrants from some arid nations where water is scarce might bathe less frequently than those from countries where water is more abundant.

People in most cultures in the United States and Canada make a great effort to disguise their natural body odors by bathing frequently, using douches, or applying antiperspirants, colognes, and/or perfumes with scents that are deemed to be desirable. These practices may mask the symptoms of some diseases and infections. There are 148 diseases associated with odors of the breath, skin, urine, stool, penis, and vagina (Mayo Clinic, n.d.a). During the assessment, the nurse should:

- Note the nature of breath odor—sweet may suggest diabetic ketoacidosis (sickly sweet smell), alcoholism (distinctive), liver failure (a sweet smell), or maple syrup urine disease; unpleasant or foul may suggest renal failure (urine or fishlike breath due to ammonia) and infections of the mouth, nose, pharynx, or chest (putrid odor).
- Examine state of teeth and teeth hygiene and note whether the teeth are real or false—loose-fitting teeth may be responsible for mouth ulcers or decayed teeth, which may cause halitosis (bad breath odor).
- Check the following tests results for indications of abnormalities:
  - Blood tests such as full blood count and the erythrocyte sedimentation rate will be helpful in determining the presence of infection.

Interdisciplinary Team Approach to Chronic Pain Management

The purpose of this study was to identify ethnic differences in interdisciplinary pain treatment outcome for clients from diverse ethnic backgrounds experiencing chronic pain. The study was a retrospective chart review of prospective data. Participant data were obtained from medical record of clients who had been assessed, evaluated, and subsequently treated using an interdisciplinary pain management program in the Chicago area. Clients participated in either full- or half-day programs that included individual pain psychology, physical therapy, occupational therapy, biofeedback, relaxation training, vocational counseling, and medical management. In addition to the individual sessions, all clients participated in the following groups: psychology (e.g., pain cycles and cognitive restructuring); relaxation training; physical therapy (e.g., conditioning and core strengthening exercises); Feldenkrais (a movement-based therapy); occupational therapy (e.g., body mechanics and community outing); pool therapy; vocational counseling; and nursing lectures (e.g., sleep hygiene and use of laughter). The investigators assessed a sample of 116 White, African American, and Latino/Latina clients with chronic pain who participated in a 4-week interdisciplinary pain treatment program. The outcome measure consisted of pre- and posttreatment and change scores on the Multidimensional Pain Inventory, Pain Anxiety Symptoms Scale, Chronic Pain Acceptance Questionnaire, Coping Strategies Questionnaire—Revised, and Center for Epidemiologic Studies Depression Scale—short form.

Ethnic minorities differed from whites on a number of treatment outcome measures at pre- and posttreatment. At pretreatment, Latinos/Latinas reported greater levels of pain-related anxiety, pain severity, and pain catastrophizing than White counterparts experiencing chronic pain. Both Latinos/Latinas and African Americans reported greater use of prayer at pre- and posttreatment, with Whites showing the greatest decrease in the use of prayer in response to treatment. At posttreatment, African American clients had a slightly greater level of anxiety than Whites. There was a significant difference in levels of depression at posttreatment with African Americans having higher levels of depression than Whites or Latinos/Latinas. There was a significant ethnic difference in the use of pain catastrophizing at pretreatment with Latinos/Latinas compared to Whites. There were also significant ethnic differences pre- and posttreatment with both Latinos/Latinas and African Americans using prayer as a coping strategy more than Whites. There was significant ethnicity effect for pain severity at pretreatment with both African Americans and Latinos/Latinas reporting a significantly greater level of pain severity than Whites. There was also significant posttreatment ethnicity effect for general activity level with Whites having a significantly higher level of activity than African Americans.

Clinical Implications:

Although the researchers reported that ethnic minority groups have a greater level of distress when experiencing chronic pain when compared to Whites, African American, Latino/Latina, and White clients with chronic pain who participated in the study all demonstrated a significant reduction in emotional distress, pain-related anxiety, use of maladaptive coping strategies such as catastrophizing, and perception of pain severity when they participated in a 4-week interdisciplinary team intervention to manage their pain. An integral part of the interdisciplinary team, nurses have a key role to play in assisting clients from diverse ethnic backgrounds to effectively manage chronic pain. Nurses should seek opportunities to collaborate with health professionals from other disciplines to plan, implement, and evaluate interdisciplinary interventions such as the one described in this study in order to help clients manage their chronic pain.

Reference: Gagon, C. M., Matsura, J. T., Smith, C. C., & Stanos, S. P. (2013). Ethnicity and interdisciplinary pain treatment. *Pain and Practice, 14*(6), 532–540.

- Renal function tests may suggest renal failure as cause of breath odor.
- Liver function tests may suggest hepatic coma as cause of breath odor.
- Blood sugar may suggest diabetic ketoacidosis as a cause of breath odor.
- Blood alcohol level to establish if alcoholism may be the cause of the breath odor.
- Urine analysis
  - Glucose and ketones present may suggest diabetic ketoacidosis as cause of breath odor.
  - Urine microscopy and culture may detect urinary tract infection.
- Culture of the mouth, gums, and nasopharynx may be necessary to diagnose anaerobic infections that may be the cause of breath odor.
- Sputum microscopy and culture
- Vaginal or penile discharge swab for culture, if appropriate
- Stool tests
  - Stool microscopy for ova, parasites, and culture for bacteria
  - Giardia antigen
  - Twenty-four-hour stool analysis of fecal fat—if **steatorrhea** is present (i.e., fatty, pale-colored, extremely smelly stools that float in the toilet and are difficult to flush away due to excess fat in the stool)
- Radiological investigations
  - X-ray or CT scan of chest or sinuses—if suspect respiratory infection as a cause of breath odor
  - Esophagogram will help detect a diverticulum (a pouch opening from the esophagus) that may cause bad breath odor (Mayo Clinic, n.d.b).

Biocultural Variations in Skin

An accurate and comprehensive examination of the skin of clients from culturally diverse backgrounds requires knowledge of biocultural variations and skill in recognizing color changes, some of which might be subtle. Awareness of normal biocultural differences and the ability to recognize the unique clinical manifestations of disease are developed over time as the nurse gains experience with clients with various skin colors.

The assessment of a client's skin is subjective and is highly dependent on observational skill, the ability to recognize subtle color changes, and repeated exposure to individuals having various gradations of skin color. *Melanin* is responsible for the various colors and tones of skin observed in different people. Melanin protects the skin against harmful ultraviolet rays—a genetic advantage accounting for the lower incidence of skin cancer among darkly pigmented Black and Native American clients (Everett, Budescu, & Sommers, 2012).

Normal skin color ranges widely. Some health care practitioners have attempted to describe the variations by labeling their observations with some of the following adjectives: *copper, olive, tan,* and various shades of *brown* (*light, medium, and dark*). In observing pallor in clients, the term *ashen* is sometimes used. Of greatest clinical significance, particularly for clients whose health condition might be linked to changes in skin color, is the ability to establish a reliable description of a baseline color and subsequently recognize when variations occur in an individual (Kaminska-Winciorek & Spiewak, 2012).

Mongolian Spots

Mongolian spots are irregular areas of deep blue pigmentation usually located in the sacral and gluteal areas but sometimes occurring on the abdomen, thighs, shoulders, or arms. During embryonic development, the melanocytes originate near the embryonic nervous system in the neural crest. They then migrate into the fetal epidermis. Mongolian spots are embryonic pigment that has been left behind in the epidermal layer during fetal development. The result looks like a bluish discoloration of the skin.

Mongolian spots are a normal variation in children of African, Asian, or Latin descent. By adulthood, these spots become lighter but usually remain visible. Mongolian spots are present in 90% of Blacks, 80% of Asians and Native Americans,

and 9% of Whites (Jarvis, 2015; Overfield, 1995). To the unfamiliar eye, Mongolian spots can be confused with bruises. Recognition of this normal variation is particularly important when dealing with children who might be erroneously identified as victims of child abuse, causing much anguish to the parents or guardians.

Vitiligo

Vitiligo, a condition in which the melanocytes become nonfunctional in some areas of the skin, is characterized by unpigmented, patchy, milky white skin patches that are often symmetric bilaterally. Vitiligo affects an estimated 2 to 5 million Americans. There is no greater prevalence among dark-skinned individuals, although the disorder may cause greater psychosocial stress in these groups because it is more visible (Buttaro, Trybulski, Polgar Bailey, & Sandberg-Cook, 2013). People with vitiligo have a statistically higher-than-normal risk for pernicious anemia, diabetes mellitus, and hyperthyroidism. These factors are believed to reflect an underlying genetic abnormality.

Hyperpigmentation

Other areas of the skin affected by hormones and, in some cases, differing for people from certain ethnic backgrounds are the sexual skin areas, such as the nipples, areola, scrotum, and labia majora. In general, these areas are darker than other parts of the skin in both adults and children, especially among African American and Asian clients. When assessing these skin surfaces on dark-skinned clients, observe carefully for erythema, rashes, and other abnormalities because the darker color might mask their presence.

Cyanosis

A severe condition indicating a lack of oxygen in the blood, **cyanosis** is the most difficult clinical sign to observe in darkly pigmented persons. Because peripheral vasoconstriction can prevent cyanosis, be attentive to environmental conditions such as air conditioning, mist tents,

and other factors that might lower the room temperature and thus cause vasoconstriction. For the client to manifest clinical evidence of cyanosis, the blood must contain 5 g of reduced hemoglobin in 1.5 g of methemoglobin per 100 mL of blood (Overfield, 1995). Only severe cyanosis is apparent in skin. It is best to check the conjunctivae, oral mucosa, and nail beds rather than to rely on the assessment of the skin, which will appear dull and lifeless in darkly pigmented people.

Given that most conditions causing cyanosis also cause decreased oxygenation of the brain, other clinical symptoms, such as changes in the level of consciousness, will be evident. Cyanosis usually is accompanied by increased respiratory rate, use of accessory muscles of respiration, nasal flaring, and other manifestations of respiratory distress. Exercise caution when assessing persons of Mediterranean descent for cyanosis because their circumoral region is normally dark blue.

Jaundice

In both light- and dark-skinned clients, **jaundice** is best observed in the sclera. When examining culturally diverse individuals, exercise caution to avoid confusing other forms of pigmentation with jaundice. Many darkly pigmented people, for example, African Americans, Filipinos, and others, have heavy deposits of subconjunctival fat that contain high levels of carotene in sufficient quantities to mimic jaundice. The fatty deposits become denser as the distance from the cornea increases. The portion of the sclera that is revealed naturally by the palpebral fissure is the best place to accurately assess color. If the palate does not have heavy melanin pigmentation, jaundice can be detected there in the early stages (i.e., when the serum bilirubin level is 2 to 4 mg/100 mL). The absence of a yellowish tint of the palate when the sclerae are yellow indicates carotene pigmentation of the sclerae rather than jaundice. Light- or clay-colored stools and dark golden urine often accompany jaundice in both light- and dark-skinned clients. To distinguish between carotenemia and jaundice, it is necessary

to inspect the posterior portion of the hard palate using bright daylight or good artificial lighting. Also, check the palms and soles for a yellow-orange color (Jarvis, 2015; Overfield, 1995). The ingestion of large amounts of carotene-rich foods may mimic jaundice; therefore, ask if the person recently ingested significant amounts of sweet potatoes, carrots, dark green leafy vegetables, butternut squash, or romaine lettuce.

Pallor

Assessing for **pallor** in darkly pigmented clients can be difficult because the underlying red tones are absent. This is significant because these red tones are responsible for giving brown or black skin its luster. The brown-skinned individual will manifest pallor with a more yellowish brown color, and the black-skinned person will appear ashen or gray. Generalized pallor can be observed in the mucous membranes, lips, and nail beds. The palpebrae, conjunctivae, and nail beds are preferred sites for assessing the pallor of anemia. When inspecting the conjunctiva, lower the lid sufficiently to see the conjunctiva near the inner and outer canthi. The coloration is often lighter near the inner canthus.

In addition to changes seen on skin assessment, the pallor of impending shock is accompanied by other clinical manifestations, such as increasing pulse rate, oliguria, apprehension, and restlessness. Anemia, particularly chronic iron deficiency anemia, might be manifested by the characteristic "spoon" nails, which have a concave shape. A lemon-yellow tint of the face and slightly yellow sclerae accompany pernicious anemia, which is also manifested by neurologic deficits and a red, painful tongue. Also, fatigue, exertional dyspnea, rapid pulse, dizziness, and impaired mental function accompany the most severe anemia (Jarvis, 2015; Overfield, 1995).

Erythema, Petechiae, and Ecchymoses

Erythema (redness) can also be difficult to assess in darkly pigmented clients because the contrast between white and red is more pronounced than it is when the skin color is darker. Erythema is frequently associated with localized inflammation and is characterized by increased skin temperature. The degree of redness is determined by the quantity of blood in the subpapillary plexus, whereas the warmth of the skin is related to the rate of blood flow through the blood vessels. In the assessment of inflammation in dark-skinned clients, it is often necessary to palpate the skin for increased warmth, tautness, or tightly pulled surfaces that might indicate edema and hardening of deep tissues or blood vessels. The dorsal surfaces of the fingers are the most sensitive to temperature sensations and should be used to assess for erythema.

The erythema associated with rashes is not always accompanied by noticeable increases in skin temperature. Macular, papular, and vesicular skin lesions are identified by a combination of palpation and inspection. In addition, it is important to listen to the client's description of symptoms. For example, persons with macular rashes will usually complain of itching, and evidence of scratching will be apparent. When the skin is only moderately pigmented, a macular rash might become recognizable when the skin is gently stretched. Stretching the skin decreases the normal red tone, thus providing more contrast and making the macules appear brighter. In some skin disorders with a generalized rash, the rash is most readily visible on the hard and soft palates.

Petechiae are best visualized in the areas of lighter melanization, such as the abdomen, buttocks, and volar surface of the forearm. When the skin is black or very dark brown, petechiae cannot be seen in the skin. Most of the diseases that cause bleeding and the formation of microscopic emboli, such as thrombocytopenia, subacute bacterial endocarditis, and other septicemias, are characterized by petechiae in the mucous membranes and skin. Petechiae are most easily seen in the mouth, particularly the buccal mucosa, and in the conjunctiva of the eye (Jarvis, 2015).

Ecchymoses caused by systemic disorders are found in the same locations as petechiae, although their larger size makes them more apparent on dark-skinned individuals. When differentiating

petechiae and ecchymoses from erythema in the mucous membrane, pressure on the tissue will momentarily blanch erythema but not petechiae or ecchymoses.

Addison's Disease

The cortisol deficiency characteristic of **Addison's disease** causes an increase in melanin production, which turns the skin a bronze color that resembles sun tan. The nipples, areola, genitalia, perineum, and pressure points such as the axillae, elbow, inner thighs, and buttocks look bronze. Addison's disease is very difficult to recognize in people with darkly pigmented skin; therefore, laboratory tests and other clinical manifestations of the disease should be used to corroborate the skin changes (Jarvis, 2015).

Uremia

Uremia is the illness accompanying kidney failure characterized by unexplained changes in extracellular volume, inorganic ion concentrations, or lack of known renal synthetic products. Uremic illness is due largely to the accumulation of organic waste products, not all identified, that are normally cleared by the kidneys. Renal failure causes retained urochrome pigments in the blood to turn the skin of a person with uremia gray or orange-green. In people with darkly pigmented skin, it may be difficult to visualize the skin color changes; therefore, skin manifestations of uremia are often masked. Laboratory tests and other clinical findings are needed to corroborate the observation of skin color change when assessing a person with suspected uremia.

Albinism

The term **albinism** refers to a group of inherited conditions. People with albinism have little or no pigment in their eyes, skin, or hair. They have inherited altered genes that do not make the usual amounts of the pigment melanin. One person in 17,000 in the United States has some type of albinism. Albinism affects people from all races. Most children with albinism are born to parents who have normal hair and eye color for their ethnic backgrounds. Sometimes, people do not recognize that they have albinism. There are different types of albinism, and the amount of pigment in the eyes varies. Although some individuals with albinism have reddish or violet eyes, most have blue eyes, whereas others have hazel or brown eyes.

Vision problems are associated with all forms of albinism. People with albinism always have impaired vision (not correctable with eyeglasses) and many have low vision. Low vision refers to impaired vision in which there is a significant reduction in visual function that cannot be corrected by conventional glasses, but which may be improved with special aids or devices. The degree of vision impairment varies with the type of albinism. Many people with albinism are legally blind due to abnormal development of the retina and abnormal patterns of nerve connections between the eye and the brain. The presence of these eye problems defines the diagnosis of albinism. Therefore, the main test for albinism is an eye examination. People with albinism need to take precautions to avoid damage to the skin caused by the sun, such as wearing sunscreen lotions, hats, and sun-protective clothing (National Organization for Albinism and Hypopigmentation, 2014; Seibert & Darling, 2013).

Normal Age-Related Skin Changes

Although aging is accompanied by the growing presence of wrinkles in all cultures, Blacks, Asian Americans, American Indians, and Eskimos wrinkle later in life than their Anglo-American counterparts. Light skin shows the effects of sun damage more than dark skin, regardless of race or ethnicity, and the area of the skin that is exposed to the sun shows the effects of aging more than protected skin, such as those parts covered by clothing. **Café au lait spots**, tan to light brown irregularly shaped oval patches with well-defined borders, are caused by increased

melanin pigment in the basal cell layer of the skin (Kaminska-Winciorek & Spiewak, 2012).

Regardless of climate, dry skin is inevitable in individuals older than 70 years of age. Transepidermal water loss will result in a dry, tight, and often inflamed-looking appearance. It gives an impaired acid mantle and impaired immune response, impacting and compromising the skins structural integrity. Examples of severe transepidermal water loss are eczema or psoriasis. These conditions occur when vital fluids evaporate and the skin becomes very dry and inflamed. Restoring free water levels and thickening the matrix of the skin is an integral part of returning the skin back to a healthy functional state. African Americans have a significantly higher transepidermal water loss than Whites, which correlates with the water content of the stratum corneum layer of the skin (Kaminska-Winciorek & Spiewak, 2012).

Moles occur when cells in the skin grow in a cluster instead of being spread throughout the skin. These cells are called melanocytes, and they make the pigment that gives skin its natural color. Moles may darken after exposure to the sun, during the teen years, and during pregnancy. Because the number of moles increases with age, they are thought to be the result of long-term exposure to the sun. People with lighter skin have more moles than those with darkly pigmented skin. Whites have more moles than Asian Americans or African Americans. Most moles are benign; however, moles that are more likely to be cancer are those that look different than other existing moles or those that first appear after age 30. If nurses notice changes in a mole's color, height, size, or shape, they should consult with a dermatologist. Any client who has a mole that bleeds, oozes, itches, or becomes tender or painful should be referred immediately to a dermatologist (Jarvis, 2015; Kaminska-Winciorek & Spiewak, 2012).

Nurses and other health care providers often overestimate or underestimate age when dealing with clients whose cultural heritage is different from their own. Whites tend to underestimate the age of Africans, Asians, and American Indians, whereas African Americans, Asians, and American Indians tend to overestimate the age of White clients (Gunn et al., 2013).

Biocultural Variations in Sweat Glands

The *apocrine* and *eccrine sweat glands* are important for fluid balance and thermoregulation. Approximately 2 to 3 million glands open onto the skin surface through pores and are responsible for the presence of sweat. When glands are contaminated by normal skin flora, odor results. Most Asians and Native Americans have a mild to absent body odor, whereas Whites and African Americans tend to have strong body odor.

Eskimos have made an environmental adaptation whereby they sweat less than Whites on their trunks and extremities but more on their faces (Taylor & Machado-Moreira, 2013). This adaptation allows for temperature regulation without causing perspiration and dampness of their clothes, which would decrease their ability to insulate against severe weather and would pose a serious threat to their survival.

The amount of chloride excreted by sweat glands varies widely, and African Americans have lower salt concentrations in their sweat than Whites do. A study of Ashkenazi Jews (of European descent) and Sephardic Jews (of North African and Middle Eastern descent) revealed that those of European origin had a lower percentage of sweat chlorides (Levin, 1966). This variation might be significant in the care of clients with renal or cardiac conditions or of children with cystic fibrosis (Gunn et al., 2013; Taylor & Machado-Moreira, 2013).

Biocultural Variation in the Head

Nurses will notice marked, biocultural variations when examining the hair, eyes, ears, and mouths of clients from diverse racial and ethnic backgrounds. The ability to distinguish normal variations from abnormal ones could have serious implications as some variations are associated with systemic sometimes life-threatening conditions.

Hair

Perhaps one of the most obvious and widely variable cultural differences occurs with assessment of the hair. African American hair varies widely in texture. It is very fragile and ranges from long and straight to short, spiraled, thick, and kinky. The hair and scalp have a natural tendency to be dry and require daily combing, gentle brushing, and the application of oil. By comparison, clients of Asian backgrounds generally have straight, silky hair.

Obtaining a baseline hair assessment is significant in the diagnosis and treatment of certain disease states. For example, hair texture is known to become dry, brittle, and lusterless with inadequate nutrition. The hair of black children with severe malnutrition, as in the case of marasmus, frequently changes not only in texture but also in color. The child's hair often becomes straighter and turns a reddish copper color. Certain endocrine and genetic disorders are also known to affect the amount, thickness, and texture of the client's hair (Macbeth & Harries, 2012).

Although gray hair correlates with age for both men and women, there are cultural differences in the rate of hair graying. Whites gray significantly faster than any other group; 66% of fair-haired individuals, compared to 37% of dark-haired persons, have fully white by age 60 (Overfield, 1995). Among Asian Americans, graying might be delayed significantly, with some in their eighth or ninth decade of life showing little or no graying.

Eyes

Biocultural differences in both the structure and the color of the eyes are readily apparent among clients from various cultural backgrounds. Racial differences are evident in the palpebral fissures. Persons of Asian background are often identified by their characteristic epicanthal eye folds, whereas the presence of narrowed palpebral fissures in non-Asian individuals might be diagnostic of a serious congenital anomaly known as Down syndrome or trisomy 21.

There is culturally based variability in the color of the iris and in retinal pigmentation: Darker irises are correlated with darker retinas. Clients with light retinas generally have better night vision but can experience pain in an environment that is too light. The majority of African Americans and Asians have brown eyes, whereas many individuals of Scandinavian or northern European descent have blue eyes (Overfield, 1995).

It is clinically relevant that differences in visual acuity (clearness of vision) occur among people from different cultures. When eyeglasses are prescribed to improve visual clarity, blacks have poorer corrected visual acuity than whites. The visual acuity of Hispanic Americans is between that of Blacks and Whites (Qiu, Wang, Singh, Lin, 2014). American Indians are comparable to Whites in visual acuity; Japanese and Chinese Americans have the poorest corrected visual acuity because of a high incidence of myopia (Overfield, 1995; Qiu et al., 2014). Dutch-German Mennonites have an X chromosome disorder that causes night blindness (and low phosphate levels) (Orton, Innes, Chudley, Bech-Hansen, 2014).

Ears

Ears come in a variety of sizes and shapes. Earlobes can be freestanding or attached to the face. Ceruminous glands are located in the external ear canal and are functional at birth. Cerumen (ear wax) is genetically determined and comes in two major types: dry cerumen, which is gray and flaky and frequently forms a thin mass in the ear canal, and wet cerumen, which is dark brown and moist. Asians and Native Americans (including Eskimos) have an 84% frequency of dry cerumen. Wet cerum is found in 99% of African Americans and 97% of Whites (Overfield, 1995). The clinical significance of this occurs when examining or irrigating the ears; the presence and composition of cerumen are not related to poor hygiene, and flaky, dry cerumen should not be mistaken for the dry lesions of eczema.

Hearing loss may be genetic, congenital, or acquired through aging, injury, infection, or accident. On rare occasions, hearing loss is caused by surgery when the excision of a brain

tumor is necessary. Age-related hearing loss, or **presbycusis**, is the slow loss of hearing that occurs as people get older and the cilia (tiny hair cells) in the inner ear become damaged or die. The following factors that contribute to age-related hearing loss should be considered in the health history and physical examination: family history (age-related hearing loss tends to run in families); repeated exposure to loud noises; smoking (smokers are more likely to have hearing loss than nonsmokers); certain medical conditions such as diabetes; and some prescription medicines (e.g., the antibiotic gentamicin). Although hearing loss caused by noise and aging previously has been considered permanent, there is animal research using vitamin B_3 that offers promise for restoring hearing loss (Gladstone Institute, 2014). After age 40, men have poorer hearing than women. Blacks have better hearing at high and low frequencies; whites have better hearing at middle frequencies. Melanin pigmentation is significantly more abundant in the cochlea of African Americans than Whites. Research detailing pigmentation in the cochlea helps to explain the observed racial differences in hearing thresholds between African Americans and Whites and may be the reason that African Americans are less susceptible to noise-induced hearing loss such as that caused by loud music or occupational exposure to noise (Sun, Xin, Lin, et al., 2014).

Mouth

Oral hyperpigmentation also shows variation by race. Usually absent at birth, hyperpigmentation increases with age. By age 50, 10% of Whites and 50% to 90% of African Americans will show oral hyperpigmentation, a condition believed to be caused by a lifetime of accumulation of postinflammatory oral changes (Kliegman et al., 2011; Overfield, 1995).

Cleft uvula, a condition in which the uvula is split either completely or partially, occurs in 18% of some Native American groups and 10% of Asians (Kliegman et al., 2011). Ethnic differences exist in the incidence of cleft lip and palate with

American Indians having the highest incidence (1/300 live births), followed by Asians (1/500 live births), and Whites (1/750 live births). Blacks have the lowest incidence (1/2,500 live births) (National Institutes of Health, 2013; Kliegman et al., 2011). The incidence of cleft lip and palate rises with increased parental age; older mothers with additional parity have an increased incidence of having children with cleft palate (Tewfik & Myers, 2013).

Leukoedema, a grayish-white benign lesion occurring on the buccal mucosa, is present in 68% to 90% of blacks and 43% of whites. Care should be taken to avoid mistaking leukoedema for oral thrush or related infections that require treatment with medication (Overfield, 1995).

Teeth

Teeth are often used as indicators of developmental, hygienic, and nutritional adequacy, and there are important biocultural differences. It is rare for a White baby to be born with teeth (1 in 3,000), but the incidence is 1 in 11 among Tlingit Indian infants and 1 or 2 in 100 among Canadian Aboriginal infants. Although congenital teeth are usually not problematic, extraction is necessary for some breast-fed infants (Kliegman et al., 2011; Overfield, 1995).

The size of teeth varies widely, with the teeth of Whites being the smallest, followed by Blacks and then Asians and Native Americans. The largest teeth are found among Native Alaskans and Australian Aborigines. Larger teeth cause some groups to have prognathic (protruding) jaws, a condition that is seen more frequently in African and Asian Americans. The condition is normal and does not reflect a serious orthodontic problem.

Agenesis (absence of teeth) varies by race, with missing third molars occurring in 18% to 35% of Asians, 9% to 25% of Whites, and 1% to 11% of Blacks. Throughout life, whites have more tooth decay than blacks, which might be related to a combination of socioeconomic factors and biocultural variation. Complete tooth loss occurs

more often in Whites (51%) than in African Americans (39%) despite the higher incidence of periodontal disease in Blacks (National Institute of Dental and Craniofacial Research, 2014). There is evidence that as dental care is more advanced and accessible, both whites and blacks will retain more of their original teeth over their lifespans (National Institute of Dental and Craniofacial Research, 2014).

Dental caries or tooth decay is significant because there are known correlations between dental caries and other conditions such as cleft lip and palate, renal failure, cystic fibrosis, immunosuppression, heart defects, low birth weight, seizures, maternal illness, and rickets (Kliegman et al., 2011). The differences in tooth decay between African Americans and Whites can be explained by the fact that African Americans have harder and denser tooth enamel, which makes their teeth less susceptible to the organisms that cause caries. The increase in periodontal disease among African Americans is believed to be caused by poor oral hygiene. When obvious signs of periodontal disease are present, such as bleeding and edematous gums, a dental referral should be initiated.

Biocultural Variations in the Mammary Venous Plexus

Regardless of gender, the superficial veins of the chest form a network over the entire chest that flows in either a transverse or a longitudinal pattern. In the transverse pattern, the veins radiate laterally and toward the axillae. In the longitudinal pattern, the veins radiate downward and laterally like a fan. These two patterns occur with different frequencies in the two populations that have been studied, Whites and Navajos. The recessive longitudinal pattern occurs in 6% to 10% of White women and in 30% of Navajos. The only known alteration of either pattern is produced by breast tumor. Although this variation has no clinical significance, it is mentioned so that if nurses note its presence during physical assessment, they will recognize it as a normal variation (Overfield, 1995; Yang et al., 2012).

Biocultural Variations in the Musculoskeletal System

Many normal biocultural variations are found in clients' musculoskeletal systems. The long bones of blacks are significantly longer, narrower, and denser than those of whites. Bone density measured by race and gender shows that black males have the densest bones, accounting for the relatively lower incidence of osteoporosis and hip fractures in this population. Similarly, Black women have lower incidence of these two conditions when compared with Hispanic and White women (Jarvis, 2015; Silva, Shen, Heo, et al., 2012). Bone density in Chinese, Japanese, and Native Alaskans is below that of Whites (Overfield, 1995). In a study of men aged 65 and older, the highest prevalence of self-reported nontraumatic fracture was Whites, 17%; African Americans, 15%; Hispanics, 14%; and Asian Americans, 11%. Low bone mineral density was associated with higher prevalence of bone fracture in all groups (Shin et al., 2014).

Curvature of the body's long bones varies widely among culturally diverse groups. Native Americans and First Nation People of Canada have anteriorly convex femurs, whereas Blacks have markedly straight femurs, and Whites have intermediate femurs. This characteristic is related to both genetics and body weight. The femurs of thin blacks and whites have less curvature than average, whereas those of obese blacks and whites display increased curvatures. It is possible that the heavier density of the bones of blacks helps to protect them from increased curvature caused by obesity. Blacks tend to be wide shouldered and narrow hipped; Asians tend to be wider in the hips and narrower in the shoulders. The clavicle is a long bone that is responsible for shoulder width; therefore, taller people generally have wider shoulders than shorter people (Overfield, 1995; Silva et al., 2011).

As the largest component of adipose tissue-free body mass in humans, skeletal muscle is central to the body's nutritional, physiologic, and metabolic processes. Between the ages of 18 and

80 years, Blacks have more skeletal muscle than White, Hispanic, and Asian counterparts across the entire age range, even when adjusting for weight and height. Body composition should be interpreted according to ethnicity and gender. Different standards for skeletal muscle should be applicable for multiethnic populations (Silva et al., 2011).

Table 3-6 summarizes biocultural variations occurring in the musculoskeletal system that have been identified through observation and study of people from various cultures and subcultures.

Biocultural Variations in Illness

Researchers have abundant evidence that there is a relationship between ethnicity and the incidence of certain diseases across the lifespan, from infancy to old age. Knowledge of normal biocultural variations and those occurring during illness helps nurses to conduct more accurate, comprehensive, and thorough physical examinations of clients from diverse cultures.

Biocultural Variations in Laboratory Tests

As summarized in Table 3-7, biocultural variations occur with some laboratory tests, such as measurement of hemoglobin, hematocrit, cholesterol, serum transferrin, blood glucose, creatinine, and estimated glomerular filtration rate. There are also biocultural differences in the results of tests conducted during pregnancy. For example, the multiple marker screening test and two tests of amniotic fluid constituents are routinely used to screen pregnant women for potential fetal problems.

Table 3-6: Biocultural Variations in the Musculoskeletal System

Bone/Muscle	Remarks
Bone	
Frontal	Thicker in Black males than in White males
Parietal occiput	Thicker in White males than in Black males
Palate	Tori (protuberances) along the suture line of the hard palate
	Problematic for denture wearers
	Incidence:
	Blacks 20%
	Whites 24%
	Asians Up to 50%
	Native Americans Up to 50%
Mandible	Tori (protuberances) on the lingual surface of the mandible near the canine and premolar teeth
	Problematic for denture wearers
	Most common in Asians and Native Americans; exceeds 50% in some Eskimo groups
Humerus	Torsion or rotation of proximal end with muscle pull
	Greater degree of torsion observed in Whites than Blacks
	Torsion in Blacks is symmetric; torsion in Whites tends to be greater on right side than left side.
Radius	Length at the wrist variable

continued

Table 3-6: Biocultural Variations in the Musculoskeletal System (continued)

Bone/Muscle	Remarks
Ulna	Ulna and radius are not always of equal length; useful for assessing radial and ulnar fractures and post-op recovery of bone healing
	Equal length:
	Swedes 61%
	Chinese 16%
	Ulna longer than radius:
	Swedes 16%
	Chinese 48%
	Radius longer than ulna:
	Swedes 23%
	Chinese 10%
Vertebrae	Twenty-four vertebrae are found in 85%–93% of all people; racial and sex differences reveal 23 or 25 vertebrae in select groups.
	Vertebrae Population
	23 11% of Black females
	25 12% of Native Alaskan and Native American
	Related to lower back pain and lordosis
Pelvis	Hip width is 1.6 cm (0.6 in.) less in Black women than in White women; Asian women have significantly smaller pelvises.
Femur	Convex anterior Native American
	Straight Black
	Intermediate White
Second tarsal	Second toe longer than the great toe
	Incidence:
	Whites 8–34%
	Blacks 8–12%
	Vietnamese 31%
	Melanesians 21%–57%
	Clinical significance for joggers and athletes
Height	White males are 1.27 cm (0.5 in.) taller than Black males and 7.6 cm (2.9 in.) taller than Asian males.
	White females = Black females
Composition of long bones	Longer, narrower, and denser in Blacks than in Whites; bone density in Whites > Chinese, Japanese, and Native Alaskan
	Osteoporosis lowest in Black males; highest in White females

Table 3-6: Biocultural Variations in the Musculoskeletal System (continued)

Bone/Muscle	Remarks
Muscle	
Peroneus tertius	Responsible for dorsiflexion of foot

Muscle absent:

Asians, Native Americans, and Whites	3%–10%
Blacks	10%–15%
Berbers (Sahara desert)	24%

No clinical significance because the tibialis anterior also dorsiflexes the foot

Palmaris longus	Responsible for wrist flexion

Muscle absent:

Whites	12%–20%
Native Americans	2%–12%
Blacks	5%
Asians	3%

No clinical significance because three other muscles are also responsible for flexion

Based on data reported by Overfield, T. (1995). *Biologic variation in health and illness: Race, age, and sex differences.* New York, NY: CRC Press; Shin, M., Zmuda, J., Barrett-Connor, E., Sheu, Y., Patrick, A., Leung, P., ..., Cauley, J. (2014). Race/ethnic differences in associations between bone mineral density and fracture history in older men. *Osteoporosis International*, 25(3), 387–845.

Table 3-7: Biocultural Variations and Clinical Significance for Selected Laboratory Tests

Test	Remarks
Hemoglobin/ hematocrit	1 g lower for Blacks than other groups; Blacks < counterparts in other groups
Serum transferrin	Biocultural variation in children aged 1–3½ years
	Mean for Blacks 22 mg/100 mL > Whites
	Note: May be due to lowered hemoglobin and hematocrit levels found in Blacks
	Clinical significance: Transferrin levels increase in the presence of anemia, thus influencing the diagnosis, treatment, and nursing care of children with anemia.
Serum cholesterol	Biocultural variation across the lifespan

Birth	Blacks = Whites
Childhood	Blacks 5 mg/100 mL > Whites
Tohono O'odham (Pima) Indians 20–30 mg/100 mL >Whites	
Adulthood	Blacks < Whites
Tohono O'odham (Pima) Indians 50–60 mL/100 mL < Whites	

Clinical significance: Prevention, treatment, and nursing care of clients with cardiovascular disease

continued

Table 3-7: Biocultural Variations and Clinical Significance for Selected Laboratory Tests (continued)

Test	Remarks
High-density lipoproteins (HDLs)	Biocultural variation in adults Blacks > Whites Asians ≥ Whites Mexican Americans < Whites
Ratio of HDL to total cholesterol	Blacks < Whites
Low-density lipoproteins (LDLs)	Biocultural variation in adults Blacks < Whites *Clinical significance:* Prevention, treatment, and nursing care of clients with cardiovascular disease
Blood glucose	Biocultural variation in adults North American Indians, Hispanics, Japanese > Whites Blacks = Whites (for equivalent socioeconomic groups) *Clinical significance:* Diagnosis, treatment, and nursing care of adults and children with hypoglycemia and diabetes mellitus
Creatinine	For patients >49 years of age, the average creatinine level is 0.6–1.2 mg/dL in adult males and 0.5–1.1 mg/dL in adult females. (In the metric system, a milligram is a unit of weight equal to one-thousandth of a gram, and a deciliter is a unit of volume equal to one-tenth of a liter.) A person with only one kidney may have a normal level of about 1.8 or 1.9. Creatinine levels that reach 10.0 or more in adults indicate severe kidney impairment and the need for dialysis to remove wastes from the blood. For blacks, the normal average is 13% higher than counterparts in the general population. *Clinical significance:* Interpretation of test results for Blacks with suspected or diagnosed renal disease needs to take racial difference into account.
Estimated glomerular filtration rate (eGFR)	Blacks have more extreme rate of eGFR, followed by Hispanics, Whites, and Asians. *Clinical significance:* eGFR predicts onset of end-stage renal disease (ESRD) and need for dialysis and renal transplantation. Projected kidney failure during chronic kidney disease stages 3 and 4 was high in blacks, Hispanics, and Asians relative to whites. Mortality for those with projected kidney failure is highest in whites. Differences in eGFR decline and mortality contribute to racial disparities in ESRD incidence.
Multiple marker screening	Biocultural variations in blood levels for protein and hormones in pregnant women. Alpha-fetoprotein (AFP), hCG, and estriol levels in Black and Asian women > Whites. *Clinical significance:* High AFP levels signal that the woman is at increased risk for being delivered of an infant with spina bifida and neural tube defects, whereas low levels may signal Down syndrome; Down syndrome also is associated with low levels of estriol and high levels of hCG. Black and Asian American women have higher average levels of AFP, hCG, and estriol than White counterparts. Using a single median for women of all cultures: • Causes Black and Asian women to be falsely identified as being *at risk* for having infants with spina bifida and neural tube defects; by being classified as *high risk*, women are more likely to be subjected to invasive and expensive procedures such as amniocentesis; some may elect to abort the pregnancy based on screening test results. • Inappropriately lowers the identified Down syndrome risk for Black and Asian women.

Table 3-7: Biocultural Variations and Clinical Significance for Selected Laboratory Tests (continued)

Test	Remarks
Lecithin/ sphingomyelin ratio	Biocultural variations in amniotic fluid measures of fetal pulmonary maturity.
	Blacks have higher ratios than Whites from 23 to 42 weeks' gestation.
	Clinical significance: The ratio is used to calculate the risk of respiratory distress in premature infants: Lung maturity in Blacks is reached 1 week earlier than in Whites (34 vs. 35 weeks); racial differences should be considered in making decisions about inducing labor or delivering by caesarean section.

Table based on data from Allanson, A., Michie, S., & Matreau, T. M. (1997). Presentation of screen negative results on serum screening for Down's syndrome. *Journal of Medical Screening, 4*(1), 21–22; Chapman, S. J., Brumfield, C. G., Wenstrom, K. D., & DuBard, M. B. (1997). Pregnancy outcomes following false-positive multiple marker screening test. *American Journal of Perinatology, 14*(8), 475–478; Chan, R. L. (2014). Biochemical markers of spontaneous preterm birth in asymptomatic women. *Biomedical Research*, 2014. doi: 10.1155/2014/164081PMCID: PMC3914291; Derose, S. F., Rutkowski, M. P., Crooks, P. W., Shi, J. M., Wang, J. Q., Kalantar-Zadeh, K., …, Jacobsen, S. J. (2013). Racial differences in estimated Glomerular Filtration decline, ESDR, and mortality in an integrated health system. *American Journal of Kidney Disease, 62*(2), 236–244; O'Brien, J. E., Dvorin, E., Drugan, A., Johnson, M. P., Yaron, Y., & Evans, M. I. (1997). Race-ethnicity-specific variation in multiple-marker biochemical screening: Alpha-fetoprotein, hCG, and estriol. *Obstetrics and Gynecology, 89*(3), 355–358; National Down Syndrome Society, 2014; Overfield, T. (1995). *Biologic variation in health and illness: Race, age, and sex differences.* New York, NY: CRC Press.

Caution should be used in interpreting genetic data as population categories are not discrete and separate entities. African Americans and Latinos have complex recent ancestral histories. African Americans on average are estimated to have approximately 20% European ancestry, and this proportion varies substantially among different African American populations within North America. Genetic analysis of individual ancestry indicates that some self-identified European Americans have substantial recent African genetic ancestry. Population categories including race and ethnic groups are inadequate and misleading to fully describe the pattern and range of variation among individual clients. The more accurate assessment of disease risk is obtained by genotyping. **Genotyping** refers to the process of identifying differences in genetic makeup using biological testing rather than assuming their population affiliation as a surrogate.

Although the reasons for differences aren't always known, genetics, environment, diet, socioeconomic background, race, ethnicity, and lifestyle factors contribute to the differences in test results.

Transcultural Perspectives in Clinical Decision Making and Actions

After completing a comprehensive cultural assessment through the health history and physical examination, analyze the subjective and objective data. Leininger suggests three major modalities to guide nursing decisions and actions for the purpose of providing culturally congruent care that is beneficial, satisfying, and meaningful to clients: *cultural care preservation or maintenance, cultural care accommodation or negotiation,* and *cultural care repatterning or restructuring* (Leininger, 1991; Leininger & McFarland, 2002; McFarland & Wehbe-Alamah, 2015).

Cultural care preservation or maintenance refers to those professional actions and decisions that help people of a particular culture to retain and/or preserve relevant care values so that they can maintain their well-being, recover from illness, or face handicaps and/or death (Leininger, 1991; Leininger & McFarland, 2002; McFarland & Wehbe-Alamah, 2015). **Cultural care accommodation or negotiation** refers to professional

actions and decisions that help people of a designated culture to adapt to or to negotiate with others for beneficial or satisfying health outcomes with professional care providers (Leininger, 1991; Leininger & McFarland, 2002; McFarland & Wehbe-Alamah, 2015). **Cultural care repatterning or restructuring** refers to professional actions and decisions that help clients reorder, change, or greatly modify their lifeways for new, different, and beneficial health care patterns while respecting the clients' cultural values and beliefs and yet providing more beneficial or healthier lifeways than before the changes were coestablished with the clients (Leininger, 1991; Leininger & McFarland, 2002, 2006; McFarland & Wehbe-Alamah, 2015).

Whether the nurse uses Leininger's three modes for decisions and actions or engages in other analytic processes, the next step in the process leading to culturally competent decision making and actions is to set mutual goals with the client, develop a plan of care, confer with and make referrals to other members of the interprofessional health care team (when needed), and implement a plan of care, either alone or with others. This process is presented primarily from the nurse's vantage point, is based on the health histories and physical examinations by the nurse and other team members, and focuses on the nurse–client interaction and those aspects of the care plan that fall within the scope of practice and responsibilities of professional nurses.

Credentialed or licensed health professionals (e.g., physicians, pharmacists, social workers, dieticians, and physical, occupational, respiratory, and other therapists) have been educated to follow a similar process. Although some folk, traditional, religious, and spiritual healers may follow a comparable process, others might rely on a different approach, for example, reliance on subjective data from the client that is based on a spiritual assessment. They may prefer to practice their healing interventions with the client in private and may or may not want to collaborate with other members of the team. Be mindful that the federal Health Insurance Portability and Accountability Act (HIPAA) regulations may prohibit the sharing of some information, especially when the client is too ill to provide informed consent to release medical information with family, friends, and healers without authorization.

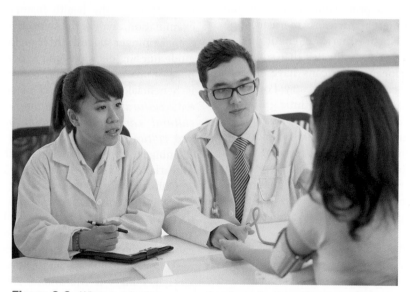

Figure 3-3. When conducting a comprehensive cultural assessment, the nurse collaborates with the client and physician as a members of an interprofessional health care team (Dragon Images/Shutterstock.com).

Once the plan has been implemented, it should be evaluated in collaboration with the client, the client's family and significant others, and with other credentialed, licensed, folk, traditional, religious, and spiritual healers who are members of the team. The evaluation includes a comprehensive analysis of the plan's effectiveness in meeting mutually established goals and desired outcomes. As indicated in Figure 3-3, nurses collaborate with clients, physicians, and other members of the health care team to determine if the care delivered was culturally acceptable, congruent and competent, safe, affordable, accessible, high quality, and based on research, scientific evidence, and best professional practices. Gather additional subjective and objective data to determine the effectiveness of the intervention(s) and the client's overall satisfaction with care delivery and outcomes. Health care facilities, home and community health agencies, and related health care organizations usually have comprehensive evaluation processes and instruments that they administer to clients or patients and then subsequently review individually and in the aggregate for the purpose of improving the quality of care.

Summary

Many biocultural variations in health and illness are apparent in the health assessment and physical examination. For example, nurses will note differences based on the client's gender, age, race, ethnicity, and/or genetic makeup. In gathering subjective and objective assessment data, note biocultural differences in body measurements, pain perception, general appearance, and symptom manifestation For example, in assessing the skin of lightly and darkly pigmented clients, there are notable differences in the manifestations of cyanosis, jaundice, pallor, erythema, petechiae, and ecchymoses. From the head to the toes, systematically use multiple techniques to gather data through observation, inspection, auscultation, palpation, and smell to conduct a comprehensive physical examination of the client. Upon completion of the health assessment and physical examination, analyze and synthesize subjective and objective findings from the assessment, review the results of laboratory tests, and collaborate with the client and other members of the health care team to develop mutual goals, make clinical decisions, plan care, implement the plan, and evaluate the care. After evaluating the care, it may be necessary to ask the client additional questions, conduct a more focused physical examination on a particular body system, and/or revise the plan of care to ensure that it provides safe, culturally acceptable, congruent, competent, affordable, accessible, high-quality care that is evidence based and reflects best professional practices.

REVIEW QUESTIONS

1. In your own words, describe the key components of a comprehensive cultural assessment.
2. Compare and contrast your approach to the assessment of light- and dark-skinned clients for cyanosis, jaundice, pallor, erythema, and petechiae.
3. Review the biocultural variations in laboratory tests for hemoglobin, hematocrit, serum cholesterol, serum transferrin, creatinine, eGFR, multiple marker screening, and amniotic fluid constituents.
4. Critically analyze the reasons for the current interest in herbal medicines by nurses, physicians, pharmacists, and other health care providers. How does knowledge of these medicines facilitate the nurse's ability to provide culturally competent and congruent nursing care?

CRITICAL THINKING ACTIVITIES

1. Critically analyze the instrument, tool, or form used by nurses when conducting an initial client or resident admission assessment at a hospital, extended care facility, or other health care agency in terms of its relevance to the health and nursing needs of persons from diverse cultures. From a transcultural nursing

perspective, identify the strengths and limitations of the admission assessment instrument. What suggestions would you make to enhance the effectiveness of the instrument in assessing the cultural needs of newly admitted clients or residents? Be sure to consider the practical constraints that nurses face in the current health care environment, such as time limitations, external forces that require nurses to care for increasingly large numbers of clients, and other constraints, before you suggest modifications to the existing instrument.

2. Using the Andrews and Boyle Transcultural Nursing Assessment Guide for Individuals and Families (Appendix A), answer the questions in each data category as they apply to you. As you write your responses to the questions, critically reflect on your own health-related cultural values, attitudes, beliefs, and practices.

3. Using the Andrews and Boyle Transcultural Nursing Assessment Guide for Individuals and Families (Appendix A), interview someone from a cultural background different from your own to assess his or her health-related cultural values, attitudes, beliefs, and practices. After you have completed the interview, compare and contrast those responses with your own responses in Question 2. Identify the ways in which you are *alike*. Critically analyze the *differences* as potential sources of cross-cultural conflict, and explore ways in which they might influence the nurse–client interaction.

4. Conduct a head-to-toe physical examination of a person from a racial background different from your own. Summarize your findings in writing. In a constructively self-critical manner, reflect on what aspects of the exam were (1) easiest and (2) most difficult for you. Try to determine the reason(s) why some aspects were relatively easy or difficult for you. What further information or skill development would assist you in gaining confidence in your ability to conduct physical examinations on people from diverse racial backgrounds?

REFERENCES

Allen, K. D., Oddone, E. Z., Coffman, C. J., Keefe, F. J., Lindquist, J. H., Bosworth, H. B. (2010). Racial differences in osteoarthritis pain and function: Potential explanatory factors. *Osteoarthritis and Cartilage, 18*, 160–167.

American Cancer Society. (n.d.). Genetics and breast cancer. Retrieved from http://www.cancer.org/cancer/breastcancer/index

American Heart Association. (2014). African Americans and heart disease, stroke. Retrieved on 10/10/14 at http://www.heart.org/HEARTORG/Conditions/More/MyHeartandStrokeNews/African-Americans-and-Heart-Disease_UCM_444863_Article.jsp

American Psychiatric Association. (2013). *Diagnostic statistical manual of mental disorders* (5th ed.) Arlington, VA: Author.

BCC Research. (2013). Botanical and plant-derived drugs [Report]. Retrieved September 2014 from http://www.bccresearch.com/market-research/biotechnology/botanical-plant-derived-drugs-markets-bio022f.html

Becares, L., Shaw, R., Nazroo, S., Stefford, M., Albor, C., & Atkin, K. (2012). Ethnic diversity effects on physical morbidity, mortality, and health behaviors: A systematic review of the literature. *American Journal of Public Health, 102*(12), e33–e66.

Becker, W. C., Starrels, J. L., Heo, M., Li, X., Weiner, M. G., & Turner, B. J. (2011). Racial differences in primary care opioid risk reduction strategies. *Annals of Family Medicine, 9*, 219–225.

Bongki, P., Jun, J. H., Jung, J., You, S., & Lee, M. S. (2014). Herbal medicines for cancer cachexia: Protocol for a systematic review. *British Medical Journal Open, 4*, e005016 doi: 10.1136/bmjopne-2014-005016. Retrieved from http://www.mayoclinic.org

Bress, A., Han, J., Patel, S. R., Desai, A. A., Mansour, I., Groo, V., ..., Cavallari, R. L. (2013). Association of Aldosterone Synthase Polymorphism (*CYP11B2* -344 T>C) and genetic ancestry with atrial fibrillation and serum aldosterone in African Americans with heart failure. *PloS One, 8*(7), e71268.

Browning, B. L., & Browning, S. R. (2013). Detecting identity by descent and estimating genotype error rates in sequence data. *American Journal of Human Genetics, 93*(5), 840–851.

Buttaro, T. M., Trybulski, J., Polgar Bailey, P., & Sandberg-Cook, J. (2013). *Primary care: A collaborative practice*. St. Louis, MO: Elsevier.

Casorbi, I., Bruhn, O., & Werk, A. N. (2013). Challenges in pharmacogenetics, *European Journal of Pharmacology, 69*(Suppl. 1), S17–S23.

Center for Disease Control and Prevention. (2013). Genetic testing. Retrieved from http://www.cdc.gov/genomics/gtesting/index.htm

Derose, S. F., Rutkowski, M. P., Crooks, P. W., Shi, J. M., Wang, J. Q., Kalantar-Zadeh K., ..., Jacobsen, S. J. (2013). Racial differences in estimated glomerular filtration decline, ESDR, and mortality in an integrated health system. *American Journal of Kidney Disease*, *62*(2), 236–244.

Dixon, B., Pena, M., & Taveras, M. (2012). Lifecourse approach in childhood obesity. *Advances in Nutrition*, *3*(1), 73–82.

Domchek, S. M. (2014). Evolution of genetic testing for inherited susceptibility to breast cancer. *Journal of Clinical Oncology*, *33*(4), 295. doi: 10.1200/JCO.2014.59.3178 *JCO December 15, 2014 JCO.2014.59.317*

Dotson, W. D., Douglas, M. P., Kolor, K., Stewart, A. C., Bowen, M. S., Gwinn, M., ..., Khoury, M. J. (2014). Prioritizing genomic applications for action by level of evidence: A horizon-scanning method. *Clinical Pharmacology and Therapeutics*, *95*(4), 394–402.

Dubay, L., & Lebrun, A. (2012). Health, behavior, and health care disparities: Disentangling the effects of income and race in the United States. *International Journal of Health Services*, *42*(4), 607–625.

Everett, J. S., Budescu, M., & Sommers, M. S. (2012). Making sense of skin color in clinical care. *Clinical Nursing Research*, *21*(4), 495–516.

Ezenwa, M. O., & Fleming, M. F. (2012). Racial disparities in pain management in primary care. *Journal of Health Disparities Research and Practice*, *5*(3), 12–26.

Ferdinand, K. C., Elkayam, U., Mancini, D., Ofili, E., Pina, I., Anand, I., Leggett, C. (2014). Use of isosorbide, dinitrate and hydralazine in African-Americans with heart failure 9 years after the African-American Heart Failure Trial. *American Journal of Cardiology*, *114*(1), 151–159.

Fuchs, F. D. (2011). Why do Blacks have a higher prevalence of hypertension? *Hypertension*, *57*, 379–380.

Gagon, C. M., Matsura, J. T., Smith, C. C., & Stanos, S. P. (2013). Ethnicity and interdisciplinary pain treatment. *Pain and Practice*, *14*(6), 532–540.

Gladstone Institute. (2014). Vitamin supplement successfully prevents noise-related hearing loss. *Science Daily*. Retrieved from http://www.sciencedaily.com/releases/2014/12/141202123840.htm

Godoy-Paiz, P., Toner, B., & Vidal, C. (2011). "Something in our hearts": Challenges to mental health among urban Mayan women in post-war Guatemala. *Ethnicity and Inequalities in Heath and Social Care*, *4*(3), 127–137. doi: 10.1108/17570981111249266.

Grossman, S., & Porth, C. (2014). *Porth's pathophysiology: Concepts of altered health states*. Philadelphia, PA: Wolters Kluwer.

Gunn, D. A., de Craen, A. J. M., Dick, J. L., Tomlin, C. C., van Heemest, D., Catt, S., ..., Westendorp, R. G. J. (2013). Facial appearance reflects human familial longevity and cardiovascular disease risk in healthy individuals. *Journals of Gerontology series A Biological Medical Sciences*, *68*(2), 145–152.

Haeok, B., Fitzpatrick, J., & Baik, S. (2013). Why isn't evidence-based practice improving health care for minorities in the United States? *Applied Nursing Research*, *26*(2013), 263–268.

Herman, W. H., & Cohen, R. M. (2012). Racial and ethnic differences in the relationship between HbA1c and blood glucose: Implications for the diagnosis of diabetes. *Journal of Clinical Endocrinology & Metabolism*, *97*(4), 1067–1072.

Hsieh, A. Y., Tripp, D. A., & Li-Jun, L. (2011). The influence of ethnic concordance and discordance on verbal and nonverbal behaviors of pain. *Pain*, *152*, 2016–2022.

Hwang, H., Zhang, J., Chung, K. A., Leverenz, J. B., Zabetian, C. P., Peskind, E. R., ..., Zhang, J. (2011). Glycoproteomics in neurodegenerative diseases. *Mass Spectrometry Review*, *29*(1), 79–125.

Institute of Medicine. (2011). *Relieving pain in America: A blueprint for transforming prevention, care, education, and research*. Washington, DC: National Academies Press.

Jarvis, C. (2015). *Physical examination and health assessment* (7th ed.). St. Louis, MO: Elsevier/Saunders.

Kaback, H. R., Smirnova, V. Nie, Y., & Zhou, Y. (2011). Alternating transport mechanism LacY. *Journal of Membrane Biology*, *239*(1–2), 9327–9335.

Kaiser Family Foundation. (2014). Poverty rate by race and ethnicity. Retrieved from http:////www.kff.org/state--category/indicator/poverty rate by ethnicity

Kaminska-Winciorek, G., & Spiewak, R. (2012). Tips and tricks in the dermoscopy of pigmented lesions. *BMC Dermatology*, *12*(14), 12–14.

Kleinman, A. (1980). *Patients and healers in the context of culture*. Berkeley, CA: University of California Press.

Kliegman, R. M., Stanton, B. F., Saint Geme, J. W., Schor, N. F., & Behrman, R. E. (2011). *Nelson's textbook of pediatrics* (19th ed.). Philadelphia, PA: Elsevier Saunders.

Koleck, T. A., Bender, C. M., Sereika, S. M., Ahrendendt, G., Jankowitz, R. C., McGuire, K. P., ..., Conley, Y. P. (2014). Apolipoprotein E genotype and cognitive function in postmenopausal women with early-stage breast cancer. *Oncology Nursing Forum*, *41*(6), E313–E325.

Kwok, W., & Bhuvanakrishna, T. (2014). The relationship between ethnicity and the pain experience of cancer patients: A systematic review. *Indian Journal of Palliative Care*, *20*(3), 194–200.

Leininger, M. M. (1991). *Culture care diversity and universality: A theory of nursing*. New York, NY: NLN Press.

Leininger, M. M., & McFarland, M. R. (2002). *Transcultural nursing: Concepts, theories, research and practices*. New York, NY: McGraw-Hill.

Leininger, M. M., & McFarland, M. R. (2006). *Culture care diversity & universality: A worldwide nursing theory*. Sudbury, MA: Jones & Bartlett.

Levin, S. (1966). Effect of age, ethnic background and disease on sweat chloride. *Israeli Journal of Medical Science*, 2(3), 333–337.

Luca, A., Jimenez-Fonseca, P., & Gascon, P. (2013). Clinical evaluation and optimal management of cancer cachexia. *Critical Reviews in Oncology/Hematology*, 88(4), 625–636.

Ludwig-Beymer, P. A. (2008). Transcultural aspects of pain. In M. M. Andrews & J. S. Boyle (Eds.), *Transcultural concepts in nursing care* (5th ed., pp. 329–354). Philadelphia, PA: Wolters Kluwer/Lippincott, Williams, & Wilkins.

Macbeth, A., & Harries, M. (2012). Hair loss in hospital medicine: A practical guide. *British Journal of Hospital Medicine*, 73(7), 372–379.

Marino, S. E., Birnbaum, A. K., Leppik, I. E., Conway, J. M., Musib, L. C., Brundage, R. C., & Cloyd, J. C. (2012). Steady-state carbamazepine pharmacokinetics following oral and stable-labeled intravenous administration in epilepsy patients: Effects of race and sex. *Clinical Pharmacology and Therapeutics*, 91(3), 483.

Mayo Clinic. (n.d.a). Causes of odor symptoms. Retrieved from http://www.rightdiagnosis.com/symptoms/odor_symptoms/causes.htm

Mayo Clinic. (n.d.b). Diagnostic tests for odor. Retrieved from http://www.rightdiagnosis.com/symptoms/odor_symptoms/tests.htm

Mayo Clinic. (n.d.c). Lactose intolerance: Symptoms. Retrieved from http://www.mayoclinic.org/diseases-conditions/lactose-intolerance/basics/symptoms/con-20027906

McCance, K. L., & Huether, S. E. (2014). *The biologic basis for disease in adults and children*. St. Louis, MO: C.V. Mosby.

McFarland, M. R., & Wehbe-Alamah, H. B. (2015). *Leininger's culture care diversity and universality: A worldwide theory of nursing* (3rd ed.). Burlington, MA: Jones & Bartlett Learning.

Meghani, S., Polomano, R. C., Tait, R. C., Vallerand, A. H., Anderson, K. O., & Gallagher, R. M. (2012). Advancing a national agenda to eliminate disparity in pain care: Directions for health policy, education, practice, and research. *Pain and Medicine*, 13(1), 5–28.

Mossey, J. M. (2011). Defining racial and ethnic minorities in pain management. *Clinical Orthopaedics and Related Research*, 469(7), 1859–1870.

Murray-Wright, M. (2014). Genetics and genomics. Personal communication, December 24, 2014.

National Cancer Institute. (2014). *National Cancer Institute Fact Sheets: Cancer types*. Bethesda, MD: National Institutes of Health. Retrieved at http://www.cancer.gov/cancer topics.Table?

National Center for Biotechnology. (2014). Genetic testing registry. Retrieved from http://www.ncbi.nlm.nih.gov/gtr/docs/help/

National Center for Complementary and Integrative Health. (2015). Herbs at a glance. Retrieved from https://nccih.nih.gov/health/herbsataglance.htm

National Down Syndrome Society. (2014). Prenatal testing. Retrieved from http://www.ndss.org/About-NDSS/Media-Kit/Position-Papers/CDC-Study-on-Prevalence-of-Down-Syndrome-/

National Football League. (2014). NFL consensus data on players' race, weight, and height. Retrieved from http://heavy.com/sports/2014/09/what-percentage-of-nfl-players-are-black-white/

National Institute of Dental and Craniofacial Research. (2014). Dental caries, race, and ethnicity. Retrieved from http://www.nidcr.nih.gov/

National Institute on Alcohol Abuse and Alcoholism. (2014). *Minority health and health disparities*. Rockville, MD: National Institutes of Health, Alcohol Research Centers. Retrieved at http://www.niaaa.nih.gov/alcohol-health/special-populations-co-occurring-disorders/diversity-health-disparities

National Institutes of Health. (2013). Cleft lip and cleft palate. Retrieved from http://www.ncbi.nlm.nih.gov/pubmedhealth/PMH0002046/?report=printable

National Organization for Albinism and Hypopigmentation. (2014). What is albinism? Retrieved from *The National Organization for Albinism and Hypopigmentation*: http://www.albinism.org/publications/what_is_albinism.html

Nicholls, P. (2014). The poverty of conservatism. *Nation*, 21(16), 3–4.

O'Brien, J. E., Dvorin, E., Drugan, A., Johnson, M. P., Yaron, Y., & Evans, M. I. (1997). Race-ethnicity-specific variation in multiple-marker biochemical screening: Alpha-fetoprotein, hCG, and estriol. *Obstetrics and Gynecology*, 89(3), 355–358.

Obeig-Odoom, F. (2012). Health, wealth, and poverty in developing countries: Beyond the state, market, and civil society. *Health Sociology Review*, 21(2), 156–162.

Orton, N. C., Innes, A. M., Chudley, A. E., & Bech-Hansen, N. T. (2014). Unique disease heritage of the Dutch-German Mennonite population. *American Journal of Medical Genetics Part A*, 146A(8), 1072–1087.

Overfield, T. (1995). *Biologic variation in health and illness: Race, age and sex differences*. New York, NY: CRC Press.

Palit, S., Kerr, K., Kuhn, B., Terry, E., DelVentura, J., Bartley, E., ..., Rhudy, J. (2013). Exploring pain processing differences in Native Americans. *Health Psychology*, 32(11), 1127–1136.

Pardasani, M., & Bandyopadhyay, S. (2013). Ethnicity matters: Experiences of minority groups in public health. *Journal of Cultural Diversity*, 21(3), 90–98.

Pedersen, D., Errazuriz, C., Kienzler, H., Lopez, V., Sharma, B., Bustamante, I., et al. (2012). *Political violence, natural disasters and mental health outcomes: Developing innovative health policies and interventions. McGill University, Douglas Mental Health University Institute*. Montreal, Quebec: Global Health Research Initiative.

Porth, C. M. (2015) *Essentials of pathophysiology: Concepts of altered health states* (4th ed.). Philadelphia, PA: Lippincott.

Qiu, M.,Wang, S. Y., Singh, K., & Lin, S. (2014). Racial disparities in uncorrected and undercorrected refraction errors in the United States. *Investigative Ophthalmological and Visual Sciences, 55*(10), 6996–7005.

Rahim-Williams, B., Riley, J., Williams, A. K., & Fillingim, R. B. (2012). A quantitative review of ethnic group differences in experimental pain response: Do biology, psychology, and culture matter? *Pain Medicine, 13*(4), 522–540.

Rotimi, C. N., & Jorde, L. B. (2010). Ancestry and disease in the age of genomic medicine. *New England Journal of Medicine, 36,* 1551–1558.

Ryder, A. G., & Chentsova-Dutton, Y. E. (2012). Depression in cultural context: "Chinese somatization," revisited. *Psychiatric Clinics of North America, 35*(1), 15–36. doi: http://libproxy.umflint.edu:2129/10.1016/j.psc.2011.11.006

Schembre, S. M., Nigg, C. R., & Albright, C. L. (2011). Racial/ethnic differences in desired body mass index and dieting practices among young women attending college in Hawai'i. *Hawaii Medical Journal, 70*(7 Suppl.), 32–36.

Seibert, D. C., & Darling T. N. (2013). Physical, psychological, and ethical issues in caring for individuals with genetic skin disease. *Journal of Nursing Scholarship, 45*(1), 89–95.

Shin, M. H., Zmuda, J., Barrett-Connor, E., Sheu, Y., Patrick, A., Leung, P., ..., Cauley, J. (2014). Race/ethnic differences in associations between bone mineral density and fracture history in older men. *Osteoporosis International, 25*(3), 837–845.

Silva, A. M., Shen, W., Heo, M., Gallager, D., Wang, Z., & Sardinha, L. B. (2011). Ethnicity-related skeletal muscle differences across the life span. *Human Biology, 22(1),* 76–82.

Simons, R. C., & Hughes, C. C. (1985). *The culture-bound syndromes: Folk illnesses of psychiatric and anthropological interest.* Dordrecht, The Netherlands: D. Reidel/Kluwer Academic.

Spokoyny, I., Barazangi, N., Jaramillo, V., Rose, J., Chen, C., Wong, C., & Tong, D. (2014). Reduced clopidogrel metabolism in a multiethnic population: prevalence and rates of recurrent cerebrovascular events. *Journal of Stroke and Cerebrovascular Diseases, 23*(4), 694–698.

Sun X., Yang C. Q., Wen T., Zeng F. C., Wang Q., Yang W. Y., & Lin H. H. (2014). Water stress enhances expression of genes encoding plastid terminal oxidase and key components of chlororespiration and alternative respiration in soybean seedlings. *Z Naturforsch C,* 69(7-8): 300–308.

Tait, R. C., & Chibnall, J. T. (2014). Racial/ethnic disparities in the assessment and treatment of pain. *American Psychologist, 69*(2), 131–141.

Taylor, N. A., & Machado-Moreira, C. A. (2013). Regional variations in transepidermal water loss, eccrine sweat gland density, sweat excretion rates, and electrolyte composition in resting and exercising humans. *Extreme Physiology and Medicine, 2*(4), 2–4.

Taylor, C., Kavanagh, P., & Zuckerman, B. (2014). Sickle cell train-neglected opportunities in the era of genomic medicine. *JAMA, 311*(15), 1495–1496.

Tewfik, T. L., & Myers, A. D. (2013). Cleft lip and palate and mouth and pharynx deformities. *Medscape.* Retrieved on October 9, 2014 at http://emedicine.medscape.com/article/837347-overview

U.S. Census Bureau. (2014a). U.S. and World Population Clock. (U.S. Department of Commerce). Retrieved October 5, 2014, from United States Census Bureau: http://www.census.gov/popclock/

U.S. Census Bureau. (2014b). Current population survey (CPS): Annual Social and Economic Supplements. Retrieved at http://www.census.gov/current population-survey2014_Annualsocialandeconomicsupplements

Wang, Y., Kennedy, J., & Caggana, M. (2013). Sickle cell disease incidence among newborns in New York State by maternal race/ethnicity and nativity. *Genetics and Medicine, 15*(3), 222–228.

Wang, L., McLeod, H. L., & Weinshilbourm, R. M. (2011). Genomics and drug response. *New England Journal of Medicine, 364,* 1144–1153.

Wells, W. (2014). A matter of life and death. *McLeans, 127*(21), 18–20.

World Health Organization. (2013). *WHO traditional medicine strategy: 2014–2023.* Geneva, Switzerland: WHO Press.

Wyatt, R. (2013). Policy forum: Pain and ethnicity. *American Medical Association Journal of Ethics, 15*(3), 449–454.

Yang, H. J., Gil, Y. C., Jin, J. D., Cho, H., Kim, H., & Lee, H. Y. (2012). Novel findings of the anatomy and variations of the axillary vein and its tributaries. *Clinical Anatomy, 25*(7), 893–902.

Yu, D. S., & Lee, D. T. (2012). Do medically unexplained somatic symptoms predict depression in older Chinese? *International Journal of Geriatric Psychiatry, 27*(2), 119–126. doi: 10.1002/gps.2692.

Ziemer, D. C., Kolm, P., Weintraub, W. S., Vaccarino, V., Rhee, M. K., Twombly, J. G., ..., Phillips, L. S. (2010). Glucose-independent, Black–White differences in hemoglobin A1c Levels: A cross-sectional analysis of 2 studies. *Annals of Internal Medicine, 152*(12), 770–777. doi:10.7326/0003-4819-152-12-201006150-00004

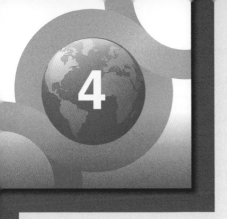

4

The Influence of Cultural and Health Belief Systems on Health Care Practices

● Margaret M. Andrews

Key Terms

Allopathic medicine
Alternative medicine
Complementary and
    integrative health
Cultural belief systems
Dietary supplements
Folk healers
Folk healing system

Health behavior
Health belief systems
Holistic paradigm
Hot/cold theory of disease
Humors
Illness behavior
Integrative health
Magico-religious paradigm
Metaphor
Mechanism

Objective materialism
Paradigm
Professional care systems
Reductionism
Scientific paradigm
Self-care
Sick role behavior
Worldview
Yin and yang

Learning Objectives

1. Describe the major cultural belief systems of people from diverse cultures.
2. Compare and contrast professional and folk healing systems.
3. Identify the major complementary and alternative health care therapies.
4. Describe the influence of culture on symptoms and illness behaviors.
5. Critically analyze the efficacy of selected herbal remedies in the treatment of health problems.

In this chapter, we examine the major cultural belief systems embraced by people from diverse cultures and explore the characteristics of three of the most prevalent worldviews, or paradigms, related to health–illness beliefs: magico-religious, scientific, and holistic. We explore self-treatment, professional care systems, and folk (indigenous, traditional, generic) care systems and their respective healers. After analyzing the influence of culture on symptoms and sick roles, as well as illness behaviors, we examine selected complementary and alternative therapies used to treat physical and psychological diseases and illnesses.

Cultural Belief Systems

Cultural meanings and **cultural belief systems** develop from the shared experiences of a social group and are expressed symbolically. The use of symbols to define, describe, and relate to the world around us is one of the basic characteristics of being human. One of the most common expressions of symbolism is **metaphor**. In metaphor, one aspect of life is connected to another through a shared symbol. For example, the phrase "what a tangled web we weave" expresses metaphorically the relationship between two normally disparate concepts—human deception and a spider's web. People often use metaphors as a way of thinking about and explaining life's events.

Every group of people has found it necessary to explain the phenomena of nature. From these explanations emerges a common belief system. The explanations usually involve metaphoric imagery of magical, religious, natural/holistic, scientific, or biological form. The range of explanations is limited only by the human imagination.

The set of metaphoric explanations used by a group of people to explain life's events and offer solutions to life's mysteries can be viewed as the group's **worldview** or major paradigm. A **paradigm** is a way of viewing the world and the phenomena in it. A paradigm includes the assumptions, premises, and linkages that hold together a prevailing interpretation of reality. Paradigms are slow to change and do so only if and when their explanatory power has been exhausted.

The worldview reflects the group's total configuration of beliefs and practices and permeates every aspect of life within the group's culture. Members of a culture share a worldview without necessarily recognizing it. Thinking itself is patterned on or derived from this worldview because the culture imparts a particular set of symbols to be used in thinking. Because these symbols are taken for granted, people do not normally question the cultural bias of their thoughts. The use in the United States of the term *American* reflects such an unconscious cultural bias. This term is understood by citizens of the United States to refer only to themselves collectively, although in reality, it is a generic term referring to people in the Americas, the combined continental landmasses of North America and South America and their islands in the Western Hemisphere, including Canadians, Mexicans, Colombians, and all others living in the Americas.

Another example of symbolism and worldview can be seen in the way nurses use terms such as *nursing care*, *health promotion*, and *illness and disease*. Nurses often take for granted that all their clients define and relate to these concepts in the same way they do. This reflects an unconscious belief that the same cultural symbols are shared by all and therefore do not require reinterpretation in any given nurse–client context. Such an assumption accounts for many of the problems nurses face when they try to communicate with others who are not members of the health profession culture.

Health Belief Systems

Generally, theories of health and disease or illness causation are based on a group's prevailing worldview. These worldviews include a group's health-related attitudes, beliefs, and practices, frequently referred to as health belief systems. People embrace three major **health belief systems** or **worldviews**: magico-religious, scientific (or biomedical), and holistic, each with its own corresponding system of health beliefs. In two of these worldviews (magico-religious and holistic), disease is thought of as an entity separate from self, caused by an agent external to the body but capable of "getting in" and causing damage. This causative agent has been attributed to a variety of natural and supernatural phenomena. Furthermore, many people sometimes adhere to or believe in aspects of two or even three of the systems at any one time. For example, a person who is ill may understand that the illness has an identified causative agent; at the same time, the person may pray to recover quickly and perhaps

embark on a sacred journey to see a vortex specialist to unite body, mind, and spirit.

Magico-Religious Health Paradigm

In the **magico-religious paradigm**, the world is an arena dominated by supernatural forces. The fate of the world and those in it, including humans, depends on the actions of God, the gods, or other supernatural forces for good or evil. In some cases, the human individual is at the mercy of such forces regardless of behavior. In other cases, the gods punish humans for their transgressions. Many Latino, African American, and Middle Eastern cultures are grounded in the magico-religious paradigm. Magic involves the calling forth and control of supernatural forces for and against others. Some African and Caribbean cultures, such as Voodoo, have aspects of magic in their belief systems. In Western cultures, there are examples of this paradigm in which metaphysical reality interrelates with human society. For instance, Christian Scientists believe that physical healing can be effected through prayer alone.

Ackernecht (1971), in an article about the history of medicine, states that "magic or religion seems to satisfy better than any other device a certain eternal psychic or 'metaphysical' need of mankind, sick and healthy, for integration and harmony." Magic and religion are logical in their own way, but not based on empiric premises; that is, they defy the demands of the physical world and the use of one's senses, particularly observation. In the magico-religious paradigm, disease is viewed as the action and result of supernatural forces that cause the intrusion of a disease-producing foreign body or health-damaging spirit.

Throughout the world, five categories of events are believed to be responsible for illness in the magico-religious paradigm. These categories, derived from the work of Clements (1932), are sorcery, breach of taboo, intrusion of a disease object, intrusion of a disease-causing spirit, and loss of soul. One of these belief categories, or any combination of them, may be offered to explain the origin of disease. Alaska Natives, for example, refer to soul loss and breach of taboo (breaking a social norm, such as committing adultery). West Indians and some Africans and African Americans believe that the malevolence of sorcerers is the cause of many conditions. *Mal ojo*, or the evil eye, common in Latino and other cultures, can be viewed as the intrusion of a disease-causing spirit.

In the magico-religious paradigm, illness is initiated by a supernatural agent with or without justification, or by another person who practices sorcery or engages the services of sorcerers. The cause-and-effect relationship is not organic; rather, the cause of health or illness is mystical. Health is seen as a reward given as a sign of God's blessing and goodwill. Illness may be seen as a sign of God's special favor insofar as it gives the affected person the opportunity to become resigned to God's will, or it may be seen as a sign of God's possession or as a punishment. For example, in many Christian religions, the faithful gather communally to pray to God to heal those who are ill or to practice healing rituals such as laying on of hands or anointing the sick with oil.

In addition, in this paradigm, health and illness are viewed as belonging first to the community and then to the individual. Therefore, one person's actions may directly or indirectly influence the health or illness of another person. This sense of community is virtually absent from the other paradigms.

Scientific or Biomedical Health Paradigm

In the **scientific paradigm**, life is controlled by a series of physical and biochemical processes that can be studied and manipulated by humans. Several specific forms of symbolic thought processes characterize the scientific paradigm. The first is **determinism**, which states that a cause-and-effect relationship exists for all natural phenomena. The second, **mechanism**, assumes that it is possible to control life processes through mechanical, genetic, and other engineered interventions. The

third form is **reductionism**, according to which all life can be reduced or divided into smaller parts; study of the unique characteristics of these isolated parts is thought to reveal aspects or properties of the whole, for example, the human genome and its component parts. The final thought process is **objective materialism,** which states that what is real can be observed and measured. There is a further distinction between subjective and objective realities in this paradigm.

The scientific paradigm considers only forces that cannot be observed and measured. Members of most Western cultures, including the dominant cultural groups in the United States, Canada, Europe, and Australia, espouse this paradigm. When the scientific paradigm is applied to matters of health, it is often referred to as the *biomedical model.*

In the biomedical model, all aspects of human health can be understood through the natural sciences, biology, chemistry, physics, and mathematics. This fosters the belief that psychological and emotional processes can be reduced to the study of biochemical exchanges. Only the observable is real and worthy of study. Effective treatment consists of physical and chemical interventions, often without regard to human relationships.

In this model, disease is viewed metaphorically as the breakdown of the human machine because of wear and tear (stress), external trauma (injury, accident), external invasion (pathogens), or internal damages (fluid and chemical imbalances, genetic or other structural changes). Disease causes illness, has a more or less specific cause, and has a predictable time course and set of treatment requirements. This paradigm is similar to the magico-religious belief in external agents, having replaced supernatural forces with infectious and genetic agents.

Using the metaphor of the machine, biomedicine uses specialists to take care of the "parts:" "fixing" a part restores the machine's ability to function. The computer is the analogy for the brain; engineering is a task for biomedical practitioners. The discovery of DNA and human genome research has led to the field of genetic engineering,

an eloquent biomedical metaphor. The symbols used to discuss health and disease reflect the US cultural values of aggression and mastery. For example, microorganisms attack the body, war is waged against the invaders, money is donated for the campaign against cancer, and illness is a struggle in which the patient must put up a good defense. The biomedical model defines health as the absence of disease or the signs and symptoms of disease. To be healthy, one must be free of all disease. By comparison, the World Health Organization defines health more holistically as "a state of complete physical, mental, and social well-being and not merely the absence of disease or infirmity" (WHO, 1948, p. 100). The definition is often cited and has not been amended since 1948.

Holistic Health Paradigm

In the **holistic paradigm**, the forces of nature itself must be kept in natural balance or *harmony*. Human life is only one aspect of nature and a part of the general order of the cosmos. Everything in the universe has a place and a role to perform according to natural laws that maintain order. Disturbing these laws creates imbalance, chaos, and disease. The holistic paradigm has existed for centuries in many parts of the world, particularly in American Indian and Asian cultures. It is gaining increasing acceptance in the United States and Canada because it complements a growing sense that the biomedical view fails to account fully for some diseases as they naturally occur.

The holistic paradigm seeks to maintain a sense of balance between humans and the larger universe. Explanations for health and disease are based on imbalance or disharmony among the human, geophysical, and metaphysical forces of the universe. For example, in the biomedical model, the cause of tuberculosis is clearly defined as the invasion of mycobacterium. In the holistic paradigm, whereby disease is the result of multiple environment–host interactions, tuberculosis is caused by the interrelationship of poverty, malnutrition, overcrowding, and mycobacterium.

The term *holistic*, coined in 1926 by Jan Christian Smuts, defines an attitude or mode of perception in which the whole person is viewed in the context of the total environment. Its Indo-European root word, *kailo*, means "whole, intact, or uninjured." From this root have come the words *hale, hail, hallow, holy, whole, heal*, and *health*. The essence of health and healing is the quality of wholeness we associate with healthy functioning and well-being.

In this paradigm, health is viewed as a positive process that encompasses more than the absence of signs and symptoms of disease. It is not restricted to biologic or somatic wellness but rather involves broader environmental, sociocultural, and behavioral determinants. In this model, diseases of civilization, such as unemployment, racial discrimination, ghettos, and suicide, are just as much illnesses as are biomedical diseases.

Metaphors used in this paradigm, such as the *healing power of nature, health foods*, and *Mother Earth*, reflect the connection of humans to the cosmos and nature. The belief system of Florence Nightingale, who emphasized nursing's control of the environment so that patients could heal naturally, was also holistic.

A strong metaphor in the holistic paradigm is exemplified by the Chinese concept of **yin and yang**, in which the forces of nature are balanced to produce harmony. The *yin* force in the universe represents the female aspect of nature. It is characterized as the negative pole, encompassing darkness, cold, and emptiness. The *yang*, or male force, is characterized by fullness, light, and warmth. It represents the positive pole. An imbalance of forces creates illness (see Evidence-Based Practice 4-1).

Illness is the outward expression of disharmony. This disharmony may result from seasonal changes, emotional imbalances, or any other pattern of events. Illness is not perceived as an intruding agent but as a natural part of life's rhythmic course. Going in and out of balance is seen as a natural process that happens constantly throughout the life cycle. Health and illness are aspects of the same process, in which the individual organism changes continually in relation to the changing environment.

In the holistic health paradigm, because illness is inevitable, perfect health is not the goal. Rather, achieving the best possible adaptation to the environment by living according to society's rules and caring appropriately for one's body is the ultimate aim. This places a greater emphasis on preventive and maintenance measures than typically occurs in biomedicine.

Another common metaphor for health and illness in the holistic paradigm is the **hot/cold theory of disease**. This is founded on the ancient Greek concept of the four body humors: yellow bile, black bile, phlegm, and blood. **Humors** are vital components of the blood found in varying amounts. The four humors work together to ensure the optimum nutrition, growth, and metabolism of the body. When the humors are balanced in the healthy individual, the state of *ecrasia* exists. When the humors are in a state of imbalance, this is referred to as dyscrasia (Osborn, 2015). The treatment of disease becomes the process of restoring the body's humoral balance through the addition or subtraction of substances that affect each of these four humors. Foods, beverages, herbs, and drugs are all classified as hot or cold depending on their effect, not their actual physical state. Disease conditions are also classified as either hot or cold. Imbalance or disharmony is thought to result in internal damage and altered physiologic functions. Medicine is directed at correcting the imbalance as well as restoring body function. Although the concept of hot and cold is itself widespread, found in Asian, Latino, Black, Arab, Muslim, and Caribbean societies, each cultural group defines what it believes to be hot and cold entities, and little agreement exists across cultures.

Health and Illness Behaviors

The series of behaviors typifying the health-seeking process have been labeled *health and illness behaviors*. These behaviors are expressed in the

Chronic Disease Self-Management and Health Literacy in Four Ethnic Groups

An interdisciplinary team of investigators studied chronic disease, self-management, and health literacy in four U.S. ethnic groups: Vietnamese, African Americans, Whites, and Latinos. The researchers defined health literacy as the wide range of skills and competencies that people develop to seek out, comprehend, evaluate, and use health information and concepts to make informed choices, reduce health risks, and improve quality of life.

The facilitators of self-management of disease included speaking and listening skills that promote better clinician–patient communication; math skills, such as sliding scales for insulin dosage based on blood glucose levels; reading skills to read educational materials about disease processes and treatment; social support from family members, such as spouse and adult children; and social support from neighbors and friends who have higher levels of literacy than the patient and, in some instances, more financial resources. For example, a Vietnamese participant with diabetes who lives in a rooming house reported that his landlord's wife buys extra vegetables for him whenever she goes shopping.

Barriers to disease self-management include confusion about the name of the diagnosis and the underlying cause of the chronic health problem(s), such as confusing certain aspects of their conditions with other conditions, for example, misunderstanding the differences among high blood pressure, high blood sugar, and high cholesterol. One Vietnamese patient stated that he thought his diabetes had been caused by imprisonment during the Vietnam War and by the poor diet and forced labor he endured more than 40 years ago. Another patient indicated that hypertension means that the blood is flowing very fast, and he stated that a complication of the rapid heartbeat is that the "heart is going to become very agitated," resulting in high cholesterol and obstruction of the veins.

Clinical Implications:

- Nurses and other members of the health care team should recognize that patients' cultural health belief systems and explanatory models are interrelated with their health and linguistic literacy, educational background, and socioeconomic status.
- Cultural health beliefs exert important influences on the self-management of chronic diseases such as diabetes and hypertension.
- Cultural health beliefs are part of internally consistent explanatory models constructed by the patient in an effort to make sense of his/her diagnosis and the clinical manifestations of the underlying cause(s) of illness.
- Sometimes the patient's yin/yang or hot/cold theories fail to align with the biomedical explanation, and the patient may decide to disregard the information and refrain from adhering to the biomedical recommendations and advice provided by nurses, physicians, and other health professionals.

Reference: Shaw, S. J., Armin, J., Torres, C. H., Orzech, K. M., & Vivian, J. (2012). Chronic disease self-management and health literacy in four ethnic groups. *Journal of Health Communication, 17*, 67–81.

roles people assume after identifying a symptom. Related to these behaviors are the roles individuals assign to others and the status given to the role players. People assume various types of behaviors once they have recognized a symptom. **Health behavior** is any activity undertaken by a person who believes himself or herself to be healthy for the purpose of preventing disease or detecting disease in an asymptomatic stage. **Illness behavior** is any activity undertaken by a person who feels ill to define the state of his or her health and discover a suitable remedy. **Sick role behavior** is any activity undertaken by a person who considers himself ill to get well or to deal with the illness.

Three sets of factors influence the course of behaviors and practices carried out to maintain health and prevent disease: (1) one's beliefs about health and illness; (2) personal factors such as age, education, knowledge, or experience with a given disease condition; and (3) cues to action, such as advertisements in the media, the illness of a relative, or the advice of friends.

A useful model of illness behavior has been proposed by Mechanic (1978), who outlines 10 determinants of illness behavior that are important in the help-seeking process (see Table 4-1). Awareness of these motivational factors can help nurses offer the appropriate assistance to clients as they work through the illness process.

Types of Healing Systems

The term *healing system* refers to the accumulated sciences, arts, and techniques of restoring and preserving health that are used by any cultural group. In complex societies in which several cultural traditions flourish, healers tend to compete with one another and/or to view their

Table 4-1: Mechanic's Determinants of Illness Behavior

Determinant	Description
Quality of symptom	The more frightening or visible the symptom, the greater the likelihood that the individual will intervene.
Seriousness of symptom	The perceived threat of the symptom must be serious for action to be taken. Often others will step in if the person's behavior is considered dangerous (e.g., suicidal behavior) but will be unaware of potential problems if the person's behavior seems natural ("he always acts that way").
Disruption of daily activities	Behaviors that are very disruptive in work or other social situations are likely to be labeled as illness much sooner than the same behaviors in a family setting. An individual whose activities are disrupted by a symptom is likely to take that symptom seriously even if on another occasion he would consider the same symptom trivial (e.g., acne just before a date).
Rate and persistence of symptom	The frequency of a symptom is directly related to its importance; a symptom that persists is also likely to be taken seriously.
Tolerance of symptom	The extent to which others, especially family, tolerate the symptom before reacting varies; individuals also have different tolerance thresholds.
Sociocognitive status	A person's information about the symptom, knowledge base, and cultural values all influence that person's perception of illness.
Denial of symptom	Often, the individual or family members need to deny a symptom for personal or social reasons. The amount of fear and anxiety present can interfere with perception of a symptom.
Motivation	Competing needs may motivate a person to delay or enhance symptoms. A person who has no time or money to be sick will often not acknowledge the seriousness of symptoms.
Assigning of meaning	Once perceived, the symptom must be interpreted. Often people explain symptoms within normal parameters ("I'm just tired").
Treatment accessibility	The greater the barriers to treatment—whether psychological, economic, physical, or social—the greater the likelihood that the symptom will not be interpreted as serious or that the person will seek an alternative form of care.

From Mechanic, D. (1978). *Medical sociology* (2nd ed.). New York, NY: The Free Press, a Division of Macmillan, Inc. Copyright © 1978 by David Mechanic. By permission.

scopes of practice as separate from one another. In some instances, however, practitioners may make referrals to different healing systems. For example, a nurse may contact a rabbi to assist a Jewish patient with spiritual needs, or a *curandero* may advise a Mexican American patient to visit a health care provider for an antibiotic when traditional practices fail to heal a wound.

Self-Care

For common minor illnesses, an estimated 70% to 90% of all people initially try **self-care** with over-the-counter medicines, megavitamins, herbs, exercise, and/or foods that they believe have healing powers. Many self-care practices

have been handed down from generation to generation, frequently by oral tradition. Self-care is the largest component of the American health care system and accounts for billions of dollars in revenue (Lillyman & Farquharson, 2013; Shaw, 2012). The use of over-the-counter medications, or nonprescription medications, is a common form of self-care. Dietary supplements such as herbs, vitamins, minerals, or other substances are very popular and used extensively in the United States. Box 4-1 shows tips for making informed decisions and evaluating information about dietary supplements. When self-treatment is ineffective, people are likely to turn to *professional* and/or *folk* (indigenous, generic, traditional) healing systems.

Box 4-1 Tips for Making Informed Decisions and Evaluating Information About Dietary Supplements

Basic Points to Consider

1. Do I need to think about my total diet?

   Yes, dietary supplements are intended to supplement your diet, not to replace the varieties of food that are important for your health

2. Should I check with my doctor or health care provider before using a supplement?

   Yes, this is a good idea. Dietary supplements are not always risk free.
   Always check with your health care provider if you are pregnant, breast-feeding, or if you have a chronic medical condition such as diabetes, hypertension, or heart disease.

   • Some supplements may interact with prescription and over-the-counter medicines.
   • Some supplements can have unwanted effects during surgery.
   • Adverse effects from the use of dietary supplements should be reported to the FDA by calling 1-800-FDA-1088.

3. Evaluate product websites and labels carefully; under the law, manufacturers of dietary

supplements are responsible for making sure their products are safe before they are marketed.

   • Who operates the website?
   • What is the purpose of the website?
   • What is the source of the information on the site and does the site have references?
   • Is the information current?

4. Think twice about believing what you read. Here are some assumptions that raise safety concerns:

   "Even if a product may not help me, it at least will not hurt me."
   "When I see the term 'natural,' it means that a product is healthful and safe."
   "A product is safe when there is no cautionary information on the product label."
   "A recall of a harmful product guarantees that all such harmful products will be immediately and completely removed from the marketplace."

5. Contact the manufacturer for more information about the specific product that you are purchasing.

From: U.S. Food and Drug Administration, Center for Food Safety and Applied Nutrition (2014).

Professional Care Systems

According to Leininger (1991, 1997; Leininger & McFarland, 2002; Leininger & McFarland, 2006), **professional care systems**, also referred to as scientific or biomedical systems, are formally taught, learned, and transmitted professional care, health, illness, wellness, and related knowledge and practice skills that prevail in professional institutions, usually with multidisciplinary personnel to serve consumers. Professional care is characterized by specialized education and knowledge, responsibility for care, and expectation of remuneration for services rendered. Nurses, physicians, physical therapists, and other licensed health care providers are examples of professionals who comprise professional care systems in the United States, Canada, Europe, Australia, and other parts of the world.

Folk Healing System

A **folk healing system** is a set of beliefs that has a shared social dimension and reflects what people actually do when they are ill versus what society says they ought to do according to a set of social standards (Andrews, Ybarra, & Matthews, 2014). According to Leininger (1991) and Leininger and McFarland (2002), all cultures of the world have had a lay health care system, which is sometimes referred to as indigenous or generic. The key consideration that defines folk systems is their history of tradition: many folk healing systems have endured over time through oral transmission of beliefs and practices from one generation to the next. A folk-healing system uses healing practices that are often divided into secular and sacred components.

Most cultures have **folk healers** (sometimes referred to as traditional, lay, indigenous, or generic healers), most of whom speak the native tongue of the client, sometimes make house calls, and usually charge significantly less than health care providers in the professional care system (Leininger, 1997; Leininger & McFarland, 2002, 2006). In addition, many cultures have lay midwives (e.g., *parteras* for Hispanic women),

doulas (support women for new mothers and babies), or other health care providers available for meeting the needs of clients. Table 4-2 identifies indigenous or folk healers for selected groups.

If clients use folk healers, these healers should be an integral part of the health care team and included in as many aspects of the client's care as possible. For example, a nurse might include the folk healer in obtaining a health history and in determining what treatments already have been used in an effort to bring about healing. In discussing traditional remedies, it is important to be respectful and to listen attentively to healers who combine spiritual and herbal remedies for a wide variety of illnesses, both physical and psychological in origin. Chapter 13 provides detailed information about the religious beliefs and spiritual healers in major religious groups.

Complementary, Integrative, and Alternative Health System

Complementary, integrative, and alternative health is an umbrella term for hundreds of therapies based on health care systems of people from around the world. Some of these therapies have ancient origins in Egyptian, Chinese, Greek, and American Indian cultures. Others, such as osteopathy and magnet therapy, have evolved more recently. **Allopathic** or biomedicine is the reference point, with all other therapies being considered complementary (in addition to), integrative (combined with selected magico-religious or holistic therapies whose efficacy has been scientifically documented), or alternative to (instead of).

Integrative health care is defined as a comprehensive, often interdisciplinary approach to treatment, prevention, and health promotion that brings together complementary and conventional therapies. The use of an integrative approach to health and wellness has grown within care settings across the United States, including hospitals, hospices, and military health facilities (National Center for Complementary and Integrative

Table 4-2: Healers and Their Scope of Practice

Culture/Folk Practitioner	Preparation	Scope of Practice
Hispanic		
Family member	Possesses knowledge of folk medicine	Common illnesses of a mild nature that may or may not be recognized by modern medicine
Curandero	May receive training in an apprenticeship; may receive a "gift from God" that enables him or her to cure; knowledgeable in use of herbs, diet, massage, and rituals	Treats almost all of the traditional illnesses; some may not treat illness caused by witchcraft for fear of being accused of possessing evil powers; usually admired by members of the community
Espiritualista or spiritualist	Born with the special gifts of being able to analyze dreams and foretell future events; may serve apprenticeship with an older practitioner	Emphasis on prevention of illness or bewitchment through use of medals, prayers, amulets; may also be sought for cure of existing illness
Yerbero	No formal training; knowledgeable in growing and prescribing herbs	Consulted for preventive and curative use of herbs for both traditional and Western illnesses
Sabador	Knowledgeable in massage and manipulation of bones and muscles	Treats many traditional illnesses, particularly those affecting the musculoskeletal system; may also treat nontraditional illnesses
Black		
"Old lady"	Usually an older woman who has successfully raised her own family; knowledgeable in child care and folk remedies	Consulted about common ailments and for advice on child care; found in rural and urban communities
Spiritualist	Called by God to help others; no formal training; usually associated with a fundamentalist Christian church	Assists with problems that are financial, personal, spiritual, or physical; predominantly found in urban communities
Voodoo priest and priestess or *Houngan* and *Mambo*	May be trained by other priests/priestesses In the United States the eldest son of a priest becomes a priest; the daughter of a priest(ess) becomes a priestess if she is born with a veil (amniotic sac) over her face	Knowledgeable about properties of herbs; interpretation of signs and omens; able to cure illness caused by voodoo; uses communication techniques to establish a therapeutic milieu like a psychiatrist; treats Blacks, Mexican Americans, and Native Americans
Chinese		
Herbalist	Knowledgeable in diagnosis of illness and herbal remedies	Both diagnostic and therapeutic; diagnostic techniques include interviewing, inspection, auscultation, and assessment of pulses
Acupuncturist	3½ –4½ years (1,500–1,800 hours) of courses on acupuncture, Western anatomy and physiology, Chinese herbs; usually requires a period of apprenticeship, learning from someone else who is licensed or certified Licensure required in the United States	Diagnosis and treatment of yin/yang disorders by inserting needles into *meridians*, pathways through which life energy flows; when heat is applied to the acupuncture needle, the term *moxibustion* is used May combine acupuncture with herbal remedies and/or dietary recommendations. Acupuncture is sometimes used as a surgical anesthetic

continued

Table 4-2: Healers and Their Scope of Practice (continued)

Culture/Folk Practitioner	Preparation	Scope of Practice
Amish		
Braucher or baruch-doktor	Apprenticeship	Men or women who use a combination of modalities including physical manipulation, massage, herbs, teas, reflexology, and *brauche*, a folk-healing art with origins in 18th and 19th century Europe; especially effective in the treatment of bedwetting, nervousness, and women's health problems; may be generalist or specialist in practice; some set up treatment rooms; some see non-Amish as well as Amish patients
Lay midwives	Apprenticeship	Care for women before, during, and after delivery
Greek		
Magissa "magician"	Apprenticeship	Woman who cures *matiasma* or evil eye; may be referred to as doctor
Bonesetters	Apprenticeship	Specialize in treating uncomplicated fractures
Priest (Orthodox)	Ordained clergy Formal theological study	May be called on for advice, blessings, exorcisms, or direct healing
Native American		
Shaman	Spiritually chosen Apprenticeship	Uses incantations, prayers, and herbs to cure a wide range of physical, psychological, and spiritual illnesses
Crystal gazer, hand trembler (Navajo)	Spiritually chosen Apprenticeship	Diviner diagnostician who can identify the cause of a problem, either by using crystals or by placing hand over the sick person; does not implement treatment

Adapted with permission from Hautman, M. A. (1979). Folk health and illness beliefs. *Nurse Practitioner, 4*(4), 23–31.

Health, 2014). The NCCIH's mission is to define, through rigorous scientific investigation, the usefulness and safety of complementary and integrative health approaches and their roles in improving health and health care. The center's research priorities include the study of complementary approaches such as spinal manipulation, meditation, and massage, to manage pain and other symptoms that are not always well-addressed by conventional biomedical treatments. The center's research also encourages self-care methods that support healthier lifestyles and uncovers potential usefulness and safety issues of natural products (National Center for Complementary and

Integrative Health, 2014). NCCIH was formerly known as the National Center for Complementary and Alternative Medicine.

Consider a client who has been diagnosed with breast cancer. Worldwide, an estimated 33% to 47% of individuals use complementary or integrative therapies to manage symptoms, prevent toxicities, and improve quality of life during cancer treatment (Hoerner, et al., 2014; Richardson, et al., 2014). An estimated 48% to 80% of North American breast cancer survivors use complementary and integrative therapies following diagnosis (Greenlee et al., 2014; Link et al., 2013). Examples of complementary or integrative

therapies that are recommended by oncologists in clinical practice guidelines on the use of integrative therapies as supportive care in patients treated for breast cancer include acupuncture, massage therapy, and biofeedback for the management of pain, nausea associated with chemotherapy, and other aspects of care for people with breast cancer. An example of an alternative therapy such as using a special diet to treat cancer instead of undergoing the treatment recommended by an oncologist is not recommended for the treatment of breast care (Greenlee et al., 2014).

Complementary Health Approaches

The National Institutes of Health categorizes complementary and integrative health approaches as follows:

1. *Alternative medical systems* are built on complete systems of theory and practice. Often these systems have evolved apart from and earlier than the conventional medical approach used in the United States or Canada. Examples of alternative medical systems that have developed in Western cultures include homeopathic medicine and naturopathic medicine. Examples of systems that have developed in Eastern cultures include traditional Chinese medicine and Ayurveda, which originated in India.

2. *Natural Products* include herbs (also known as botanicals), vitamins, minerals, and probiotics. They are often marketed to the public as *dietary supplements*. Interest in and use of natural products have continued to grow each year for the past decade. Data from the 2012 National Health Survey (Centers for Disease Control and Prevention [CDC], 2014) reveal that 17.7% of US adults reported they had used nonvitamin, nonmineral dietary supplements during 2012.

3. *Mind and body* practices include a diverse group of techniques administered by a trained practitioner or teacher that are designed to enhance the mind's capacity to affect bodily functions and symptoms. The most commonly used mind and body practices include deep breathing, meditation, massage, yoga, progressive relaxation, hypnosis, and guided imagery. In the United States, 8.4% of adults use mind and body practices (CDC, 2014).

4. *Manipulative and body-based methods* are based on manipulation and/or movement of one or more parts of the body. Some examples include chiropractic or osteopathic manipulation and massage therapy; they are used by 8.5% of US adults.

5. *Energy therapies* involve the use of energy fields in two ways:
   - *Biofield therapies* are intended to affect energy fields that surround and penetrate the human body. (The existence of such fields has not yet been scientifically proven.) Some forms of energy therapy manipulate biofields by applying pressure and/or manipulating the body by placing the hands in, or through, these fields. Examples include qigong, Reiki, and Therapeutic Touch.

   - *Bioelectromagnetic-based therapies* involve the unconventional use of electromagnetic fields, such as pulsed fields, magnetic fields, or alternating-current or direct-current fields.

Nonvitamin, nonmineral dietary supplements (17.9%), practitioner-based chiropractic or osteopathic manipulation (8.5%), yoga with deep breathing or meditation (8.4%), and massage therapy (6.8%) were the most prevalent complementary health approaches used by US adults. Regional differences exist in the use of complementary health approaches: 16.4% of adults in the West North Central region and 11.4% of adults in the Mountain region used chiropractic or osteopathic manipulation, compared to the national average of 8.5%. The Southern and Pacific regions have significantly lower use (CDC, 2014). Box 4-2 identifies and describes some of the complementary and alternative therapies most commonly used by people in the United States and Canada to promote health

Box 4-2 Selected Complementary and Alternative Therapies

Acupuncture refers to a family of procedures involving stimulation of anatomical points on the body by a variety of techniques. The acupuncture technique that has been most studied scientifically involves penetrating the skin with thin, solid, metallic needles that are manipulated by the hands or by electrical stimulation. When heat is applied to the needles, it is referred to as moxibustion.

Aromatherapy involves the use of essential oils (extracts or essences) from flowers, herbs, and trees to promote health and well-being.

Ayurveda includes diet and herbal remedies and emphasizes the use of body, mind, and spirit in disease prevention and treatment.

Chiropractic focuses on the relationship between bodily structure (primarily that of the spine) and function, and how that relationship affects the preservation and restoration of health. Chiropractors use manipulative therapy as an integral treatment tool.

Dietary supplements are products (other than tobacco) taken by mouth that contain a *dietary ingredient* intended to supplement the diet. *Dietary ingredients* may include vitamins, minerals, herbs or other botanicals, amino acids, and substances such as enzymes, organ tissues, and metabolites. *Dietary supplements* come in many forms, including extracts, concentrates, tablets, capsules, gelcaps, liquids, and powders. The United States and Canada have special requirements for labeling and regulate them as foods, not drugs.

Guided imagery refers to a wide variety of techniques, including simple visualization and direct suggestion using imagery, metaphor and story-telling, fantasy exploration and game playing, dream interpretation, drawing, and active imagination where elements of the unconscious are invited to appear as images that can communicate with the conscious mind (Academy for Guided Imagery, 2014).

Homeopathic medicine is an alternative medical system. In homeopathic medicine, there is a belief that "like cures like," meaning that small, highly diluted quantities of medicinal substances are given to cure symptoms, even though the same substances given at higher or more concentrated doses would actually cause those symptoms.

Massage therapists manipulate muscle and connective tissue to enhance function of those tissues and promote relaxation and well-being.

Naturopathy is an alternative medical system based on the premise that there is a healing power in the body that establishes, maintains, and restores health. Practitioners work with the patient with a goal of supporting this power through treatments such as nutrition and lifestyle counseling, dietary supplements, medicinal plants, exercise, homeopathy, and traditional Chinese medicine.

Osteopathic medicine is a form of conventional medicine that, in part, emphasizes diseases arising in the musculoskeletal system. There is an underlying belief that all of the body's systems work together, and disturbances in one system may affect function elsewhere in the body. Some osteopathic physicians practice osteopathic manipulation, a full-body system of hands-on techniques to alleviate pain, restore function, and promote health and well-being.

Qigong ("chee-GUNG") is a component of traditional Chinese medicine that combines movement, meditation, and regulation of breathing to enhance the flow of qi (pronounced "chee" and meaning *vital energy*) in the body, improve blood circulation, and enhance immune function.

Reiki ("RAY-kee") is a Japanese word representing *Universal Life Energy*. Reiki is based on the belief that when spiritual energy is channeled through a Reiki practitioner, the patient's spirit is healed, which in turn heals the physical body.

Therapeutic touch is based on the premise that the healing force of the therapist affects the patient's recovery; healing is promoted when the body's energies are in balance. By

passing their hands over the patient, healers can identify energy imbalances.

Traditional Chinese medicine (TCM) is the current name for an ancient system of health care from China. TCM is based on a concept of balanced qi, or *vital energy*, which is believed to flow throughout the body. Qi regulates a person's spiritual, emotional, mental, and physical balance, and is influenced by the opposing forces of yin (negative energy) and yang (positive energy). Disease is proposed to result from the flow of qi being disrupted and yin and yang becoming imbalanced. Among the components of TCM are herbal and nutritional therapy, restorative physical exercises, meditation, acupuncture, and remedial massage.

Yoga is a term derived from a Sanskrit word meaning yoke or union. Yoga involves a combination of breathing exercises, meditation, and physical postures that are used to achieve a state of relaxation and balance of mind, body, and spirit.

Source: Center for Disease Control (2014) and National Center for Complementary and Alternative Medicine (2014).

and prevent and treat disease. Figure 4-1 provides the percentage of US adults who used selected complementary health approaches in the past 12 months by type of approach.

Other mind–body techniques are still considered complementary and integrative, including meditation, prayer, mental healing, and therapies that use creative outlets such as art, music, or dance.

Efficacy of Complementary Health Approaches

Research on complementary health approaches has focused on seven main areas: medicinal plants, chiropractic and low back pain, acupuncture and pain, cell processes and diseases (e.g., cancer, asthma), the oxidative degradation of lipids, and diabetes and insulin. Research is also being done on the quality-of-life impact of complementary health approaches, including the influence of exercise and physical therapies on pain and end-of-life care (Moral-Munoz, Cobo, Peis, Arroyo-Morales, & Herrer-Viedman, 2014). For further information on evidence related to the efficacy of specific health approaches and the reliability and validity of the research conducted, you are encouraged to visit the Cochrane Library, which is the repository for the Cochrane Collaboration, a worldwide organization that prepares systematic reviews of health care therapies.

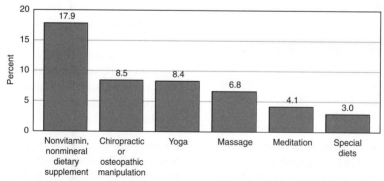

Figure 4-1. Percentage of U.S. adults who used selected complementary health approaches in the past 12 months by type of approach. (Source: CDC/NCHS, National Health Interview Survey, 2012 in Center for Disease Control. (2014). National Center for Health Statistics Data Brief: Regional variation in use of complementary health approaches. Retrieved on October 18, 2014 at http://www.cdc.gov/nchs/data/databriefs/db146.htm)

Summary

Cultural belief systems develop from the shared experiences of a social group and are expressed symbolically. The use of symbols to define, describe, and relate to the world around us is one of the basic characteristics of being human. The major cultural belief systems embraced by people of the world are the magico-religious, scientific, and holistic health paradigms or worldviews. In the magico-religious cultural belief system, a supernatural agent or agents are responsible for health and illness. Health often is seen as a reward given as a sign of blessing and goodwill by a supernatural agent, and illness may be seen as a sign of punishment by a supernatural agent or agents. Most physicians and nurses are formally educated in the scientific or biomedical belief system, in which life is controlled by a series of physical and biochemical processes that can be studied and manipulated by humans through allopathic medicine or professional care systems.

In the holistic cultural belief system, the forces of nature must be kept in natural balance or harmony. Human life is only one aspect of nature and a part of the general order of the cosmos. Disturbing the laws of nature creates imbalance, chaos, and disease. Examples of the holistic cultural belief system include the yin/yang and hot/cold theories of health and illnesses.

REVIEW QUESTIONS

1. In your own words, describe what is meant by the following terms: (a) cultural belief system, (b) worldview, and (c) paradigm.
2. What are the primary characteristics of the three major health belief systems: magico-religious, scientific, and holistic paradigms?
3. What are the differences between professional and folk care systems?
4. What is allopathic medicine?
5. What is the primary mission of the National Center for Complementary and Integrative Health (NCCIH)?
6. Identify the five major categories of complementary or integrative approaches.

CRITICAL THINKING ACTIVITIES

1. Select a complementary health approach that you would like to know more about, for example, acupuncture, chiropractic, or homeopathy. Search the Internet for information about this practice, and go to a library to conduct background research. After you have learned more about the practice, contact a healer who uses that health approach and ask the following questions:
   a. How did you prepare to be a practitioner of _____?
   b. What do you believe are the major benefits of _____ to clients or patients?
   c. What health-related conditions do you believe respond best to _____?
   d. Are there any risks to clients resulting from the use of _____?

2. According to the World Health Organization, 80% of the people in the world use complementary or integrative health approaches for the treatment of common illnesses. Select a common illness, such as upper respiratory infection, arthritis, gastrointestinal upset, or a similar condition, and identify the various complementary and integrative approaches to allopathic medicine that clients might use. What is the efficacy of each intervention that you have identified? How effective do you think the complementary and alternative practices are compared with allopathic medicine? Compare the cost of each practice as well as its efficacy.

3. Please view the video "Scientific Results of Yoga for Health and Well-being," which can be found on the NCCIH website (nccih.nih.gov, on the Training tab) as part of their Online Continuing Education Series. The presentation will help you to learn more about the use of yoga and tai chi to improve balance and prevent falls, especially in the elderly. After

viewing the video, identify the areas for which you're convinced there is adequate evidence to support incorporating yoga as a complementary health approach into your nursing practice.

4. The herb *Echinacea* is frequently used for the prevention and treatment of the common cold. If a patient asked your opinion about the use of *Echinacea*, how would you reply? Would you recommend that the patient use this herb for treatment of a cold? Explain why or why not.

5. Visit three websites in the Internet Resources list on thePoint for further information about specific types of alternative and complementary medicine. Select a disease for which you think a complementary or alternative intervention might be helpful, for example, breast cancer, hypertension, osteoarthritis, or other chronic condition. Critically analyze the potential benefits and adverse effects of the intervention on clients with this disease. Indicate whether you believe there is sufficient evidence to support recommending the intervention to a client.

REFERENCES

Academy for Guided Imagery. (2014). What is guided imagery? Retrieved from http://acadgi.com/whatisguidedimagery/index.html

Ackernecht, E. (1971). Natural diseases and rational treatment in primitive medicine. *Bulletin of the History of Medicine, 19*, 467–497.

Andrews, T. J., Ybarra, V., & Matthews, L. L. (2014). For the sake of our children: Hispanic immigrant and migrant families' use of folk healing and biomedicine. *Medical Anthropology Quarterly, 27*(3), 385–413.

Center for Disease Control (2012). National Health Interview Survey. Retrieved from http://www.cdc.gov/nchs/nhis/nhis_2012_data_release.htm

Center for Disease Control. (2014). National Center for Health Statistics Data Brief: Regional variation in use of complementary health approaches. Retrieved from http://www/cdc.gov/nchs/data/databriefs/db146.htm

Clements, F. E. (1932). Primitive concepts of disease. *University of California Publications in Archeology and Ethnology, 32*(2), 185–252.

Greenlee, H. G., Balneaves, L. G., Carlson, L. E., Cohen, M., Deng, G., Hershman, D., ..., Tripahy, D. (2014). Clinical practice guidelines on the use of integrative therapies as supportive care in patients treated for breast cancer. *Journal of the National Cancer Institute Monographs, 50*(3), 346–358.

Hautman, M. A. (1979). Folk health and illness beliefs. *Nurse Practitioner, 4*(4), 23–31.

Horner, M., Bueschel, G., Dennert, G., Less, D., Ritter, E., & Zwahlen, M. (2014). How many cancer patients use complementary and alternative medicine: A systematic review and metaanalysis. *Integrative Cancer Therapies, 11*(3), 187–203.

Leininger, M. M. (1991). *Culture care diversity and universality: A theory of nursing.* New York: National League for Nursing Press.

Leininger, M. M. (1997). Founder's focus alternative to what? Generic vs. professional caring, treatments and healing modes. *Journal of Transcultural Nursing, 91*(1), 37.

Leininger, M. M., & McFarland, M. R. (2002). *Transcultural nursing: Concepts, theories, research and practices.* New York, NY: McGraw-Hill.

Leininger, M. M. & McFarland, M. R. (2006). *Culture care diversity & universality: A worldwide nursing theory* (2nd ed.). Sudbury, MA: Jones & Bartlett, Publishers.

Lillyman, S., & Farquharson, N. (2013). Self-care management education models in primary care. *British Journal of Community Nursing, 18*(11), 556–564.

Link, A. R., Gammon, M. D., Jacobson, J. S., Abrahamson, P., Bradshaw, P., Terry, M. B., ..., Greenless, H. (*2013*). Use of self-care practitioner-based forms of complementary and alternative medicine before and after breast cancer. *Evidence-Based Complementary and Alternative Medicine, 2013*, 301549. doi: 10.1155/2013/301549

Mechanic, D. (1978). *Medical sociology* (2nd ed.). New York, NY: Free Press.

Moral-Munoz, J. A., Cobo, M. J., Peis, E., Arroyo-Morales, M., Herrer-Viedman, E. (2014). Analyzing the research in integrative and complementary medicine by means of science mapping. *Complementary Therapies in Medicine, 22*, 409–418.

National Center for Complementary and Integrative Health. (2015). Complementary, alternative or integrative medicine: What's in a name? Retrieved from https://nccih.nih.gov/health/integrative-health

Osborn, D. K. (2015). *Greek medicine: The four humors.* Retrieved from http://www.greekmedicine.net/b_p/Four_Humors.html

Richardson, J., Loyola-Sanchez, A., Sinclair, S., Harris, J., Letts, L., MacIntyre, N. J., ..., Ginnis, K. M. (2014). Self-management interventions for chronic disease: A systematic scoping review. *Clinical Rehabilitation, 28*(11), 1067–1077.

Shaw, S. J., Armin, J., Torres, C. H., Orzech, K. M., & Vivian, J. (2012). Chronic disease self-management and health literacy in four ethnic groups. *Journal of Health Communication, 17,* 67–81.

U.S. Food and Drug Administration, Center for Food Safety and Applied Nutrition. (2014). Questions and answers on dietary supplements. Retrieved from http://www.fda.gov/Food/DietarySupplements/QADietarySupplements/default.htm

World Health Organization. (1948). Preamble to the Constitution of the World Health Organization as adopted by the International Health Conference, New York, 19–22 June, 1946; signed on 22 July 1946 by the representatives of 61 States (Official Records of the World Health Organization, no. 2, p. 100) and entered into force on 7 April 1948.

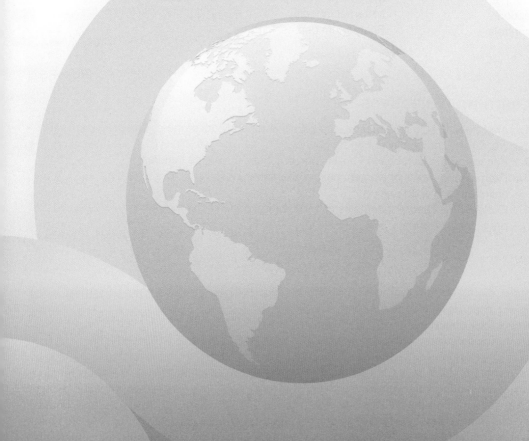

Part Two

Transcultural Nursing: Across the Lifespan

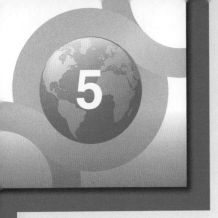

5

Transcultural Perspectives in Childbearing

● Jana Lauderdale

Key Terms

Abortion
Childbearing
Contraception
Fertility controls

Imbalance
Intimate partner violence
Intrauterine device (IUD)
Maternal morbidity
Maternal mortality
Postpartum depression

Pregnancy
Prescriptive beliefs
Restrictive beliefs
Taboos

Learning Objectives

1. Analyze how culture influences the beliefs and behaviors of the childbearing woman and her family during pregnancy.
2. Recognize the childbearing beliefs and practices of diverse cultures.
3. Examine the needs of women making alternative lifestyle choices regarding childbirth and child rearing.
4. Explore how cultural ideologies of childbearing populations can impact pregnancy outcomes.

This chapter discusses how cultural diversity influences the experience of **childbearing**. The experiences of the woman and those of her significant other during pregnancy, birth, and the postpartum period are examined. Recommendations for practice are provided in each section for nurses caring for childbearing women and their families. Also presented for the reader's consideration are discussions related to culturally specific circumstances and behaviors of the childbearing woman and her family.

Overview of Cultural Belief Systems and Practices Related to Childbearing

Pregnancy and childbirth practices in contemporary Western society have seen dramatic changes over the past three decades. As global populations become increasingly mobile, we are seeing cultures converge, which calls for a reorientation of our nursing skills and nursing behaviors.

In light of global population shifts that are likely to continue for years to come, cultural beliefs regarding childbearing and childrearing need to be examined to enable nurses to offer our patients culturally congruent care throughout their pregnancy, birth, and the early postpartum.

One aspect does remain static: Childbearing is universal and, as Chalmers (2013) notes, is a great leveler, as all women who give birth do so in one of two ways. This is also a time of transition and social celebration of central importance in any society, signaling a realignment of existing cultural roles and responsibilities, psychological and physiologic states, and social relationships. The differences in how women experience this transition lie in the cultural values and beliefs surrounding pregnancy, the birthing process, and postpartum practices.

The dominant cultural practices or rituals include formal prenatal care (including childbirth classes), ultrasonography to view the fetus, and hospital delivery. Hospital deliveries routinely involve a highly specialized group of nurses, obstetricians, perinatologists, and pediatricians who actively monitor the mother's physiologic status and the fetal status (see Figure 5-1), deliver the infant, and provide postpartum and newborn care. Routine hospital care can also include inducing labor, providing anesthesia for labor and delivery, and performing a cesarean section. There is not total cultural agreement about the value of these dominant practices, however, and some health care providers elect to offer their pregnant clients alternative health care services. These alternatives include in-hospital and free-standing birth centers (see Figure 5-2) and care by nurse practitioners and nurse midwives who promote family-centered care and emphasize pregnancy as a normal process requiring minimal technological intervention.

It is a known fact that the United States spends more money than any other country on health care and more on maternal health than any other type of hospital care; however, women in the United States have a higher risk of dying of pregnancy-related complications than those in 40 other countries. Health disparities in the United States also play a role in increased **maternal morbidity** and **maternal mortality**, although it is unclear to what extent. For example, African American women are nearly four times more likely to die of pregnancy-related complications

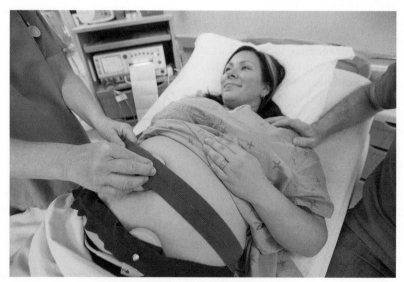

Figure 5-1. Fetal monitoring (Tyler Olson/Shutterstock.com).

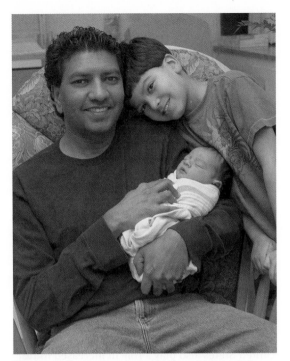

Figure 5-2. Family-oriented birth center (glenda/ Shutterstock.com).

than White women. These rates and disparities have not improved in more than 20 years (Amnesty International, USA, 2010).

Subcultures within the United States have very different practices, values, and beliefs about childbirth and the roles of women, men, social support networks, and health care practitioners. One such subculture includes proponents of the "back to nature" movement, who are often vegetarian, use lay midwives for home deliveries, and practice herbal or naturopathic medicine. Other groups that might have distinct cultural practices include African Americans, American Indians, Hispanics, Middle Eastern groups, Orthodox Jewish groups, Asians, and recent immigrants, among others. Additionally, religious background, regional variations, age, urban or rural background, sexual preference, and other individual characteristics all might contribute to cultural differences in the experience of childbirth.

Despite the great variations that can exist in relation to the social class, ethnic origin,

family structure, and social support networks of women in the United States, many health care providers mistakenly assume that pregnancy and childbirth are experienced similarly by all people. In addition, some professional nurses view some traditional cultural beliefs, values, and practices related to childbirth as "old-fashioned," "back in the day," or "old wives' tales." Although some of these customs are changing rapidly, particularly for immigrants in the United States, many women and families are attempting to preserve their own valued patterns of experiencing childbirth (see Evidence-Based Practice 5-1).

Fertility Control and Culture

The professional literature lacks information specific to cultural beliefs and practices related to the control of fertility. A woman's fertility depends on several factors, including the likelihood of sterility, the probability of conceiving, and of intrauterine mortality. In addition, the duration of a postpartum period, during which a woman is unlikely to ovulate or conceive, influences fertility. These variables are further modified by cultural and social variables, including marriage and residence patterns, diet, religion, the availability of **abortion**, the incidence of venereal disease, and the regulation of birth intervals by cultural or artificial means, all of which are influenced by cultural norms, values, and traditions. This section focuses on those societal factors that influence reproductive rights and population control.

Unintended Pregnancy

In the United States, according to Finer and Zolna's (2011) combined data study, 49% of pregnancies in 2006 were unintended—a slight increase from 48% in 2001. Among women aged 19 years and younger, more than four out of five pregnancies were unintended. The proportion of pregnancies that were unintended was highest among teens younger than age 15 years, at 98%.

Pregnancy, Childbirth, and Motherhood: A Metasynthesis of the Lived Experiences of Immigrant Women

One of the most joyous processes in human nature should be that of pregnancy, childbirth, and motherhood. However, for immigrant women resettling in a new country, pregnancy may prove to be an unsettling experience. The authors conducted a metasynthesis using the seven steps of Noblit and Hare's (1988) metaethnography. The aim of the study was to synthesize qualitative research in the area of immigrant women's perceptions of pregnancy, childbirth, and motherhood as migrants in their newly adopted country. Fifteen studies published between 2003 and 2013 were selected that represented the topic of interest. Four major themes were found to be common in all the studies: expectations of pregnancy and childbirth, experiences of motherhood, encountering confusion and conflict with beliefs, and dealing with migration challenges. The results from the study indicate immigrant women believe they have the right to receive quality and culturally congruent health care, regardless of background.

Clinical Implications:

- Provide increased emotional support to immigrant women during pregnancy as needed.

- Work to ensure that institutions provide linguistically informed and culturally congruent services to enhance antenatal visits.
- Make cross-cultural training available to providers in order to address cultural issues that could negatively impact childbirth, such as female excision.
- Maximize involvement of lay community outreach workers with the same cultural background, to inform women of available reproductive services.
- Respect and consider traditional practices in the women's care to improve health outcomes for both mother and child.
- Learn as much as possible about the cultural belief systems of your patients in order to build an environment of trust and open communication to improve the childbearing experience.

Reference: Benza, S., & Liamputtong, P. (2014). Pregnancy, childbirth and motherhood: A meta-synthesis of the lived experiences of immigrant women. *Midwifery, 30,* 575–584.

The largest increases in unintended pregnancy rates were among women with low education, low income, and cohabiting women. Mosher, Jones, and Abma (2012) reported similar findings in data from the National Survey of Family Growth, which indicated no significant decline in the overall proportion of unintended births between the 1982 and the 2006 to 2010 surveys. The proportion of births that were unintended did decline during these years among married, non-Hispanic White women. Women more likely to experience unintended births included unmarried women, black women, women who are socioeconomically disadvantaged, and those with less education. The public cost of births

resulting from unintended pregnancies has been reported to be $8 billion; for teens, the average cost was even higher, topping out at $9.1 billion (Sonfield, Kost, & Gold, 2011). Figure 5-3 illustrates a teenager's reaction to an unintended pregnancy.

Women's attitudes related to pregnancy, contraception, fertility, and childbearing have had limited exploration. Rocca and Harper (2012) used 2009 data from the National Survey of Reproductive and Contraceptive Knowledge to specifically investigate if contraceptive attitudes and knowledge explain disparities in method used. Using mediation analysis and regression models, they reported that Blacks and Latinas believe the

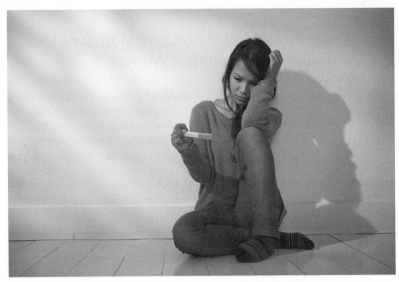

Figure 5-3. Pregnant teenager (Diego Cervo/Shutterstock.com).

government encourages contraceptive use to limit minority population growth. They also indicated that although Blacks and Latinas used less effective methods than Whites, their attitudes did not explain the disparities in method used. For example, lower contraceptive knowledge only partially explained Latinas' use of less effective methods. The investigators concluded that "other" variables needed study, including provider behavior and health system features.

Unintended pregnancy can have numerous negative effects on the mother and the fetus, including a delay in prenatal care, continued or increased tobacco and other drug use, as well as increased physical abuse during pregnancy; any of these factors can lead to preterm labor or low-birth-weight (LBW) infants (Finer & Zolna, 2011). Consideration must also be given to what is *influencing* unintended pregnancy, which includes changes in social mores sanctioning motherhood outside of marriage, **contraception** availability including abortion, earlier sexual activity, and multiple partners. In addition to increasing access to contraception and targeting high-risk groups, programs aimed at reducing or preventing unintended pregnancy must build on the cultural meaning of the problem and focus on the processes women and their partners use to make fertility decisions.

The United States has established family planning goals in *Healthy People 2020* aimed at improving pregnancy planning, spacing, and preventing unintended pregnancy. An objective is to *increase* the proportion of pregnancies that are *intended* to 56%. Family planning efforts that can help reduce unintended pregnancy include increasing access to contraception, particularly to the more effective and longer-acting reversible forms, and increasing correct and consistent use of contraceptive methods overall (U.S. Department of Health and Human Services, 2014). As of this printing, this goal has yet to be achieved.

Contraceptive Methods

Commonly used methods of contraception in the United States include hormonal methods, **intrauterine devices (IUDs)**, permanent sterilization, and, to a lesser degree, barrier and "natural" methods. Natural methods of family planning are based on the recognition of fertility through signs and symptoms and abstinence during periods of fertility. The religious beliefs of some cultural groups might affect their use

of **fertility controls** such as abortion or artificial regulation of conception; for example, Roman Catholics might follow church edicts against artificial control of conception, and Mormon families might follow their church's teaching regarding the spiritual responsibility to have large families and promote church growth (Andrews & Hanson, 2012). Negative outcomes of religious family planning teachings have recently been studied. Pritchard, Roberts, and Pritchard (2013) analyzed WHO data from two continents sharing religious–cultural views on suicide and family planning those being Western European Catholic and Latin American Catholic countries. He reported that in Latin American female youth (15 to 24 years of age), less access to contraception contributed to unintended pregnancies and higher suicide rates.

The ability to control fertility successfully also requires an understanding of the menstrual cycle and the times and conditions under which pregnancy is more or less likely to occur—in essence, an understanding of bodily functions. When these functions change, the woman might perceive the changes as abnormal or unhealthy. Because the use of artificial methods of fertility control might alter the body's usual cycles, women who use them might become anxious, consider themselves ill, and discontinue the method. American Indian women monitor their monthly bleeding cycles closely and believe in the importance of monthly menstruation for maintaining harmony and physical well-being. Contraceptives such as the IUD are generally better accepted by American Indian women than hormonal methods because of the normal or increased flow associated with the IUD. Because the mechanism of action of an IUD might include the expulsion of a fertilized ovum, some women in this group oppose the use of the IUD for religious reasons.

Refugees and Reproductive Health

Since the Rwandan crisis in 1994, an estimated 26 million individuals have been displaced across international borders (as of mid-2013) as part of a mass exodus from their homes due to war, ethnic and civil unrest, and political instability (UNHCR, 2013). Women and children account for approximately 80% of the world's refugees, and displaced women are extremely vulnerable to poor reproductive illness and outcomes (CDC, Division of Reproductive Health, National Center for Chronic Disease Prevention and Health Promotion, 2014). The CDC has developed a refugee program with a focus on refugee reproductive health. The goals for the program are presented in Box 5-1. Women living in refugee situations encounter many barriers to contraceptive use,

---

Box 5-1 CDC Refugee Reproductive Health Activities Goals

1. Initiate epidemiologic studies to evaluate the reproductive health status of women in refugee and IDP settings to better provide information to improve service, quality, and accessibility.
2. Design, implement, and evaluate reproductive health rapid assessment tools and behavioral and epidemiologic surveillance systems appropriate to refugee settings.
3. Design, recommend, and evaluate interventions and "best practices" identified through epidemiologic research, rapid assessment, and surveillance.
4. Strengthen the capacity of the refugee/IDP community, as well as the agencies providing health services, to collect and use data to improve reproductive health status and services.
5. Translate and communicate study findings and best practices to refugees and supporting agencies.

CDC, Division of Reproductive Health, National Center for Chronic Disease Prevention and Health Promotion, Atlanta, GA. (2006). Retrieved from http://www.cdc.gov

and even with the development of programs that target refugee women in the United States, sponsored refugee women continue to experience barriers to reproductive health. For example, Somali Bantu women relocated to Hartford, CT, reported that a major barrier to unmet health needs was the ethnic distinction/language barrier (Gurnah, Khoshnood, Bradley, & Yuan , 2011). The authors attributed this finding to the interpreter translation being conducted in a Somali language that the Somali Bantu did not understand.

Religion and Fertility Control

The influence of religious beliefs on birth control choices varies within and between groups, and adherence to these beliefs may change over time. Cultural practices tend to arise from religious beliefs, which can influence birth control choices. For example, the Hindu religion teaches that the right hand is clean and the left is dirty. The right hand is for holding religious books and eating utensils, and the left hand is used for dirty things, such as touching the genitals. This belief complicates the use of contraceptives requiring the use of both hands, such as a diaphragm (Bromwich & Parsons, 1990).

In many cases, birth control is seen as an act of God. Purnell and Selekman (2008) describe the Muslim belief that abortion is "haram" unless the mother's life is in danger; consequently, unintended pregnancies are dealt with by praying a miscarriage will occur. A fact that is perhaps of greater significance to fertility in Muslim women is that a woman's sterility can be reason for abandoning or divorcing her. The authors go on to say that Islamic law forbids adoption; infertility treatment is allowed, but is limited to artificial insemination using the couple's own sperm and eggs. A pregnant Muslim woman is shown in Figure 5-4.

According to Orthodox Jewish beliefs, infertility counseling and intervention such as sperm and egg donation (from the couple) meet with religious approval; adoption is viewed as a last resort (Washofsky, 2000). The use of condoms and birth control pills are acceptable; abortion and sterilization are the least-supported birth

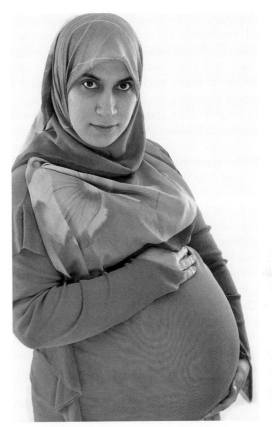

Figure 5-4. Pregnant woman (ZouZou/Shutterstock. com).

control methods. However, in cases where the mother's life is in jeopardy, abortion is not opposed (Kolatch, 2000).

In some African cultures, there are strongly held beliefs and practices related to birth spacing. Because postpartum sexual activity has traditionally been taboo, some women leave their home for as long as 2 years to avoid pregnancy (Miller, 1992). See Figure 5-5 for a photo of an African woman and her children.

Cultural Influences on Fertility Control

It is common for health professionals to have misconceptions about contraception and the prevention of pregnancy in cultures different from their own. A qualitative study by Eckhardt and Lauderdale (2013) sought to identify and

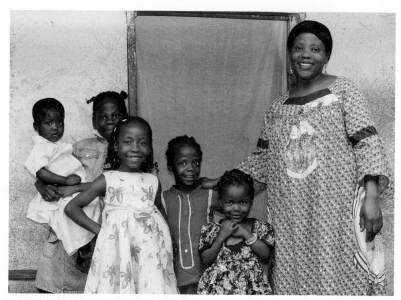

Figure 5-5. Traditional African mother and children (Sylvie Bouchard/Shutterstock.com).

describe the barriers to family planning in North Kamagambo, Kenya, to understand the cultural context in which they exist. Since the Lwala Community Hospital's opening in the North Kamagambo region of Kenya in 2007, the number of patients seeking contraceptives and family planning counseling has increased. However, maternal mortality remains high and the culture expects women to bear many children. Although this places a large burden on women's health and increases a lifetime risk of maternal mortality, cultural and religious hesitance toward family planning persists. See Evidence-Based Practice 5-2.

Nurses providing family planning services must take care to be culturally sensitive so that women can be assisted in examining their own attitudes, beliefs, and sense of gynecologic well-being regarding fertility control.

Pregnancy and Culture

All cultures recognize **pregnancy** as a special transition period, and many have particular customs and beliefs that dictate activity and behavior during pregnancy. Recent reports of childbirth customs in the United States have focused on accounts of differing beliefs and practices relative to pregnancy among various ethnic and cultural groups. This section describes some of the biologic and cultural variations that might influence nursing care during pregnancy.

Biologic Variations

Knowledge of certain biologic variations resulting from genetic and environmental backgrounds is important for nurses who care for childbearing families. For example, pregnant women who have the sickle cell trait and are heterozygous for the sickle cell gene are at increased risk for asymptomatic bacterial and urinary tract infections such as pyelonephritis. This places them at greater-than-normal risk for premature labor as well. Although heterozygotes are found most commonly among African Americans (8% to 14%), individuals living in the United States and Canada who are of Mediterranean ancestry, as well as those of Germanic and Native North American descent,

The Impact of Culture on Knowledge, Attitude, and Practice of Family Planning Methods in Rural North Kamagambo, Kenya

The purpose of the study was to explore how culture impacts knowledge, attitude, and practice regarding family planning in order to design an effective family planning education program tailored to the needs of Lwala and surrounding communities. This exploratory, descriptive, qualitative study employed six focus groups to collect data and included local men, women, Umama Salamas (lay community birth attendants), maternal child health workers, religious community leaders, and Lwala hospital family planning clinic staff. Data were collected using an open-ended interview guide. Constant comparative analysis was used for analyzing interview data. Five themes emerged: preparing the ground (education), cultural barriers and beliefs regarding family planning, health care system issues and health care access, protecting our women and ourselves, and "war" of contradictions and fears.

The findings suggest the community is open to learning and engaging in family planning. Furthermore, the community will likely benefit from this education, as misconceptions of side effects and myths regarding family planning were similar across groups.

Clinical Implications:

- Tailor family planning education based on cultural/community needs as well as education/literacy level.
- Train educators as needed.
- Ensure the privacy of women seeking family planning in the hospital.
- Show respect for differing family planning beliefs.
- Standardize information communicated by health care providers to improve consistency.
- Target men for education to decrease burden of secrecy for women seeking care.
- Discuss with women and men the societal, cultural, and religious hesitance toward male condom use.
- Identify alternative methods for contraception when government contraceptive supply is low.

Reference: Eckhardt, S., & Lauderdale, J. (2013). The impact of culture on knowledge, attitude, and practice of family planning methods in rural North Kamagambo, Kenya. Unpublished study.

might also carry the trait (Overfield, 1985; Perry, 2000). If both parents are heterozygous, there is a one-in-four chance that the infant will be born with sickle cell disease.

Another important biologic variation relative to pregnancy is diabetes mellitus. The incidence of non–insulin-dependent and gestational diabetes is much higher than normal among some American Indian groups—a problem that increases maternal and infant morbidity. Illnesses that are common among European Americans might manifest themselves differently in American Indian clients. For example, an American Indian woman might have a high blood sugar level but be asymptomatic for diabetes mellitus. The mortality rate in pregnant American Indian women with diabetes is higher than in White European American women. Diabetes during pregnancy, particularly with uncontrolled hyperglycemia, is associated with an increased risk of congenital anomalies, stillbirth, macrosomia, birth injury, cesarean section, neonatal hypoglycemia, and other problems.

Because long-term studies have been conducted among the Pima Indians of Arizona, we know that, for the last 40 years or so, they have a very high incidence of gestational diabetes and other health problems during pregnancy (Pettitt, Baird, Aleck, Bennett, & Knowler, 1983). Because some of the children born to Pima mothers after the studies began are now 30 to 40 years old, we

Childbirth Postexcision

Excision has been described by the WHO (2010) as a complete or partial removal of the clitoris and the labia minora, with or without the labia majora. Although communal advantages and some personal benefits have been cited in the literature for female excision, deleterious outcomes have been noted to occur, including psychological stress, adverse obstetric and perinatal outcomes such as postpartum hemorrhage, and newborn risks of stillbirth, death, need for resuscitation at birth, and LBW (United Nations Children's Fund, 2005; WHO, 2008). In order to understand the impacts of excision on childbirth, hermeneutic phenomenology was used to analyze the narratives of four women who had been excised.

Clinical Implications:

- Break the "taboo of silence." The women prefer an open, respectful discussion regarding their excision.

- Share explicit care plans to identify and share each woman's wishes regarding her excision, particularly when multiple providers are involved.
- Provide language/dialect interpreters when sharing information to prevent frustration for the women.
- Ensure that the provider's approach to excised women is as respectful as it is for any other woman seeking maternity care. Remember, the woman in front of you is a "woman who has been excised" versus an "excised woman."

Reference: d'Entremont, M., Smythe, L., & McAra-Couper, J. (2014). The sounds of silence: A hermeneutic interpretation of childbirth post excision. *Health Care for Women International*, *35*, 300–319.

---

can see how a mother's diabetes can influence her child's health in adulthood. Researchers have found that the children of women with diabetes during pregnancy have a higher risk of becoming obese and getting diabetes earlier in life than those born to mothers who had normal blood sugar (Chamberlain, n.d.; The Pima Indians: Obesity and Diabetes, 2010).

Pregnant American Indians and Alaskan Native women with type 2 diabetes are at an increased risk of having babies born with birth defects. Gestational diabetes increases the baby's risk for problems such as macrosomia (large body size) and neonatal hypoglycemia (low blood sugar). Although the blood glucoses of American Indian and Alaskan Native women usually return to normal after childbirth, these women have an increased risk of developing gestational diabetes in future pregnancies. In addition, studies show that many women with gestational diabetes will develop type 2 diabetes later in life (The Diabetes Monitor, 2011).

Cultural Variations Influencing Pregnancy

Several cultural variations may influence pregnancy. Those highlighted in this section include alternative lifestyle choices, nontraditional support systems, cultural beliefs related to parental activity during pregnancy, and food taboos and cravings. Nurses must be able to differentiate among beliefs and practices that are harmful and those that are benign. Few cultural customs related to pregnancy are dangerous and many are health promoting. However, one practice that is dangerous is female excision. This cultural practice occurs in approximately 28 African countries and affects 100 to 140 million girls and women (WHO, 2008). The emotional and psychological impact of this practice on childbirth is important to recognize when providing childbearing care for women having undergone this procedure. See d'Entremont, Smythe, McAra-Couper's (2014) study description in Evidence-Based Practice 5-3.

Alternative Lifestyle Choices

Although the dominant cultural expectation for North American women remains motherhood within the context of the nuclear family, recent cultural changes have made it more acceptable for women to have careers and pursue alternative lifestyles. Changing of cultural expectations has influenced many middle-class North American women and couples to delay childbearing until their late 20s and early 30s and to have small families. Many of today's women are career oriented, and they may delay childbirth until after they have finished college and established their career. Some women are making choices regarding childbearing that might not involve the conventional method of conception and childrearing.

Lesbian childbearing couples are a distinct subculture of pregnant women with special needs (see Figure 5-6). Randi (2012) reports that the way intake forms are completed needs to be re-evaluated in light of these social changes. How the patient became pregnant is one such example. Instead of assuming she became pregnant via intercourse, Randi suggests asking the patient to tell you "the story" of how she became pregnant, thus keeping the interview less threatening and nonjudgmental. The author underscores the need to be aware of the language used in the first encounter with a pregnant woman in order to set the tone for future provider–patient encounters. The most common fear reported by lesbian mothers is the fear of unsafe and inadequate care from the practitioner once the mother's sexual orientation is revealed. Reluctance to disclose sexual orientation to one's health care provider can act as a barrier to a woman receiving appropriate services and referrals (Snowden, 2011).

In their review of the literature, McManus, Hunter, and Rennus (2006) found four areas that are significant in regard to lesbians considering parenting: (1) sexual orientation disclosure to providers and finding sensitive caregivers, (2) conception options, (3) assurance of partner involvement, and (4) how to legally protect both the parents and the child. Lesbian and heterosexual pregnancies have many similarities. Issues of sexual activity, psychosocial changes related to attaining the traditionally defined maternal tasks of pregnancy (Rubin, 1984), and birth education all need to be addressed with lesbian couples. Special needs of the lesbian couple requiring

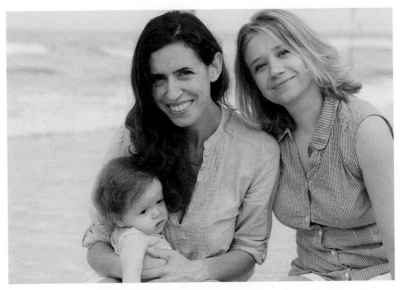

Figure 5-6. Couple with child (Dubova/Shutterstock.com).

Vulnerable and Strong: Lesbian Women Encountering Maternity Care

Phenomenology was used to interpret pregnant lesbian couples' descriptions of their maternity experiences. Vulnerability, responsibility, and caring were woven throughout the narratives, which reveal that pregnant lesbian women who disclose their sexuality to their health care provider risk judgment and discrimination. The findings highlighted three themes: being open, being exposed, and being confirmed.

Clinical Implications:

- Understand that being pregnant and living in a lesbian relationship increase visibility, thus enhancing vulnerability.
- Couples may take responsibility for acts of caring as they are accustomed to health care providers being uncertain and anxious regarding their relationship.

- Lesbian pregnant couples prefer that health care providers not focus on their sexuality, but rather treat them as any other laboring couple.
- The need to be accepted, cared for, and communicated with are essential with this group of women.
- Not using words such as "lesbian" or "partner" can be viewed as discriminating and reinforce a feeling of invisibility.
- Comprehend the responsibility of ethical caring for patients different than themselves.

Reference: Spidsberg, B. D. (2007). Vulnerable and strong- lesbian women encountering maternity care. *Journal of Advanced Nursing*, 60(5), 478–486.

assessment include social discrimination, family and social support networks, obstacles in becoming pregnant (i.e., coitus versus artificial insemination), maternal role development, legal issues of adoption by the partner, and coparenting roles (Spidsberg, 2007).

Buchholz's (2000) qualitative study was one of the first to examine the childbirth experiences of lesbian couples. The researcher focused on the positive aspects of the experience and the reasons why they were positive for the mother. Preparation of the nursing staff before the couple's arrival in the delivery area was seen by the couples as helpful. This preparation assisted the staff with the execution of the couple's birth plan and helped identify, ahead of time, nurses who would prefer not to work with the couple. The nurses' inclusion of the mother's partner in the labor and delivery process, by acknowledging their approaching parenthood and allowing the partner to assist with newborn care after

delivery, was seen as positive. The nursing staff conveyed support by using comforting gestures, checking with the couple frequently, answering questions, and just "being there" for them (Buchholz, 2000).

Buchholz's study identified two major concerns of lesbian couples. The first centered on legal issues, such as power of attorney, visiting restrictions for the partner, and birth certificate information (father identification). The second concern dealt with the couple's attention to nurses' behavioral cues and questioning whether "busyness" on the part of the nurses might somehow equate to discomfort with the situation. To further illustrate the issues surrounding nursing care and lesbian childbearing needs, a study by Spidsberg (2007) used a phenomenological hermeneutical approach to describe the meaning given to the maternity care experience by lesbian couples. See Evidence-Based Practice 5-4.

Health care providers, policy makers, and the public need to be mindful of research findings and exercise increased sensitivity when providing care and establishing evidence-based practice standards and policies, in order to meet the needs of the expanding view of "family."

Maternal Role Attainment

Maternal role attainment is often taken for granted in Western culture. If you give birth and become a mother, the assumption is that you automatically become "maternal" and successfully care for and nurture your infant. However, many factors can affect maternal role attainment, including separation of mother and infant in cases such as illness, incarceration, or adoption, to name only a few.

An example of successful maternal role attainment superimposed with a chronic illness is described in a phenomenological study that explored factors affecting maternal role attainment in HIV-positive Thai mothers selected for their successful adaptation to the maternal role. The results indicated six internal and external factors used to assist in attainment: (1) setting a purpose of raising their babies; (2) keeping their HIV status secret; (3) maintaining feelings of autonomy and optimism by living as if nothing were wrong, that is, normalization; (4) belief of quality versus quantity of support from husbands, mothers, or sisters; (5) hope for a cure; and (6) belief that their secret is safe with their health care providers. The study results indicated that while the diagnosis of HIV created challenges in attaining the mothering role, the women's feelings of shame of infection (seen as a disease of prostitutes in Thai culture) were buffered by their will to live and their love of and hope for a future with their children. The researcher notes that in Thai society, women are the major agents of socialization in a child's life. As such, the knowledge gained by studying how HIV-positive Thai mothers managed the dual demands of survival and the attainment of the maternal role will help health care providers as they work to care for and provide support to women in similar circumstances (Jirapaet, 2001).

Nontraditional Support Systems

A cultural variation that has important implications is a woman's perception of the need for formalized assistance from health care providers during the antepartum period. Western medicine is generally perceived as having a curative rather than a preventive focus. Indeed, many health care providers view pregnancy as a physiologic state that at any moment will become pathologic. Because many cultural groups perceive pregnancy as a normal physiologic process, not seeing pregnant women as ill or in need of the curative services of a doctor, women in these diverse groups often delay seeking, or even choose not to seek, prenatal care.

Pregnant women and their partners have been placing increased emphasis on the quality of pregnancy and childbirth for some time, with many childbearing women relying on nontraditional support systems. For couples who are married, white, middle class, and infrequent users of their extended family for advice and support in childbirth-related matters, this kind of support might not be crucial. However, for other, more traditional cultural groups, including African Americans, Hispanics, Filipinos, Asians, and Native Americans, the family and social network (especially the grandmother or other maternal relatives) may be of primary importance in advising and supporting the pregnant woman.

A number of factors influence childbearing practices for Filipino women including cultural beliefs, socioeconomic factors, and, in recent years, Western medicine. Approximately 41% of Filipino births are supported by indigenous attendants called *hilots*. The attendants act as a consultant throughout the pregnancy. During the postpartum period, the *hilot* performs a ritualistic sponge bath with oils and herbs, which is believed to have both physical and psychological benefits. The extended family is involved in the care of the baby, mother, and the household. Breast-feeding

is encouraged and hot soups are encouraged to increase milk production (Pacquiao, 2008).

In Arab countries, labor and delivery is considered the business of women. Traditionally, *dayahs* and midwives presided over home deliveries. The *dayahs* provide support during the pregnancy and labor and are considered by traditional Arab women to be most knowledgeable due to their experience in caring for other pregnant women. Hospital births are on the rise in most Arab countries, with a decrease in the number of traditional home births (Purnell, 2012).

A thorough cultural assessment to ascertain a pregnant woman's use of nontraditional support systems and/or Western health care during her pregnancy is essential. Once this assessment is complete and a trusting relationship has been established, the woman's pregnancy can be managed with consideration given to all the components that both she and the nurse believe are important for a successful outcome. Support during labor is known to have positive effects, such as reduced labor pain, reduced stress, shorter duration of labor, less medication need, increased maternal satisfaction, and a positive attitude going into motherhood (Chalmers & Wolman, 1993; Gordon et al., 1999). The decision for the type of support desired by a woman often has cultural underpinnings and must be explored in order to make appropriate cultural accommodations in care when possible.

Cultural Beliefs Related to Activity During Pregnancy

Cultural variations also involve beliefs about activities during pregnancy. A belief is something held to be actual or true on the basis of a specific rationale or explanatory model. **Prescriptive beliefs**, which are phrased positively, describe what should be done to have a healthy baby; the more common **restrictive beliefs**, which are phrased negatively, limit choices and behaviors and are practices/behaviors that the mother should *not* do in order to have a healthy baby. **Taboos**, or restrictions with serious supernatural

consequences, are practices believed to harm the baby or the mother. Many people believe that the activities of the mother—and to a lesser extent of the father—influence newborn outcome. Box 5-2 describes some traditional prescriptive and restrictive beliefs and taboos that provide cultural boundaries for parental activity during pregnancy. These beliefs are attempts to increase a sense of control over the outcome of pregnancy.

Negative or restrictive beliefs are widespread and numerous. They include activity, work, and sexual, emotional, and environmental prescriptions. Taboos include the Orthodox Jewish avoidance of baby showers, divulgence of the infant's name before the infant's official naming ceremony, and laws, customs, and practices during labor and delivery (Noble, Rom, Newsome-Wicks, Engelhardt, & Woloski-Wruble, 2009). One Hispanic taboo involves the traditional belief that an early baby shower will invite bad luck, or *mal ojo*, the evil eye (Spector, 2008).

Positive beliefs often involve wearing special articles of clothing, such as the *muneco* worn by some traditional Hispanic women to ensure a safe delivery and prevent morning sickness. Other beliefs and practices involve ceremonies and recommendations about physical and sexual activity.

A cultural belief may cause harm if there is a poor neonatal outcome and the mother blames herself. For example, the mother whose fetus has died as a result of a cord accident, and who believes that hanging laundry caused the cord to encircle the baby's neck or body, might experience severe guilt. The nurse who is sensitive to the mother's anguish might say, "Many people say that if you reach over your head during pregnancy, it will cause the cord to wrap around the baby's neck. Have you heard this belief?" Once the woman responds, the nurse can explore her feelings about the practice. Do others in her family or social support network share her belief? The nurse might share her own views by saying, "I have not read in any medical or nursing books that this practice is related to cord problems, although I know many people share your belief." The discussion can then continue focusing on the

Box 5-2 Cultural Beliefs Regarding Activity and Pregnancy

Prescriptive Beliefs

- Remain active during pregnancy to aid the baby's circulation (Crow Indian)
- Keep active during pregnancy to ensure a small baby and an easy delivery (Mexican and Cambodian)
- Remain happy to bring the baby joy and good fortune (Pueblo and Navajo Indian, Mexican, Japanese)
- Sleep flat on your back to protect the baby (Mexican)
- Continue sexual intercourse to lubricate the birth canal and prevent a dry labor (Haitian, Mexican)
- Continue daily baths and frequent shampoos during pregnancy to produce a clean baby (Filipino)

Restrictive Beliefs

- Avoid cold air during pregnancy to prevent physical harm to the fetus (Mexican, Haitian, Asian)
- Do not reach over your head or the cord will wrap around the baby's neck (African American, Hispanic, White, Asian)
- Avoid weddings and funerals or you will bring bad fortune to the baby (Vietnamese)
- Do not continue sexual intercourse or harm will come to you and baby (Vietnamese, Filipino, Samoan)

- Do not tie knots or braid or allow the baby's father to do so because it will cause difficult labor (Navajo Indian)
- Do not sew (Pueblo Indian, Asian)

Taboos

- Avoid lunar eclipses and moonlight or the baby might be born with a deformity (Mexican)
- Do not walk on the streets at noon or 5 o'clock because this might make the spirits angry (Vietnamese)
- Do not join in traditional ceremonies like Yei or Squaw dances or spirits will harm the baby (Navajo Indian)
- Do not get involved with persons who cast spells or the baby will be eaten in the womb (Haitian)
- Do not say the baby's name before the naming ceremony or harm might come to the baby (Orthodox Jewish)
- Do not have your picture taken because it might cause stillbirth (African American)
- During the postpartum period, avoid visits from widows, women who have lost children, and people in mourning because they will bring bad fortune to the baby (South Asian Canadian)

Information on Cambodian Canadian, Asian, Iranian Canadian, Japanese, South Asian Canadian, Vietnamese, and Haitian cultures from Waxler-Morrison, N., Andrews, J., & Richardson, E. (1990). *Cross-cultural caring: A handbook for health professionals*. Vancouver, BC: University of British Columbia Press.

feelings and perceptions of the event as experienced by the woman and her family.

Food Taboos and Cravings

Many cultures traditionally believed that the mother had little control over the outcome of pregnancy except through the avoidance of certain foods. Another traditional belief in many cultures is that a pregnant woman must be given the food that she smells to eat; otherwise, the fetus will move inside of her and a miscarriage will result (Spector, 2008). Spicy, cold, and sour foods are often believed to be foods that a pregnant woman should avoid during pregnancy.

Some pregnant women experience pica: the craving for and ingestion of nonfood substances, such as clay, laundry starch, or cornstarch. Some Hispanic women prefer the solid milk of magnesia that can be purchased in Mexico, whereas other women eat the ice or frost that forms inside refrigerator units. The causes of pica are poorly

understood, but there are some cultural implications because women from certain ethnic or cultural groups experience this disorder more frequently than others. In the United States, pica is common in African American women raised in the rural South and in women from lower socioeconomic levels. It is not uncommon to see small balls of clay in plastic bags sold in country stores in the rural South. The phenomenon of pica has also been described in other countries including Kenya, Uganda, and Saudi Arabia (Boyle & Mackey, 1999).

Cultural Issues Impacting Prenatal Care

Mexican American childbearing women seem to represent a healthy model for preventing LBW infants. However, acculturation to US lifestyle may put them at an increased risk for poor birth outcomes, according to a study conducted by Martin et al. (2004). An ethnographic study in California examined the influence of acculturation on pregnancy beliefs and practices of Mexican American childbearing women. Lagana (2003) reported that "selective biculturalism" emerged as a protective approach to stress reduction and health promotion. The women interviewed indicated that regardless of the level of acculturation to US culture, during pregnancy, they returned to traditional Mexican practices. Such practices include a low-fat, high-protein, natural diet (eat right—*come bien*); exercise for well-being (walk—*camina*); and avoidance of worry or stress, which could have a negative effect on the pregnancy outcome (don't worry— *no se preocupe*). The women described the family as a major support during pregnancy, but also valued the economic and personal freedom available to women in the United States. These conflicting values lead to the adoption of a "selective bicultural perspective." This perspective allowed the women to maintain or reject cultural practices as needed. The fact that the women in this study lived in a largely Latino town might have limited their bicultural stress; pregnant Mexican

women living in a more heterogeneous environment might experience higher levels of stress related to cultural conflicts. The author suggests, "It is likely that some cultural traits protective of pregnancy are lost through the process of acculturation" (Lagana, 2003, p. 123). This statement indicates that health care providers need to not only consider the support from family and social support networks but also explore the impact of stress from cultural conflicts on pregnancy outcomes. Some research has shown that preventive and health-promoting behaviors in pregnant minority women can be used to encourage healthy lifestyles and optimal utilization of health services and to obtain better outcomes of pregnancy (Feng, Zhang, & Owen, 2007).

Cultural Interpretation of Obstetric Testing

Many women do not understand the emphasis that Western prenatal care places on urinalysis, blood pressure readings, and abdominal measurements. For traditional Islamic women from the Middle East, the vaginal examination can be so intrusive and embarrassing that they avoid prenatal visits or request a female physician or midwife. For women of other cultural groups, common discomforts of pregnancy might be managed with folk, herbal, home, or over-the-counter remedies on the advice of a relative (generally the maternal grandmother) or friends (Spector, 2008). Health care providers can attempt to meet the needs of women from traditional cultures by explaining health regimens so that they have meaning within the cultural belief system. However, such explanations are only an initial step. Nursing visits can be made to the home, or group prenatal visits might be made based on self-care models instituted by nurses in local community centers. Additionally, nurses can incorporate significant others into the plan of care. During prenatal visits, nurses can provide information on normal fetal growth and development, and they can discuss how the health and behavior of the mother and those around her can influence fetal outcome.

Cultural Preparation for Childbirth

Women from diverse cultural backgrounds often use culturally appropriate ways of preparing for labor and delivery. These methods might include assisting with childbirth from the time of adolescence, listening to birth and baby stories told by respected elderly women, or following special dietary and activity prescriptions during the antepartal period. Most commonly in American culture, pregnant women and their significant others attend childbirth classes/or get pregnancy information from the Internet.

Preparation for childbirth can be developed through programs that allow for cultural variations, including classes during and after the usual clinic hours in busy urban settings, teen-only classes, single-mother classes, group classes combined with prenatal checkups at home, classes on rural reservations, and presentations that incorporate the older "wise women" of the community. In addition, nurses can organize classes in languages other than English and conduct these classes in community settings that are culturally appropriate and welcoming to women.

Birth and Culture

Beliefs and customs surrounding the experience of labor and delivery can vary, despite the fact that the physiologic processes are basically the same in all cultures. Factors such as cultural attitudes toward the achievement of birth, methods of dealing with the pain of labor, recommended positions during delivery, the preferred location for the birth, the role of the father and the family, and expectations of the health care practitioner might vary according to the degree of acculturation to Western childbirth customs, geographic location, religious beliefs, and individual preference.

Traditionally, cultures have viewed the birth of a child in one of two very different ways. For example, the birth of the first son may be considered a great achievement worthy of celebration, or the birth may be viewed as a state of defilement or pollution requiring various purification ceremonies. Western culture generally views birth as an achievement. This achievement is not always attributed solely to the mother, but extends to the medical staff as well. Gifts and celebrations are often centered on the newborn rather than the mother. Increasingly, pregnant women and their partners are assuming more active roles in the management of their own health and birth experiences. Playing an active role, however, does not always ensure the desired outcome. For example, some women who have prepared themselves for a "natural" childbirth might ultimately require analgesia or a cesarean section, potentially causing feelings of disappointment or a sense of failure.

Traditional Home Birth

All cultures have an approach to birth rooted in a tradition of home birth, being within the province of women. For generations, traditions among the poor included the use of "granny" midwives by rural Appalachian Whites and southern African Americans and *parteras* by Mexican Americans. A dependence on self-management, a belief in the normality of labor and birth, and a tradition of delivery at home might influence some women to arrive at the hospital in advanced labor. The need to travel a long distance to the closest hospital might also be a factor contributing to arrival during late labor or to out-of-hospital delivery for many American Indian women living on rural, isolated reservations.

Liberian women are reluctant to share information about pregnancy and childbirth as these subjects are taboo to talk about with others. Husbands or male elders are the ones who make decisions about allowing a woman to seek care at a clinic or hospital when she is experiencing a difficult and arduous labor. Further complicating this situation, women are reluctant to seek professional health care at clinics or hospitals because they are more comfortable in their own homes with traditional (but untrained) birth attendants (Lori & Boyle, 2011). These findings highlight that the influence of culture on childbirth extends beyond the birth experience itself, often affecting the outcome.

The literature offers another recent example of the impact culture has on childbearing care

Reproductive Health in Indigenous Chihuahua: Giving Birth "Alone Like the Goat"

Chopel (2014) examined the beliefs and practices of an indigenous, reclusive group of women in Chihuahua, Mexico. The women are from four ethnic groups collectively called the Tarahumaras. Due to their remote location, there is limited information regarding their reproductive health outcomes, risks, protective factors, and beliefs and behaviors. They provide for themselves through farming and goat herding. Using a qualitative, mixed methods approach, the author describes health inequities, health care barriers, and contextual issues that must be considered when developing interventions for indigenous women like the Tarahumaras. In-depth interviews ($n = 31$) were conducted with local health agents, key state officials, indigenous community leaders, traditional doctors, and indigenous trained *parteras empiricas*. Focus groups ($n = 16$) were also conducted with female and male community members along with participant observation and field notes. Analysis was aided by using the open source coding software, TAMS. Major concepts included disparities in biomedical knowledge, trust between nonindigenous providers and the patient, and structural issues impacting medical access.

Clinical Implications:

- Include key community leaders and indigenous healers when developing, implementing, and evaluating interventions.
- Assist in increasing safe births and decreasing unplanned pregnancies by making a broad choice of family planning options available at every health encounter.
- Increase "safe birth" practices; encourage women to deliver their babies in a hospital or local clinic while simultaneously preparing for an emergency home birth.
- Advocate for solar electricity for local clinics, health houses, or health centers to improve proper lighting for births and radio communications with the nearest hospital.
- Advocate for "holistic hospitals," which can provide both indigenous and medical assistance.
- Promote Kangaroo care for mothers and babies to enhance exclusive breast-feeding and bonding.

Reference: Chopel, A. (2014). Reproductive health in indigenous Chihuahua: Giving birth 'alone like the goat'. *Ethnicity & Health, 19*(3), 270–296.

practices of a remote population of women in Mexico (see Evidence-Based Practice 5-5). These findings indicate that as health care groups working with indigenous populations strive to design programs to improve health outcomes, integrating cultural beliefs into Western health care education might ultimately improve client satisfaction and health outcomes.

Support During Childbirth

Despite the traditional emphasis on female support and guidance during labor, women from diverse cultures report a desire to have husbands or partners present for the birth. Spouses or partners are now encouraged and even expected to make important contributions in supporting pregnant women during labor. Unfortunately, some US hospitals still enforce rules that limit the support person from attending the birth unless he or she has attended a formal childbirth education program. A description of the effects of Turkish fathers' attendance during labor and delivery on the experience of childbirth is presented in Evidence-Based Practice 5-6.

Many women also wish to have their mother or some other female relative or friend present during labor and birth. Because many hospitals have rules limiting the number of persons present, the mother-to-be might be forced to make a difficult choice among the persons close to her.

Effects of Fathers' Attendance to Labor and Delivery on the Experience of Childbirth in Turkey

This study was planned to experimentally determine the effects of fathers' attendance to labor and delivery on the experience of childbirth. The concept of allowing a partner's attendance in labor and delivery has not been popular in Turkey because of cultural and religious reasons, hospital policies, and environmental conditions in delivery units. Partner attendance has increased in recent years, but the opportunity is still limited and only available in a few hospitals.

The study recruited 50 primigravida low-risk women and their partners, assigning half of the women and their partners to an experimental group and half to a control group. The Perception of the Birth Scale was used to measure women's attitudes about the labor and delivery experience; the Father Interview Form was used to describe fathers' participation styles and experiences in labor and delivery. Women in the control group did not have their husbands in the labor and delivery rooms where they received routine care.

The fathers attending the labor indicated they were there "to support their wives." All the fathers adopted active roles in supporting their wives with breathing, relaxation techniques, and emotional support; however, at the time of delivery, 44% of the fathers-to-be chose to leave the delivery room, while the other 56% stayed and continued supporting their wives. Wives whose husbands adopted an active support role through the labor and birth reported more positive perceptions about their delivery experience and were more aware of events during the birth. The researchers concluded that the fathers' presence and support had positive effects on all aspects of childbirth. This study supports other research that provides powerful evidence of improved outcomes such as shorter labors, less analgesia use, less operative vaginal delivery, or cesarean section when mothers are supported in labor.

Clinical Implications:

- Support childbirth education and preparation for both fathers and mothers when culturally acceptable and appropriate.
- Encourage and support fathers to adopt an active role in childbirth.
- Work to change hospital policies and cultural myths that exclude fathers' involvement in pregnancy, birth, and the postpartum period.

Reference: Gunger, I., & Beji, N. K. (2007). Effects of fathers' attendance to labor and delivery on the experience of childbirth in Turkey. *Western Journal of Nursing Research*, 29, 213–231.

For reasons of modesty, an Orthodox Jewish woman in labor may choose a woman from the community as a labor support person (Noble et al., 2009). The spouse may elect to stay in the labor room, provided the mother's private parts are covered. Similar findings are reported from women of Islamic, Chinese, and Asian Indian backgrounds. Practices followed by these groups might include strict religious and cultural prohibitions against viewing the woman's body by *either* the husband or any other man. Labor practices are explicit for Orthodox Jewish women. Men are expected to not touch their wife or view their wife's genital area; they may offer verbal support. The culturally sensitive nurse will make every effort to cover or drape the woman appropriately and to provide the husband with the opportunity to excuse himself during the delivery without fear of being viewed as being insensitive (Purnell & Selekman, 2008). Other noteworthy considerations when caring for laboring Orthodox Jewish couples include keeping the laboring mother's head covered at all times, perhaps by providing her with a surgical cap, and allowing an Orthodox man to pick up his newborn directly

Box 5-3 Intrapartum Nursing Care for Culturally Diverse Women

1. If you are unable to speak the woman's language, make every effort to arrange for an interpreter.
2. If your nursing agency commonly cares for culturally diverse clients, find out whether other nurses have had experiences with similar clients. Share resources and your expertise with staff members.
3. Attempt to gain as much information as possible by completing a cultural assessment. (See Appendix A for the Andrews/Boyle Transcultural Nursing Assessment Guide for Individuals and Families.)
4. Elicit the mother's expectations about her labor and delivery experience.
5. Ask if she wants a support person with her. If so, have her identify that person.
6. Explore with her any cultural rituals she wants incorporated into her plan of care. If requests are manageable, honor them.
7. Be patient, draw pictures, gesture. Identify key words from family or the interpreter that you will need to be able to express yourself to her, for example, push, blow, pant, and stop.

from the crib versus having a female nurse or physician hand him the newborn; practicing Orthodox men are not allowed contact with adult women other than their spouses (Noble et al., 2009).

Nurses must determine how much personal control and involvement are desired by a woman and her family during the birth experience. It is always best practice for the nurse to ask patients directly about their cultural beliefs and preferences so that hospital practices can be aligned with individual needs.

Economically disadvantaged women from culturally diverse backgrounds have few birth options; most labor and give birth in large public hospitals. Routine patterns of care and decreased individualization are common in these institutions. These and other problems, such as language barriers, make the provision of culturally competent care during the birth process a challenge. However, any special provisions or attempts to understand the client from her perspective will be received with cooperation and gratitude. Recommendations for intrapartum nursing care of the culturally diverse pregnant woman are presented in Box 5-3.

Cultural Expression of Labor Pain

Although the pain threshold is remarkably similar in all persons, regardless of gender or social, ethnic,

or cultural differences, these differences play a definite role in a person's perception and expression of pain. Pain is a highly personal experience, dependent on cultural learning, the context of the situation, and other factors unique to the individual (Ludwig-Beymer, 2008). In the past, it was commonly believed that because women from Asian and Native American cultures were stoic, they did not feel pain in labor (Bachman, 2000). In addition to the physiologic processes involved, cultural attitudes toward the normalcy and conduct of birth, expectations of how a woman should act in labor, and the role of significant others influence how a woman expresses and experiences labor pain.

Callister and Vega (1998) reported that Guatemalan women in labor tend to vocalize their pain. Coping strategies include moaning or breathing rhythmically and massaging the thighs and abdomen. Japanese, Chinese, Vietnamese, Laotian, and other women of Asian descent maintain that screaming or crying out during labor or birth is shameful; birth is believed to be painful but something to be endured (Bachman, 2000).

Birth Positions

Numerous anecdotal reports in the literature describe "typical" birth positions for women of diverse cultures, from the seated position in a

birth chair favored by Mexican American women to the squatting position chosen by Laotian Hmong women. The choice of positions is influenced by many factors other than culture, and the socialization that occurs when a woman arrives in a labor and delivery unit might prevent her from stating her preference.

Cultural Meaning Attached to Infant Gender

The meaning that parents attach to having a son or daughter varies from culture to culture. Historically in the United States, families saw males as being the preferred gender of the firstborn child for reasons including male dominated inheritance patterns, carrying on the family name, and becoming the "man" of the family should the need arise. However, modern societies report a preference for a gender mix. Although the "structural" conditions in which son preference was originated have eroded, the related "cultural" idea of boys providing higher utility for the family, etc., may have survived. Arnold (1997) found a high persistence of son preference even in the face of rapid modernization in developing countries. In undeveloped countries, depending on the population and the cultural belief system in place, sons continue to be desired as the firstborn.

As a long tradition in Asian culture, the preferred sex of the firstborn child is male. One question related to gender preference that has not been studied until recently is, if a mother does *not* have the preferred firstborn sex, does this increase the likelihood of postpartum depression (PPD) or negatively impact mother–infant bonding? Pham and Hardie (2013) completed a study whose aim was to evaluate the association of a commonly reported cultural belief that there is a relationship between a mother's mood and the gender of an Asian woman's firstborn child. The authors used secondary analysis to address the aim of the study. The sample was obtained from the Pregnancy Risk Assessment Monitoring System (PRAMS) of 40 states in the United States and included 1,310 women of Asian origin who

delivered their first children during the prior 2 to 4 month period. Based on data from the PRAMS survey mailed 2 to 4 months postpartum, participants were selected who had given birth to their first children and were of Chinese, Japanese, Filipino, or other Asian origin. Chi-squared analyses and an independent sample test were used to assess the relationship between the child's sex and the mother's response to three PRAM mood questions; a single score was generated by summing the responses to the three questions.

The analysis of each of the three questions found there were no significant differences between Asian women whose firstborn children were female or male in their reports of feeling depressed or sad. The hypothesis that the birth of a firstborn female child would have a measurable effect on the Asian mother's mood was not supported. The practical implications, to provide care to detect symptoms of PPD in all women, remain the "pillar of care" (Pham & Hardie, 2013). For culturally competent care of Asian childbearing women, signs of impending depression may be more subtle such as constant physical complaints. Also, many Asian women may not be comfortable expressing their feelings regarding mood, and, as their cultural beliefs dictate, they may remain in bed for up to 1 month, to assist in healing. These practices should not be taken as signs of depression but rather as a trigger for nurses to learn more about their childbearing cultural belief system.

Culture and the Postpartum Period

Western medicine considers pregnancy and birth the most dangerous and vulnerable time for the childbearing woman. However, other cultures place much more emphasis on the postpartum period. Many cultures have developed special practices during this time of vulnerability for the mother and the infant in order to mobilize support and strengthen the new mother for her new role (Lee, Yang, & Yang, 2013).

In a study by Igarashi, Horiuchi, and Porter (2013), the researchers investigated what influenced Japanese women's postpartum experience either positively or negatively. Interestingly, the research revealed that lack of Japanese health literacy was more likely to obstruct positive communication between the patient and health care providers while in the hospital setting, leading to loneliness. When women felt loneliness, they rated their care satisfaction low. These findings underscore the need for nurses to include the patient's health literacy level as part of their regular assessment and make culturally appropriate adjustments to ensure proper patient education and participation in care.

Postpartum Depression

Postpartum depression (PPD) is reported worldwide. However, identifying and reporting of PPD in non-Western cultures may be delayed by culturally unacceptable labeling of the disorder, varying symptoms, or differences in treatments from culture to culture (American Psychiatric Association, 2013; Committee on Cultural Psychiatry, 2002; Yoshida, Yamashita, Ueda, & Tashiro, 2001). Insights provided by the literature suggest nurses should assess new mothers for culture-specific signs of PPD with the understanding that not all cultures recognize PPD as a medical disorder. Symptoms we associate with PPD are viewed differently in other cultures, for example, as a sign of "spirit possession," as in some traditional Muslim cultures.

"Jinn" possession, as reported in a study conducted in the United Kingdom by Hanely and Brown (2014), includes possession by an evil spirit that has a negative power over the mind and the body. Symptoms include anxiety, crying, mood swings, and emotional instability, all of which are symptoms of PPD. However in this particular culture, the symptoms are not associated with PPD but are believed to be caused by the Jinn's influence. The purpose of the study was to explore the maternal experience of Jinn possession compared with Western interpretations

of PPD. The study, which took place in an Arabian Gulf state in a Muslim community, included 10 women who had recently given birth and identified themselves as experiencing Jinn possession. Data were collected using open-ended interviews in the Arabic language. Data analysis consisted of recorded interviews being transcribed verbatim, with coding, category development, and finally the identification of themes. The four major themes included shared knowledge of Jinn possession, symptoms of possession, risk factors for possession, and preventing and treating Jinn possession. The results confirmed that the symptoms of Jinn possession align with PPD symptoms.

In Western culture, treatment for PPD typically follows a pharmaceutical approach. However, drug treatment may be culturally inappropriate for Muslim women experiencing such symptoms. Culturally appropriate care may instead include support through family and community (Hanely & Brown, 2014). Clinical implications include the importance of nurses acknowledging the illness and the feelings the woman expresses and allowing her to choose the treatment that she feels is right for her.

Hot/Cold Theory

Central to the belief of perceived imbalance in the mother's physical state is adherence to the hot/cold theories of disease causation. Pregnancy is considered a "hot" state. Because a great deal of the heat of pregnancy is thought to be lost during the birth process, postpartum practices focus on restoring the balance between the hot and cold, or yin and yang. Common components of this theory focus on the avoidance of cold, in the form of air, water, or food. This real fear of the detrimental effects of cold air and water in the postpartum period can cause cultural conflict when the woman and infant are hospitalized. In order to avoid conflict, some women may pretend to follow the activities suggested by nurses, for example, pretending to shower. Nurses must assess the woman's beliefs regarding bathing and other self-care practices in a nonjudgmental manner.

The common use of perineal ice packs and sitz baths to promote healing can be replaced with the use of heat lamps, heat packs, and anesthetic or astringent topical agents for those who prefer to avoid cold influences. The routine distribution of ice water to all postpartum women is another aspect of care that can be modified to meet a woman's cultural needs. Offering women a choice of water at room temperature, warm tea or coffee, broth, or another beverage should satisfy most women's needs for warmth, along with the offering of additional bed blankets. It is always appropriate to discuss cultural practices with the new mother to elicit her concerns, needs, and preferences.

Postpartum Dietary Prescriptions and Activity Levels

Dietary prescriptions are also common in this period. The nurse might note that a woman eats little "hospital" food and relies on family and friends to bring food to her while she is in the hospital. If there are no dietary restrictions for health reasons, this practice should be respected. Fruits and vegetables and certainly cold drinks might be avoided because they are considered "cold" foods. Indeed, the nurse should assess what types of food are being eaten by the woman and document them as appropriate to ensure the foods are nutritious and not harmful.

Regulation of activity in relation to the concept of disharmony or **imbalance** includes the avoidance of air, cold, and evil spirits. Hispanic women are encouraged to stay indoors and avoid strenuous work. Since pregnancy and birth are believed to cause a "hot" state, the woman should avoid "hot" activities such as excessive exercise, including sex, strenuous household chores, quarrelling, or crying (Sein, 2013) in order to achieve the balance between hot and cold. Some women from traditional cultural groups view themselves as "sick" during the postpartal lochia flow. They might avoid heavy work, showering, bathing, or washing their hair during this time. Cultural prescriptions vary regarding when women can

return to full activity after childbirth: Many traditional cultures suggest that a woman can resume normal activities in as little as 2 weeks; others suggest waiting up to 4 months.

Postpartum Rituals

Placental burial rituals are part of the traditional Hmong culture, and with the continued growth in the number of Hmong Americans emigrating from California to different areas of the United States, cultural conflicts are common, especially in the areas of reproductive health (Clemings, 2001). In an effort to assimilate, many Hmong have continued to use animistic ceremonies and herbal remedies in addition to using Western medicine. Helsel and Mochel's (2002) study explored Hmong Americans' attitudes regarding placental disposition, cultural values affecting those attitudes, and perceptions of the willingness of Western providers to accommodate Hmong patients' wishes regarding placental disposal. The Hmong believe the placenta is the baby's "first clothing" and must be buried at the family's home, in a place where the soul can find the afterlife garment once the person is deceased. If the soul is unable to find the placental "jacket," it will not be able to reunite with its ancestors and will spend eternity wandering. Helsel and Mochel's study (2002) suggests that even though Hmong immigrants have embraced Western culture, traditional Hmong beliefs about placental burial remain an important cultural belief. These beliefs should be respected and the staff should make every effort to accommodate their request.

Cultural Influences on Breast-Feeding and Weaning Practices

Culturally, breast-feeding and weaning can be affected by a variety of values and beliefs related to societal trends, religious beliefs, the mother's work activities, ethnic cultural beliefs, social support, access to information on breast-feeding, and the health care provider's personal beliefs and experiences regarding breast-feeding and/or

weaning practices, to name a few. The World Health Organization and UNICEF (2010) recommend children worldwide be breast-fed exclusively for the first 6 months of life followed by the addition of nutritional foods, as they continue to breast-feed for up to 2 years, with no defined upper limit on the duration. Physiologically, children can successfully breast-feed for the first several years of life. While this is common in other cultures, few women in the United States participate in extended breast-feeding (longer than 3 years) for fear of disapproval; if prolonged breast-feeding does occur, it is often concealed from family, friends, and health care providers. Dettwyler's work (2004) in this area reports segments of the country where relatively large groups of women nurse longer than 3 years. These areas include Seattle, WA; Salt Lake City, UT; College Station, TX; and Wilmington, DE.

Cartagena et al. (2014) support this view reporting that Hispanic mothers are more likely to practice nonexclusive breast-feeding, initiate early introduction of solid foods including ethnic foods, and perceive plumper infants as healthy infants. Cultural norms driving family influences and socioeconomic factors do play a role in the feeding practices of this population.

For breast-feeding women from traditional backgrounds, it is important for nurses to be aware of factors that have been shown to affect the quality and duration of the breast-feeding experience, along with factors impacting weaning practices. Wambach and Cohen's (2009) qualitative study examined breast-feeding experiences of urban adolescent mothers. English-speaking adolescent mothers, between the ages of 13 and 18, who were currently breast-feeding or had breast-fed their infants within the past 6 months, were invited from teen obstetric clinics at two urban university-affiliated medical centers. Twenty-three teens completed the study. The findings indicated that adolescent mothers chose breast-feeding mainly for infant health reasons, closeness, and bonding. Among those who weaned, problems, such as perceptions of insufficient milk supply, nipple/breast pain, time

demands of school or work, problems with pumping, embarrassment, lack of support, and feeling overwhelmed and frustrated led to weaning. Many who weaned did not seek help and reported regret about weaning earlier than planned. Those who continued breast-feeding beyond 6 weeks reported significant emotional and informational support from family, friends, school, and their babies. The findings indicate a need for tailoring interventions based on the mother's developmental stage in life and a need to educate and support teens to help prevent early weaning.

McKee, Zayas, and Jankowski (2004) examined predictors of successful breast-feeding initiation and persistence in a sample of low-income African American and Hispanic women in the urban Northeast. The findings indicated that those women with a strong cultural identification and cultural social support tended to initiate breast-feeding and continue with breast-feeding longer than those in the groups who did not have strong cultural identification. Adolescent African American and Latina mothers in Chicago were interviewed to explore the teens' perceptions of breast-feeding and what influenced their infant-feeding decisions and practices. Reported influences included perceptions of breast-feeding benefits (bonding, baby's health), perceptions of the problems with breast-feeding (pain, embarrassment, no experience with the act of breast-feeding), and respected, influential people (Hannon, Willis, Bishop-Townsend, Martinez, & Scrimshaw, 2000).

Researchers have studied ethnicity, cultural beliefs or practices, and social mores as a way to understand the influences on infant-feeding practices. However, one group, in particular—the Native American population—has been studied less closely. Breast-feeding among indigenous populations (e.g., Aboriginal/Alaska Native and American Indian women) declined with the advent of infant formula availability. However, there has been a push from within Native American communities to a return to infant feeding "the natural way." There has also been research suggesting that breast-feeding may have

a significant impact on the development of diabetes in later life. A program that targets promotion of breast-feeding among Native women as a type 2 diabetes prevention intervention promotes the use of elders and family for support (Murphy & Wilson, 2008). Banks (2003) describes how breast-feeding is being successfully promoted among the Kanesatake, a rural Mohawk community in Quebec, Canada, using culturally competent community-based interventions. The promotion strategies include educating extended family on breast-feeding benefits; teaching the nutritional merits of breast-feeding, particularly to the maternal grandmother; addressing the social, emotional, and spiritual aspects of breast-feeding; using the oral tradition as a way to share information; setting the stage for cooperative and interactive learning; and creating teaching methods that avoid conventional courses, lectures, or written materials on infant-feeding practices, as native women are not attracted to or affected by these methods.

In the Kanesatake project, a respected elder volunteered to promote breast-feeding in her community. After completing a training session, she chose to use subtle teaching encounters at banks, grocery stores, and social gatherings as a way to promote breast-feeding. Support groups or "talking circles" were organized for extended family and grandmothers of pregnant women where breast-feeding issues were discussed openly and freely, led by the elder. This approach is a good example of how community strengths, incorporation of culturally specific learning styles, and cultural sensitivity can be used as the foundation for successful program development.

Prior to the industrialized age, women always breast-fed or, if they were of "royal" blood or upper class, they used "wet nurses," women who had recently had a baby themselves and breast-fed other women's babies. Midwives attended births. They had a variety of names: aunties, medicine women, midwives, doulas, or grandmothers (grannies), but whatever their names, they were women that have and still are providing the support necessary for successful birthing and breast-feeding experiences. As immigrants continue to pour into the United States and American-born women adhering to their traditional cultural heritage attempt to make informed decisions regarding infant-feeding practices, it is imperative as nurses to examine specific cultural norms and practices that influence breast-feeding outcomes as we work to develop successful strategies.

Cultural Issues Related to Intimate Partner Violence During Pregnancy

Domestic violence has emerged as one of the most significant health care threats for women and their unborn children. Numerous transcultural factors influence the prevalence of and response to domestic violence, including a history of family violence, sexual abuse experienced as a child, alcohol and drug abuse by the mother or significant other, shame associated with abuse, fear of retaliation by the abuser, or fear of financial implications if the mother leaves the abuser, to cite a few. Outcomes of abuse shared by abused women of all cultures include stress (physical and emotional), poor lifestyle health practices, delayed prenatal care, and lack of support.

A study by Shadigian and Bauer (2005) identified homicide as a leading cause of pregnancy-associated death and suicide also as an important cause of death among pregnant and recently pregnant women. Health care providers must acknowledge and understand that homicide is a leading cause of pregnancy-associated death and commonly is a result of **intimate partner violence** (IPV). Screening for both partner violence and suicidal ideation is an essential component of comprehensive health and nursing care for women during and after pregnancy.

It has been well documented (Bewley & Gibbs, 1994) that physical abuse during pregnancy is often focused on the abdomen, breasts, and/or genitals, which puts both the mother and her unborn child at risk. Physical abuse often has psychological consequences for the victim, including possible addiction to drugs and alcohol, stress,

Prenatal Care Delays Related to Battering

This study evaluated patterns of abuse during the pregnancies of 132 African American, 208 Hispanic, and 162 White American women from low-income clinics in large metropolitan cities in the West. The researchers found that the incidence of abuse did not vary significantly among ethnic groups and that the abused women from these groups sought prenatal care 6.5 weeks later than did the nonabused group. In this study, one in four women reported that they had been physically abused since their current pregnancy began, with African American women experiencing the most severe and most frequent abuse.

Clinical Implications:

- Include questions about abuse in every routine history taken during pregnancy in order to identify abused women.

- Offer information about abuse and available community resources. Women reporting abuse will need further screening with specific tools. Nurses should be aware of subtle signs of abuse. For example, psychosomatic complaints, injuries inconsistent with the explanation, failure to keep clinic appointments, and overprotective partners might be indications of abuse.

- Become familiar with community resources for referrals.

Reference: Taggart, L., & Mattson, S. (1996). Delay in prenatal care as a result of battering in pregnancy: Crosscultural implications. *Health Care for Women International*, *17*, 25–34.

and depression. These factors can also affect both the mother's health and potentially affect the future health of the newborn and later as the child develops.

Information regarding women in abusive situations is scarce, partly because of underreporting. We do know, however, that abused women are less likely to seek health care because their abuser limits access to resources and that battering occurs more frequently during pregnancy. It is estimated by the CDC (2009) that 324,000 pregnant women are victims of IPV each year.

An abused pregnant woman has a greater risk of delivering an LBW infant. One of the associations between abuse and LBW is delay in obtaining prenatal care. Indeed, findings from studies conducted during the past two decades have clearly shown that physical and sexual abuse predicts poor health during pregnancy and the postpartum period (Leserman, Stewart, & Dell, 1999). Taggart's and Mattson's (1996) study of the relationship between battering and prenatal care is still pertinent for nurses who care for pregnant women. Evidence-Based Practice 5-7 discusses this study and its importance in identifying delays in obtaining prenatal care as a result of IPV.

The legacy of patriarchy, which is still deeply embedded in our culture, undoubtedly contributes to violence against women as do other factors, especially alcohol and drug abuse. Kita, Yaeko, and Porter's (2014) study of intimate partner violence (IPV) in Japan reported risk factors associated with IPV during pregnancy, which included pregnant women over 30 years old, multiparous, previous abortion experience, and having a male partner under 30 years old.

This discussion focuses on three culturally different groups of women who may experience IPV during pregnancy: Hispanic, African American, and American Indian pregnant women. What links these groups of pregnant women are shared ideologies or characteristics that influence their behavior and have profound effects on their pregnancy outcomes. Ideologies

of each group are examined and recommendations are identified for nurses working with pregnant women in these unique circumstances. Recommendations for health care providers will follow each discussion and will emphasize the importance of culturally competent care to these at-risk clients.

Hispanic Pregnant Women

Although there are many different Hispanic groups, most share some important commonalities, for example, religion, customs, and language. As with any cultural group, differences do exist among the members. The incidence of spouse abuse among pregnant Hispanic women is not clear in the literature. Access to health care for pregnant Hispanic women is problematic. Barriers to prenatal health care include lack of health care insurance, language barriers, and low levels of education, all of which may encourage the use of traditional healers and remedies and might foster mistrust of health care professionals, leading to noncompliance. Many Hispanic women tend to be in low-paying jobs whose annual earnings are considerably less than those of non-Hispanic women. They may also have less education than White women and live in large, extended households, often made up of several children and extended family members. The literature concurs, reporting the health status of Hispanic pregnant women may be affected by their economic level as economic status has been shown to limit access to care (Center for American Progress Action Fund, 2010; Suarez & Ramirez, 1999).

These factors place Hispanic women at a distinct disadvantage for accessing prenatal care. Furthermore, these same factors tend to discourage the pregnant Hispanic woman from disclosing a situation of abuse and violence. Her choices are the same as other women in abusive situations: She can try to make the relationship work, or she can leave her abuser. Charles and Perreira (2007) investigated IPV during pregnancy and 1 year postpartum. Findings indicated that Hispanic women who are no longer romantically involved with their children's fathers were likely to experience IPV during pregnancy. Less educated women, women who reported that they or their spouses used substances (i.e., alcohol or illicit drugs), and women who reported that their pregnancy was unplanned were also at high risk of IPV both during and after their pregnancy. Pregnancy outcomes included preterm birth and LBW infants. The authors of this study noted that violence during pregnancy strongly predicted violence after pregnancy. Shneyderman and Kiely (2013) added to these findings, reporting women at highest risk in their study for pregnancy risk factors, were those participating in reciprocal violence or fighting back. Providers should consider both perpetration and victimization whenever women arrive for care, noting interventions that need to be developed according to the form of IPV presenting.

The Hispanic pregnant woman who chooses to leave her abuser must often face language barriers, a poor economic situation, no insurance, and perhaps leaving her traditional family support network. These same factors inhibit the seeking of information regarding resources available to abused women. Even when faced with death, some abused women find it very difficult to expose their private situation to someone outside their cultural circle. Furthermore, certain groups of Hispanic women, such as migrants, are at higher risk because they are separated from family support systems in addition to confronting barriers related to poverty and language.

Nurses and other health practitioners in prenatal clinics are in an ideal position to facilitate a trusting relationship with an abused woman. Good assessment skills are crucial, because the first sign of abuse might not be an admission of abuse but physical findings of trauma. It is also helpful that the nurses have strong interpersonal skills and a genuine interest in Hispanic culture. In this situation, a Spanish-speaking health care provider might be able to form a trusting relationship more quickly, enabling the woman to share information about domestic violence.

Recommendations for providing assistance to abused pregnant Hispanic women include working with and mobilizing support, using the family and kinship structure, educating the abused woman regarding available resources for abused women, encouraging the woman's inner strength, and assisting in the development of skills necessary to mobilize resources.

African American Pregnant Women

Many cultural values of African Americans emphasize the larger Black society rather than focusing on individuals, making "all" collectively responsible for one another (Hine & Thompson, 1998). Therefore, many African American women exist in a social context supported by social connectedness versus that of autonomy (see Figure 5-7).

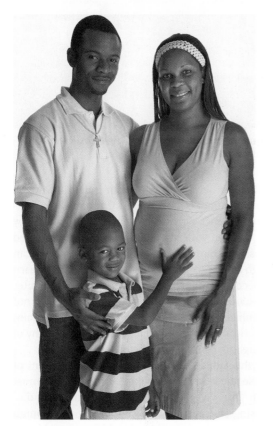

Figure 5-7. Pregnant family (Jaimie Duplass/Shutterstock.com).

It is difficult to understand the specific factors related to IPV among African American women because of the lack of information. However, poor economic conditions might be a primary reason why violence occurs in African American families; domestic violence is often related to social and economic resources. The risk of wife abuse appears to increase when the woman has a higher educational status than her partner or when the man is unemployed or has trouble keeping a job—situations that are common in African American male–female relationships (Barnes, 1999).

One of the most difficult barriers confronting African American abused women who attempt to get help from police or from the legal system is the stereotypical view that violence among African Americans is normal. This view could cause African American victims' claims of abuse to be dismissed or ignored.

Again, the nurse in the prenatal setting is in an ideal position to gather information and initiate a trusting relationship. The abused pregnant African American woman might not be willing to incriminate her spouse or significant other because she already sees him as a "victim of society." The nurse might need to rely heavily on her assessment and history-taking skills, being particularly alert to instances of trauma and problems with past pregnancies. Patient education must stress that although a woman may see her man as a "victim," that does not mean she must tolerate abuse. The nurse can identify shelter facilities in the woman's neighborhood and other areas. If the woman feels uncomfortable going outside her neighborhood (and many do for fear they will not be understood outside their culture), the nurse can encourage her to go to members of her extended family, a situation that might be more acceptable within African American culture. What is most important is that she has a plan of what to do, where to go, and whom to call for help the next time she is afraid for her own safety. Last, the nurse must realize that in most instances, African American women believe that it is the responsibility of the woman to maintain

the family, regardless of other factors. Therefore, African American women may be more likely to stay in an abusive relationship.

American Indian Pregnant Women

Violence within families has not always been part of American Indian society. Traditionally, American Indian cultures were based on harmony and respect. Many activities Western culture has ascribed to one sex were shared in American Indian society, including the roles of warrior and hunter. As Indian communities strive to maintain their cultural heritage, the concepts of spirituality (balance, harmony, oneness), passive forbearance (humility, respect, circularity, connection, honor), and behaviors that promote harmonious living are reinforced in daily living (Nichols, 2004). Historically, cruelty to women and children resulted in public humiliation and loss of honor. Cultural disintegration, poverty, isolation, racism, and alcoholism are just a few of the problems that have fostered violence in American Indian cultures. Nevertheless, cruelty to women and children continues to be viewed by American Indians as a social disgrace (Green, 1996).

In a study by Bohn (2002), the complicating factor of lifetime abuse events was shown to be a significant contributor to preterm birth and LBW infants. This means that the nurse should not only assess for current abuse by the spouse or significant other but also evaluate the other types of abuse inflicted over the mother's lifetime, such as alcohol or drug abuse. Since the 1970s, American Indian tribes have made an effort to develop programs to meet the many needs of their communities. However, violence against women has not been addressed adequately because of the male-dominated leadership, other needs of the tribes, and the shame associated with abuse (Bohn, 1993). This trend is changing gradually as Indian communities have recognized that domestic abuse is a significant social problem and are taking measures to address it (see Figure 5-8).

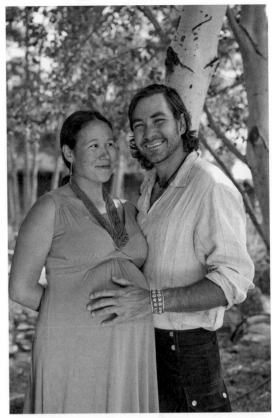

Figure 5-8. Native American couple (Mona Makela/ Shutterstock.com).

In interviews with American Indian women, a sense of humor is most helpful. Culturally, it is common for American Indians to use humor when they are dealing with stress, especially health-related stress, and they view someone with whom they can laugh as easy to talk to. The nurse should also learn to become comfortable with periods of silence after questions. This does not mean that clients are not listening but rather just the opposite. Culturally, American Indians think all questions are worthy of thoughtful consideration before answering.

Once abuse has been identified, the extent of abuse must then be evaluated. The nurse must then intervene by providing information, discussing alternatives, and supporting the woman in her decision. Options should focus on Native American resources because such resources have

usually been designed to be culturally sensitive. If only non-Indian resources are available, the nurse should follow through within these agencies.

Abuse within American Indian culture is traditionally handled within the family first. The abused woman might be reluctant to go outside of the family for help because this might cause both families (hers and her spouse's or significant other's) to ostracize her. It is important to know that American Indian women generally consider it a virtue to stay with your mate no matter what the circumstance, especially if the marriage was performed or "blessed" by a traditional medicine man or woman. A woman who chooses to stay with her abuser might do so out of loyalty to her culture. As with all women attempting to leave an abusive relationship, she must know that her health care provider cares about and views her safety and that of her unborn baby as the priority (Hellmuth, Gordon, Stuart, & Moore, 2013).

Summary

Culture, as it relates to pregnancy and childbirth, was discussed from many vantage points. As the United States becomes home to immigrants and refugees from around the world, and as once considered traditional societal norms are changing, so too must nurses adapt their care in ways that consider and are respectful of beliefs different from their own. These cultural and biologic variations have created opportunities for health care providers to learn about and incorporate evidence and traditional beliefs into current health care practices, improving pregnancy and birth experiences for all women of differing backgrounds.

Cultural beliefs and practices are continuously evolving, making it necessary for the nurse to acknowledge and explore the meaning of childbearing with each family with whom he/she has contact. It is also important to remember that behavior must be evaluated from within each person's cultural context and based on evidence, when available, so that the care provided is not only evidence based but also meaningful. It is always important for the culturally competent nurse to demonstrate genuine concern, interest, and respect for the patient's differing backgrounds. Only when these aspects are fully realized can we develop and provide culturally congruent care for childbearing women and their families.

REVIEW QUESTIONS

1. How will the biologic variations discussed impact the nursing care of the childbearing woman and her family?
2. Describe the special needs of lesbian couples during the childbearing process. What are common prejudgments about lesbian mothers and how can they affect care?
3. Compare traditional Western medical support for pregnant women with nontraditional support, and describe why both might be critical for successful pregnancy outcomes in women from diverse backgrounds.
4. Why is it important to understand the differences between prescriptive and restrictive beliefs of a mother's behavior during pregnancy?
5. How can nursing interventions for the pregnant American Indian woman presenting for IPV care be made more culturally congruent?

CRITICAL THINKING ACTIVITIES

1. Critically analyze and describe the culturally competent nursing interventions for a Hispanic woman after fetal demise from a cord accident.
2. Discuss the responses the culturally competent postpartum nurse should initiate when an Asian woman refuses to get out from under her bedding.
3. Discuss and compare the cultural differences in the expression of labor pain. Critically

analyze how you would respond to your Hispanic labor patient's expression of pain versus your Native American labor patient's manifestation of pain. Why the different approaches?

4. Describe and analyze how the nurse might alter her care approach to an Orthodox Jewish husband who has followed his cultural traditions and refuses to accept his newborn from a female nurse.

REFERENCES

American Psychiatric Association. (2013). *Diagnostic and statistical manual of mental disorders* (5th ed., text revision). Washington, DC: Author.

Amnesty International, USA. (2010). Deadly delivery: The maternal health care crises in the USA. AMR 51/007/2010.

Andrews, J.M., & Hanson, P.A. (2008). Religion, culture and nursing. In M.M. Andrews, & J.S. Boyle (Eds.)

Andrews, M. M., & Hanson, P. A. (2012). Religion, culture and nursing. In M. M. Andrews & J. S. Boyle (Eds.), *Transcultural concepts in nursing* (5th ed., pp. 351–402). Philadelphia, PA: Lippincott Williams & Wilkins.

Arnold, F. 1997. *Gender preferences for children. Demographic and Health Surveys Comparative Studies No. 23.* Calverton, MD: Macro International Inc.

Bachman, J. A. (2000). Management of discomfort. In D. L. Lowdermilk, S. E. Perry, & I. M. Bobak (Eds.), *Maternity and women's health care* (7th ed., pp. 463–487). St. Louis, MO: Mosby.

Banks, J. W. (2003). Ka'nistenhsera Teiakotihsnie's: A native community rekindles the tradition of breastfeeding. *AWHONN Lifelines, 7*(4), 340–347.

Barnes, S. Y. (1999). Theories of spouse abuse: Relevance to African Americans. *Issues in Mental Health Nursing, 20,* 357–371.

Benza, S., & Liamputtong, P. (2014). Pregnancy, childbirth and motherhood: A meta-synthesis of the lived experiences of immigrant women. *Midwifery, 30*(2014), 575–584.

Bewley, C., & Gibbs, A. (1994). Coping with domestic violence in pregnancy. *Nursing Standard, 8*(50), 25–28.

Bohn, D. K. (1993). Nursing care of Native American battered women. *AWHONN's Clinical Issues in Perinatal and Women's Health Nursing, 4*(3), 424–436.

Bohn, D. K. (2002). Lifetime and current abuse, pregnancy risks, and outcomes among Native American women. *Journal of Health Care for the Poor and Underserved, 13*(2), 184–198.

Boyle, J. S., & Mackey, M. (1999). Pica: Sorting it out. *Journal of Transcultural Nursing, 10*(1), 65–68.

Bromwich, P., & Parsons, T. (1990). *Contraception: The facts* (2nd ed.). Oxford, UK: Oxford University Press.

Buchholz, S. (2000). Experiences of lesbian couples during childbirth. *Nursing Outlook, 48*(6), 307–311.

Callister, L. C., & Vega, R. (1998). Giving birth: Guatemalan women's voices. *Journal of Obstetric, Gynecologic, and Neonatal Nursing, 27,* 289–295.

Cartagena, D. C., Ameringer, S. W., McGrath, J., Jallo, N., Masho, S. W., & Myers, B. J. (2014). Factors contributing to infant overfeeding with Hispanic mothers. *Journal of Obstetric, Gynecologic, and Neonatal Nursing, 43,* 139–159.

CDC. 2007. Unintended pregnancy prevention, home. Retrieved January 5, 2007, from http://www.cdc.gov/reproductivehealth/UnintendedPregnancy/index.htm

CDC, Division of Reproductive Health, and the National Center for Chronic Disease Prevention and Health Promotion. (2014). Retrieved June 30, 2014, from http://www.cdc.gov

Center for Disease Control and Prevention. (2009). Intimate partner violence during pregnancy: A guide for clinicians. Available at: http://www.cdc.gov/reproductivehealth/violence/intimatepartnerviolence/sld001.htm#2

Chalmers, B. (2013). Commentary, cultural issues in perinatal care. *Birth, 40*(4), 217–220.

Chalmers, B., & Wolman, W. (1993). Social support in labour—A selective review. *Journal of Psychosomatic Obstetrics and Gynaecology, 14,* 1–15.

Chamberlain, J. (n.d.). The Pima Indians: The vicious cycle. Retrieved January 3, 2007, from *National Institutes of Health, National Institute of Diabetes and Digestive and Kidney Diseases Web site*: http://diabetes.niddk.nih.gov/dm/pubs/pima/vicious/vicious.htm

Charles, P., & Perreira, K. M. (2007). Intimate partner violence during pregnancy and 1-year post-partum. *Journal of Family Violence, 22*(7), 609–619.

Chopel, A. (2014) Reproductive health in indigenous Chihuahua: Giving birth 'alone like the goat'. *Ethnicity & Health, 19*(3), 270–296.

Clemings, R. (2001). Fresno's Hmong leave for new lives. *Fresno Bee,* A1–A12.

Committee on Cultural Psychiatry. (2002). *Cultural assessment in clinical psychiatry.* Washington, DC: American Psychiatric Publishing.

d'Entremont, M., Smythe, L., & McAra-Couper, J. (2014). The sounds of silence: A hermeneutic interpretation of childbirth post excision. *Health Care for Women International, 35,* 300–319.

Dettwyler, K. A. (2004). When to wean: Biological versus cultural perspectives. *Clinical Obstetrics and Gynecology, 47*(3), 712–723.

Diabetes Monitor. (2011). Health problems in American India/Alaska native women: Diabetes. Retrieved July 6, 2014 from http://www.diabetesmonitor.com/b350.htm

Eckhardt, S., & Lauderdale, J. (2013). The impact of culture on knowledge, attitude, and practice of family planning methods in rural North Kamagambo, Kenya. Unpublished study.

Feng, D., Zhang, Y., & Owen, D. (2007). Health behaviors of low-income pregnant minority women. *Western Journal of Nursing Research, 29*, 284–300.

Finer, L. B., & Zolna, M. R.(2011). Unintended pregnancy in the United States: Incidence and disparities, 2006. *Contraception, 84*(5), 478–485.

Gordon, N. P., Walton, D., McAdam, E., Derman, J., Gallitero, G., & Garrett, L. (1999). Effects of providing hospital based doulas in health maintenance organization hospitals. *Obstetrics & Gynecology, 98*, 756–764.

Green, K. (1996). *Family violence in aboriginal communities: An aboriginal perspective.* Ottawa, ON: National Clearing House on Family Violence.

Gurnah, K., Khoshnood, K., Bradley, E., & Yuan, C. (2011). Lost in translation: Reproductive health care experiences of Somali Bantu women in Hartford, Connecticut. *Journal of Midwifery & Women's Health, 56*(4), 340–346.

Hanely, J., & Brown, A. (2014). Cultural variations in interpretation of postnatal Illness: Jinn possession amongst Muslim communities. *Community Mental Health Journal, 50*, 348–353.

Hannon, P. R., Willis, S. K., Bishop-Townsend, V., Martinez, I. M., & Scrimshaw, S. C. (2000). African-American and Latina adolescent mothers' infant feeding decisions and breastfeeding practices: A qualitative study. *Journal of Adolescent Health, 26*(6), 399–407.

Hellmuth, J., Gordon, K., Stuart, G., & Moore, T. (2013). Women's intimate partner violence perpetration during pregnancy and postpartum. *Maternal and Child Health Journal, 17*, 1405–1413.

Helsel, D., & Mochel, M. (2002). Afterbirths in the afterlife: Cultural meaning of placental disposal in a Hmong American community. *Journal of Transcultural Nursing, 13*(4), 282–286.

Hine, D. C., & Thompson, K. (1998). *A shining thread of hope.* New York, NY: Broadway Books.

Igarashi, Y., Horiuchi, S., & Porter, S. (2013). Immigrants' experiences of maternity care in Japan. *Journal of Community Health, 38*(4), 781–790.

Jirapaet, V. (2001). Factors affecting maternal role attainment among low-income, Thai, HIV-positive mothers. *Journal of Transcultural Nursing, 12*(1), 25–33.

Kita, S., Yaeko, K., & Porter, S. E. (2014). Prevalence and risk factors of intimate partner violence among pregnant women in Japan. *Health Care for Women International, 35*, 442–457.

Kolatch, A. (2000). *The second Jewish book of why.* Middle Village, NY: Jonathan David.

Lagana, K. (2003). Come bien, camina y no se preocupe— Eat right, walk and do not worry: Selective biculturalism during pregnancy in a Mexican American Community. *Journal of Transcultural Nursing, 14*(2), 117–124.

Lee, S., Yang, S., & Yang, Y. (2013). Doing-In-Month ritual among Chinese and Chinese-American. *Journal of Cultural Diversity, 20*(2), 94–99.

Leserman, J., Stewart, J., & Dell, D. (1999). Sexual and physical abuse predicts poor health in pregnancy and postpartum. *Psychosomatic Medicine, 61*, 92.

Lori, J. R., & Boyle, J. S. (2011). Cultural childbirth practices, beliefs, and traditions in post-conflict Liberia. *Health Care for Women International, 32*(6), 1–20.

Ludwig-Beymer, P. (2008). Transcultural aspects of pain. In M. M. Andrews & J. S. Boyle (Eds.), *Cultural aspects of nursing care* (pp. 329–354). Philadelphia, PA: Wolters Kluwer Health/Lippincott Williams & Wilkins.

Martin, J.A., Hamiliton, B.E.,Suton, P.D., Ventura, S.J., Menacker, F., & Munson, M.L. (2004). Births: Final date for 2002 [Data file]. National Vital Statistics Reports, 52(10). Available from CDC website, http://www.cdc.gov.

McKee, M. D., Zayas, L. H., & Jankowski, K. R. B. (2004). Breastfeeding intention and practice in an urban minority population: Relationship to maternal depressive symptoms and mother–infant closeness. *Journal of Reproductive and Infant Psychology, 22*(3), 167–181.

McManus, A. J., Hunter, L. P., & Renn, H. (2006). Lesbian experiences and needs during childbirth: Guidance for health care providers. *Journal of Obstetric, Gynecologic, and Neonatal Nursing, 35*(1), 13–23.

Miller, M. A. (1992). Contraception outside North America: Options and popular choices. *NAACOG's Clinical Issues in Perinatal and Women's Health Nursing, 3*(2), 253–265.

Mosher, W. D., Jones, J., & Abma, J. C.. (2012). Intended and unintended births in the United States: 1982–2010. *National Health Statistics Reports: U.S. Department of Health and Human Services, 55.*

Murphy, S., & Wilson, C. (2008). Breastfeeding promotion: A rational and achievable target for a type 2 diabetes prevention intervention in Native American communities. *Journal of Human Lactation, 24*(2), 193–198.

Nichols, L. A. (2004). The infant caring process among Cherokee mothers. *Journal of Holistic Nursing, 22*(3), 1–28.

Noble, A., Rom, M., Newsome-Wicks, M., Engelhardt, K., & Woloski-Wruble, A. (2009). Jewish laws, customs, and practice in labor, delivery and postpartum care. *Journal of Transcultural Nursing, 20*, 323–333.

Noblit, G. W., & Hare, R. D. (1988). *Meta-ethnography: Synthesizing qualitative studies.* Newbury Park, CA: Sage.

Overfield, T. (1985). *Biologic variation in health and illness.* Menlo Park, CA: Addison-Wesley.

Pacquiao, D. F. (2008). People of Filipino heritage. In L. Purnell & B. Paulanka (Eds.), *Transcultural health care: A culturally competent approach* (3rd ed., pp. 175–195). Philadelphia, PA: F.A. Davis Co.

Perry, S. E. (2000). Medical-surgical problems in pregnancy. In D. L. Lowdermilk, S. E. Perry, & I. M. Bobak (Eds.),

Maternity and women's health care (7th ed., pp. 887–911). St. Louis, MO: Mosby.

Pettitt, D. J., Baird, H. R., Aleck, K. A., Bennett, P. H., & Knowler, W. C. (1983). *New England Journal of Medicine, 308*, 242–245.

Pham, A., & Hardie, T. (2013). Does a first-born female child bring mood risks to new Asian American mothers? *Journal of Obstetric, Gynecologic, and Neonatal Nursing, 42*, 471–476.

Pritchard, C., Roberts, S., & Pritchard, C. (2013). Giving a voice to the unheard'? Is female youth (15–24 years) suicide linked to restricted access to family planning? Comparing two Catholic continents. *International Social Work, 56*, 798–815.

Purnell, L.,& Selekman, J. (2008). People of Jewish heritage, In: L. Purnell, & B. Paulanka (Eds.) *Transcultural health care: A culturally competent approach* (3rd ed., pp. 278–292). Philadelphia: F.A. DavisCo.

Purnell, L. (2012). *Transcultural health care: A culturally competent approach* (4th ed.). Philadelphia, PA: F.A. Davis Co.

Randi, B. S. (2012). Improving prenatal care for pregnant lesbians. *International Journal of Childbirth Education, 27*(4), 37–40.

Rocca, C., & Harper, C. (2012). Do racial and ethnic differences in contraceptive attitudes and knowledge explain disparities in method use? *Perspectives on Sexual and Reproductive Health, 44*(3), 150–158.

Rubin, R. (1984). *Maternal identity and the maternal experience*. New York, NY: Springer.

Sein, K. (2013). Beliefs and practices surrounding postpartum period among Myanmar women. *Midwifery, 29*, 1257–1263.

Shadigian, E. M., & Bauer, S. T. (2005). Pregnancy-associated death: A qualitative systematic review of homicide and suicide. *Obstetrical and Gynecological Survey, 60*(3), 183–190.

Shneyderman, Y., & Kiely, M. (2013). Intimate partner violence during pregnancy: Victim or perpetrator? Does it make a difference? *BJOG, 120*, 1375–1385.

Sonfield, A., Kost, K., & Gold, R. B (2011). The public costs of births resulting from unintended pregnancies: National and state-level estimates. *Perspectives on Sexual and Reproductive Health, 43*(2), 94–102.

Spector, R. (2008). *Cultural diversity in health and illness* (7th ed.) Upper Saddle River. NJ: Prentice Hall Health.

Spidsberg, B. D. (2007). Vulnerable and strong-lesbian women encountering maternity care. *Journal of Advanced Nursing, 60*(5), 478–486.

Suarez, L., & Ramirez, A. G. (1999). Hispanic/Latino health and disease. In R. M. Huff & M. V. Kline (Eds.), *Promoting health in multicultural populations* (pp. 115–136). Thousand Oaks, CA: Sage.

Taggart, L., & Mattson, S. (1996). Delay in prenatal care as a result of battering in pregnancy: Crosscultural implications. *Health Care for Women International, 17*, 25–34.

The Pima Indians: Obesity and Diabetes. 2010. Retrieved April 25, 2010, from http://diabetes.niddk.nih.gov/dm/pubs/pima/obesity.htm

U.S. Department of Health and Human Services. 2014. Healthy People 2020 topics & objectives. HealthyPeople.gov. [Accessed June, 2014] http://www.healthypeople.gov/2020/topicsobjectives2020/objectiveslist.aspx?

UNHCR Mid-Year Refugee Trends. (2013). Retrieved July 2, 2014 from http://www.unhcr.org/52af08d26.html

United Nations Children's Fund (UNICEF). (2005). *Changing a harmful social convention: Female genital mutilation/cutting. Innocenti Digest.* Florence, Italy: Author.

Wambach, K. A., & Cohen, S. M. (2009). Breastfeeding experiences of urban adolescent mothers. *Journal of Pediatric Nursing, 24*(4), 244–254.

Washofsky, M. (2000). *Jewish living: A guide to contemporary reform practice*. New York, NY: UAHC (Union of American Hebrew Congregations) Press.

World Health Organization (WHO). (2008). *Eliminating female genital mutilation: An interagency statement: OHCHR, UNAIDS, UNDP, UNECA, UNESCO, UNFPA, UNHCR, UNICEF, UNIFEM, WHO.* Geneva, Switzerland: Author.

World Health Organization (WHO). (2010). *Global strategy to stop health-care providers from performing female genital mutilation: UNAIDS, UNDP, UNFPA, UNICEF, UNIFEM, WHO, FIGO, ICN, IOM, WCPT, WMA, MWIA.* Geneva, Switzerland: Author.

World Health Organization and UNICEF. (2010). *Global strategy for infant and young child feeding*. Geneva, Switzerland: Switzerland World Health Organization.

Transcultural Perspectives in the Nursing Care of Children

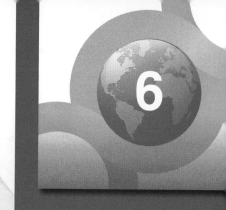

6

Margaret M. Andrews and Barbara C. Woodring

Key Terms

Bed sharing
Blended family

Conjugal family
Cosleeping
Curandero
Extended family

Infant attachment
Nuclear family
Parent-child relationship
Premasticate

Learning Objectives

1. Understand the composition of children as a population across cultures in the United States and Canada.
2. Explore childrearing practices, both specific and universal across cultures, and their impact on the development of children.
3. Analyze the impact of selected cultural beliefs and practices on the development of children.
4. Examine the biocultural aspects of selected acute and chronic conditions affecting children.
5. Synthesize the transcultural concepts and evidence-based practices that support the delivery of culturally competent care for children and adolescents.

Children in a Culturally Diverse Society

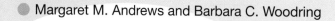

Cultural survival depends on the transmission of values and customs from one generation to the next; this process relies on the presence of children for success. This interdependent nature of children and society reinforces the need for the greater society to nurture, care for, and socialize members of the next generation. In this chapter, the composition of children as a population, the effect of childrearing practices both specific and universal across cultures, and the cultural influences on child growth, development, health, and illness are be examined as well as an understanding

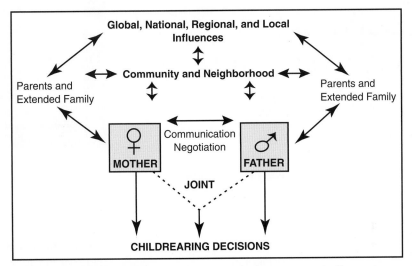

Figure 6-1. Model depicting the interrelation of culture, communication, and parental decisions about childrearing practices.

of how transcultural concepts and evidence-based practices support the delivery of culturally competent care for children and adolescents. Figure 6-1 provides a visual representation of the interrelationship among culture, communication, and parental decisions/actions during child rearing. This schematic representation also serves as a model for understanding culturally significant decisions that affect the care of children and, therefore, will be evident throughout this chapter.

Most children are cared for by their natural or adoptive parents. In this chapter, the term *parent* refers to the primary care provider whether natural, adoptive, relational (grandparents, aunts, uncles, cousins), or those who are unrelated but who function as primary providers of care and/or parent surrogates for varying periods of time. In some cases, the primary provider of care looks after the infant, child, or adolescent for a brief time, perhaps for an hour or two, while the parents are unable to do so. In other cases, this person might function as a long-term or permanent parent substitute even though legal adoption has not occurred. For example, a grandparent might assume responsibility for a child in the event of parental death, illness, disability, or imprisonment. The same factors influencing the

parents' cultural perspectives on childrearing also influence others who might assume the care of the child (Chen & Eisenberg, 2012).

Children as a Population

When defining children as a population, it is important to consider various elements that shape this population as a whole, such as its racial and ethnic makeup, the impact of poverty on this population, and the health status of children and adolescents in the United States and Canada. Other important considerations when examining this population are cross-cultural differences in growth and development, infant attachment, and crying.

Racial and Ethnic Composition

According to the U.S. Census Bureau (2013), there are 74.2 million people under the age of 18 who live in the United States; of these, 67.9% are White, 24.1% Hispanic (of any race), 14.2% Black, and 5.7% Asian/Pacific Islander/Native American/ Alaska Native. The number of Hispanic children has increased faster than that of any other group (U.S. Census Bureau, 2013). It is estimated that

by 2020, 40% of school-aged children in the United States will represent federal minority groups. More than 3.5 million children in the United States are foreign-born, and millions more are the children of recent immigrants. Many of these children constitute the more than 10.9 million school-age children who speak a language other than English at home (Ryan, 2013). Approximately two-thirds of these children come from Spanish-speaking homes, and a large percentage of the remainder speaks a variety of Asian languages. Many children of immigrants live in linguistic isolation in the 5.9% of households where no member age 14 or older speaks English "very well" (U.S. Census Bureau, 2013).

Although immigrants and their children are found throughout the United States and Canada, they tend to cluster in certain geographic areas. California, New York, Texas, Florida, New Jersey, Illinois, and Massachusetts are homes for almost two-thirds of all foreign-born children. Georgia, Virginia, Washington, Arizona, and Maryland also have relatively high numbers of children whose parents recently immigrated to the United States (U.S. Census Bureau, 2013). In Canada, most immigrants reside in one of the major metropolitan areas: Toronto, Vancouver, and Montreal are home for the majority of children of recent immigrants (Statistics Canada, 2015).

Poverty

The impact of poverty on children's health is cumulative throughout the life cycle, and disease in adulthood frequently is the result of early health-related episodes that become compounded over time. For example, when poverty leads to malnutrition during critical growth periods, either prenatally or during the first 2 years of life, the consequences can be catastrophic and irreversible, resulting in damage to the neurologic and musculoskeletal systems. If the brain fails to receive sufficient nutrients during critical growth periods, the child is likely to experience diminished cognitive development, leading to poor academic performance and later poorer job performance, lower pay, and thus perpetuation of the cycle of poverty and poor health.

Child poverty in the United States continues to grow; one in five children (16.1 million) was poor in 2012, 40% of whom lived in extreme poverty at less than half of the federal poverty level. More than two-thirds of poor children live in families with a working adult (Centers for Disease Control and Prevention, 2014a). In 2014, the Children's Defense Fund reported that two-thirds of children in poverty lived in working family households of US citizens, and more than 7.2 million children under 19 were uninsured in 2012. A disproportionate number of children in poverty are from African American and Latino backgrounds. Children in mother-only families are nearly four times as likely to be in poverty as those in married-couple families. Research links poverty to numerous risks and disadvantages for children, including increased abuse, neglect, lower reading scores, overall less success in the classroom, failure, delinquency, malnutrition, and violence (Centers for Disease Control and Prevention, 2014a; Children's Defense Fund, 2014; Carlson, McNulty, Bellair, & Watts, 2014; Singh & Lin, 2013). One out of every ten Canadian children lives in poverty, and among children from Aboriginal heritage, a group that comprises 4% of the total Canadian population, 25% of children are poor (Statistics Canada, 2015).

Children's Health Status

Indicators of child health status include birth weight, infant mortality, and immunization rates. In general, children from diverse cultural backgrounds have less favorable indicators of health status than their white counterparts. Health status is influenced by many factors, including access to health services. There are numerous barriers to quality health care services for children, such as poverty, geography, lack of cultural competence by health care providers, racism, and other forms of prejudice. Families from diverse cultures might have trouble in their interactions with nurses and other health care providers, and these difficulties might have an adverse impact on the delivery of health care. Because ethnic minorities are

underrepresented among health care professionals, parents and children often have different cultural backgrounds from their health care providers.

Growth and Development

Although the growth and development of children are similar in all cultures, important racial, ethnic, and gender differences can be identified. For example, there is cross-cultural similarity in the sequence, timing, and achievement of developmental milestones such as smiling, separation anxiety, and language acquisition. However, from the moment of conception, the developmental processes of the human life cycle take place in the context of culture. Throughout life, culture exerts an all-pervasive influence on the developing infant, child, and adolescent. Developmental researchers who have worked in other cultures have become convinced that human functioning cannot be separated from the cultural and more immediate context in which children develop (Chen & Eisenberg, 2012). For example, during a study of children aged 0 to 6 years from three different Aboriginal groups in Canada, researchers discovered that although the participants' gross motor developmental milestones were achieved earlier when compared to the general population of Canadian children, language skills were developed later (Findlay, Kohen, & Miller, 2014).

Although it is difficult to separate nongenetic from genetic influences, some populations are shorter or taller than others are during various periods of growth and in adulthood. African American infants are approximately three-fourths of an inch shorter at birth than Whites. In general, African American and White children are tallest, followed by Native Americans; Asian children are the shortest. Children of higher socioeconomic status are taller in all cultures. Data on African American and White children between 1 and 6 years old show that at age 6, African Americans are taller than Whites. Around age 9 or 10 years, white boys begin to catch up in height. White girls catch up with their African American counterparts around 14 or 15 years of age. African American children have longer legs in proportion to height than

other groups (Overfield, 1995). During puberty, growth in African American children begins to slow down, and White children catch up so that the two races achieve similar heights in adulthood.

The growth spurt of adolescence involves the skeletal and muscular systems, leading to significant changes in size and strength in both sexes but particularly in boys. White North American youths age 12 to 18 years are 22 to 33 pounds heavier and 6 inches taller than Filipino youths the same age. African American teenagers are somewhat taller and heavier than White teens up to age 15 years old. Japanese adolescents born in the United States or Canada are larger and taller than Japanese adolescents who are born and raised in Japan, primarily due to differences in diet, climate, and social milieu (Overfield, 1995). To provide consistent comparisons of height and weight of children, the WHO (2010) has developed universally approved benchmarks for age-appropriate height/weight measures for children up to age 5 years based on data from 11 million children in 55 different countries or ethnic groups. Based on the wide variation in head circumference data gathered in the study, no global standards were recommended in an effort to avoid misdiagnosis of microcephy or macrocephy (Natale & Rajagopalan, 2014).

Certain growth patterns appear across cultural boundaries. For example, regardless of culture, neuromuscular activities evolve from general to specific, from the center of the body to the extremities (proximal-to-distal development), and from the head to the toes (cephalocaudal development). Adult head size is reached by the age of 5 years, whereas the remainder of the body continues to grow through adolescence. Physiologic maturation of organ systems, such as the renal, circulatory, and respiratory systems, occurs early, whereas maturation of the central nervous system continues beyond childhood. Tooth eruption occurs earlier in Asian and African American infants than in their White counterparts.

In terms of child development, many developmental theories are based on observations of Western children and, therefore, may not have cross-cultural generalization. Investigations of the

universality of the stages of development proposed by Piaget, the family role relations emphasized by Freud, and patterns of mother–infant interaction suggested by Bowlby to indicate security of attachment have resulted in modifications of the theories to reflect newer cross-cultural data.

Other growth and development patterns seem to be specific to cultural groups. For example, in some cultures, the standard Western mobility pattern of sitting—creeping—crawling—standing—walking—squatting is not followed. The Balinese infant goes from sitting to squatting to standing. Hopi (Native American) children begin walking 1 to 2 months later than Anglo-American children.

Infant Attachment

Cross-cultural differences are apparent when examining **infant attachment**, the relationship that exists between a child and their primary caregiver, which provides "a secure base from which to explore and, when necessary, as a haven of safety and a source of comfort" (Benoit, 2004, p. 1). Researchers have discovered that German and Anglo-American mothers expect early autonomy in the child and have fewer physical interventions as the child plays, thus encouraging exploration and independence (Dewar, 2014). Japanese children are seldom separated from their mother, and there is close physical interaction with the child (Dewar, 2014). Similarly, Puerto Rican and Dominican mothers display close mother–child relationships with more verbal and physical expression of affection than European American parents. Anglo-American mothers tend to give greater emphasis to qualities associated with individualism such as autonomy, self-control, and activity (Dewar, 2014). Puerto Rican mothers describe children in terms congruent with Puerto Rican culture: emphasis is placed on relatedness (e.g., affection, dignity, respectfulness, responsiveness to mother) and proximity seeking (Dewar, 2014). The development of African children is strongly related to the nutritional status of the child: those who tend to be malnourished have lessened attachment (Dewar, 2014).

Studies suggest that differences in infant attachment are linked to cultural variations in parenting behavior and life experiences. Parental socialization, values, beliefs, goals, and behaviors are determined in large measure by how a culture defines good parenting and preferred child behaviors for each gender. Other factors include the move from rural to urban residences and the associated social, economic, and lifestyle changes that shift children to more independent and autonomous behaviors. Some researchers argue that contemporary urbanization has created complex and highly technological societies that simultaneously foster children's autonomous, cooperative, and prosocial behavior (Chen & Eisenberg, 2012; Keller, 2013).

Crying

Cultural differences exist in the way mothers perceive, react, and behave in response to their infants' cues, behaviors, and demands. Knowledge of cultural differences in parental responses to crying is relevant for nurses because assessment of the severity of an infant's distress is often based on the parent's interpretation of the crying. The seriousness of a problem may be overestimated or underestimated because of cultural variations in perception of the infant's distress. The degree of parental concern toward an infant may be misinterpreted if one's cultural beliefs and practices differ from those of the parent (Dewar, 2013). For example, in Asian and Latino cultures, the male child is expected to maintain strong control over his emotions, and not cry in the presence of others; therefore, a child crying in pain may be interpreted one way by a nurse and dismissed as inappropriate gender-related behavior by a parent.

Culture-Universal and Culture-Specific Child Rearing

The values, attitudes, beliefs, and practices of one's culture affect the way parents and other providers of care relate to a child during various

developmental stages. In all cultures, infants and children are valued and nurtured because they represent the promise of future generations. Figure 6-2 presents a model summarizing the cultural factors that influence parental beliefs and practices related to child rearing. Influences on the parents include cultural and socioeconomic factors, educational background, political and legal considerations, religious and philosophical beliefs, environmental factors, contemporary technologies, personal attributes, and individual preferences. These influences, in turn, shape and form parental beliefs about normal growth and development; nutrition and diet; sleep; toilet training; communication patterns; and parent–child interactions and relationships, including beliefs and practices concerning parental authority. Beliefs and practices also influence discipline and culturally appropriate relationships with siblings, extended family members, nurses, physicians, teachers, law enforcement and other authority figures, and peers. Similarly parental cultural beliefs and practices influence behaviors and interventions that promote the child's health (immunizations, foods, exercise/activity) and the manner in which he/she is cared for during illness, how parents know when their child is sick or injured, the perceived seriousness of the illness or injury (and the need for primary, secondary, or tertiary care), type(s) of healers and interventions used to cure or heal the child. Lastly, factors inherent in the child, such as genetic and acquired conditions, gender, age, and related characteristics.

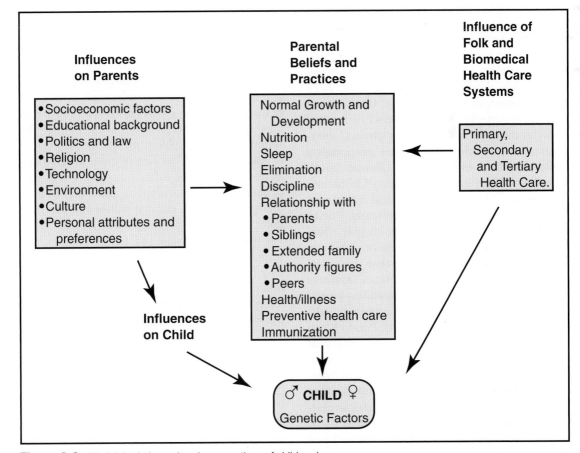

Figure 6-2. Model depicting cultural perspectives of childrearing.

Throughout infancy, childhood, and adolescence, girls and boys undergo a process of socialization aimed at preparing them to assume adult roles in the larger society into which they have been born or to which they have migrated. As children grow and develop, their communications and interactions occur within a cultural context. That which is considered acceptable is strongly influenced by parental education, social expectation, religious background, and cultural ties. However, all parents want their children to treat them respectfully and to show respect toward others, thus becoming a source of pride and honor to their family and cultural heritage.

There are many universal childrearing practices, but most research has focused on specific cultural differences rather than on similarities. It is important to distinguish between cultural practices and those that reflect the economic well-being of the family, for example, the stereotypes that suggest that teenage pregnancy is more common and more acceptable among African Americans than among counterparts in other cultures. When socioeconomic factors are considered, the myth is shattered. Although African American adolescents from the lower socioeconomic groups have higher rates of teen pregnancy, this is not true for middle- and upper-income African Americans (Aruda, 2011; Bresnahan, et al., 2014; Carlson et al., 2014).

Although not an exhaustive review of childrearing customs, the following discussion focuses on clinically significant childrearing behaviors among families from diverse cultures. These include nutrition, sleep, elimination, menstruation, parent–child relationships and discipline, and child abuse. Cross-cultural differences concerning gender are also discussed in this section.

Nutrition: Feeding and Eating Behaviors

In many cultures, breast-feeding is traditionally practiced for varying lengths of time ranging from several weeks to several years. The growing availability and convenience of extensively marketed prepared formula have resulted in a decrease in the number of women who attempt to breast-feed, especially among recent migrants to the United States who may culturally find it inappropriate to breast-feed in public. Many nursing mothers immigrating to the United States or Canada may be separated from female family members who could assist them with successful breast-feeding, and lack of an interpreter during prenatal and postnatal visits with health professionals can become a barrier to breast-feeding (Schmied et al., 2012).

Some cultural feeding practices might result in threats to the infant's health. The practice of propping a bottle filled with milk, juice, or carbonated beverages to quiet a child or lull them to sleep is known in many cultures and can result in dental caries; this practice should be discouraged. In some cultures, mothers **premasticate**, or chew, food for young children in the belief that this will facilitate digestion. This practice, most frequently reported among Black and Hispanic mothers, is of questionable benefit and may transmit infection from the mother's mouth to the baby (Centers for Disease Control and Prevention, 2014b; Rakhmanina et al., 2011).

Health status is dependent in part on nutritional intake, thus integrally linking the child's nutritional status and wellness. Although the United States is the world's greatest food-producing nation, nutritional status has not been a priority for many people in this country. An estimated 1% of children in the United States are malnourished (John Hopkins Children's Center, 2015). Malnutrition is described as undernutrition (not enough essential nutrients or nutrients excreted too rapidly) or overnutrition (eating too much of the wrong food or not excreting enough food) (WHO, 2010). Malnutrition may be serious enough to interfere with neuro- and musculoskeletal development.

Malnutrition is not exclusive to children from poor, lower socioeconomic groups. By definition, many middle- and upper-income families have obese children who are also malnourished. Obesity frequently begins during infancy, when some mothers succumb to cultural pressures to overfeed (Moreno, Johnson-Shelton, & Boles, 2013). For example, among many who identify

themselves as Filipino, Vietnamese, Somali, Hispanic American, and Mexican, to name a few cultures, fat babies generally are considered healthy babies (Bresnahan, Zhuang, & Park, 2014; Cachelin & Thompson, 2014; Cartagena et al., 2014; Centers for Disease Control and Prevention, 2014b). Among some African tribes, such as the Igbo and Yoruba in Nigeria, overweight babies are considered healthy, and mild to moderate obesity in children is considered a sign of affluence. Similar beliefs have been identified among Somali and Berber women (Liamputtong, 2011) as well as some Hispanic mothers who subscribe to a long-standing cultural belief that "a chubby baby is a healthy baby" (Children's Defense Fund, 2014). Evidence-Based Practice 6-1 describes racial and ethnic differences in childhood obesity.

The popularity of fast-food restaurants and "junk" foods has resulted in a high-calorie, high-fat, high-cholesterol, and high-carbohydrate diet for many children. Parents and children are frequently involved in numerous activities outside the house and have less time for traditional tasks such as cooking or seating the family together for a meal. Because fast foods have some intrinsic nutritional value, their benefit should be evaluated based on age-specific requirements. Poverty forces some parents to provide inexpensive substitutes for the expensive, often unavailable, essential nutrients. These lower nutrients, high-fat, high-calorie foods are referred to as "empty calories" and have led to the epidemic of childhood obesity. The prevalence of childhood obesity among various cultural and ethnic groups within the United States was described by Ogden, Carroll, Kit, and Flegal (2014). The reported weight-for-age imbalance among preschool, school-age, and adolescent African American and Hispanic children was especially disturbing and purports serious complications of hypertension, diabetes, and cardiovascular disease for young Black and Hispanic adults (see Figure 6-3).

The extent to which families retain their cultural practices at mealtime varies widely. However, when a child is hospitalized, their recovery might be enhanced by familiar foods, and nurses should assess the influence of culture on eating habits. For example, most Asian parents believe that children should be fed separately from adults and that they should acquire "good table manners" by the time they are 5 years old; these practices can be supported during hospitalization. For hospitalized children, nurses can foster an environment that closely simulates the home (e.g., use of chopsticks rather than silverware). Family members can be encouraged to visit during mealtime to encourage the child to eat. As the child's condition allows, food may be brought from home, and/or the family can be encouraged to eat with the child if this is appropriate.

In many cultures, illness is viewed as a punishment for an evil act, and fasting (abstaining from solid food and sometimes liquids) is viewed as penance for evil. A situation may become dangerous, and even deadly, should a parent view the child's illness as an "evil" event and consequently withhold food and/or water. Dehydration occurs rapidly and malnutrition may quickly follow. These dangerous issues may require legal intervention to protect the child and may produce difficult, culturally insensitive outcomes. Nurses must be vigilant to support cultural eating habits and be prepared to educate parents and children about the prevention of and intervention for malnutrition and dehydration.

Safe drinking water is not always available in many regions of the world. Contaminated water is found in all countries at some time and in some countries at all times. Children die daily from waterborne diseases that could be prevented with a few drops of bleach or a safe water supply. Weather-related disasters, earthquakes, famine, and war typically escalate the water crises. In cases of vomiting, diarrhea, and dehydration, contaminated water supplies should always be investigated as a possible source.

Sleep

Although the amount of sleep required at various ages is similar across cultures, differences in sleep patterns and bedtime rituals exist. The sleep

Racial and Ethnic Differences in Childhood Obesity

The World Health Organization warns that the increasing prevalence of obesity in children during the past 30 years has reached epidemic levels. A global problem affecting many low- and middle-income countries, obesity affected more than 42 million children under the age of 5 in 2013. Nearly 31 million of these children live in urban parts of developing countries and are at risk for remaining obese into adulthood, at which time they are more likely to develop diabetes and cardiovascular diseases (World Health Organization, 2014). Children at highest risk for obesity live in the United States, United Kingdom, and Mexico.

Measuring Overweight and Obesity in Children

It is difficult to develop one simple index for the measurement of overweight and obesity in children and adolescents because their bodies undergo a number of physiologic changes as they grow. Measurement is further compounded by the child's race; African Black children carry less body fat than White counterparts, and Hispanic and Asian children typically have a higher percentage of body fat. Given the wide variation in the level and distribution of body fat between different racial and ethnic groups, different benchmarks for defining overweight and obesity are used in different countries. Cowie (2014) reports on various tools and strategies used to measure and assess overweight and obesity in children and identifies what is currently considered to be the most reliable and effective. Different methods to measure a body's healthy weight, depending on the age, are available from the World Health Organization. In the United States, the Centers for Disease Control's reference data are based on a sample of boys and girls aged 2 to 20 years (CDC, 2010).

Factors Contributing to Obesity in Early Childhood

Weden, Brownell, and Rendall (2012) studied differences in the likelihood of early childhood obesity between Black and White US children using data from the Early Childhood Longitudinal Study directed by the National Center for Education Statistics. The sample consisted of a nationally representative cohort with $n = 1,515$ children and their mothers (age 14 to 21 years) who were assessed in waves at 9 months, 2 years, 4 years, and upon entry into kindergarten using computer-assisted, in-home interviews with children, mothers, fathers, or guardians. The investigators examined differences in Black and White children's prevalence of socioeconomic, prenatal, perinatal, and early life risk and protective factors relative to their likelihood of obesity in early childhood. Black children's mothers were only one-third as likely as White children's mothers to have completed high school, a strong indicator of socioeconomic disadvantage. Black children were 3 to 3.5 times as likely as White children to live in a family or household whose annual income was below $25,000, and their mothers were three to four times as likely to be unmarried. In analyzing prenatal and perinatal risk factors, almost half of Black children's mothers, compared to one-third of White children's mothers, were overweight or obese before pregnancy. Prepregnant obesity was the strongest risk factor for early childhood obesity, with Black children's mothers being more likely to be obese than White counterparts, thus perpetuating "a troubling cycle of intergenerational transmission of racial disparities in body mass index" (Weden et al., 2012, p. 2062). The investigators also studied racial differences in protective factors that would decrease the likelihood of early childhood obesity, for example, long-duration breast-feeding (>8 months), frequency and quality of meals, children's television viewing, and exercise/physical activity care (Bresnahan, et al., 2014; Cachelin & Thompson, 2014; Kirby, Liang, Hsin-Jen, & Wang et al., 2012; Moreno et al., 2013).

Protective Factors Contributing to Prevention of Obesity in Early Childhood

Among early life protective factors to reduce the likelihood of obesity, Black children were less

(continued)

Racial and Ethnic Differences in Childhood Obesity (continued)

likely than White children to be breast-fed for 1 to 7 months and only one-third as likely to be breast-fed for 8 months or longer. Black children were also less likely than White children to have daily family meals. Twice as many Black children as White children watched television for 4 or more hours per day during the daytime at 4 years of age. Black children's mothers were more likely to be employed full time than White children's. Black children also were more likely to be cared for by relatives or in a day care center and less likely to be cared for by a nonrelative or exclusively by their parents. In the statistical analyses, it was revealed that younger children's television watching was not correlated with obesity, as has been reported elsewhere in the literature, perhaps because television-related sedentary behavior is a more critical determinant in obesity at older ages.

Clinical Implications

The study findings provide insights into potentially modifiable determinants of racial disparities in early childhood obesity among Black and White pre-school-aged children. Disparities among Black children are concerning because early childhood obesity often develops into adult obesity, which, in turn, has implications for adult cardiovascular disease and diabetes, the leading causes of premature death in African Americans. Eliminating Black–White differences in early childhood obesity provides an opportunity to reduce racial disparities in the overall health and longevity of both Black and White populations.

The study findings also have implications for nurse midwives, obstetric nurses, obstetricians, doulas, and others who assist with deliveries and engage in parent education programs about the benefits of breast-feeding, proper nutrition, and exercise/activity; for employers who establish workplace policies related to breast-feeding; for teachers responsible for exercise and activity programs in preschools and kindergartens; for dieticians who are responsible for nutrition and diet education programs for the parents and other care givers for preschool-aged children; and for federal, state, foundation, and corporate funding for the prevention of childhood obesity.

References

Cowie, J. (2014). Measurement of obesity in children. Primary Health Care, 24(7), 18–23

Kirby, J. B., Liang, L., Hsin-Jen, C., & Wang, Y. (2012). Race, place, and obesity: The complex relationships among community racial/ethnic composition, individual race/ethnicity, and obesity in the United States. American Journal of Public Health, 102(8), 1572–1578

Moreno, G., Johnson-Shelton, D., & Boles, S. (2013). Prevalence and prediction of overweight and obesity among elementary school children. Journal of School Health, 83(1), 157–163

Weden, M. M., Brownell, P., & Rendall, M. S. (2012). Prenatal, perinatal, early life, and sociodemographic factors underlying high body mass index in early childhood. American Journal of Public Health, 102(11), 2057–2065

World Health Organization. (2014). Global strategy on diet, physical activity: Childhood overweight and obesity. Retrieved on 11-5-14 at http://www.who.int/dietphysicalactivity/childhood/en/

practices in a family household reflect some of the deepest moral ideals of a cultural community. Nurses working with families of young children in both community and inpatient settings frequently encounter cultural differences in family sleeping behaviors.

Community health, psychiatric, and pediatric nurses who work with young children and their families often assess the family's sleep and rest patterns. **Bed sharing** is the practice of a child sleeping with another person on the same sleeping surface for all or part of the night. Although bed sharing may be born out of financial necessity, it is a cultural phenomenon in many societies that emphasize closeness, togetherness, and interdependence (Jain, Romack, & Jain, 2011). Globally, bed sharing prevalence ranges widely, from 6% to 70%; an estimated 15% of US children

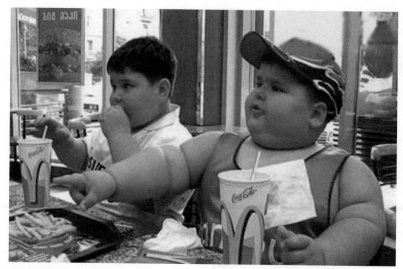

Figure 6-3. Childhood obesity is often initiated or reinforced through diets of "fast foods."

bed share. Among children in households with an annual income less than $20,000/year, bed sharing is 1.5 times more likely than those with incomes greater than $20,000/year. On the issue of family cosleeping, nurses traditionally have taken a rigid approach that excludes this common cultural practice. Although some degree of **cosleeping**—the practice of parents and children sleeping together in the same bed for all or part of the night—is common in families with young children, there are marked cultural differences in the proportion that regularly implement this practice (Barajas, Martin, Brooks-Gunn, & Hale, 2011; Jain et al., 2011; Lujik, Mileva-Seitz, Jansen et al., 2013; Salm Ward, 2014).

Research has found that the majority of parents bring their children into bed with them at some time. Parents bring their children into bed with them to facilitate breast-feeding, to comfort the child, to improve the child's sleep or parent's sleep, to monitor the child, to improve bonding or attachment, and for other reasons; the constellation of reasons for bed sharing depends largely on the culture of the family (Huang et al., 2013; Salm Ward, 2014).

Cosleeping is more common and occurs most frequently among African American families (Luijk, Mileva-Seitz, Jansen, et al., 2013). Most White middle-class North American and European families believe that infants and children should sleep alone. There are no negative associations between cosleeping during the toddler years and behavior and cognition at 5 years of age (Barajas et al., 2011).

The type of bed in which a child sleeps might vary considerably. In a traditional American Samoan home, infants sleep on a pandanus mat covered with a blanket, and sometimes, a pillow is used. The cradleboard is used by several Native American nations. Constructed by a family member, a cradleboard is made of wood and might be decorated in various ways depending on the affluence of the family and tribal customs (see Figure 6-4). The cradleboard helps the infant feel secure and is easily moved while the family engages in work, travel, or other activities. Although cradleboards have been blamed for exacerbating hip dysplasia in Native American infants, diapering counterbalances this by causing a slight abduction of the hips (Kliegman, Stanton, Saint Geme, Schor, & Behrman, 2011).

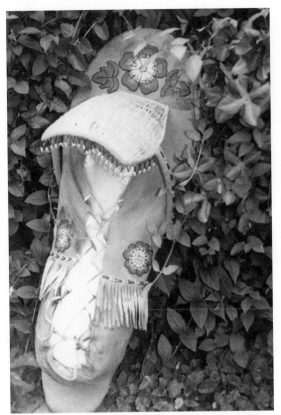

Figure 6-4. The cradleboard, created many centuries before the car seat, helps to promote infant mobility and safety and its use is still prevalent among some Native Americans.

In the United States and Canada, the common developmental milestone of sleeping for 8 uninterrupted hours by age 4 to 5 months is regarded as a sign of neurologic maturity. In many other cultures, however, the infant sleeps with the mother and is allowed to breast-feed on demand with minimal disturbance of adult sleep. In such an arrangement, there is less parental motivation to enforce "sleeping through the night," and infants continue to wake up every 4 hours during the night to be fed (Huang et al., 2013). Thus, it appears that this developmental milestone, in addition to its biologic basis, is a function of context.

A common transition from sleeping in a crib to a bed without side rails is a developmental marker that is important to the child. This transition usually occurs during preschool years, depending upon the physical space in the home, the parental attitude toward the child's independence, and the child's neuromuscular development/coordination. For the hospitalized child, caregivers need to identify the child's usual bedtime routines. For example, once children have gained the independence of leaving a crib, it may be emotionally traumatic for them to be placed into a hospital bed with side rails of any kind. Health care providers need to be sensitive to this situation and reassure both child and parent that any regressive behavior that occurs as a result of reverting to a bed with side rails will be short-lived. Bedtime routines and preparation for sleep might include a snack, prayers, and/or a favorite toy or story. Common bedtime routines should be continued in the hospital as much as possible.

Homelessness presents many problems, one of which is the lack of a consistent place for a child to sleep. Although nomadic tribes have for centuries moved their habitat on a daily basis, even they generally had a consistent tent or covering. Today, approximately 1.6 million of children experience homelessness each year and daily face the issues of not having a permanent, safe, or secure place in which to lay their head (The National Center on Family Homelessness, 2015). Whether because of poverty, disease, war, or disaster, children with or without families nightly wander without a safe place to sleep. The toll of the massive number of homeless children that are the result of recent natural disasters, war, and famine has yet to be estimated. Lack of a safe place to sleep is only one of many issues to be considered (see Figure 6-5).

Elimination

Elimination refers to ridding the body of wastes. It is a function that is accomplished by the combined work of the gastrointestinal, genitourinary, respiratory, and integumentary systems of the body. Of primary concern to parents of toddlers and preschoolers is bowel and bladder control. Toileting or toilet training is a major developmental milestone and is taught through a variety of cultural patterns.

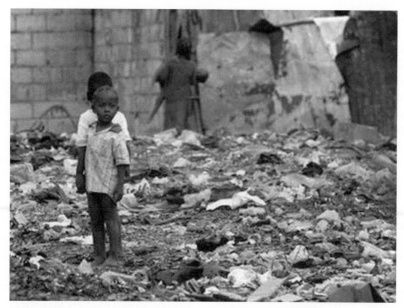

Figure 6-5. A Haitian child stands amidst earthquake rubble without clean water, food, or a place to sleep.

Most children are capable of achieving dryness by 2½ to 3 years of age. Bowel training is more easily accomplished than bladder training. Daytime (diurnal) dryness is more easily attained than nighttime (nocturnal) dryness. Some cultures start toilet training a child before his or her first birthday and consider the child a "failure" if dryness is not achieved by 18 months. Often, there is significant shaming, blaming, and embarrassment of the child who has not achieved dryness by the culturally acceptable timetable. The nurse should remember that due to spinal cord/nerve development, maintenance of dryness is not physiologically possible until the child is able to walk without assistance. In some cultures, children are not expected to be dry until 5 years of age. Generally speaking, "Girls typically acquire bladder control before boys, and bowel control typically is achieved before bladder control" (Kliegman et al., 2011, p. 71). Constipation in a child is a persistent concern among parents who expect a ritualistic daily pattern of bowel movements. In some cultures, infants are given herbs aimed at purging them when they are a few days, weeks, or months old to remove evil spirits from the body.

Parents should be advised against using purgatives in infants because fluid and electrolyte imbalance occurs, and dehydration can ensue rapidly.

The role of the nurse is to acknowledge that toilet training can be taught through a variety of cultural patterns but that physical and psychosocial health are promoted by accepting, flexible approaches. A previously toilet-trained child might become incontinent as a result of the stress of hospitalization, but will generally regain control quickly when returned to the familiar home environment. Parents should be reassured that regression of bowel and bladder control frequently occurs when a child is hospitalized; this is normal and is expected to be a short-term occurrence.

Menstruation

Ethnicity is the strongest determinant of the duration and character of menstrual flow, although diet, exercise, and stress are also known to influence menstruation in women of all ages. In most cultures globally, menarche signals that a girl's body is physiologically becoming ready for motherhood.

The age at which it is culturally appropriate for a young woman to bear children is highly variable (Davis, Farage, & Miller, 2011). As indicated in Figure 6-6, in some cultures, motherhood occurs in the early teens, which results in children parenting children, often with encouragement and support from an extended family, including other wives in polygamous cultures. In other cultures, adolescent pregnancy is discouraged.

Attitudes toward menstruation are often culturally based, and the adolescent girl might be taught many folk beliefs. For example, in traditional Mexican American families, girls and women are not permitted to walk barefooted, wash their hair, or take showers or baths during menses. In encouraging hygienic practices, respect

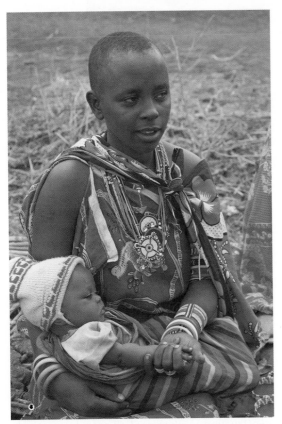

Figure 6-6. Menarche sets the developmental stage for girls to become mothers: children parenting children (Giancana/Shutterstock.com).

cultural directives by encouraging sponge bathing, frequent changing of sanitary pads or tampons, and other interventions that promote cleanliness (Davis et al., 2011). Some Mexican Americans believe that sour or iced foods cause the menstrual flow to thicken, and some Puerto Rican teenagers have been taught that drinking lemon or pineapple juice will increase menstrual cramping. The nurse should be aware of these beliefs and should respect personal preferences concerning beverages. The teenager might have been taught the folk practices by her mother or by another woman in her family who might be watchful during the girl's menstrual periods. If menstruation coincides with hospitalization, nurses should respect the teenager's preferences and reassure the mother or significant other that cultural practices will be respected.

Many cultural groups treat menstrual cramping with herbs and a variety of home remedies. Health care providers should ask the adolescent whether she takes anything special during menstruation or in the absence of menstrual flow. Verify the amount and type of home remedies used to determine possible interactive effect with prescribed medications.

Adolescent girls of Islamic religious backgrounds have cultural and/or religious prohibitions and duties during and after menstruation. In Islamic law, blood is considered unclean. The blood of menstruation, as well as blood lost during childbirth, is believed to render the female impure. Because one must be in a pure state to pray, menstruating girls and women are forbidden to perform certain acts of worship, such as touching the Koran, entering a mosque, praying, and participating in the feast of Ramadan. During the menstrual period, sexual intercourse is forbidden for both men and women. When the menstrual flow stops, the girl or woman performs a special washing to purify herself. In Islam, sexual pollution applies equally to men and women. For men, sexual intercourse and the discharge of semen is an act that renders a man impure and requires a ritual washing before being able to perform the prayer. Buddhist and Hindu women do not enter the kitchen and may sleep in separate/special rooms during menses (Davis et al., 2011).

Parent–Child Relationships and Discipline

In some cultures, both parents assume responsibility for the care of children, whereas in other cultures, the relationship with the mother is primary and the father remains somewhat distant. With the approach of adolescence, the gender-related aspects of the **parent–child relationship** might be modified to conform to cultural expectations.

Some cultures encourage children to participate in family decision making and to discuss or even argue points with their parents. Some African American families, for example, encourage children to express opinions verbally and to take an active role in all family activities. Many Asian parents value respectful, deferential behavior toward adults, who are considered experienced and wise; therefore, children are discouraged from making decisions independently. The witty, fast reply that is viewed in some US, Canadian, European, and Australian cultures as a sign of intelligence and cleverness might be punished in some non-Western circles as a sign of rudeness and disrespect.

The use of physical acts, such as spanking or various restraining actions, is connected with discipline in many groups, but can sometimes be interpreted by those outside the culture as inappropriate and/or unacceptable. Physical punishment of Native North American children is rare. Instead of using loud scolding and reprimands, Native North American parents generally discipline with a quiet voice, telling the child what is expected. During breast-feeding and toilet training, or toilet learning, Native North American children are typically permitted to set their own pace, and parents tend to be permissive and nondemanding. Some African American parents tend to point out negative behaviors of a child and may use spanking and physical punishment as a strategy to quickly gain the child's attention and rapidly get him or her to behave, especially in public (Whaley, 2013).

With the approach of adolescence, parental relationships and discipline generally change.

Teens are usually given increasing amounts of freedom and are encouraged to try out adult roles in a supervised way that enables parents to retain considerable control. In many cultures, adolescent boys are permitted more freedom than girls of the same age. Among some religious groups, such as the American Amish, adolescents are given a period of time (a month to a year) of a more independent lifestyle prior to commitment to specific religious life rules.

Child Abuse

Child abuse and neglect have been documented throughout human history and are evident across cultures. International attention to child maltreatment emerged in the late 1970s, and the International Society for the Prevention of Child Abuse and Neglect (ISPCAN) held an international congress to explore physical abuse and neglect, molestation, child prostitution, nutritional deprivation, and emotional maltreatment from a cross-national perspective. This congress led to the formation of a multicountry study of child maltreatment/abuse and the United Nations–WHO joint publication "Enhancing the Rights of Adolescent Girls" (WHO, 2010).

Cross-cultural variability in childrearing beliefs and practices has created a dilemma that makes the establishment of a universal standard for optimal child care, as well as definitions of child abuse and neglect, extremely difficult. In defining child maltreatment across cultures, the WHO and UNICEF have included Korbin's (1991) classic three characteristics: (1) cultural differences in childrearing practices and beliefs, (2) departure from one's culturally acceptable behavior, and (3) harm to children.

Practices that are acceptable in the culture in which they occur may be considered abusive or neglectful by outsiders; some examples follow. In many Middle Eastern cultures, despite warm temperatures, infants are covered with multiple layers of clothing and might be observed to sweat profusely because parents believe that young children become chilled easily and die of exposure to

the cold. Many African nations continue to practice rites of initiation for boys and girls, usually at the time of puberty. In some cases, ritual circumcision—of both boys and girls—is performed without anesthesia, and the ability to endure the associated pain is considered to be a manifestation of the maturity expected of an adult. In the United States and Canada, some Southeast Asian folk healing practices such as coining, cupping, and burning that produce marks on the body are used for treatment of upper respiratory illnesses, pain relief, and various other illnesses. In some Middle Eastern and Mexican societies, fondling of the genitals of infants and young children is used to soothe them or encourage sleep; however, such fondling of older children or for the sexual gratification of adults falls outside of acceptable cultural behaviors.

Although African American children are three times more likely than White children to die of child abuse (Lanier, Maguire, Tova, Drake, & Hubel, 2014), there is considerable disagreement about whether race differences exist in the prevalence of child abuse independent from socioeconomic factors such as income, education, and employment status. Health care providers need to become knowledgeable about folk beliefs, childrearing practices, and cultural variability in defining child maltreatment.

Gender Differences

From the moment of birth, differentiation between the sexes is recognized. Physical differences between boys and girls appear early in life and form the basis for adult roles within a culture. Normal newborn boys are larger, more active, and have more muscle development than newborn girls. Normal newborn girls react more positively to comforting than do newborn boys.

Physiologically, adult men differ from adult women in both primary and secondary sex characteristics. On average, men have a higher oxygen-carrying capacity in the blood, a higher muscle-to-fat ratio, more body hair, a larger skeleton, and greater height.

Behaviorally, there are also differences between the two sexes, especially in the division of labor. The early differentiation of gender roles is manifested in gender-specific tasks, play, and dress. For children, gender differences can be identified cross-culturally in six classes of behavior: nurturance, responsibility, obedience, self-reliance, achievement, and independence (Barry, Bacon, & Child, 1967). Variability in gender role behavior is common. Most people in a society adopt common behaviors defined as appropriate to their biologic sex, but there are many exceptions. Gender roles are themselves highly variable by age, social class, religious orientation, and sexual preference. The stringency of expectations also varies: girls and women in the United States, Canada, Australia, Israel, and many parts of Europe can violate gender role norms with fewer explicit sanctions than their counterparts in other regions of the world.

Health and Health Promotion

The concept of health varies widely across cultures. Regardless of culture, most parents desire health for their children and engage in activities that they believe to be health promoting. Because health-related beliefs and practices are such an integral part of culture, parents might persist with culturally based beliefs and practices even when scientific evidence refutes them, or they might modify them to be more congruent with contemporary knowledge of health and illness.

Illness

The family is the primary health care provider for infants, children, and adolescents. It is the family that determines when a child is ill and when to seek help in managing an illness. The family also determines the acceptability of illness and sick-role behaviors for children and adolescents. Societal and economic trends influence the cultural beliefs that are passed from generation to generation. Health, illness, and treatment (care/cure) are part of every child's cultural heritage.

Every society has an organized response to defined health problems. Certain people are designated as being responsible for deciding who is sick, what kind of sickness the person has, and what kind of treatment is required to restore the person to health.

Research has consistently demonstrated that African American and Hispanic children are less likely to have seen a physician than are Whites. They also have a lower average number of ambulatory visits than their White counterparts. Even when children are hospitalized, minorities receive fewer services than do Whites (Federal Interagency Forum on Child and Family Statistics, 2006; Statistics Canada, 2009; Children's Defense Organization, 2009).

Health Belief Systems and Children

Among many cultural groups, traditional health beliefs coexist with Western medical beliefs. Members of a cultural group choose the components of traditional (Western) medicine, Eastern medicine, or folk beliefs that seem appropriate to them. A Mexican American family, for example, might take a child to a physician and/or a traditional healer (curandero). After visiting the physician and the **curandero**, the mother might consult with her own mother and then give her sick child the antibiotics prescribed by the physician and the herbal tea prescribed by the traditional healer. If the problem is viral in origin, the child will recover because of his or her own innate immunologic defenses, independent of either treatment. Thus, both the herbal tea of the *curandero* and the penicillin prescribed by the physician might be viewed as folk remedies; neither intervention is responsible for the child's recovery.

Belief systems about specific symptoms are culturally unique. These are referred to as cultural illnesses. In Hispanic culture, *susto* is caused by a frightening experience and is recognized by nervousness, loss of appetite, and loss of sleep. Mexican American babies must be protected from these experiences. *Pujos* (grunting) is an illness manifested by grunting sounds and protrusion of the umbilicus. It is believed to be caused by contact with a woman who is menstruating or by the infant's own mother if she menstruated sooner than 60 days after delivery.

The evil eye, *mal ojo*, is an affliction feared throughout much of the world. The condition is said to be caused by an individual who voluntarily or involuntarily injures a child by looking at or admiring him or her. The individual has a desire to hold the child, but the wish is frustrated, either by the parent of the infant or by the reserve of the individual. Several hours later, the child might become listless, cry, experience fever, vomiting, and/or diarrhea. The most serious threat to the infant with *mal ojo* is dehydration; the nurse encountering this problem in the community setting needs to assess the severity of the dehydration and plan for immediate fluid and electrolyte replacement. Parents should be taught the warning signs and the potential seriousness of dehydration. A simple explanation of the causes and treatment of dehydration should be provided. If the parents adhere strongly to traditional beliefs, respect their desire for the *curandera* to participate in the care. Parents or grandparents might wish to place an amulet, talisman, or religious object such as a crucifix or rosary on the child or near the bed.

For the Mexican American family, *caida de la mollera*, or fallen fontanel, can be attributed to a number of causes such as failure of the midwife to press preventively on the palate after delivery, falling on the head, abruptly removing the nipple from the infant's mouth, and failing to place a cap on the infant's head. The signs of this condition include crying, fever, vomiting, and diarrhea. Given that health care providers frequently note the correspondence of these symptoms with those of dehydration, many parents see *deshidratacion* (dehydration) or *carencia de agua* (lack of water) as synonymous with *caida de la mollera*. Although regional differences exist, parental treatment usually is directed at rehydration, thus raising the fontanel.

Empacho is a digestive condition believed by Mexicans to be caused by the adherence of

undigested food to some part of the gastrointestinal tract. This condition causes an "internal fever," which cannot be observed but which betrays its presence by excessive thirst and abdominal swelling believed to be caused by drinking water to quench the thirst. Children who are prone to swallowing chewing gum are believed to experience *empacho*, but it can affect persons of any age.

Among some Hindus from northern India, there is a strong belief in ghost illness and ghost possession. These culture-bound syndromes, or folk illnesses, are based on the belief that a ghost enters its victim and tries to seize the soul. If the ghost is successful, it causes death. Illness and the supernatural world are linked by the concepts of fever and the ghost, which is a supernatural being discussed in Hindu sacred scriptures. One sign of ghost illness is a voice speaking through a delirious victim; this may occur in children and adults. Other signs are convulsions and body movements, indicating pain and discomfort, and choking or difficulty breathing. In the case of an infant, incessant crying is a sign. The psychological state of the parents is often involved in the diagnosis, and some believe that ghosts might be cultural scapegoats for the illness and death of children. When an infant or small child becomes ill and dies, a mother or father might be relieved of psychic tension from feelings of personal guilt by transferring the blame for the death to a ghost.

Biocultural Influences on Childhood Disorders

Children may be born with genetic traits inherited from their biologic parents, who have inherited their own genetic compositions. The child's genetic makeup affects his or her likelihood of both contracting and inheriting specific conditions. In both children and adults, genetic composition has been demonstrated to affect the individual's susceptibility to specific diseases and disorders. It is often difficult to separate genetic influences from socioeconomic factors such as poverty, lack of proper nutrition, poor hygiene, and environmental conditions such as lack of ventilation, sanitary facilities, and heat during cold weather, and clothing that is insufficient to provide protection during the various seasons. Other factors responsible for differing susceptibilities to specific conditions are variations in natural and acquired immunity, intermarriage, geographic and climatic conditions, ethnic background, race, and religious practices. Some studies have attempted to explain differences in susceptibility solely on the basis of cultural heritage, but they have not succeeded in doing so. This section examines some common conditions in which genetic constitution seems to be a factor influencing child health.

Immunity

Perhaps one of the most frequently cited examples of the connection between immunity and race is that of malaria and the sickle cell trait in Africans. Black Africans possessing the sickle cell trait are known to have increased immunity to malaria, a serious endemic disease found in warm, moist climates. Thus, blacks with the sickle cell trait survived malarial attacks and reproduced offspring who also possessed the sickle cell trait.

The transfer of immunity to many contagious diseases via injection/ingestion of live or attenuated viruses has been a major factor in decreasing childhood deaths. However, there is no evidence of culture-bound positive or negative effects where vaccines are available. Some religious groups refuse immunizations and often experience outbreaks of preventable communicable diseases within their community. Other parents refuse immunizations based on the belief of a connection between childhood autism and vaccines, which has not been supported by clinical research to date.

Intermarriage

Intermarriage among certain cultural groups has led to a wide variety of childhood disorders. For example, there is an increased incidence of ventricular septal defects (VSDs) among the Amish, amyloidosis among Indiana/Swiss and Maryland/German families, and intellectual disability in several other groups (Kliegman et al., 2011).

Ethnicity

Although the role of socioeconomic factors in tuberculosis—such as overcrowding and poor nutrition—cannot be disregarded, ethnicity also appears to be a factor in this disease. Groups with a relatively high incidence of tuberculosis are Native North Americans living in the Southwest United States and in northern and prairie regions of Canada, Mexican Americans, and Africans and refugees from third world countries. Ethnicity is also linked to several noncommunicable conditions such as Tay–Sachs disease, a neurologic condition affecting Ashkenazi Jews of Northeastern European descent, and phenylketonuria (PKU), a metabolic disorder primarily affecting Scandinavians (Kliegman et al., 2011).

Race

Race has been linked to the incidence of a variety of disorders of childhood. For example, the endocrine disorder cystic fibrosis primarily affects White children, and sickle cell anemia has its primary influence among Blacks and those of Mediterranean descent. Black children are known to be at risk for inherited blood disorders, such as thalassemia, G-6-PD deficiency, and hemoglobin C disease. In addition, an estimated 70% to 90% of black children have an enzyme deficiency that results in difficulty with the digestion and metabolism of milk (Coutts, 2013).

Beliefs Regarding the Cause of Chronic Illnesses and Disabilities

Chronic illnesses and disabilities in children and adults have become the dominant health care problem in North America and are the leading causes of morbidity and mortality (Agency for Healthcare Research, and Quality, 2014; Centers for Disease Control and Prevention, 2014). Illness is viewed by many cultures as a form of punishment. The child and/or family with a chronic illness or disability might be perceived to be cursed by a supreme being, to have sinned, or to have violated a taboo. In some cultural groups, the affected child is seen as tangible evidence of divine displeasure, and its arrival is accompanied throughout the community by prolonged private and public discussions about what wrongs the family might have committed.

Inherited disorders and illnesses are frequently envisioned as being caused by a family curse that is passed along from one generation to the next through blood. Within such families, the nurse's desire to determine who is the carrier for a particular gene might be interpreted as an attempt to discover who is at fault and might be met with family resistance.

Folk beliefs mingled with eugenics have resulted in the realization that many chronic conditions, particularly intellectual disability, are the products of intermarriage among close relatives (Agency for Healthcare Research and Quality, 2014; Centers for Disease Control and Prevention, 2014b). The belief that a chronically ill or disabled child might be the product of an incestuous relationship can further complicate attempts to encourage parents to seek assistance.

Among those who believe that chronic illness and disability are caused by an imbalance of hot and cold (as in Latino cultures) or yin and yang (as in Southeast Asian cultures), the cause and potential cure lie within the individual. He or she must try to reestablish equilibrium through regaining balance. Unfortunately for those with permanent disabilities who cannot be fully healed, their community might perceive them as living in a continually impure or diseased state.

Traditional beliefs can be tenacious and tend to remain even after genetic inheritance or physiologic patterns of chronic disease progression are explained to the family. However, new information is quickly integrated into the traditional system of folk beliefs more often, as is evidenced by the addition of currently prescribed medications to the hot/cold classification system embraced by many Hispanic families. An explanation of the genetic transmission of disease might be given to a family, but this does not guarantee that the older, traditional belief in a curse or "bad blood" will disappear.

When disability is seen as a divine punishment, an inherited evil, or the result of a personal state of impurity, the very presence of a child with a disability might be something about which the family is deeply ashamed or with which they are unable to cope. In addition to suffering from public disgrace, some parents or families, especially immigrant groups from Eastern Europe and Southeast Asia, also fear that disabled children will be taken away and institutionalized against their will.

Some cultural explanations of the cause of chronic disease or disability are quite positive. For example, some Mexican American parents of chronically ill children believed that a certain number of ill and disabled children would always be born into the world. Many Mexican American parents who embrace Roman Catholicism believe that God has singled them out for the role because of their past kindnesses to a relative or neighbor who was disabled and view the birth of the disabled infant as God's will.

The number of chronically ill children in industrialized nations has increased markedly over the past decade, particularly those from minority and low-income households who are at high risk for health disparities (Agency for Healthcare Research and Quality, 2014; Centers for Disease Control and Prevention, 2014a; Schreirer & Chen, 2013). This increase is primarily due to dramatic changes in obesity, environmental pollutants responsible for asthma and other respiratory illnesses, accidents, and injuries. Adolescent pregnancy among low-income populations is often accompanied by poor nutrition before and during pregnancy, failure to seek prenatal care (or waiting until the third trimester to do so), and low-birth-weight infants who are at high risk for respiratory illnesses and failure to thrive (Kliegman et al., 2011; Upadhya & Ellen, 2011). In the United States, extensive medical resources are used to save the lives of very low-birth-weight infants; however, the lifesaving efforts often leave a child with multiple chronic illnesses; in countries with fewer medical resources, such as Uganda and Haiti, these same very-low-birth-weight babies will not survive infancy (see Figure 6-7).

Special Health Care Needs of Adolescents

There are approximately 23 million adolescents in the United States and Canada (Laughlin, 2014; Statistics Canada, 2015; U.S. Census Bureau, 2014).

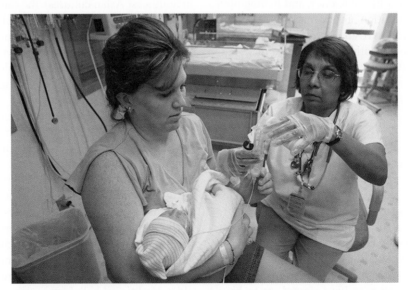

Figure 6-7. Many low-birth-weight infants are "saved" by the availability of hi-tech health care, only to experience multiple chronic illnesses later in life.

Teenagers are in a process of evolving from childhood to adulthood, and they belong not only to the cultural groups that have formed the basis for their values, attitudes, and beliefs but also to the subculture of adolescents. This subculture links the adolescent with other adolescents through a system of socially transmitted behaviors and belongings, such as brand-named clothing, music, and status symbols. The adolescent subculture has its own set of values, beliefs, and practices that may or may not be in harmony with those of the cultural group that previously guided their behaviors.

The adolescent subculture is vaguely structured and lacks formal written rules or codes. Conformity with the peer group behavior is expected. One of the most outstanding characteristics of the adolescent subculture is preoccupation with clothing, hairstyles, and grooming. Clothing mirrors the personal feelings of the adolescent and facilitates identity with the peer group.

Some young men and women prefer to dress in traditional clothing. In the hospital setting, gowns might stifle the individual's sense of identity, so the adolescent should be permitted to wear familiar clothing whenever the style does not interfere with safety, comfort, or hygiene. In a clinical setting, there is no harm in allowing a reasonable amount of makeup, jewelry, or other items of apparel that might be important to the adolescent. Body piercing, prominent in some culture for years, has become widely accepted to the adolescent subculture worldwide. The nurse must assess the placement of the piercing to determine whether it may safely remain in place or must be removed. Piercing of the tongue may prove a hygienic issue and must be discussed with the teen before requiring removal.

There is a relationship between some diseases and socioeconomic status; consequently, low-income teenagers may have a wide range of diagnosed and undiagnosed diseases. During the transition from dependent children to independent adults, some disorders might interfere with the adolescent's development of a positive body image, sexual and personal identity, and value system. The entrance of HIV/AIDS as a global health issue has caused adolescents and adults worldwide to seriously evaluate their sexual behavior. The U.S. Agency for International Development, in collaboration with the World Bank, has completed a 13-nation study of adolescent health in Asia and the Near East in which the key educational tool for adolescents was teaching the ABCs of sex: **A**bstinence, **B**e Faithful, and use **C**ondoms. However, condoms are not always used, and unplanned pregnancies and/or unwanted diseases such as HIV, AIDS, pelvic inflammatory disease, chlamydia, and others often follow in adolescents globally (Centers for Disease Control and Prevention, 2014; U.S. Agency for International Development, 2012). Evidence-Based Practice 6-2 identifies effective ways to assist Latina adolescents prevent rapid repeat births.

Culturally Competent Nursing Care for Children and Adolescents

A few principles of care for specific cultural groups have been provided to illustrate the practical ways in which culturally competent nursing care should be provided. The examples are intended to be illustrative, not exhaustive.

Nursing Assessment of the Family

When assessing the family of a child or adolescent in a clinical setting, nurses should consider the cultural background of the family, the belief systems of the family, as well as the relationship between the child and their family. Each of these components plays a vital role in the cultural assessment of the family and their ability to provide culturally competent care.

Cultural Background

Culture, like language, is acquired early in life, and cultural understanding is typically established by age 5. Every interaction, sound, touch, odor, and experience has a cultural component

Preventing Rapid Repeat Births Among Latina Adolescents: The Role of Parents

Nationally, an estimated 20% of adolescent mothers become pregnant again within 24 months of a previous birth; this is known as a *rapid repeat birth*. Latina adolescents have the highest rate of rapid repeat births in the United States. Although not all adolescent births have adverse outcomes for the Latina mother, they have been associated with an increased rate of sexually transmitted infections and HIV, reduced educational attainment, and decreased financial independence. Adolescent childbearing can also influence future generations. Children born to adolescent mothers have lower levels of cognitive development in childhood, experience less academic achievement, and face a statistically higher probability of becoming adolescent parents themselves, thereby perpetuating a cycle of rapid repeat births among the Latino community.

Several effective pregnancy prevention and parent-based interventions to prevent rapid repeat births among Latino youths from engaging in risky sexual behavior have been developed:

- National Campaign to Prevent Teen and Unplanned Pregnancy
- National Council of La Raza
- Families Talking Together
- Familias Unidas (Families United)
- Cuidalos (Take Care of Them)
- Rompe el Silencio (Break the Silence)

In a national random-digit dial telephone survey of greater than 1,000 adolescents age 12 to 19 years, investigators found that the majority of Latino youths (55%) identified their parents as the greatest influence on their sexual decision making, a proportion significantly greater than reported by their White (42%) and African American (50%) peers. Among pregnant and parenting Latina adolescents, parents are often the primary source of social, emotional, and financial support, and most adolescent parents live at home after giving birth to a child. Research reveals that parents can influence a range of significant behaviors and outcomes among pregnant and parenting teens, including participation in prevention programs, encouragement to pursue higher education, improved contraception knowledge and use, and reduced likelihood of future pregnancies.

Clinical Implications:

- Latina adolescent parents are an underserved population with complex reproductive and sexual health needs.
- Nurses should recognize the importance of the Latino family in guiding adolescent sexual behavior.
- Parent-based interventions should take into account that adolescents have already engaged in sexual activity and are likely to do so again.
- Interventions should examine the pregnancy intentions of pregnant and parenting Latina adolescents, specific issues in having a partner who is older, various forms of effective contraceptive use, integration of secondary prevention with sexually transmitted infections and HIV prevention, and support for further education and/or pursuit of a career or technical training that will enable the adolescent to be financially self-sufficient.

Reference: Bouris, A., Guiliamo-Ramos, V., Cherry, K., Dittus, P, Michael, S., & Gloppen, K. (2012). Preventing rapid repeat births among Latina adolescents. *American Journal of Public Health*, *102*(10), 1842–1847.

that is absorbed by the child even when it is not taught directly. Lessons learned at such early ages become an integral part of thinking and behavior. Table manners, the proper behavior when interacting with adults, sick role behaviors, and the rules of acceptable emotional response are anchored in culture. Many beliefs and behaviors learned at an early age persist into adulthood.

Over time, culture has influenced family functioning in many ways, including marriage forms and ceremonies; choice of mates; postmarital residence; family kinship system; rules governing inheritance, household, and family structure; family obligations; family–community dynamics; and alternative family formations. These traditions have given families a sense of stability and support from which members draw comfort, guidance, and a means of coping with the problems of life, including physical and mental illness, handicaps, disabilities, dying, and death.

Each family modifies the culture of the larger group in ways that are uniquely its own. Some beliefs, practices, and customs are maintained, whereas others are altered or abandoned. Although it is helpful for you to have a basic knowledge of children's cultural backgrounds, it is also necessary to view each family on an individual basis. Assumptions or biased expectations cannot be allowed to replace accurate assessment. It is essential for the nurse to remember that not all members of a cultural group behave in the same fashion. For example, although many Chinese North American children behave in a manner congruent with the stereotype—showing respect for authority, polite social behavior, and a moderate-to-soft voice—some are disrespectful, impolite, and boisterous, and illness only exaggerates the differences. Individual differences, changing norms over time, the degree of acculturation, the length of time the family has lived in a country, and other factors account for variations from the stereotype.

Family Belief Systems

The behavior of children and adolescents is influenced by childrearing practices, parental beliefs about involvement with children, and the type and frequency of disciplinary measures. Although both parents exert an influence on the child's orientation to health, research indicates that a wide cultural variability exists, with the mother being the most influential parent in many cultural groups; this is easily verified in most single-parent households and also very visible in matriarchal societies of African and African American families. Identifying the attitudes, values, and beliefs about health and illness held by the parents and other providers of child care is an important part of the cultural assessment of the family.

Mothers' attitudes toward health and illnesses are related to their educational level. Mothers with little formal education tend to be more fatalistic about illness and less concerned with detecting clinical manifestations of disease in their children than are well-educated mothers. The former are also less likely to follow up on precautionary measures suggested by health care providers. A mother who believes that people have no control over whether they become sick is more likely to seek care in an emergency facility and less likely to have a preventive approach to health. She is also less likely to seek preventative education and might not comply with recommended immunization schedules. Nursing interventions with a mother who believes that there is much a person can do to keep from becoming ill will be different with regard to the nature of health education and counseling provided.

Assessment data related to the belief system(s) of the family provide the nurse with facts from which to choose approaches and priorities. For a mother who is not oriented to prevention of illness or maintenance of health, focusing energies on teaching might not be productive; it might be more useful to spend time designing family follow-up care or establishing an interpersonal relationship that invites the parent to follow recommended immunization schedules, well-child care, and other aspects of health promotion.

Family Structures

Families have become increasingly diverse and complex in recent decades, and there are many ways that social scientists have classified them. One out of every five children in the United States lives with at least one foreign-born parent, and the population is projected to become even more

ethnically diverse in the future (Laughlin, 2014; U.S. Census Bureau, 2014). The number of children under age 18 living in **nuclear** or **conjugal families**, those with two married biologic parents and one or more children, is 46.7 million or 63% of all children (Laughlin, 2014; U.S. Census Bureau, 2014). Among families worldwide, the nuclear family is a rarity. In only 6% of the world's societies are families as isolated and nuclear as in the United States and Canada. Approximately 18 million children, or 24% of all US children, live in a **single-parent family**, most of whom live with a single female parent. An additional 3.8 million children, or 5% of children, live with two unmarried parents. 3.3 million children (5% of children) do not live with either parent; rather, they reside with a guardian, such as another relative or nonrelative acting as a guardian for the child in the absence of a parent. Fifty-five percent of children (1.83 million) who do not live with a parent live with a grandparent or other extended family member. If children coreside with members of their mother's family, this is referred to as a matrifocal family constellation; if the children coreside with members of their father's family, it is called a patrifocal family constellation.

Blended families include children from a previous marriage of the wife, husband, or both parents, or families formed outside of marriage. Lastly, there are **extended families** in which parents and children coreside with other members of one parent's family. The extended family is far more universally the norm. Kin residence sharing, for example, has long been acknowledged as characteristic of many African American, Chinese American, Mexican American, Amish, and other groups (Laughlin, 2014; U.S. Census Bureau, 2014).

Early in the nurse–parent relationship, it is necessary to identify members of the family who play a significant role in the care of the child. In societies where the extended family is the norm, parents—particularly those who married at a young age—might be considered too inexperienced to make major decisions on behalf of their child. In these groups, key decisions are frequently made in consultation with more mature relatives such as grandparents, uncles, aunts, cousins, or other kin. Sometimes, nonkin is considered to be part of the extended family. In many religions, the members of one's church, synagogue, temple, or mosque are viewed as extended family members who might be relied on for various types of support, including child care. Not coincidentally, members of some congregations refer to one another as brothers and sisters. The Amish family pattern is referred to as *friendscraft*, or three-generational family structure. Amish parents know that they can rely on the support of their entire church community. For example, a young Amish couple might turn to that community for assistance with decision making, finances, and emotional and spiritual support when a child is ill. The nurse should ask the parents if anyone else will be participating in the decision making that affects their child. Once that information is known, the person(s) identified by the parents should be included in the child's plan of care.

The influence of the extended family or the social support network on the child's development becomes particularly important when the number of single-parent families in some culturally diverse groups is considered. The nuclear family is the unit for which most health care programs are designed. Consider the implicit message about the family when two or three chairs for visitors are placed in hospital rooms, physician or nurse practitioner offices, and other health care settings, for example. Although a handful of rural hospitals make special accommodations for the extended and church family of clients, few provide a place for the Amish to hitch their horses and buggies adjacent to the facility. With the advent of Family-Centered Care in the United States, all children's hospitals provide more flexible visiting hours and extend visiting privileges to include siblings, extended family, and friends (see Evidence-Based Practice 6-3).

When Health Care Provider Decisions Clash with Parental Preference

Each year, health care research unravels the mystery of previously unknown diseases and conditions; recently, expanded knowledge about Proteus syndrome has been revealed. This rare congenital and progressive disorder causes soft tissue overgrowth (nonmalignant tumors), resulting in swelling that compresses nerves, vessels, and organs. Asymmetrical growth of skeletal and soft tissue also produces spinal deformities and respiratory compromise. It was a 12-year-old with Proteus syndrome who attracted the attention of the health care team. Turner (2010) provides unique insight into 2 years in the life of this child. These 2 years reflected a situation in which the care perceived necessary for the longevity of the child was in direct conflict with the traditional cultural beliefs of a Chinese family who immigrated to the United States. Over several years, the child deteriorated from attending school regularly to a nonverbal, agitated child exhibiting self-injurious behavior (head banging, scratching, and banging of extremities); she was hospitalized seven times. The mother had difficulty physically managing the child; the family had limited financial resources, lived in a small apartment that could not accommodate needed care equipment, was unable to communicate in English, and had no extended family available; the parents voluntarily placed the child in medical foster care.

Over nearly 2 years in foster care, the child improved significantly. Consistent pain management helped to eliminate the self-injurious behavior; mobility improved; she demonstrated the understanding of simple words and began smiling. Since the course/progression of Proteus syndrome is unknown and hospitalizations were becoming more frequent, the primary medical team requested a palliative care consultation.

To determine the outcome of the ethical dilemma, the health care team utilized a four-quadrant ethical decision-making tool taking into consideration medical indications (principles of beneficence and nonmalfeasance), patient preference (respect for autonomy), quality of life (principles of beneficence, nonmalfeasance, and autonomy), and contextual features (loyalty and fairness). When the decisions were made and presented to the parents, they determined it was their familial duty to take the child out of foster care and back to their home to provide a dignified death. The health care team was severely divided about this decision: Some felt, for the child's well-being, she should return to the foster care home where she was showing emotional improvement, and others believed it was a parental decision related to the care of a minor child. This dilemma was taken to the hospital ethics committee for decision. The committee determined that the rights of the parents superseded the other factors and the child was discharged to the parental home with a home care and pain management plan.

This was clearly a difficult decision; however, the solution has ended being a correct one. Once again in her home environment, the child began to thrive, smile, make eye contact with her family, and even walk as few feet. She has been at home for 2 years and her parents seemed quite comfortable with the results: Supported by strong cultural ties, her mother never stops smiling.

Reference: Turner, H. N. (2010). Parental preference or child well-being: An ethical dilemma. *Journal of Pediatric Nursing*, 25(1), 58–63.

Nursing Interventions

Care of the hospitalized child's body is the primary domain of the nurse. Principles related to personal hygiene, including bathing, shaving, and hair care, apply to children of all racial and ethnic backgrounds, but the specific manner in which care is given might vary widely. Despite its importance, hair care is sometimes omitted for

Black children because White, Hispanic, Asian, and Native American nurses might be unfamiliar with proper care. The hair of black children varies widely in texture and is usually fragile. Hair might be long and straight or short, thick, and kinky. The hair and scalp have a natural tendency to be dry and to require daily combing, gentle brushing, and application to the scalp of a light oil such as Vaseline or mineral oil. The hair might be rolled on curlers, braided, or left loose, according to personal preference. Bobby pins or combs might be used to keep the hair in place. If an individual has cornrow braids or shaved, sculptured hair, the scalp might be massaged, oiled, and shampooed without unbraiding the hair. Some blacks prefer straightened hair, which might be obtained chemically or thermally. Hair that has been straightened with a pressing comb will return to its naturally kinky state when exposed to moisture or humidity or when hair growth occurs. Children of Asian descent tend to have straight hair that does not require the same amount of care as the hair of most African Americans or Whites.

Textural variations also are found in the facial hair of culturally diverse boys and men during adolescence and adulthood. Many Asian teenage boys have light facial hair and require infrequent shaving, whereas African American boys and men tend to have a heavy growth of facial hair requiring regular attention. Some black teenage boys have tightly curled facial hair, which, when shaved, curls back upon itself and penetrates the skin. This may result in a local foreign-body reaction on the face that can lead to the formation of papules, pustules, and multiple small keloids. Some African American teens and men might prefer to grow beards rather than shave, particularly when they are ill. Before shaving a teen, determine his usual method of facial grooming and attempt to shave or apply depilatories (agents that remove hair) in a similar manner. When using depilatories, protect the skin from irritation by keeping the chemical from contacting the client's nose, mouth, eyes, and ears. Straight and safety razors are contraindicated when depilatories are used because they can cause local irritation to the skin.

Nurses should ask the child's parent or extended family member how personal hygiene is carried out at home if in doubt. Children might feel more secure if a parent or close family member actually provides the care. If you determine that the child would benefit from care by a familiar caregiver from home, the rationale for requesting family intervention should be explained. Comments that the nursing staff is too busy or uninterested in providing personal hygiene or hair care should be avoided; rather, the benefit to the child's security and sense of well-being should be emphasized.

When bathing a client, remember that the washcloth removes some parts of the outermost skin layer. Such sloughed skin, which will be evident on the washcloth and in the bathwater, will vary in color depending on the ethnic group of the person being bathed. The sloughed skin of a darkly pigmented child, for example, will be a brownish black color. This does not mean that the child was dirty; the normal sloughing of skin is simply more evident in darkly pigmented people when compared with lightly pigmented groups. The more melanin that is present, the darker the skin color will be. Because dryness is more evident on darkly pigmented skin, Vaseline, baby oil, lanolin cream, and lotions can be applied after the bath to give the skin a shiny, healthy appearance.

Communicating with the Hospitalized Child and Family

Communicating with the child and the family is a key component in a successful hospitalization and recovery. Verbal communication is especially difficult when the child–family–health care provider do not speak the same language. The nurses may obtain the services of an interpreter, although they should be aware of gender- and age-related customs before doing so. For instance,

an adolescent girl might be uncomfortable with an older male interpreter, and an older boy might prefer a friend to translate rather than an interpreter connected to the health agency. Attention should also be paid to the correct national origin of the child before seeking an interpreter; for example, an individual from Southeast Asia may speak Vietnamese, Cambodian, or Laotian—vastly different languages. Approximately 15% of migrant/immigrant families speak English in the home; this factor should be included in the nursing assessment. Most children and adolescents involved in the American school system learn English quickly and may serve as interpreters for family members. Even in families who have mastered English as a second language, the stress of illness and hospitalization may cause them to have difficulty communicating with English. Therefore, using a formal or informal interpreter is recommended.

Nonverbal expressions can be powerful communication tools. Nurses should take their cues from observing the family interactions. Some Italian parents/families are very demonstrative with facial expressions and arm/hand gestures while the children may remain quiet. On the other hand, Asian parents and children both remain quiet and often wear "masked faces" showing very little emotional expression. Nurses must be aware of their own nonverbal expressions or actions, as they are often interpreted as disrespect or dislike of the individual rather than a situation.

Evaluation of the Nursing Care Plan

Obtaining a thorough cultural assessment, including use of folk remedies, during the initial encounter with the child/adolescent and parents is essential. It is upon this basis that the plan of care is developed, negotiated, and evaluated. To evaluate the effectiveness of the nursing care plan in providing culturally competent care, first ask a few probing questions to determine whether the plan was successful in achieving the desired outcomes, including the

mutual goals established with the child and parents. Second, if the goals were not met, ask a few probing questions to determine the reasons for failure. Were the child and parents included in the planning and implementation of the nursing care? Were extended family members included in the plan? Did the true decision maker in the family participate in the care plan? Third, if the goals were met, the reasons for their success should be evaluated and communicated to other members of the health care team for future reference.

Application of Cultural Concepts to Nursing Care

Two case studies are presented here to demonstrate the application of transcultural nursing concepts, theories, and research findings to clinical nursing practice. The first, Case Study 6-1, focuses on a very young child from an American Amish family and the second, Case Study 6-2, on a dying child from a Buddhist family. Each case exemplifies the need for involvement of extended families of varying types. Each also reflects how the response of the nursing team affected the end result of the child's care. In addition, a specific, individualized plan of care for the Amish family is presented. As shown, the nursing issues in each case are complex and multifaceted. The interconnectedness of the various components of the child's situation with the larger system is often minimized or disregarded. The values and beliefs of both the nurses within the health care delivery system and the family's extended social network must be considered. For the purpose of analysis, some fundamental conflicts in values and beliefs have been identified. Similarities and differences also have been indicated in the nursing plan of care.

In the case involving the Amish child, the young nurse was clearly advocating for a patient, in a situation requiring change in hospital practice, if not policy. It is assumed that this facility

CASE STUDY 6-1

Presence of Immediate and Extended Family

A rural Amish community is located about 50 miles from an urban medical center, the only facility available for care of an acutely ill child. An enthusiastic new RN emphatically presents her case to allow the presence of family/**extended family** of a 6-month-old Amish child who has been admitted for the repair of a cardiac VSD. The nurse is passionate about the issue, rational in her approach, and assured that she can prevail to change existing visitation policies.

The problem of overnight accommodation for the extended community family has become a topic of debate among the nursing staff. Sensitive to the cultural practices and beliefs of the Amish child and his family, the new RN begins stating her position on behalf of the family's right to adhere to Amish cultural practices to her supervisor. The supervisor listens impatiently and quickly interrupts with her decision. "These people are such a nuisance. The child wouldn't even have the VSD if they didn't insist on intermarriage within their own community. Then they come here in droves and think we have to give them a place to sleep. This isn't a hotel. They can just go back to their horses and buggies and old-fashioned ways. The answer is NO! The natural, biologic mother and father may spend the night. Everyone else is to go home. And that's final."

The nurse leaves the discussion with her supervisor feeling dejected; however, she completes her data collection. Using Leininger's transcultural model (1991), she examines the underlying attitudes, values, and beliefs among the Amish parents and those of the health care providers and then develops an individualized, culturally congruent, plan of care. Prior to discharge, the nurse, in collaboration with the parents and other significant members of the extended family, evaluates the effectiveness of the nursing care from a transcultural nursing perspective. The young nurse must also review the process in which change can be accomplished within the agency. She needs to determine what parts of the system can/should be manipulated to bring about desired change and who are the formal and informal leaders who can effect change.

Outcome: There are no definitive solutions or answers for this dilemma. The case study is intended to demonstrate the complexity of the cross-cultural issues and to emphasize the necessity for thoughtful analysis of various facets of the problem. The ability to synthesize information from previous learning—psychology, anthropology, religion and theology, history, economics, sociology, principles of leadership, and others—to the nursing care of children from culturally diverse backgrounds is invaluable.

The cultural assessment is the foundation of excellent transcultural care and cannot be overlooked even in the face of major obstacles of attitudes of others or limited time. A cultural assessment must become an integral part of the admission assessment of all children and adolescents, thus enabling excellent, individualized, family-centered care.

---

had not yet implemented principles of family-centered care, which are common practice in most agencies that care for children. Given the negative response of the nursing supervisor, it would seem the nurse needs to reassess her approach to the problem. She would be wise to first gather data from her colleagues to help her understand the immediate, inflexible response of the supervisor, and then determine whether there are possible compromises that would be acceptable to both family and supervisor. She will need to present the risk versus benefits of having the extended family remain with the child: Consider factors from agency perspective, the legal perspective, perspective of other patients, and the child/family perspective (see Box 6-1). A review of the literature will reveal significant data that support involvement of extended family in hastening recovery of the child by supporting the entire family.

CASE STUDY 6-2

End-of-Life Care for a Buddhist Adolescent

Ving, 16 years of age, was born in Vietnam and immigrated to Australia with her family 15 years ago. She is a devout Buddhist. Ving was born hepatitis B positive, which is now complicated by advanced liver cancer. Over the past few weeks, Ving's pain has become unmanageable at home, and her family has her admitted to the hospital for better pain management. Her family is concerned that appropriate preparations be made for her death.

In collaboration with Buddhists monks, the nurses of the inpatient unit agree that Ving would be cared for through the final hours of her life with minimal noise and minimal activity in her room; this was to ensure that her soul was as untroubled as possible. Her family remained with Ving around the clock and agreed to notify the nurses when she died; the health care team agreed not to touch the body until the family agreed it was appropriate.

Outcome: On the day of her death, family, close friends, and spiritual advisors were present to oversee the process. Eight hours after her death, it was determined that Ving's consciousness had departed; she was then examined by the health care team, and the time of death was documented.

Adapted with permission from The Royal Australian College of General Practitioners from Clark, K., & Phillips, J. End of life care—The importance of culture and ethnicity. (2010). *Australian Family Physician*, 39(4), 210 -213. Available at www.racgp.org.au/afp/2010/april/end-of-life-care-%E2%80%93-the-importance-of-culture-and-ethnicity

Box 6-1 Nursing Plan of Care: Hospitalization of an Amish Child: Conflicting Cultural Values

Goal: Child's recovery and ultimate discharge from the hospital (return to parents) in an optimal state of health. This is a mutual goal of the Amish child's parents and of the health care providers within the health care system. In order to plan care for this child, the nurse needs to examine the underlying attitudes, values, and beliefs of the two groups that are in conflict. Points on which there is agreement must be identified as well.

Amish–Rural, Agricultural Lifestyle	Urban Health Care Providers
Family	
Large families, extended sociocultural–religious network of community members who assist the natural parents	Small family units, urban lifestyle, nuclear family
Cooperation and support among extended family, especially in stressful "crisis" times such as hospitalization of a child	Individual responsibility by members of a nuclear family; mother and father primarily responsible
Child generally not left alone when away from community; someone from the community visits or stays in absence of parents.	Visiting by grandparents and siblings accepted but only two at any given time and only parents can remain over night.
Concept of family includes "nonblood relatives."	Concept of family includes only biologically related persons.
Parental Obligations	
Children are a part of a larger cultural group; adult members of the larger community have various relationships and obligations to the children and parents even though they are not biologically related.	Mother and father are responsible for children; only they may stay with the child overnight. Physical size of hospital facilities does not allow for a large number of visitors, who clutter rooms, violate fire safety rules by blocking doorways, and hinder delivery of care. Responding to requests for information from every visitor is time consuming and violates HIPAA policies.

(continued)

Economic Considerations

Communal sharing of resources; hospital bill is paid from a common fund; entire bill is paid in cash upon discharge.	Rely on private or state subsidized health insurance coverage for payment of all costs related to patient care; sense of anonymity and impersonal involvement

Traditional and Religious Values

Religious values permeate all aspects of daily living; time set aside daily for prayer and reading of scripture.	Religion is important and adherence to practices often vary based on severity of illness; worship usually limited to a single day of the week, such as Saturday or Sunday.
Belief that illness afflicts both the "just" and the less righteous and is to be endured with patience and faith	Illness is part of a cause–effect relationship; science and technology will one day conquer illness.
Protestant work ethic (in an agricultural, rural sense)	Protestant work ethic (in an urban sense)
Dress is according to 19th-century traditions; specific colors and styles indicate marital status.	Fashions occur in trends; wide range of "acceptable" dress.
Married men wear beards; single men are clean-shaven.	Whether a man shaves is a matter of personal preference.
Simple, rural lifestyle; family-oriented living. For religious reasons, avoid "modern" conveniences such as electricity; use candles/kerosene lights, outdoor sanitary facilities.	Use hi-tech electronic equipment, electricity, and nuclear energy. Indoor plumbing is the norm; autoflush toilets and water that runs with the wave of a hand are "ordinary."

Summary

Culture exerts an all-pervasive influence on infants, children, and adolescents and determines the nursing interventions appropriate for the individual child, parents, and extended family members. Knowledge of the cultural background of the child and family is necessary for the provision of excellent transcultural nursing care. Cross-cultural communication must convey genuine interest and allow for expression of expectations, concerns, and questions.

Culture influences the child's physical and psychosocial growth and development. Basic physiologic needs such as nutrition, sleep, and elimination have aspects that are culturally determined. Parent–child relationships vary significantly among families of different cultures, and individual differences among those with the same background add to the complexity. Cultural beliefs and values related to health and illness influence health-seeking behaviors by parents and determine the nature of care and cure expected.

Regardless of the cultural background of an adolescent, the transition from childhood to adulthood must be accomplished. This can be complicated when the adolescent's values, beliefs, and practices conflict with traditional cultural values or with those of the dominant culture in which the teenager lives. Acculturation of an adolescent presents multiple issues for the family as well as for the teen.

REVIEW QUESTIONS

1. Compare and contrast the childrearing practices of three cultural groups. For each of the three groups, also discuss the role of extended family members in raising children, and describe the ways in which extended family members can assist parents during a child's illness.

2. Critically examine the perceived causes of chronic illness and disability in children from diverse cultures. Describe how the parental philosophic and religious beliefs affect their reaction to and explanations for the child's chronic illness and/or disability.

3. Describe the symptoms associated with the following Hispanic cultural illnesses affecting children:

   a. *Pujos* (grunting)
   b. *Mal ojo* (evil eye)
   c. *Caida de la mollera* (fallen fontanel)
   d. *Empacho* (a digestive disorder)

CRITICAL THINKING ACTIVITIES

1. Arrange for an observational experience in a culturally diverse classroom. Compare and contrast the behaviors observed. Does the student–teacher interaction vary according to cultural background? What culturally based attitudes, values, and beliefs are reflected in the children's behaviors? The teacher's attitude? Ask the teacher(s) to describe the cultural similarities and differences in the classroom.

2. When caring for a child from a cultural background different from your own, spend time talking with the child's parents or primary provider of care, and discuss the childrearing beliefs and practices specifically related to the child's nutrition, sleep, elimination, parent–child relationship, discipline, growth, and development. Compare and contrast the parental responses with your own beliefs and practices.

3. When assigned to the pediatric unit, observe the number and relationship of visitors for children from various cultures. Who visits the child? If nonrelated visitors come, how do they interact with the child? With the parent(s)?

4. When caring for a child from a cultural background different from your own, ask the parent(s) or primary provider(s) of care to tell you what they believe causes the child to be healthy and unhealthy. To what cause(s) do they attribute the current illness or hospitalization? What interventions do they believe will help the child to recover? Are there any healers outside of the professional health care system (e.g., folk, indigenous, or traditional healers) whom they believe could help the child return to health?

REFERENCES

Aruda, M. M. (2011). Predictors of unprotected intercourse for female adolescents measured at their request for a pregnancy test. *Journal of Pediatric Nursing, 26*(3), 216–223. doi: 10.1016/j.pedn.2010.02.005

Agency for Healthcare Research and Quality. (2014). *2013 National Healthcare Disparities Report.* U.S. Department of Health and Human Services (AHRQ Publication No. 14–0006. Rockville, MD: Author.

Barajas, R. G., Martin, A., Brooks-Gunn, J., & Hale, L. (2011). Mother-child bed-sharing in toddlerhood and cognitive and behavioral outcomes. *Pediatrics, 128*(2), e339–e347. doi: 10.1542/peds.2010-3300.

Barry, H., Bacon, M. K., & Child, I. L. (1967). Definitions, ratings, and bibliographic sources of child-training practices of 110 cultures. In C. S. Ford (Ed.). *Cross-cultural approaches* (pp. 293–331). New Haven, CT: HRAF Press.

Benoit, D. (2004). Infant-parent attachment: Definition, types, antecedents, measurement and outcome. *Paediatrics & Child Health, 9*(8), 541–545.

Bresnahan, M., Zhuang, J., & Park, S. (2014). Cultural differences in the perception of health and cuteness of fat babies. *The International Journal of Communication and Health* (4), 52–58.

Cachelin, F. M., & Thompson, D. (2014). Impact of Asian American mothers' feeding beliefs and practices on child obesity in a diverse community sample. *Asian American Journal of Psychology, 5*(3), 223–229.

Carlson, D. L., McNulty, T. L., Bellair, P. E., & Watts, S. (2014). Neighborhoods and racial/ethnic disparities in adolescent sexual risk behavior. *Journal of Youth and Adolescence, 43*(9), 1536. doi: 10.1007/s10964-013-0052-0

Cartagena, D. C., Ameringer, S. W., McGrath, J., Jallo, N., Masho, S. W., & Myers, B. J. (2014). Factors contributing to infant overfeeding with Hispanic mothers. *Journal of Obstetric, Gynecologic, and Neonatal Nursing, 43*(2), 139. doi: 10.1111/1552-6909.12279.

Centers for Disease Control and Prevention. (2014a). Strategies for reducing health disparities: Selected

CDC-sponsored interventions, United States, 2014. *Morbidity and Mortality Weekly Report, Supplement, 63*(1), 1–47.

Centers for Disease Control and Prevention. (2014b). Infant Feeding Practices Study II and its year six follow-up. Retrieved from Centers for Disease Control and Prevention: http://www.cdc.gov/ifps/index.htm

Chen, X., & Eisenberg, N. (2012). Understanding cultural issues in child development: Introduction. *Child Development Perspectives, 6*(1), 1–4.

Children's Defense Fund. (2014). *The state of America's children.* Washington, DC: Children's Defense Fund. Retrieved from http://www.childrensdefense.org

Clark, K., & Philips, J. (2010). End of life care: The importance of culture and ethnicity. *Australian Family Physician, 39*(4), 210–213.

Coutts, D. (2013). Lactose intolerance: Causes, effects, diagnosis, and symptoms. *Gastrointestinal Nursing, 11*(2), 18–21.

Cowie, J. (2014). Measurement of obesity in children. *Primary Health Care, 24*(7), 18–23.

Davis, A., Farage, M. A., & Miller, K. W. (2011). Cultural aspects of menstruation and menstrual hygiene in adolescents. *Expert Review of Obstetrics & Gynecology, 6,* 127–13. Retrieved from http://libproxy.umflint.edu:2166/ps/i.do?id=GALE%7CA252101667&v=2.1&u=lom_umichflint&it=r&p=HRCA&sw=w&asid=911f2622653592b7ac0bf2bde25ef26e

Dewar, G. (2013). Infant crying, fussing, and colic: An anthropological perspective on the role of parenting. Retrieved from Parenting Science: http://www.parentingscience.com/infant-crying.html

Dewar, G. (2014). The science of attachment parenting. Retrieved from Parenting Science: http://www.parenting-science.com/attachment-parenting.html

Federal Interagency Forum on Child and Family Statistics. (2006). America's children in brief: Key national indicators of well-being, 2006. Retrieved from http://www.childstats.gov/americaschildren

Findlay, L., Kohen, D., & Miller, A. (2014). Developmental milestones among Aboriginal children in Canada. *Paediatrics & Child Health, 19*(5), 241–246.

Huang, Y., Hauck, F. R., Signore, C., Yu, A., Raju, T. N., Huang, T. T., & Fein, S. B. (2013). Influence of bedsharing activity on breastfeeding duration among U.S. mothers. *JAMA Pediatrics, 137*(11), 1038–1044. doi: 10.1001/jamapediatrics.20132632.

Jain, S., Romack, R., & Jain, R. (2011). Bed sharing in school-age children: Clinical and social implications. *Journal of Child and Psychiatric Nursing, 24,* 185–189.

John Hopkins Children's Center. (2015). Malnutrition. Retrieved January 11, 2015 from http://www.hopkinschildrens.org/Malnutrition.aspx

Keller, H. (2013). Attachment and culture. *Journal of Cross-Cultural Psychology, 44*(2), 175–194.

Kirby, J. B., Liang, L., Hsin-Jen, C., & Wang, Y. (2012). Race, place, and obesity: The complex relationships among community racial/ethnic composition, individual race/ethnicity, and obesity in the United States. *American Journal of Public Health, 102*(8), 1572–1578.

Kliegman, R. M., Stanton, B. F., Saint Geme, J. W., Schor, N. F., & Behrman, R. E. (2011). *Nelson textbook of pediatrics* (19th ed.). Philadelphia, PA: Elsevier Saunders.

Korbin, J. E. (1991). Cross-cultural perspectives and research directions for the 21st century. *Child Abuse and Neglect, 15*(Suppl. 1), 67–77.

Lanier, P., Maguire, K., Tova, J., Drake, B., & Hubel, G. (2014). Race and ethnic differences in early childhood maltreatment in the United States. *Journal of Developmental and Behavioral Pediatrics, 35*(7), 419–430.

Laughlin, L. (2014). *A child's day: Living arrangements, nativity, and family transitions: 2011 (selected indicators of child well-being), Current Population Reports, P70-139.* Washington, DC: U.S. Census Bureau.

Leininger, M. M. (1991). *Culture care delivery and universality: A theory of nursing.* New York, NY: National League for Nursing Press.

Liamputtong, P. (2011). *Infant feeding practices: A cross-cultural perspective.* New York, NY: Springer Science + Business Media.

Luijk, M. P., Mileva-Seitz, V. R., Jansen, P. W., van IJzendoorn, M. H., Jaddoe, V. W., Raat, H., et al. (2013). Ethnic differences in prevalence and determinants of mother-child bedsharing in early childhood. *Sleep Medicine, 14,* 1092–1099.

Moreno, G., Johnson-Shelton, D., & Boles, S. (2013). Prevalence and prediction of overweight and obesity among elementary school children. *Journal of School Health, 83*(1), 157–163.

Natale, V., & Rajagopalan, A. (2014). Worldwide variation in human growth and the World Health Organization growth standards: A systematic review. *British Medical Journal Open, 8*(1), e003735. Retrieved at http://www.pubfacts.com/detail/24401723/Worldwide-variation-in-human-growth-and-the-World-Health-Organization-growth-standards:-a-systematic

The National Center on Family Homelessness. (2015). "Children." Retrieved January 11, 2015 from http://www.familyhomelessness.org/children.php?p=ts

Ogden, C. L., Carroll, M. D., Kit, B. K., & Flegal, K. M. (2014). Prevalence of childhood and adult obesity in the United States, 2011–2012. *JAMA, 311*(8), 806.

Overfield, T. (1995). *Biologic variation in health and illness: Race, age and sex differences* (2nd ed.). New York, NY: CRC Press.

Rakhmanina, N., Hader, S., Denson, A., Gaur, A., Mitchell, C., Henderson, S., Paul, M., Barton, T., Herbert-Grant, M., Perez, E., Malachowski, J., Dominguez, K, Danner, S., & Nesheim, S. (2011). Premastication of food by caregivers of HIV-exposed children—Nine US sites, 2009–2010. *Morbidity and Mortality Weekly Report, 60*(9), 273–275.

Ryan, C. (2013). *Language use in the United States: 2011.* U.S. Department of Commerce, U.S. Census Bureau. Washington, DC: U.S. Census Bureau.

Salm Ward, T. C. (2014). Reasons for mother-infant bed sharing: A systematic narrative synthesis of the literature and implications for future research. *Maternal and Child Health Journal, 19*(3), 675–690. doi: 10.1007/s10995-014-1557-1.

Schmied, V., Olley, H., Burns, E., Duff, M., Dennis, C., & Dahlen, H. G. (2012). Contradictions and conflict: A meta-ethnographic study of migrant women's experience with breast feeding in a new country. *Biomedical Central Pregnancy and Childbirth, 12,* 163–174.

Schreirer, H. M. C., & Chen, E. (2013). Socioeconomic status and the health of youth: A multi-level, multi-domain approach to conceptualizing pathways. *Psychological Bulletin, 139*(3), 606–654.

Singh, G. K., & Lin, S. C. (2013). Marked ethnic, nativity, socio-economic disparities in disability and health insurance among U.S. children and adults: American Community Survey. *Biomedical Research International,* 2013, 627412. doi: 10.1155/2013//627412

Statistics Canada. (2015). http://www5.statcan.gc.ca/subject-sujet/subtheme-soustheme?pid=20000&id=20005&lang=eng&more=0

Steinman, L., Doescher, M., Keppel, G. A., Pak-Gorstein, S., Graham, E., Haq, A., Johnson, D. B., & Spicer, P. (2010). Understanding infant feeding beliefs, practices and preferred nutrition education and health provider approaches: An exploratory study with Somali mothers in the USA. *Maternal & Child Nutrition, 6*(1), 67–88. doi: 10.1111/j.1740-8709.2009.00185.x

Turner, H. N. (2010). Parental preference or child well being: An ethical dilemma. *Journal of Pediatric Nursing, 25*(1), 58–63.

U.S. Census Bureau. (2013). American fact finder. Retrieved from U.S. Census Bureau: http://factfinder2.census.gov/faces/nav/jsf/pages/index.xhtml

U.S. Census Bureau. (2014). Income and poverty in the United States: 2013. *Current Population Reports, P60-249,* 1–72. Retrieved from http://www.census.gov/content/dam/Census/library/publications/2014/demo/p60-249.pdf

Upadhya, K. K., & Ellen, J. M. (2011). Social disadvantages as a risk for first pregnancy among adolescent females in the United States. *Journal of Adolescent Health, 49,* 538–541. doi: 10.1016/j.jadohealth.2011.04.011

Weden, M. M., Brownell, P., & Rendall, M. S. (2012). Prenatal, perinatal, early life, and sociodemographic factors underlying high body mass index in early childhood. *American Journal of Public Health, 102*(11), 2057–2065.

Whaley, A. (2013). Sociocultural differences in the developmental consequences of the use of physical discipline during childhood. *Cultural Diversity and Ethnic Minority Psychology, 6*(1), 5–12.

World Health Organization. (2010). *Enhancing the rights of adolescent girls.* Geneva, Switzerland: WHO.

World Health Organization. (2014). Global strategy on diet, physical activity: Childhood overweight and obesity. Retrieved on 11-5-14 from http://www.who.int/dietphysicalactivity/childhood/en/

7

Transcultural Perspectives in the Nursing Care of Adults

● Joyceen S. Boyle

Key Terms

Adulthood
Caregiving
Developmental crises
Developmental tasks
Generativity
Health/illness situational crises

Health/illness situational
transitions
"High blood"
HIV/AIDS
Middle adulthood
Midlife crisis
"Nerves"
Physiologic development

Psychosocial development
Sandwich generation
Social age
Social roles
Stroke belt
Transitions of adulthood
Young adulthood

Learning Objectives

1. Evaluate how culture influences adult development.
2. Explore how health-related situational crises or transitions might influence adult development.
3. Analyze the influences of culture on caregiving in the African American culture.
4. Analyze the influences of culture on women's development in the African American family.
5. Evaluate cultural influences in adulthood that assist individuals and families to manage during health-related situational crises or transitions.
6. Explain how gender and specific religious beliefs and practices might influence an adult's health and/or illness during situational crises or transitions.

This chapter discusses transcultural perspectives of health and nursing care associated with developmental events in the adult years. The focus is primarily on **young and middle adulthood**. The first section of this chapter presents an overview of cultural influences on **adulthood**, with an emphasis on how **health/illness situational crises or transitions** might be influenced by

cultural variations. The second section provides the context for and gives an example of a health-related situational crisis. The influences of culture on individual and family responses to health problems, caregiving, and health/illness transitions and crises are discussed.

Health/illness transitions have been referred to in the past as **developmental tasks**, those transitions that occur in a normal successful adulthood. A **health/illness situational crisis** refers to changes or turmoil as individuals struggle to cope with a sudden life-threatening illness. Erikson (1963), who studied adult development, used the term "developmental tasks" or "developmental crises" to describe those times in an individual's life when changes occur, such as marriage or the birth of a child. Meleis, Sawyer, Im, Hilfinger Messias and Schumacher (2000) chose the term "**transitions**" as they believe that term more adequately describes life changes and is a conceptually more appropriate term for nursing theory. Nomenclature or terminology about changes and experiences in adulthood can be confusing as the terms are changing. In this chapter, *transitions* refer to those health or illness events that occur within adulthood and require an individual to make modifications in his/her lifestyle. Transitions can occur gradually over a period of time or they may be preceded by a situational crisis. A situational crisis includes more turmoil and anxiety and is more threatening to an individual and family. An example of a health/illness situational crisis might be a sudden myocardial infarction experienced by a 48-year-old man. Until his condition is stabilized, both he and his family will be in a crisis situation, worried and very anxious about his life. When his condition stabilizes and is no longer life threatening, both he and his family members will experience a more gradual health/illness transition. This transition will include changes in his behavior such as appropriate exercises, changes in diet that might include weight reduction, and the addition of daily medications. Whether the client experiences a crisis or a transition, he or she will need culturally competent and contextually meaningful nursing care.

Overview of Cultural Influences on Adulthood

Health/illness crises and/or transitions during adulthood are of interest to nursing because they include responses to health and illness. In addition, health/illness transitions influence how individuals respond to health promotion and wellness by shaping individual lifestyles including eating habits, exercise, work, and leisure activities. Consider, for example, how pregnancy (a transition into motherhood) influences many young adult women to improve their diet, begin moderate exercises, abstain from alcohol, and, in general, take better care of themselves so their baby will be healthy.

The adult years are a time when gradual physical and psychosocial changes occur. These changes are usually gradual and reflect the normal processes of aging. These physical changes, or **physiologic development**, are evident in the hormonal changes that take place in adulthood in both men and women. **Psychosocial development**, or the development of personality, may be more subtle but is equally important. Both physiologic development and psychosocial development are influenced by cultural values and norms, and they occur throughout a lifetime.

Physiologic Development During Adulthood

Women undergo menopause, one of the more profound physiologic changes that results in a gradual decrease in ovarian function with subsequent depletion of progesterone and estrogen. While these physiologic changes occur, self-image and self-concept (psychosocial terms) change also. The influence of culture is relevant because women learn to respond to menopause within the context of their families and culture. The *perception* of menopause and *aspects* of the experience of menopausal symptoms appear to vary across cultures. It has sometimes been assumed that non-Western women do not experience the

menopausal problems seen in Western society because their status increases as they age; however, this assumption has been challenged. In Western cultures, such as Canada and the United States, youth and beauty are valued and aging is viewed with trepidation. Western medicine has tended to treat the symptoms of menopause with hormone replacement therapy, surgical interventions, and/or pharmaceutical products. Although there are not many studies on the perimenopausal transition across cultural groups, there seem to be cultural differences in the reporting of symptoms associated with treatments for menopausal symptoms. One recent study has shown that such factors as length of time spent in the United States and social–economic status were significant predictors of number and severity of menopausal symptoms among immigrant women (Im, Lee, & Chee, 2010). This reinforces an earlier statement that women (as well as others) learn to respond to menopause and aging within the context of their families and culture.

Men also have physical and emotional changes from the decreased levels of hormones. Loss of muscle mass and strength and a possible loss of sexual potency occur slowly. However, developmental differences among both adult men and women have not been extensively examined cross-culturally, and most existing theoretical and conceptual models of adult health do not provide insight into cultural variations. The cultural belief that aging, however gradual, is a normal process and not a cause for medical and/or surgical intervention may be more apparent in diverse cultural groups.

Psychosocial Development During Adulthood

Adulthood was termed the "empty middle" by Bronfenbrenner (1977). A noted developmental psychologist, his use of this term was an indication of Western culture's lack of interest in the adult years. Traditionally, these years were viewed as one long plateau that separates childhood from old age. It was assumed that decisions affecting marriage and career were made in the late teens and that drastic changes in developmental processes seldom occurred afterward. For many years, most developmental theorists saw adulthood as a period to adapt to and come to terms with aging and one's own mortality. Western thinking has changed considerably since Bronfenbrenner's observations. Psychosocial development in middle age is now viewed as a vigorous and changing stage of life involving many challenges and transformations.

Sociocultural factors in Western society have precipitated tremendous changes, producing crises, change, and other unanticipated events in adult lives. Divorce, remarriage, career changes, and increased mobility, as well as other societal changes (the sexual revolution, the women's movement), have had a profound impact on the adult years. Many middle-aged adults may be caught in the **sandwich generation**—still concerned with older children (and sometimes grandchildren) while also increasingly concerned with the care of aging parents. Middle life can be a time of reassessment, turmoil, and change. Society acknowledges this with common terms such as **midlife crisis** or even *empty nest syndrome*, along with other terms that imply stress, dissatisfaction, and unrest. However, adulthood is not always a tumultuous, crisis-oriented state; many middle-aged persons welcome the space, time, and independence that middle age often brings. Midlife can be a time of challenge, enjoyment, and satisfaction for many persons. We now tend to view a "midlife crises" as a time of transition that can be a positive experience, including the mastery of new skills and behaviors that helps an individual to change and grow in response to a new environment (Meleis et al., 2000).

Chronologic Standards for Appropriate Adult Behavior

Much of the work on adult development was done in the 1960s and 1970s by developmental psychologists such as Bronfenbrenner (1977); Havighurst (1974); and Neugarten (1968), all of who proposed

different theories about adult development. We still rely on some of this early work as we attempt to understand the complexities of adult development. Neugarten (1968) observed that each culture has specific chronologic standards for appropriate adult behavior and that these cultural standards prescribe the ideal ages at which to leave the protection of one's parents, choose a vocation, marry, have children, and, in general, get on with life. The events associated with these standards do not necessarily precipitate crises, but they do bring about change. What is more important is the timing of these events. As a result of each culture's sense of social time, individuals tend to measure their accomplishments and adjust their behavior according to a kind of social clock. Awareness of the social timetable is frequently reinforced by the judgments and urging of friends and family, who say, "It's time for you to ..." or "You are getting too old to ..." or "Act your age."

Problems often arise when social timetables change for unpredictable reasons. An example is the recent trend of adult children, frequently divorced, unemployed, or both, returning to live with their parents, often bringing along their own children. Grandparents caring for grandchildren is now a common phenomenon in Western society. Being widowed in young adulthood or losing one's job at age 50 due to an economic downturn are examples of events in adulthood that are likely to cause stress and conflict because they occur outside of the acceptable social timetable.

Culture exerts important influences on human development in that it provides a means for recognizing stages in the continuum of individual development throughout the lifespan. It is culture that defines social age, or what is considered an appropriate behavior in each stage of the life cycle. In nearly all societies, adult role expectations are placed on young people when they reach a certain age. Several cultures have defined rites of passage that mark the line between youth and adulthood; in the United States, markers of beginning adulthood include reaching the legal age to obtain a driver's license, to drink alcohol, or to join the military forces.

Menarche is a milestone in a young girl's physiologic development and a psychologically significant event that provides a rather dramatic demarcation between girlhood and womanhood. However, this is not an event that is celebrated openly in Western culture; most girls are too embarrassed to talk openly about it with anyone but their mothers or close friends. There are no definitive boundaries that mark adulthood for either young girls or young boys, although legal sanctions confer some rights and responsibilities at the ages of 18 and 21 years. There is no single criterion for the determination of when young adulthood begins, given that different individuals experience and cope with growth and development differently and at different chronologic ages. A young boy who joins the military forces at age 18 and serves in Iraq or Afghanistan may "grow up" more quickly than the 18-year-old who lives with his parents, has a part-time job, and attends a local community college.

Adulthood is usually divided into **young adulthood** (late teens, 20s, and 30s) and **middle adulthood** (40s and 50s), but the age lines can be fuzzy. Generally, a **young adult** in his or her late teens and early 20s struggles with independence and issues related to intimacy and relationships outside the family. Role changes occur when the young adult is pursuing an education, experiencing marriage, starting a family, and establishing a career. A **middle adult** most often concentrates on career and family matters. However, as previously mentioned, adulthood is not necessarily an orderly or predictable plateau. Experiences at work have a direct bearing on the middle-aged adult's development through exposure to job-related stress, levels of physical and intellectual activity, and social relations formed with coworkers. "Recareering" or changing careers during middle adulthood is also becoming more common. At home, family life can be chaotic, with role changes and other developmental transitions occurring with dizzying frequency. Often, adults are faced with the realization that they are getting older and feel like they have made the wrong choices or have left many things still undone.

Some life changes can lead to **developmental crises.** According to Erikson (1963), a developmental crisis occurs when an individual experiences normal and expected challenges that are age appropriate. For example, a young adult may have difficulties separating from his or her parents and establishing independence. This is usually resolved as "homesickness" and dissipates as the young adult gains the ability to adjust to a new lifestyle such as college, the military, or employment away from home. A health/illness situational crisis is often focused and specific and can occur at any time. Sometimes, a situational crisis can be precipitated by an illness, such as a diagnosis of type 2 diabetes or the death of an infant. A situational health/illness crisis usually is time limited, although additional transitions may occur. How well individuals cope with and manage the challenges of health/illness crises and transitions in adulthood is influenced by cultural values, traditions, and backgrounds.

Developmental Tasks

Throughout life, each individual is confronted with **developmental tasks** (Erikson, 1963), those responses to life situations encountered by all persons experiencing physiologic, psychological, spiritual, and sociologic changes. Although the developmental tasks of childhood are widely known and have long been studied, the developmental tasks of adulthood are less familiar to most nurses.

Several theorists have studied and defined the developmental or *midlife* tasks of adulthood. Many personality theorists—for example, Freud, Erikson, and Fromm—cite maturity as the major criterion or task of adulthood. These various theories have implications for how we define "development," "maturity," and "wisdom." According to Erikson (1963), the major developmental task of middle adulthood is the resolution of generativity versus stagnation. Resolution of the "crises" or conflict between these two conflicting forces results in attainment of the first attribute, in this case generativity. **Generativity** is accomplished through parenting, working in one's career,

participating in community activities, or working cooperatively with peers, spouse, family members, and others to reach mutually determined goals. Mature adults have a well-developed philosophy of life that serves as a basis for stability in their lives. Individuals in adulthood assume numerous **social roles**, such as spouse, parent, child of aging parent, worker, friend, organization member, and citizen. Each of these social roles involves expected behaviors established by the values and norms of society. Through the process of socialization, the individual is expected to learn the behaviors appropriate to the new role. It is important to note that many developmental theories have connotations of stability and blandness associated with adulthood, although this probably is not the case. The constellation of characteristics enumerated by Erikson and other theorists has been attributed to predominantly White Anglo-Saxon Protestant (WASP) views and behaviors. For many cultural groups in Western society, the mastery of Erikson's developmental tasks is not easily managed and is not always applicable, and in some cases, it may even be undesirable. For some groups, developmental tasks may be accomplished through culturally defined patterns that are different from or outside of the norm of what is expected in the dominant culture.

Evidence-Based Practice 7-1 discusses how an observant Jewish woman and her family, in labor, delivery, and postpartum, should have nursing care that allows her to abide by Jewish laws, customs, and practices that influence everyday life as well as those that pertain to childbearing. Childbearing is a special time for most cultures, and there are cultural prescriptions to ensure the well-being of both the mother and the child. Childbearing that occurs in young and middle adulthood is a prime example of the interface between culture, religion, childbearing practices, and transcultural nursing care.

Studies focusing on the developmental experiences of women have led several authors (Belenky, McVicker, Clinchy, Goldberger, & Tarule, 1997) to suggest that developmental stages and the

Jewish Laws, Customs, and Practice in Labor, Delivery, and Postpartum Care

This article provides a comprehensive and thorough guide to specific laws, customs, and practices of traditionally, religious observant Jews that assist the transcultural nurse or midwife to provide culturally congruent and sensitive care during labor, delivery, and the postpartum period. Providing culturally congruent care includes cultural knowledge, in this case, the nurse or midwife needs to understand the Jewish laws, customs, and practices that guide everyday life, as well as those that pertain to childbearing. These cultural issues include adherence to the laws that influence intimacy issues between husband and wife, or *niddah*; dietary laws, or *kashrut*; and observance of the Sabbath. Detailed tables are provided that list the following: (1) observant Jewish customs, laws, and practices during labor, delivery, and postpartum; (2) annual Jewish holidays and fast days; (3) a cultural assessment for Jewish clients in labor, delivery, and postpartum. Case studies are presented that describe cultural competence challenges for nurses who want to learn about the Jewish culture and how to provide culturally competent care to Jewish women during childbirth.

Clinical Implications

- Recognize that observant Jewish couples are committed to maintaining their religious laws, customs, and practices as much as possible throughout the labor, delivery, and postpartum experiences.
- Understand that childbirth is a time that is highly influenced by cultural values and beliefs.
- The religious laws, customs, and practices that will be most apparent during labor, delivery, and postpartum will pertain to prayer, communication between husband and wife, dietary laws, the Sabbath, modesty issues, and labor and birth customs.
- The culturally competent nurse follows the cues of the religious family, tailoring his or her health and nursing care in a manner that allows the family to practice their traditions in their specific designed manner while employing professionalism and creativity in providing quality patient care.

Reference: Noble, A., Rom, M., Newsome-Wicks, M., Englehardt, K., & Woloski-Wruble, A. (2009). Jewish laws, customs, and practice in labor, delivery and postpartum care. *Journal of Transcultural Nursing, 20,* 323–333.

---

associated developmental tasks of adulthood have been derived primarily from studies of men. These authors suggest that women experience adult development differently. Women's traditional location of responsibility was in the home, nurturing children and husbands as well as parents. Belenky et al. point out that this view is changing, prompted by societal changes and informed by scholars who are addressing women's psychosocial development in new ways.

Culture and Adult Transitions

More recent theories of adulthood (Demick & Andreoletti, 2003; McCrae & Costa, 2003) suggest that development is an evolutionary expanse involving different eras and transitions. These life transitions have triumphs, costs, and disruptions. Within nursing, Meleis et al. (2000) proposed a framework to study life transitions. They focus on transitions that are developmental and situational, including those brought about by an illness.

The next section discusses several important adult life transitions and examines how culture and life events influence adult growth and change during these transitions. The successful progression through developmental tasks and/or life transitions may occur slowly over many years and are important in terms of quality of life and life satisfaction. Culture influences these transitions, and it is important that nurses be able to

evaluate their adult clients and help them adjust and change in culturally appropriate ways. These adult life transitions are often based on what we could call "middle-class, White American culture." Diverse cultures may experience different life transitions or experience life transitions in different ways depending on the cultural group (Baird, 2012; Baird & Boyle, 2012). The following section focuses on various cultural groups and how they might experience adult life transitions. The terms "transitions" and "developmental tasks or goals" are used interchangeably and refer to selected activities at a certain period in life that are directed toward a goal. Unsuccessful achievement of this goal is thought to lead to inability to perform tasks associated with the next period or stage in life.

Developmental Transitions: Achieving Career Success

Many persons in traditional Western culture define career success in financial terms, while others may see it as providing service or making a contribution to the lives of their fellow citizens. Achieving success in one's career—and that includes adequate financial renumeration as well as satisfaction and enjoyment—is considered an important developmental task or goal in adulthood. However, there are many groups who struggle to attain this goal. Immigrants to the United States, Canada, or Europe may find it is very difficult to find employment that pays an adequate salary or offers opportunities for advancement or job satisfaction. North America and Europe, as well as other parts of the world, have experienced a tremendous influx of immigrants and refugees from Southeast Asia, Latin America, Eastern Europe, the Middle East, Africa, and other geographical areas. Although immigrants and refugees may aspire to career success or to earn a higher salary, those may be difficult goals to attain. They may have difficulty with the language, with the skills and educational level required, as well as other factors necessary for holding a good job in their new country.

Other factors, such as gender, also influence the attainment of satisfaction in career choices.

More women are working outside of the home, and there may be a different division of time and energy for both spouses that pose challenges. Women's presence in the work force has increased dramatically, from 30.3 million in 1970 to 72.7 million during 2006 to 2010, and this has had a significant impact on childcare and family finances. Although women have made significant gains in certain occupations, many women continue to be employed in low-paying jobs with little chance for advancement. Many are employed in occupations that have been traditionally oriented toward women (Huffington Post, April 12, 2014), and the salaries are less than men earn in similar positions. Working in a low-paying job that does not offer opportunities for advancement or intellectual challenges does not lead to career success or recognition from one's peers.

Many immigrant and refugee families experience role conflict and stress as gender roles begin to change during contact with Western culture. For example, sometimes, the male head of household who has immigrated is unable to find employment; if he was a professional in his former country, he may be reluctant to accept the menial jobs that are traditionally filled by immigrants or refugees when they first migrate to another country. Frequently, low-status jobs are more available to immigrant women, yet their traditional roles are closely tied to the home and family. When an immigrant or refugee woman begins to work outside of the home, her role changes and those changes alter the traditional power structure and the roles within the family. The lack of adequate social supports, such as affordable daycare for children and adequate compensation for work, and the additional physical and emotional stress result in an unacknowledged toll on immigrant and refugee families. Box 7-1 lists some characteristics of immigrant and refugee families.

At present, to expect members of certain groups, such as poor or ethnic minorities, newly arrived immigrants or refugees, the homeless, the mentally ill, or the unemployed, to achieve satisfaction from jobs that interest them or from status derived from succeeding in a career is unrealistic

Box 7-1 Some Characteristics of Immigrant and Refugee Families

1. Traditional family values are evident; for example, roles of men and women are differentiated. Women's role is in the home, with the family. Men are heads of the household and family providers.
2. Families tend to be extended; if members do not actually live in the same household, they visit and contact each other frequently. New immigrants and refugees tend to keep in fairly close contact with family members in the home country.
3. Many immigrants come to the United States because they already have family members here.
4. Most immigrants and refugees are poor and struggle to earn an adequate income. Often, men in refugee communities have been professionals in their home country but are unable to be employed in the same capacity in their new host country. Women are often more easily employed outside of the home,

and they often find employment as domestic or service workers. For many refugee or immigrant women, working outside of the home is a new experience for them. To earn a salary and provide for their families can be very empowering for these women.
5. Refugees may be fleeing war and political persecution. Many may experience symptoms of posttraumatic stress syndrome.
6. Traditional health and illness beliefs may influence behavior. Immigrant and refugee families may combine traditional health practices with modern Western health care. The use of traditional practices is fairly common in some groups.
7. Language is a significant barrier for the first few years that immigrants and refugees live in the United States and Canada. Children tend to learn English and become acculturated faster than their parents.

and indicates a lack of sensitivity to the problems faced by these groups. Thus, although the work role is valued in American society, the attainment of a successful career that includes financial success and personal fulfillment may not be realistic for some minority groups, immigrants, or even certain individuals within the majority culture, some of whom are returning to school in the hope of preparing for a second career.

Developmental Transition: Achieving Social and Civic Responsibility

Social and civic responsibilities are in part culturally defined. Generally speaking, American and Canadian cultures value the voluntary contributions of their citizens in various agencies and organizations that contribute services to the community or society in general. For this discussion, achieving social and civic responsibilities can be viewed as participation in those activities in adulthood that contribute to the "good of society."

Usually, this means activities and commitments outside of the immediate family. It can vary considerably, from serving as a board member for a community agency, such as a homeless shelter, to volunteering to teach in a literacy program or donating blood at the local blood bank. Not all members of dominant Western cultures value achieving an elected office in, for example, the local Parent–Teacher Association (PTA) or Rotary Club; other cultures may find these goals baffling and, instead, emphasize activities and contributions within the cultural group. For example, in some groups, religious obligations are given priority over civic responsibilities. Usually, traditional religious groups have not encouraged the emergence of women in leadership roles within the church structure or the wider society, although this is now being challenged by women within several religious groups.

Sometimes within traditional cultures, women who seek roles outside the family are criticized

because recognition and acknowledgment outside the family group may conflict with the traditional role of women. Some religious and ethnic or cultural groups believe that a woman's place is in the home, and women who attempt to succeed in a career or participate in activities outside the home or group are frowned on by other members of the group. Civic responsibilities that relate to children or domestic matters may be viewed as more appropriate for women to assume, whereas other civic activities may be viewed as more within the province of men. Middle Eastern and Southeast Asian cultures emphasize and value responsibilities and contributions to the extended family or clan rather than to the wider society. Numerous researchers (Baird, 2012; Baird & Boyle, 2012) have reported that refugee women in the United States continue to socialize almost exclusively with other refugee women, often extended family/clan or tribe members. They are more comfortable with others who not only share their traditional culture and language and life events, but who are also going through similar situational transitions (the immigrant experience).

Many refugee women are single or widowed with children. Women whose husbands have been killed or have stayed behind to fight in various conflicts are often forced to flee with children and/or elderly family members. Women refugees carry a substantial burden during the migration process and are essential in helping the family members settle into a new country. Coping with life in a new country becomes the focus of their daily lives. Finding a job, getting children into school, learning English, and other resettlement activities become challenging transitions for them. Many refugee women are justifiably very proud of their accomplishments. They learn new job skills, a new language, how to drive a car, all accomplishments that are not always recognized by members of their new society. For the refugee women and her family, these are significant achievements; however, they can be quite stressful. Often, informal social networks, such as having family members and friends nearby, are very helpful and supportive. The social and

civic responsibilities that we have associated with adulthood in Western cultures may not be appropriate for many other cultural groups. Concepts such as social connectedness and integration, resilience, and strength (described by Baird, 2012 and Baird & Boyle, 2012) might help us better understand adult development and transitions in refugee and immigrant families.

Developmental Transition: Marriage and Raising Children to Adulthood

Marriage and raising children usually take place in early to middle adulthood. The age at which young persons marry and become independent varies by custom or cultural norm, as well as by socioeconomic status. Generally speaking, in Western culture, young adults of lower socioeconomic status leave school, begin work, marry, and become parents and grandparents at earlier ages than middle-class or upper-class young adults. Indeed, many North American families encourage early independence by urging their children to attend college or to find employment away from home. Other cultural groups, such as those from the Middle East and Latin America, place more emphasis on maintaining the extended family. Even after marriage, a son and his new wife may choose to live very close to both families and to visit relatives several times each day. Families from some cultural groups, such as Hispanics, or traditional religious groups, such as the Hutterites or the Amish, may be reluctant to allow their young daughters to leave home until they marry. In many Muslim families, girls do not leave home until they are married.

Increased mobility in American and Canadian societies has impacted family life as many young families now live far away from grandparents, and the traditional influences of grandparents on young grandchildren are decreasing. Sometimes because of geographical distance, grandparents barely know their grandchildren, although digital photos via home computers, cell phones, Skype, and other technological devices are helping to keep grandparents up to date with the growth and activities of their grandchildren.

Changes in terms of women's participation in the workforce began in the 1970s when a single-income household could no longer support a comfortable, middle-class lifestyle (Huffington Post, April 9, 2014). In addition, many young women attend college or universities and want to become established in their careers before they marry or have children. With both mothers and fathers working, children are often placed in childcare facilities. These factors have had a tremendous impact on men and women's roles and responsibilities within the marriage and on how children are raised.

Developmental Transition: Changing Roles and Relationships

Relationships between marriage partners, between and among genders, within social networks of family and friends, and between parents and children and the roles men and women play within these relationships are all influenced by cultural norms and traditions. In Western culture, the relationship between a wife and husband is often enhanced in middle adulthood, although divorce at this time is not infrequent in the United States. The frequent need for both spouses to work may conflict with traditional roles and cause feelings of guilt on the part of both the husband and wife. Some women continue to assume all responsibility for domestic chores while working outside the home, and they experience considerable stress and fatigue as a result of multiple role demands. If either or both spouses are working in low-paying jobs and still struggling to make ends meet, or if the jobholder is laid off or loses his or her job, adulthood may not be a time of enjoyment and leisure activities. Some adults may experience what is known as a "midlife jolt," a particularly dramatic life event such as an accident, divorce, death of a spouse, or other life-changing event. The struggle to adjust to such an event and make meaning out of it often inspires profound and lasting personal growth and change. Of course, not everyone experiences transformative growth after a traumatic event; for some individuals, such an event might trigger depression, a sense of despair, and a downward trajectory in terms of quality of life.

The relationship between married adults can vary considerably by culture. For example, not all cultures emphasize an emotionally close interpersonal relationship between spouses. In some Hispanic cultures, women develop more intense relationships or affective bonds with their children or relatives than with their husbands. Latin men, in turn, may form close bonds with siblings or friends—ties that meet the needs for companionship, emotional support, and caring that in other cultures might be expected from their wives.

Gender roles and how men and women go about establishing personal ties with either sex are heavily influenced by culture. Touch between men (walking arm in arm) and between women is acceptable in many societies. In contemporary American society, women are more likely to have intimate, self-disclosing friendships with other women than men have with other men; a man's male friends are likely to be working, drinking, or playing "buddies." In Southern Europe and the Middle East, men are allowed to express their friendship with each other with words and embraces; expressions of affection between men are less common in American culture or might be attributed to homosexuality.

Affiliation and friendship needs in adulthood and the satisfaction of these needs are facilitated or hindered by cultural expectations. Social support, family ties, and friendship needs can be met through the extended family and kinship system or through other culturally prescribed groups such as churches, singles bars, work, and civic associations. Social networking websites are an increasingly popular way to connect with friends and family as well. An individual's health may be affected by these social ties: persons who have a reliable set of close friends and an extensive network of acquaintances are usually healthier—emotionally and physically—than persons without supportive networks and close friends. Facebook, LinkedIn, and other Internet sites might meet social needs of younger persons, or even older adults.

Roles and relationships change between adult children and their parents as both become older. Caring for and launching their own children and caring for their own aging parents place some middle-age adults between the demands of caregiving from parents and those from children. Primarily, caregivers have been women, and the stress resulting from the demands of caregiving places them at increased risk of health problems (National Alliance for Caregiving & AARP, 2009). In traditional cultures that value and maintain extended family networks, the responsibilities of caring for both children and older parents can be shared with other family members (see Figure 7-1). This decreases the responsibilities being placed on any one family member.

Adjusting to the aging of parents and the associated responsibilities, as well as finding appropriate solutions to problems created by aging parents, is a challenge created by situational, developmental, and even health–illness transitions. Placing an aged mother or father in a nursing home or extended care facility may be a decision made with reluctance and only when all other alternatives have been exhausted. Such actions may be totally unacceptable to some members of other cultural groups, in which family and community networks would facilitate the complex care required by an aged ill person. Such cultural norms would exert a great deal of social pressure on an adult son, or especially a daughter, who failed in this obligation.

Cultural values also influence professional health care roles and relationships. How individuals are approached and greeted as well as the kind and type of relationship established may be closely tied to cultural expectations and norms. A casual, first-name basis has become the norm in many health care situations, with medical receptionists (and often other health professionals as well) calling patients by their first names. While this may be appropriate at the check-in desk because of HIPPA regulations, it can be inappropriate in other instances. Health care professionals should always inquire about the appropriate manner to use in approaching clients and their family members. Table 7-1 provides some suggestions and guidelines to use in approaching clients and using their names in professional relationships.

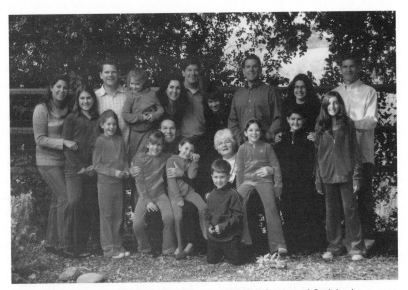

Figure 7-1. The extended family of Teresa and Neil Cooper of Carlsbad, California. This family is multiethnic in each generation, yet maintaining close family ties is a priority that has continued through three generations.

Table 7-1: Guidelines for Names

Culture	Guidelines
Arab	Both male and female children are given a first name. The father's first name is used as the middle name; the last name is the family name. Usually, a person is called formally by the first name, such as Mr. Mohammed or Dr. Anwar.
Chinese	The family name is stated or written first followed by the given name (the opposite of European and North American tradition). Only very close friends use the given name. Politeness and formality are stressed; always use the whole name or family name. Use only the family name to address men, for example, if the family name is Chin and the man's given name is Wei-jing, address the man as Chin. Women in China do not use their husband's name after marriage.
	Many Chinese take an English name that they use in their North American host country. Use the title Mr. or Mrs. preceding the English name; using only the first name is considered rude.
Latin American	The use of surnames may differ by country. Many Latin Americans use two surnames, representing the mother's and father's sides of the family. "Maria Cordoba Lopez" indicates that her father's name is Cordoba and her mother's surname is Lopez. When Maria marries, she will retain her father's name and add the last name of her husband, becoming Maria Cordoba de Recinos.
	Many Latin American immigrants drop their mother's surnames after they immigrate to the United States because having two last names can be inconvenient. In approaching clients of traditional Latin cultures, it is appropriate to use the Spanish terms *señor* or *señora*, followed by the primary surname (the husband's), if the nurse is comfortable with those terms.
Native North American	Native North American names differ by tribal affiliation. Many tend to follow the dominant cultural norms. In the Navajo culture, a health care provider may call an older Navajo client "grandfather" or "grandmother" as a sign of respect. In the past, some tribes have tended to convert traditional names into English surnames, for example, Joe Calf Looking and Phyllis Greywolf.

The above-mentioned examples are very general. If in doubt, always ask: it can be embarrassing for both the nurse and the client if the nurse uses a name in an inappropriate manner. Generally speaking, it is *always best and most appropriate* to be formal and to use the surname with the appropriate title of Mr. or Mrs. (or other culturally appropriate titles) preceding the name, unless the client has indicated that he/she prefers to be called by his/her first name.

Adapted from Purnell, L. D., (2014). *Transcultural health care: A culturally competent approach* (4th ed.). Philadelphia, PA: F.A. Davis.

Health-Related Situational Crises and Transitions

Situational transitions often occur when a serious illness is diagnosed or other traumatic events occur to individuals and their families. Some developmental theorists refer to the initial period as a "situational crisis" when a serious illness is diagnosed or traumatic event occurs. Such a diagnosis or event often leads to fear and anxiety in the client and family members. As clients and family members learn more about the precipitating condition, they realize that many of their fears are unfounded as they gain more confidence in managing the illness condition. The "crisis" dissipates but still the illness remains and must be managed appropriately. The client and family must "transition" to living with a chronic illness. It is not uncommon for a situational transition, precipitated by an illness event, to occur in middle age or late adulthood. The leading causes of death in the United States are heart disease, cancer, cerebrovascular disease, respiratory disease, accidents, and diabetes, and they are usually diagnosed in adults (Centers for Disease Control and Prevention [CDC], National Center for Health Statistics, 2010). These conditions affect individuals, but they also occur within a family system and affect children, spouses, aging parents, and other close relatives. Because middle-aged adults may be caring for aging parents, adult children, and even grandchildren, the illness of any one individual must be evaluated carefully for the myriad of ways in which it affects all members of the family. Evidence-Based Practice 7-2 describes the experiences of Latina wives as their husbands

Purposeful Normalization When Caring for Husbands Recovering from Prostate Surgery

This study describes the experiences of Latina women as their husbands recovered from radical proctectomies. Purposeful normalization can be viewed as a situational transition. The women's lives changed dramatically when their husbands were diagnosed with cancer. Cultural beliefs related to gender roles and sexual functioning are some of the strongest values and traditions within a cultural system. The husbands' depression, irritability, and erectile dysfunction posed special challenges to the Latina women in this study.

Prostrate cancer is the most frequently diagnosed noncutaneous cancer in men in the United States.

Despite high incidence rates, overall survival rates are very high and increasing all of the time. Issues such as postsurgical incontinence and erectile dysfunction, along with the fact that many prostrate survivors are married men, have prompted many to describe prostate cancer as a *couple's disease*. Partnered men have significantly better mental health, lower symptom distress, and less urinary problems than unpartnered men. Still, many wives experience significant distress when faced with their partner's diagnosis and treatment. This study interviewed 28 partners of *Latino* men who had a radical prostatectomy. The primary aim was to describe the experiences of low-income *Latinas* as their husbands recovered from radical prostatectomies. The overarching process was identified as normalization with some themes working against normality while others worked toward it.

Working Against Normality: Threats to normality of the women's lives began immediately when their husbands were diagnosed with cancer. Some concerns diminished with time, such as the initial shock and fear and dealing with the side effects. They feared losing their husband. Dealing with the symptoms and the side effects caused the women to feel anxious and frustrated. The husbands' depression and irritability, as well as erectile dysfunction, posed special challenges.

Working Toward Normality: The Latina women described many themes that kept them feeling a sense of "normal." They worked hard to conceal their own emotions and to show their husbands that they had everything under control. They tried to move forward, putting changes brought about by their husband's illness behind them. They tried to make dietary changes that they believed were helpful—such as eating more vegetables and fruits and cutting down on sugar. Their families were supportive with the grown children visiting and making frequent phone calls. Grandchildren visited and were a source of joy and comfort. Women found great support in their religious faith that helped them make changes in a positive way.

Clinical Implications

- Understand that caregiving can be extremely stressful and that caregivers need support, understanding, and help in this role. Simply acknowledging the emotional impact of both the illness itself and of caring for the patient can be helpful.
- Talk to wives/caregivers about actively shaping the emotional responses they feel and how they can help their husbands deal with the changes they are is experiencing.
- Encourage caregivers to contribute to recovery by empowering them to make healthy changes in their lifestyle, such as eating healthy food, getting appropriate amounts of sleep, and perhaps simple exercise such as walking short distances together with their husband.
- Become comfortable when discussing symptoms such as erectile dysfunction and helping clients and their partners consider alternative forms of intimacy.
- Actively encourage family members to visit and to telephone frequently. Help clients plan for grandchildren to spend the night.

Reference: Williams, K. C., Hicks, E. M., Chang, N., Connor, S. E., & Maliski, S. L. (2014). Purposeful normalization when caring for husbands recovering from prostate surgery cancer. *Qualitative Health Research 24*(3), 306–316.

recovered from radical proctectomies. The shock of the cancer diagnoses and the long-term effects of the surgery precipitated a situational transition that affected both husbands and wives.

Cultural beliefs and values influence health promotion, disease prevention, and the treatment of illness. Families influence the health-related behavior of their members because definitions of health and illness, and reactions to them, form during childhood within the family context. When an illness has social and/or cultural connotations, or involves sexual issues, shame, and/or stigma, the response from the client and the family may be more pronounced. Sexual education has sometimes been a "flash point" in numerous communities, and many parents have objected to such programs in the school setting. Shambley-Ebron (2009) conducted

a study with preadolescent African American girls and included their mothers. A targeted 8-week educational program tapped into the cultural and gender beliefs and practices to educate girls about HIV/AIDS prevention. Input for educational intervention was solicited from women in the community, including the mothers of the young girls. The findings from this study indicate that culture and gender influences play a critical role in how young African American girls develop culturally appropriate strategies to deal with sexuality and healthy womanhood. This study is also an example of how education about sensitive topics such as HIV/AIDS prevention can be conducted.

The content in this section provides the context for and gives an example of a health-related situational crisis (which is detailed in Case Study 7-1).

CASE STUDY 7-1

Mrs. Ernestine Pollard, a 57-year-old African American woman, lives in a small town in rural Georgia. Mrs. Pollard cares for her older sister, Ethel, who is now 65 years old. Mrs. Pollard explains that her sister "can't talk, and her mind's not good." Mrs. Pollard says that even as a little girl, she knew that Ethel would be her special responsibility, and when she (Mrs. Pollard) married, Ethel came to live with her and her new husband. Mr. Pollard died a few years ago following a stroke. Recently, Ethel's health has been deteriorating because of a series of what Mrs. Pollard calls "little strokes." Additionally, just a few months ago, Mrs. Pollard's 26-year-old daughter, Tywanda, returned home to live with her. Tywanda was living and working in New Jersey, where she had become ill. She was taken by friends to the emergency department and admitted to a local hospital. During this hospitalization, she tested positive for HIV. Tywanda has been a great worry to her mother for a number of years; Mrs. Pollard has suspected that Tywanda was occasionally using drugs. Although Mrs. Pollard welcomed Tywanda home again, she worried about her past high-risk behaviors and hoped

they would not continue. When Tywanda told her mother about her HIV status, Mrs. Pollard was very upset and worried.

Mrs. Pollard explains that sometimes with the stress of caregiving for Ethel and worrying about Tywanda, her "pressure goes sky high." She tells the nurse that she has had **"high blood"** for several years. Her physician prescribed medication for her blood pressure, and she tries to take it on a regular basis, but sometimes, she forgets. Other times, she decides that she just does not have the money for medication. Lately, Tywanda has been staying away from home and acting secretively, so Mrs. Pollard is not sleeping well and she is worried that Tywanda may be taking drugs again. She told her doctor that she has bad **"nerves"** and explained that she is unable to sleep at night. The physician prescribed sleeping pills for her, but Mrs. Pollard is unwilling to take them because she fears that she will not hear Ethel if she gets up during the night. Ethel seems to be getting more confused and disoriented, especially at night. Mrs. Pollard's other grown children, two daughters, live in Atlanta, several hours' drive from the small town where Mrs. Pollard lives. Mrs. Pollard is experiencing a health/illness situational crisis resulting from the stress of caregiving, the challenges of managing ongoing chronic diseases, and anxiety about her young adult daughter who is HIV positive and engages in risky behaviors.

The influences of culture on individual and family responses to health problems, caregiving, and health/illness transitions and crises are discussed.

Caregiving

Caregiving occurs when an unpaid person, usually a family member, helps another family member who has a chronic illness or disease. Many caregivers are women who are caring for their aged and ill parents or husbands. Assuming the role of caregiver often predisposes women to interrupted employment and limited access to health care insurance and pension and retirement plans.

Caregiving, as used in this chapter, implies the provision of long-term help to an impaired family member or close friend. Caregiving is usually labor intensive, time consuming, and stressful; the exact effects on the physical and emotional health of caregivers are still being documented. Although positive outcomes, such as feelings of reward and satisfaction, do occur for caregivers, caregivers still experience negative psychological, emotional, social, and physical outcomes (Family Caregiver Alliance, 2006). When caregiving for other family members takes place during middle adulthood, the roles for both the caregiver and the recipient may change as new challenges emerge. The caregiver may be forced to quit his or her job as caregiving responsibilities increase when the person being cared for becomes more infirm or ill and the need for assistance in tasks of daily living increases.

Culture fundamentally shapes how individuals make meaning out of illness, suffering, and dying. Cultural beliefs about illness and aging influence the interpretation and management of caring for the ill and aged, as well as the management of the trajectory of caregiving. Family members provide care for the vast majority of those in need of assistance. The demands of caregiving can result in negative emotional and physical consequences for caregivers. How they cope with stress, social isolation, anxiety, feelings of burden, and the challenges of caregiving will all be influenced by cultural values and traditions.

Shambley-Ebron and Boyle (2006a, 2006b) have documented that these general problems and characteristics of caregivers are compounded for African American women by the special circumstances of their lives and the lives of the men and children for whom they care. In the case of African American caregivers, prejudice, discrimination, health disparities, and poverty often all interact to increase stress and pose challenges that frequently result in poor health. Like other caregivers, African American caregivers are mostly female; most recipients of care from African American caregivers are females as well (e.g., daughters caring for their mothers) (National Alliance for Caregiving & AARP, 2009).

Culture and ethnicity can influence beliefs, attitudes, and perceptions related to caregiving, including how often individuals engage in self-care versus seeking formal health services, how many medications they take, how often they rest and exercise, and what types of foods they consume when ill. Ethnic and/or cultural differences have rarely been analyzed in caregiver research; only recently have nurse researchers and others focused on specific cultural groups to study caregiving (Family Caregiver Alliance, 2006) and the ethnocultural factors that are so important in planning support for caregivers (Crist, Kim, Pasvogel, & Velazquez, 2009).

Studies of African American caregivers have found that they tend to use religious beliefs and/or spirituality to help them cope with the stress of caregiving; Giger, Appel, Davidhizar, and Davis (2008) found that a major source of support for Black caregivers was their personal relationships with "Jesus," "God," or "the Lord." These authors suggest that spirituality is both personal and empowering for some African Americans and is related to the deepest motivations in life. Spirituality is often expressed in the context of the daily life of Black caregivers, not necessarily by formal attendance at religious events. Numerous researchers have noted that the specific nature of the religion–health connection among African Americans is of great interest to health professionals as it holds promise for integrating church-based health interventions.

The Context of HIV/AIDS and the African American Community

HIV/AIDS disproportionately affects African Americans and has had a devastating effect on African American communities. According to CDC data, at every stage—from HIV diagnosis through the death of persons with AIDS—the hardest-hit racial or ethnic group is African Americans. Even though African Americans make up only approximately 13% of the US population, 44% of the estimated new cases of HIV/AIDS diagnoses in the United States in 2010 were in African Americans (CDC, HIV among African Americans Fact Sheet, 2014; CDC, HIV/AIDS Surveillance report, 2008).

In 2014, women accounted for about one in four new HIV/AIDS cases in the United States. Of these newly infected women, about two in three are African American. Most of these women contracted HIV from having unprotected sex with a man. The rate of AIDS diagnosis for African American women was 20 times the rate of White women by the end of 2006 (National Alliance of State and Territorial AIDS Directors [NASTAD], 2008). AIDS was the fifth leading cause of death for African American females, ages 25 to 34, in 2010 (CDC, 2010. Mortality Tables, National Center for Health Statistics, Leading Causes of Death by Age Group, Black Females, United States).

Prevention Challenges

From a public health standpoint, preventive education about HIV/AIDS has been hindered by an unwillingness to talk frankly about behaviors surrounding sex and drug use, and this has been a substantial barrier in effective HIV preventive programs. In essence, the AIDS epidemic has forced society to examine and attempt to alter cultural behaviors and values that were largely ignored in the past. And, as a society, we have not always been comfortable with this frankness. Over the past three decades in the United States, the practice of high-risk HIV behaviors has changed from selected populations of White homosexual men with no history of drug use

to heterosexuals having multiple sex partners and/or using drugs. HIV/AIDS disproportionately affects selected groups, especially Blacks and Hispanics, and risk patterns are different for men and women. African American women (adolescents and adults) are especially at risk.

The CDC points out that the African American community faces numerous barriers that impact HIV prevention efforts. Among these factors are biological vulnerabilities as well as the unique characteristics and nuances of heterosexual relationships in African American culture. Also contributing to increased HIV transmission in African American communities are poverty, unemployment, substandard education, and incarceration (CDC, HIV among African Americans Fact Sheet, 2014; Womenshealth.gov, 2011). Implementing intervention programs has proven extremely difficult. Evidence-Based Practice 7-3 describes a study with African American mothers to understand how they talked to their young daughters about sexual health. This knowledge is helpful when developing culturally relevant prevention programs for sexual health, including the prevention of HIV/AIDS.

Influential Factors

Numerous explanations have been offered about the factors that influence the high rate of HIV/AIDS in African American communities. Poverty is a major factor. Denial, drug use, and homophobia and concealment of homosexual behavior also influence HIV/AIDS rates.

Poverty

The poverty rate is higher among African Americans than other racial/ethnic groups as African Americans, generally speaking, have lower incomes than other Americans. The poverty rate for all African Americans in 2012 was 28.1%, an increase from 25.5% in 2005. Black families with children under 18 headed by a single mother have the highest rate of poverty, at 47.5%, compared to only 8.4% of married-couple Black families (BlackDemographics.com. (n.d.)). The socioeconomic issues associated with poverty—including

Cultural Preparation for Womanhood in Urban African American Girls: Growing Strong Women

Poor sexual health is a significant contributor to morbidity in young African American women. Human immunodeficiency virus/acquired immune deficiency syndrome (HIV/AIDS) and other sexually transmitted infections (STIs) are tragic and costly in all populations; however, African Americans bear an excess burden of poor health due to these conditions. Understanding how knowledge about sexual health is transmitted to African American girls is needed to develop effective and culturally relevant preventive interventions.

This study explored the ways that African American mothers transmitted sexual values and information to their daughters. The author interviewed 14 mothers who had young daughters, 8 to 16 years of age. The data were qualitatively analyzed, and three major themes about *Growing Strong Black women* were identified: truth-telling, building strength through self-esteem, and spirituality as helper.

Helping their daughters grow into strong, successful, and healthy women was viewed by the mothers as a task that was primarily their responsibility. This responsibility was enacted through an ongoing process of providing truthful answers and open communication, helping their daughters develop a healthy self-esteem that would promote independence, and providing a foundation of spirituality and religious beliefs to enable their daughters to deal with the societal issues that face young African American girls and women. Mothers were honest with their daughters with regard to sexuality, their changing bodies, and relationships with men. Sometimes, mothers told their daughters painful stories of their own experiences. Other times, they sought out literature to explain how their bodies worked or how STIs occurred. Mothers reinforced their daughters' self-esteem and helped them develop confidence in their own abilities to be successful in life. They encouraged them to become active in church and school activities, to develop a faith and belief in God, and to participate in religious practices such as prayer and attendance at religious services.

Clinical Implications

- Supportive networks for young African American girls can be broadened and strengthened by involving teachers, nurses, and women from their church groups as support persons to help them achieve their goals relative to age-appropriate relationships and sexual behaviors.
- African American mothers (indeed, all mothers) of teenage girls need accurate information about sexual health and STIs. Nurses can work with churches and various community groups to provide information and support to parents.
- Culture and gender are unique and distinct aspects of the lives of young African American girls and must be taken into account when planning preventive interventions for health and well-being.
- Nursing interventions that focus on building self-esteem and supporting the future aspirations of young African American girls can be useful to reinforce parental teachings and help young girls move into adulthood successfully.
- The use of spirituality and religiosity appears consistently in the literature as ways to help young African American girls deal appropriately with life experiences.

Reference: Shambley-Ebron, D., Dole, D., & Karikari, A. (2014). Cultural preparation for womanhood in urban African American girls: Growing strong women. *Journal of Transcultural Nursing.* Online 6 May 2014. doi: 10:1177/1043659614531792

limited access to high-quality health care, housing, and HIV prevention education—directly and indirectly increase the risk for HIV infection. The CDC (HIV among African Americans Fact Sheet, 2014) suggests that these factors may explain why African Americans have worse outcomes on the HIV continuum of care, including lower rates of linkage to care, retention in care, prescription HIV treatment, and viral suppression. CDC data from 2010 indicate that 75% of HIV-infected African Americans aged 13 or older are linked to care, 48% are retained in care, 46% are prescribed antiretroviral therapy, and only 35% are virally suppressed (CDC, HIV among African Americans Fact Sheet, 2014). Accessing health care services is a problem if an individual does not have health insurance, and not all health departments offer high-quality care and follow-up for clients.

In addition, for many African Americans, day-to-day living activities (long working hours, low pay, family responsibilities) often take precedence over whether an individual has the time and energy to access educational information about HIV and AIDS. Poverty or lack of money, stigma, and lack of access to high-quality health care influence access to HIV testing and state-of-the-art treatment if an individual is diagnosed with HIV. Often, stigma, racism, and fear are associated with poverty, and they too play a part in delaying appropriate up-to-date treatment, complying with medication regimens and other appropriate care. Delay in diagnosis late in the course of HIV infection is too common for African Americans, and this delay results in missed opportunities for early medical intervention and prevention of transmission to others (CDC, HIV among African Americans Fact Sheet, 2014; Black Womens Health Imperative, n.d.).

Denial

Denial and lack of awareness of HIV/AIDS have frequently led to late diagnoses and treatment for many rural African Americans. They know that HIV/AIDS is a problem in Atlanta or New York City, or even in Florida, but they find it hard to believe that HIV/AIDS is a problem in rural Georgia or Alabama. This lack of awareness of HIV presence can affect HIV rates within communities. Talking

about HIV/AIDS may be met with disapproval as some African Americans may feel that it is not an appropriate subject for discussion. Talking frankly about sexual behavior with new partners and insisting on the use of condoms may be very difficult for African American women. They may be afraid to ask a male partner about his sexual history or his use of or experience with drugs for fear of abruptly ending their relationship. The nuances of African American male–female relationships are rarely understood by health care providers. Shambley-Ebron and Boyle (2006a, 2006b) suggest that problematic relationships between Black males and females are complex in nature and are reflections of institutional racism, political and economic oppression, and internalization of negative stereotypes on the parts of both men and women. These disabling relationships often lead to denial about HIV; this may be why many African Americans who are HIV infected do not seek early testing and do not know they are HIV positive. Persons who do not know that they are HIV infected are more likely than those with a diagnosis to engage in risky behavior and to unintentionally transmit HIV to others (CDC, A Heightened National Response to the HIV/AIDS Crises among African Americans, 2007). The denial of risks of HIV/AIDS can affect HIV rates. Approximately one in five adults and adolescents in the United States living with HIV do not know their HIV status. This translates to about 116,750 African Americans. Late diagnosis of HIV infection is common; this creates missed opportunities to obtain early medical care and prevent transmission to others. The sooner an individual is diagnosed and linked to appropriate care, the better the outcome (Womenshealth.gov, 2011).

Drug Use

Most new HIV infections among African American women (87% or 5,300) are attributed to heterosexual contact (CDC, HIV among African Americans Fact Sheet, 2014). Injecting drugs is the second leading cause of HIV infection for African American women and the third leading cause of HIV infection for African American men. In addition to the danger from contaminated needles, syringes, and other drug paraphernalia, persons who use drugs

are more likely to take other risks, such as unprotected sex, while under the influence of drugs (CDC, HIV among African Americans Fact Sheet, 2014). An early study of HIV-infected women found that women who used drugs, compared with women who did not, were also less likely to take their antiretroviral medicines exactly as prescribed or to attend clinic appointments on a regular basis (Sharpe, Lee, Nakashima, Elam-Evans, & Fleming, 2004).

Homophobia and Concealment of Homosexual Behavior

Homophobia and stigma can cause some homosexual African American men to identify themselves as heterosexual or to not disclose their sexual orientation, presenting challenges to prevention programs (Millett, Peterson, Wolitski, & Stall, 2006). The CDC indicated that in 2010, African American gay, bisexual, and other men who have sex with men represented an estimated 72% of new infections among all African American men and 36% of an estimated 29,800 new HIV infections among all gay and bisexual men (CDC, HIV Among African Americans Fact Sheet, 2014). It is extremely important to involve African American community stakeholders in developing and implementing programs to address sensitive topics and behaviors associated with homosexual sex. Confronting homophobia is necessary to achieve significant reductions in HIV/AIDS and ultimately to end this epidemic among African Americans. Involving community stakeholders will mobilize African American communities to become more aware of the need to develop strategies that address broader social and cultural factors such as homophobia, drug use, stigma, and denial (CDC, HIV among African Americans Fact Sheet, 2014).

Adult Development in an African American Family: The Convergence of Developmental and Health Illness Situational Transitions

Case Study 7-1 provides an example of a middle-aged African American woman who provides care to her developmentally delayed sister and to her 26-year-old daughter, who has HIV/AIDS. This case study points out the complex situation of three adult women, each facing significant life changes brought about by health/illness situational crises. Issues related to caregiving, aging, chronic diseases, drug use, and HIV are described. Each woman faces difficult issues that require different kinds of responses to stabilize and improve their health as they are experiencing myriad transitions that are significantly influencing their lives. Culturally appropriate ways in which the nurse might implement nursing care are suggested.

Health Promotion Interventions for Health/Illness Situational Crises

African American women are at high risk for cardiovascular diseases, particularly hypertension and stroke. Mrs. Pollard lives in that area of the South known as the **stroke belt** because morbidity and mortality from cardiovascular diseases (especially among African Americans) are quite high in this region (Mortality Tables, 2010). The nursing management priorities for Mrs. Pollard will be to support her caregiving role and provide health promotion strategies to control her blood pressure and help reduce the stress she is currently experiencing. In terms of blood pressure management, a nurse might advise Mrs. Pollard to lose weight by incorporating changes in eating habits and regular exercise into her lifestyle. However, social and cultural factors, as well as the caregiving situation, may compromise these health goals. Nurses can become more sensitive to cultural norms and values of clients like Mrs. Pollard by listening carefully, being empathetic, recognizing the client's self-interest and needs of her family members, being flexible, having a sense of timing, appropriately using the client's and family's resources, and giving relevant information at the appropriate time.

Although Mrs. Pollard does have a private physician and tries to seek care when appropriate, she considers Ethel's and Tywanda's needs before her own. Mrs. Pollard does not have health

insurance and therefore access to quality care is compromised. Tywanda attends an infectious disease clinic about 50 miles from where her mother lives. Her medications are provided through the Ryan White HIV/AIDS Program, a federal program focused exclusively on HIV/AIDS care. The program is for those who do not have sufficient health care coverage or financial resources for coping with HIV disease (U.S. Department of Health and Human Services, HIV/AIDS Bureau, n.d.). Mrs. Pollard does not accompany Tywanda when she visits the clinic because Tywanda acts as if she does not want her mother to go with her and Mrs. Pollard does not wish to leave her sister alone. The nurses at the clinic wonder if anyone in Tywanda's family really cares about her because she always comes alone to the clinic appointments. However, Tywanda does not always attend the clinic, nor does she tell her mother when she misses an appointment. Mrs. Pollard does not know about the medications that Tywanda takes for HIV/AIDS. Tywanda does not readily disclose information, and Mrs. Pollard tries to be sensitive to her daughter's wishes.

Mrs. Pollard is concerned about Ethel's appetite because she believes that the proper food will promote and enhance her health. Like many other adults, Mrs. Pollard has fairly definite preferences about food and the way it is prepared and served. The Pollard family frequently eats foods that are high in fat; for example, they enjoy servings of bacon or fatback for breakfast once or twice during the week. Breakfast is an important meal for them. They prefer their vegetables cooked with bacon, fatback, or ham for flavoring. Symbolism is attached to food in every culture, and Mrs. Pollard believes that both Ethel and Tywanda's health will improve by eating what Mrs. Pollard considers "healthy" foods. With her concern for Tywanda and the time she spends with her sister, Mrs. Pollard neglects her own diet or eats whatever is convenient, often "fast foods" or those high in fat, cholesterol, and sodium.

Mrs. Pollard needs to be gently reminded by the nurse that it is important for her to pay attention to her own nutrition also. The nurse could initiate a discussion about the kinds of nutritious foods that would be appropriate for the three of them and the different ways of preparing food. For example, vegetables can be cooked without the addition of fatback. Young-Mason (2009) suggested that understanding the art and culture of food of those we seek to help is paramount to being and becoming an astute and learned nurse. Campinha-Bacote (2013) observed that food can have many roles, in addition to providing physical nourishment. For example, food can serve as a means of enhancing interpersonal relationships or communicating love and caring. Historically, African American rites revolve around food. Being able to prepare food that her daughter and sister will eat and enjoy is a source of satisfaction for Mrs. Pollard and a reinforcement of her successful role as caregiver. It is an act of caring and love for her to prepare a meal for her family. At the same time, she must maintain her own health to continue to provide care for Tywanda and her sister.

Nurses providing care to clients like Mrs. Pollard will need to consider other cultural factors that ultimately influence the nursing goals. Rural African Americans often have cultural ways to view health and illness; these patterns of beliefs and behaviors can be viewed as culture-bound syndromes. Many of these patterns are indigenously considered to be "illnesses" or at least afflictions and most have local names. **"High blood"** is an illness condition or affliction that is associated with African American culture in the rural South. Many health care professionals make the wrong assumption that "high blood" is the same as high blood pressure, and although there are similarities, the cultural explanation of "high blood" is different from the biomedical explanation of high blood pressure. "High blood" is conceptualized in terms of blood volume, blood thickness, or even elevations of the blood in the body (e.g., "blood rushes to your head").

"High blood" is believed to be caused primarily by factors that "run blood up," such as salt, fat, meats, and sweets. This condition can result in an increased "pressure" or high blood pressure.

Sometimes, "high blood" leads to a feeling of faintness that may cause the afflicted person to "fall out" or faint. Other causal factors that result in "high blood" are emotional upsets, troubling experiences, or prolonged stress. Sometimes, it is thought to be caused by a falling out with God or by eternal forces such as enemies putting a "hex" on someone. Many older African American clients believe that eating slightly acidic foods, such as collard greens with vinegar or dill pickles, will lower "high blood." Thus, although there are similarities between "high blood" and high blood pressure, the explanations and treatments are not always the same in the cultural prescriptions as in the biomedical model.

Mrs. Pollard tries to be conscientious about taking her blood pressure medication, but she sometimes forgets to take it and sometimes does not get around to promptly renewing the prescription, so she might go without her medication for several days or a couple of weeks. The nurse should acknowledge Mrs. Pollard's active involvement in her own health promotion, encourage her to take her blood pressure medication as prescribed, and remind her to renew it promptly before she is completely out of medication. The nurse can also discuss "high blood" with Mrs. Pollard, and if there are no contraindications, she can encourage her to eat collard greens with vinegar or dill pickles. She can listen carefully to Mrs. Pollard's explanation of "high blood," and if Mrs. Pollard believes she has somehow offended God, the nurse should encourage her to talk with her church pastor.

"Nerves" or even **"bad nerves,"** while not unique to the rural South, are commonly described by many Southerners. "Bad nerves" are often equated with anxiety and worry but may refer to something as serious as a "mental breakdown" or severe emotional disorder. Mrs. Pollard uses the term to refer to her worry, concern, and anxiety about Tywanda and Ethel. Sometimes, she has "crying spells" that she describes as "just crying and crying, and not being able to stop." She gets up several times at night to answer her sister's call or to check on Tywanda and make certain that they are sleeping well. Lack of sleep and continued worry and anxiety accelerate her psychological distress. Again, recognition and acknowledgment from the nurse that she is providing excellent care for her sister and her daughter will be reassuring for her. She should be encouraged to rest and should be assured that crying and feeling sad are normal reactions to her sister's deteriorating condition and Tywanda's HIV/AIDS.

Because of a lack of economic resources, African American midlife women are likely to be subjected to many stressful life events, such as job and marital instability, lack of male companions as heads of households, erratic income, and frequent changes and relocations (Hine, 1998). Because she has worked in small local businesses (dry cleaners, restaurants) most of her life, Mrs. Pollard lacks health insurance. She has experienced many life stresses related to the lack of economic resources. Mrs. Pollard was working as a clerk in a local dry cleaning establishment when Tywanda returned home and told her mother that she had HIV/AIDS. However, as Ethel's health deteriorated and Tywanda's risky behaviors became more obvious and problematic, Mrs. Pollard decided to stop working for a while, thinking that if she stayed home, she could provide closer supervision and care to Ethel and be available to Tywanda when she needed her mother. Mrs. Pollard faces numerous situational crises: Tywanda's illness and high-risk behaviors, the poor health and aging of her sister, and economic hardship because she is the family provider and is not working at the present time. Her own health is also a concern.

Stress and anxiety are normal reactions in the lives of middle-aged adults like Mrs. Pollard. However, limited resources and lack of access to high-quality health care compound the stress and complicate a situational crisis. Mrs. Pollard's physician prescribed sleeping medication for her, assuming that would take care of her inability to sleep. The nurse can reinforce Mrs. Pollard's decision not to take this medication and explore with her how to set aside time during the day when she

might be able to take a nap. Mrs. Pollard's anxiety and inability to sleep well are directly related to the stress of caregiving. Some ways to support and help Mrs. Pollard deal with stress and anxiety may be family support and participation in religious activities. The nurse might suggest that Mrs. Pollard set aside some time during the day to quietly read the Bible or other appropriate reading material and listen to religious music. Mrs. Pollard told the nurse that she used to enjoy crocheting; she could be encouraged to try crocheting again.

Close family and spiritual ties within the African American family and community support the caregiving role. Extended and nuclear family members willingly care for sick persons and assume these roles without hesitation. Mrs. Pollard's two daughters try to help their mother and Tywanda as much as possible, but they live several hours' drive away. They try to visit one weekend each month and bring their children with them. Tywanda enjoys the company of her sisters, and Mrs. Pollard notices that on weekends when one of the sisters is expected, Tywanda's mood seems improved as she obviously looks forward to the visit. Ethel is always excited to see her nieces and looks forward to their visits. While Mrs. Pollard's daughters know that Tywanda has been diagnosed with HIV/AIDS, they are reluctant to disclose the diagnosis to others outside the family because the stigma of disclosure in a small community can affect all members of the family. Mrs. Pollard's minister is aware of Tywanda's condition, as are a few members of Mrs. Pollard's "church family." One of the primary stressors of women during the midlife years is the loss of relationships and friendship networks, often because of competing demands on time. Caregivers, like Mrs. Pollard, have very little time for their own needs. It is extremely important for Mrs. Pollard's health and coping abilities that she continue to participate in church activities as much as possible and to maintain those friendships and networks.

Spiritual beliefs form a foundation for Mrs. Pollard's daily life. Like other African Americans who live in the same rural community, Mrs. Pollard attends a small Protestant church whose membership is exclusively African American. Many, but not all, African Americans strongly believe in the use of prayer for all situations they may encounter. They use prayer and reading the Bible as a means of dealing with everyday problems and concerns. Mrs. Pollard relies a great deal on prayer, and her religious beliefs and practices provide her with support and strength in her caregiving role. Encouraging Mrs. Pollard to take even 15 minutes each day to read familiar biblical verses or listen to religious music might be one of the most helpful interventions the nurse could suggest.

Mrs. Pollard has a lifetime of experience with her church; the church has been the center of activities for African Americans for decades (Campinha-Bacote, 2013). Mrs. Pollard's religious beliefs are integrated into her daily life as a caregiver, and her belief in God enhances her ability to care for Ethel and Tywanda. She, like many other African Americans, has a personal relationship with God and is able to share her worries and concerns through prayer. Her traditional spirituality and church support provide a foundation for an active approach to coping with problems.

Adult Health Transitions and Nursing Interventions

Mrs. Pollard is distressed about the deterioration of her sister's physical condition and Tywanda's diagnosis of HIV/AIDS and drug use. In addition, Mrs. Pollard is dealing with several health problems of her own. While there are certain "crisis dimensions" to this situation, the conditions are not life threatening. Overtime, the crises lessen and the situation slowly develops a transitory nature. The health/illness transitions occur over a longer period of time. They can best be dealt with by the provision of culturally relevant health promotion and risk reduction strategies. The health teaching and nursing interventions provided to the Pollard family should focus on wellness and health promotion. In addition to the nursing interventions that are important for health promotion, there are several interventions that will

help Mrs. Pollard navigate the transitions and changes of caregiving.

An important priority of nursing care for Mrs. Pollard and her family is to help them understand and adjust to the impact of HIV disease. This includes urging Tywanda to seek help for her drug use. The nurse can refer Mrs. Pollard to the social services available for patients who have HIV/AIDS and their family members. Mrs. Pollard may want to talk to a mental health counselor about the fears and concerns she has about Tywanda and drug use. In addition, the nurse can encourage Tywanda to keep clinic appointments and to seek appropriate counseling and follow-up, not only for her HIV status but also for the use of illicit drugs. While the nurse is not a trained mental health counselor, she or he can recommend that Tywanda seek mental health services, and the nurse can be supportive and encourage health-seeking behaviors. Medications now available for treating HIV can lower viral counts and transmission of the virus to others; helping Tywanda find appropriate services and follow-through treatment is a priority in providing nursing care for this family. Of particular concern is the timing of Tywanda's illness. A serious health condition in a young, previously healthy adult child will cause unique trauma and conflict because of society's expectations that young adults will outlive their older parents. In addition, as a person diagnosed with HIV/AIDS, Tywanda has a condition that often generates shame and stigma. It is important that these issues be acknowledged by both Mrs. Pollard and Tywanda.

Achieving career success is one of the developmental transitions that Western culture emphasizes. Mrs. Pollard has worked successfully outside the home most of her adult life; because rural African American culture does not place the same kind of value on work and career as does the larger culture, career "success" is not necessarily viewed as an important accomplishment. Family ties and providing for her family are highly valued in African American culture and are emphasized over women's successful careers outside the home. Mrs. Pollard's ties of love and

affection to Tywanda and to her sister, Ethel, are reinforced by African American cultural values. In a historical study of African American women in America, Hine and Thompson (1998) suggested that Black women have always been the financial providers in Black families and that women's work roles have been culturally viewed as an inherent part of Black motherhood, not as individual careers. Mrs. Pollard has always been proud that she was able to take care of her family and that she could "make do" with very little. These values are important to family integrity and they can be positively reinforced by the nurse.

Many African American women of Mrs. Pollard's generation obtain meaning in their lives by caring for family members. Their feelings, behaviors, and attitudes go beyond a simple sentiment of affection or of family ties. In explaining why she cares for her older developmentally challenged sister, Mrs. Pollard says, "We were little girls together. I always knew that I was going to take care of her." In many societies, women disproportionally provide caregiving services and social policies and home-based programs are organized around the assumption of women's availability and willingness to provide care. At the same time, it is important to understand that Mrs. Pollard values the traditional caregiving role, and she needs support and assistance in providing the care she believes her family members need. It is important for the nurse to acknowledge that Mrs. Pollard is valued, recognized, and respected for her competence and expertise as a caregiver and as a caring and generous sister.

The nurse could begin by including Mrs. Pollard, Tywanda, and her sisters in developing mutual goals for Tywanda's progress and care. At the same time, they can discuss Ethel's deteriorating condition and the realistic expectations for her future. Mrs. Pollard should be encouraged in her role of providing help and care to family members and in promoting the health of her daughter and sister. It is also important that her attention be directed toward her own needs on occasion, considering that she tends to focus on meeting the needs of Tywanda and Ethel before her own.

Social and civic responsibilities among rural, older African Americans in the South are met almost entirely at the level of the extended family and the African American church. These ties and associations are very strong, are often complex, and are not readily understood by outsiders. African American pastors are key players in the lives of their congregants and in their communities. Mrs. Pollard should be encouraged to attend church services and to seek the help and support available to her through this important cultural resource. Mrs. Pollard sings in the church choir and tries to attend choir practice every Wednesday evening. Tywanda has agreed to stay home with her Aunt Ethel on Wednesday evenings while Mrs. Pollard is away for the evening. This should be positively reinforced by the nurse. The Black church has been a traditional source of support, and congregations are frequently made up of middle-aged or older adults. Coping strategies such as prayer, singing, or reading the Bible and resources such as family and church support may help mediate Mrs. Pollard's reaction to stressful situations. A culturally competent nurse understands that spirituality is a traditional cultural value that can be supportive during a health crisis.

Mrs. Pollard's life revolves around her family and church. The nurse must acknowledge and support cultural ties with kin and others. It is not uncommon for adult African Americans to cope with little social support from others, relying instead on internal spiritual resources. However, the support provided by close personal relationships is crucial when health conditions deteriorate or an illness develops and is necessary for successful health promotion and maintenance in caregiving activities. Mrs. Pollard's Atlanta-based daughters are crucial for support and assistance during this stressful time. The nurse should actively seek to meet them and acknowledge and encourage their contributions. They should be encouraged to participate in mutual goal setting with the members of the Pollard family.

The nurse can continue to encourage Mrs. Pollard to attend church services because her social life is derived from her participation in the activities of her church. Providing positive reinforcement for Tywanda's decision to stay with her aunt Ethel while Mrs. Pollard attends church services and choir practice would be appropriate. It is the church family who will be instrumental in providing emotional support and help as Ethel's condition continues to decline, as well as the opportunity for Mrs. Pollard to find meaning and to cope with her loss and grief if Ethel predeceases her. If Tywanda continues risky drug and sexual behavior, Mrs. Pollard will need continued support and counseling from health care professionals to continue her caregiving role. Nursing interventions at the individual and family level are extremely important in maintaining and extending quality of life.

Summary

All individuals are confronted with life transitions, crises, and/or changes. All cultures have acceptable and defined ways of responding to these life situations. Adulthood is a busy and productive time and should no longer be considered a stable "slide" toward old age. A situational health transition was presented: an African American woman, Mrs. Pollard, who cared for her developmentally delayed sister, Ethel, and her 26-year-old daughter who has HIV/AIDS. Ethel's health was deteriorating and Mrs. Pollard was fearful that her daughter was using illicit drugs. Mrs. Pollard's own health problems were exacerbated by this situational transition, and her normal development through adulthood was disrupted. How nurses can understand such situations and provide culturally appropriate care was described.

REVIEW QUESTIONS

1. Describe examples of health transitions in your family members and friends. Which types of transitions can you identify in your clients/patients? Do you think it is helpful to think of "transitions" as opposed to "developmental tasks or stages?" Why?

2. How does culture influence transitions of adulthood? For example, explain how a woman from a traditional culture such as those in the Middle East might experience adulthood differently.
3. Discuss how gender might influence adult development in a White, middle-class family.
4. Describe how social factors such as mobility, increased education, and changes in the economy have influenced adult development in American and Canadian cultures.
5. How might caregiving for a family member bring about a situational transition for a middle-aged adult? Would this differ in cultural groups such as Chinese Americans or Mexican Americans? How?
6. Describe how culture influences the role of the caregiver in some African American cultures. What can you find in the literature about caregiving in other cultural groups?

CRITICAL THINKING ACTIVITIES

1. Interview a middle-aged colleague, a client, or a person from another cultural group. Ask about adult roles within the family and how they are depicted. How are these role descriptions typical of traditional roles that are described in the literature? If not, how are they different? What are some of the reasons why they have changed?

2. Interview a middle-aged client from another cultural group. Ask about the client's experiences within the health care system. What were the differences the client noted in health beliefs and practices? Ask the client about his or her health needs during middle age.

3. Using the Andrews/Boyle Transcultural Nursing Guide for Individuals and Families provided in Appendix A, conduct a cultural assessment of a middle-aged client of another cultural group. Critically analyze how the client's culture affects the client's role within the family and the timing of developmental transitions. How might the assessment data differ if the client were older? Younger?

4. Review the literature on Mexican American culture. Describe the traditional Mexican American family. What are the cultural characteristics of Mexican Americans to consider in assessing the developmental transitions of adulthood in this group?

5. You are assigned a new patient, a 24-year-old man from El Salvador named Jose Calderon. At morning report, you learn that he has been a gang member in El Salvador, and because he wanted to stop all gang-related activities, his life was threatened. He fled to the United States and has been granted political asylum. You are told that he has extensive tattoos on his body. What do you know about gang membership in Central America? In the United States? How does membership in a gang address the needs of adolescents? What are the cultural factors that are important to consider when you are planning nursing care for a patient like Jose? For example, how do you view body tattoos? What are the issues related to political asylum, immigration, and the like? How might you assist Jose to meet his developmental needs? What might be the problems he will encounter in the US society or in our health care system?

REFERENCES

Baird, M. B. (2012). Well-Being in refugee women experiencing cultural transition. *Advances in Nursing Science, 35*(3), 240–263.

Baird, M. B., & Boyle, J. S. (2012). Well-Being in Dinka refugee women of Southern Sudan. *Journal of Transcultural Nursing, 23*(1), 14–21.

Belenky, M. F., McVicker, B., Clinchy, B. M., Goldberger, N. R., & Tarule, J. M. (1997). *Women's ways of knowing: The development of self, voice, and mind.* New York, NY: Basic Books.

BlackDemographics.com. (n.d.). Retrieved from http://blackdemographics.com/households/kpoverty/

Black Women's Health Imperative. (n.d.). Retrieved from http://blackwomenshealth.org/issues-and-resources/black-women-and-hiv-aids/

Bronfenbrenner, U. (1977). Toward an experimental ecology of human development. *American Psychologist, 32*, 513–531.

Campinha-Bacote, J. (2013). People of African American heritage. In L. D. Purnell, (Ed.), *Transcultural health care: A culturally competent approach* (pp. 91–114). Philadelphia, PA: F. A. Davis Company.

Centers for Disease Control and Prevention. (2007). A heightened national response to the HIV/AIDS crises among African Americans. U.S. Department of Health and Human Services. Retrieved from http://www.cdc.gov/hiv/topics/aa/resources/reports/heightenedresponse.htm

Centers for Disease Control and Prevention (2014). HIV among African Americans Fact Sheet. Department of Health and Human Services, retrieved from: http://www.cdc.gov/hiv/risk/racialethnic/aa/facts/index.html

Centers for Disease Control and Prevention. (2008). *HIV/AIDS surveillance report, 2008.* (Vol. *18*, pp. 1–54). Atlanta, GA: US Department of Health and Human Services. Retrieved from http://www.cdc.gov/hiv/topics/surveillance/resources/report/pdf/2006SurveillanceReport.pdf

Centers for Disease Control and Prevention, National Center for Health Statistics. (2010). In Leading causes of death. Retrieved from http://cdc.gov/nchs/deaths.htm

Centers for Disease Control and Prevention. (2010). Leading causes of death by age group, black females-United States, 2010. Retrieved from Mortality Tables at http://www.cdc.gov/nchs/nvss/mortality_tables.htm

Crist, J. D., Kim, S., Pasvogel, A., & Velazquez, J. H. (2009). Mexican American elders' use of home care services. *Applied Nursing Research, 22*(1), 26–34.

Demick, J., & Andreoletti, C. (Eds.). (2003). *Handbook of adult development.* New York, NY: Kluwer Academic/Plenum.

Erikson, E. (1963). *Childhood and society* (2nd ed.). New York, NY: Norton.

Family Caregiver Alliance. (2006). Retrieved from http://caregiver.org

Giger, J. N., Appel, S. J. Davidhizar, R., & Davis, C. (2008). Church and spirituality in the lives of the African American community. *Journal of Transcultural Nursing, 19*(4), 375–83.

Havighurst, R. J. (1974). *Developmental tasks and education.* New York, NY: David McKay.

Hine, D.C. (1994). Hine Sight: Black Women and the Re-construction of American History. Bloomingdale & Indianapolis: Indiana University Press.

Hine, D. C., & Thompson, K. (1998). *A shining thread of hope: The history of Black women in America.* New York, NY: Broadway Books.

Huffington Post. (April 9, 2014). Women in the workforce: What changes have we made? Retrieved from http://www.huffingtonpost.com/mehroz-bair/women-in-the-workforce-wh_b_4462455.html

Im, E. O., Lee, S. H., & Chee, W. (2010). Subethnic differences in the menopausal symptom experiences, acculturation and menopause among midlife minority women. *Journal of Transcultural Nursing, 21*(2), 123–133.

McCrae, R. R., & Costa, P. T. (2003). *Personality in adulthood: A five-factor theory perspective* (2nd ed.). New York, NY: Guilford Press.

Meleis, A. I., Sawyer, L. M., Im, E. O., Hilfinger Messias, D. K., & Schumacher, K. (2000). Experiencing transitions: An emerging middle-range theory. *Advances in Nursing Science, 23*(1), 12–28.

Millett, G. A., Peterson, J. L., Wolitski, R. J., & Stall, R. (2006). Great risk for HIV infection of black men who have sex with men: A critical literature review. *American Journal of Public Health, 96*, 1007–1019.

Mortality Tables. (2010). Retrieved from http://www.cdc.gov/nchs/nvss/mortality_tables.htm

National Alliance for Caregiving & AARP. (November 2009). Caregiving in the U. S.: A focused look at those caring for someone age 50 or older. Executive summary. Retrieved from www.caregiving.org/data/FINALRegularExSum50plus.pdf

National Alliance of State & Territorial AIDS Directors (NASTAD). (May 2008). The landscape of HIV/AIDS among African American women in the United States. African American Women, Issue Brief No. 1, 444 North Capital Street, NW, Suite 339 Washington, DC.

Neugarten, B. (1968). *Middle age and aging: A reader in social psychology.* Chicago, IL: University of Chicago Press.

Noble, A., Rom, M., Newsome-Wicks, M., Englehardt, K., & Woloski-Wruble, A. (2009). Jewish laws, customs, and practice in labor, delivery, and postpartum care. *Journal of Transcultural Nursing, 20*, 323–333.

Purnell, L. D. (2014). *Transcultural health care: A culturally competent approach* (3rd ed.). Philadelphia, PA: F.A. Davis.

Shambley-Ebron, D., Dole, D., & Karikari, A. (2014). Cultural preparation for womanhood in urban African American girls: Growing strong women. *Journal of Transcultural Nursing.* Online 6 May 2014. doi: 10:1177/1043659614531792

Shambley-Ebron, D. (2009). My sister, myself: A culture- and gender-based approach to HIV/AIDS prevention. *Journal of Transcultural Nursing, 20*, 28–36.

Shambley-Ebron, D., & Boyle, J. S. (2006a). In our grandmothers' footsteps: Perceptions of being strong in African American women with HIV/AIDS. *Advances in Nursing Science, 29*(3), 195–206.

Shambley-Ebron, D., & Boyle, J. S. (2006b). Self-care and the cultural meaning of mothering in African American women with HIV/AIDS. *Western Journal of Nursing Research, 28*, 42–60.

U.S. Department of Health and Human Services, HIV/AIDS Bureau. (n.d.). The HIV/AIDS program: Legislation. Retrieved from http://hab.hrsa.gov/law/leg.htm

Williams, K. C., Hicks, E. M., Chang, N., Connor, S. E., & Maliski, S. L. (2014). Purposeful normalization when caring for husbands recovering from prostate surgery cancer. *Qualitative Health Research, 24*(3), 306–316.

Womenshealth.gov (2012). Minority Women's Health, HIV/AIDS. Office on Women's Health, US. Department of health and Human Services. Retrieved from http://womenshealth.gov/minority-health/african-americans/hiv-aids.html

Young-Mason, J. (2009). Understanding culture: The art of food from the Annuals of the Caliph's Kitchens. *Clinical Nurse Specialist. CNS, 23*, 175–176.

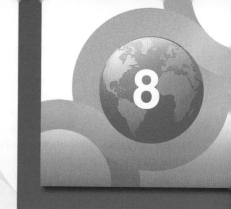

Transcultural Perspectives in the Nursing Care of Older Adults

8

Margaret A. McKenna

Key Terms

Chronic conditions
Formal support

Health behavior
Illness behavior
Informal social support
Long-term care

Self-care
Traditional medicine or
    practices

Learning Objectives

1. Demonstrate knowledge of the sociodemographic shift in the older adult population that affects the demand and roles for nurses and other health professionals.
2. Identify how socioeconomic factors, including income level, as well as community resources will influence the interactions of older adults in the health care system.
3. Integrate concepts of informal and formal support systems and culturally influenced patterns of caregiving to plan appropriate nursing care of the older adult residing in the community.
4. Develop nursing interventions for older adults in a variety of health care contexts that will be perceived as culturally acceptable.
5. Analyze factors affecting the needs of diverse older adults in a continuum of services from health promotion community-based services through care in long-term care facilities.

Nurses and other health professionals are caring for increasing proportions of older adults who are seeking health services in community health sites and health care facilities. Two major factors contributing to this larger population of older adults are longer lifespans and the growing numbers of aging baby boomers who were born between 1946 and 1964. Approximately 10,000 Americans will celebrate their 65th birthday on each and every day through 2030 (Pew Research Center, 2014).

The population of Americans aged 65 years or older will account for approximately 20% of the population by 2030 (Centers for Disease Control & Prevention, 2013). According to the World Health Organization, most of the developed world countries have applied the age of 65 years to refer to an older person, since this is associated with the age when an individual is likely to be eligible to receive pension benefits. However, there is no universal agreement on the age at which a person becomes old; indeed, an individual might be a tribal elder at the age of 50 or may not self-define as being old until well past 70 years of age.

Not only is the US population dramatically aging but we are also seeing increases in racial and ethnic diversity among older adults. Between 2010 and 2030, the percent of adults aged 65 years or older who are non-Hispanic White will decline from 80% to 71% (Ortman, Velkoff, & Hogan, 2014). By 2030, older Hispanics will make up 12% of the population, non-Hispanic Blacks 10%, and older Asians 5.4% (Federal Interagency Forum on Aging-related Statistics, 2012). The proportion of racial and ethnic minorities is estimated to grow to 41% in 2050 (Ortman et al., 2014). The older adult population is also diverse in terms of gender, sexual identity, language, education, socioeconomic status, acculturation, and other factors.

Social and cultural influences will contribute to diverse patterns of help-seeking behavior among older adults who access health care services, necessitating health care practitioners to provide culturally competent care to meet the patients' needs and to achieve positive health outcomes. While culture is not the sole determinant of behavior, it is a critical dimension in understanding the interactions of older clients within their families, the encompassing societal context, and health care settings. Therefore, the older clients' cultural traditions and values will influence how they interact with the health care system and their preferences for their residence, lifestyles, and choice of caregivers. The availability of resources in the community will affect any older client's options for care and the individual's movement on a continuum of care.

These community resources include retirement facilities, **long-term care** institutions typically referred to as nursing homes or skilled nursing facilities, funding for community services, as well as national, state, and local policies. Social and economic factors, including acculturation, influence the retention of traditional cultural values and practices.

In assessing older adults, nurses must consider individuals in these multiple contexts—such as whether they operate as caregivers within their own families—to assess and determine the families' strengths, resources, and capacities for care of aging family members. The context for delivering culturally appropriate care to clients is set by how available and affordable national, state, and local health care resources are for older adults. States, and even rural and urban locations, differ in the range of information and referral sources, acute and extended care facilities, and community-based services that are available to older adults to support their quality of life. Box 8-1 highlights multiple factors that will interact and shape the context for older adult clients who seek care or use health care services.

This chapter is organized in three sections that follow an ecological model, which recognizes that an older adult is a participant in an encompassing societal context, a local community setting, and also interacts in an interpersonal setting that includes family roles. Each of these areas influences the older adult's help-seeking behavior:

1. The encompassing social and economic factors affect the affordability and accessibility of health care options for acute, chronic, and long-term care.
2. The older adult's cultural values, practices, patterns of caregiving, as well as available community resources (informal and formal sources of help) will influence when and where older clients interact in the biomedical health care system or other systems.
3. The older adult is also influenced by his or her nuclear and extended family evident in diverse lifestyles and patterns of health-promoting or

Box 8-1 Factors that Influence Older Adults' Responses in Seeking Health Care

At the Societal Level

- Social and economic factors affect eligibility for Medicare and state medical assistance programs, which can limit older adults in receiving preventive care, acute care, or health care maintenance in the health care system.
- Changes to control Medicare expenditures force shorter hospital stays.
- Gaps in health care services put greater burdens on older patients for home and community-based care.

At the Cultural Level

- Cultural values, acculturation, access to traditional sources of health medicine, and logistical factors including language and transportation can all interact in determining when and where older adults will access the biomedical health care system.
- Different cultural traditions have values that influence patterns in caring for older adult family members as they age and require more assistance.
- Younger family members become acculturated and change traditional behaviors that may differ from older adults' expectations to be cared for at home.

At the Individual Level

- Younger adult family members who are more accustomed to the range of health care options and services may differ in their preferences and health care practices, which can conflict with older adult parents.
- Female family members who were once expected to be primary caregivers for older family members may be engaged in the workforce and unavailable as caregivers.
- Families' economic situations, proximity to the older adult, and sources of formal support in the community will determine options for residence and care needs of the older adult.

risk-taking behavior, coping behavior to manage acute and **chronic conditions**, and decision making about care and services. Chronic conditions may include diabetes, hypertension, arthritis, and other illnesses that require medication, diet modification, or symptom monitoring.

The Older Adult in Contemporary Society: Factors Affecting Health Care

This section addresses the encompassing context that surrounds and influences older adult clients: demographic factors of the aging population, socioeconomic conditions, and the theoretical frameworks that shape how older adults in Western society perceive growing older.

Changing Demographics

Many older adults are interested in remaining healthy as they age, and there are abundant opportunities for nurses working in health care facilities and in the community to interact with older clients and educate them about healthy lifestyles and health-promoting behavior. With advances in the medical community that contribute to adults reaching old age, nurses and other health care professionals can be active in creating health-promoting environments to meet and sustain healthy outcomes for older adults (Waites, 2012).

Some older adults will experience risks for heart disease and conditions including stroke, chronic respiratory diseases, Alzheimer's, and diabetes. There are 2 to 4 million Americans aged 60 years or older who are historically disadvantaged, including individuals who have been

marginalized and have very low incomes and who more frequently have higher levels of disability (CDC, 2013). One study also identified that older lesbian, gay, bisexual, and transgender (LGBT) adults continue to have higher levels of illness, disability, and premature death (Fredriksen-Goldsen & Muraco, 2012). Older adults with chronic health conditions may have a decreased ability to independently complete activities of daily living, such as managing money or taking prescribed medications. When their functioning status declines, nearly one in five older adults may lose their ability to perform their activities of daily living including bathing, toileting, and dressing. Older adults with chronic conditions that increase with age, such as arthritis, diabetes, and cardio-vascular disease (CVD), are more likely to experience physically unhealthy days or even physical distress, which is defined as 14 or more physically unhealthy days annually (CDC, 2013). In individuals 65 years and older, 40% report having at least one disabling condition (Chale, Unanski, & Liang, 2012). Two of three older Americans have multiple chronic conditions, and treatment for this population accounts for two-thirds of the country's health care budget (USDHHS, 2010). Over 1.3 million older adults are in long-term care facilities; half of these residents are 85 years or older and typically have severe impairments including cognitive impairments or dementia.

At all ages, the health status of Hispanics, Asian Americans, African Americans, Native Americans/Alaska Natives, and Native Hawaiians/Other Pacific Islanders has long lagged behind that of non-Hispanic Whites. CVD affects black adults much more consistently than other racial groups, regardless of differences in socioeconomic status (see Figure 8-1). Older African Americans have the highest rates of hypertension compared to other racial groups and higher rates of diabetes compared to Whites and Asian Americans (Gallant, Spitze, & Grove, 2010). Older adults who are African American, Hispanic (non-White), and American Indian/Alaska Native suffer a higher prevalence of CVD and diabetes than do White (non-Hispanic) populations. The rate

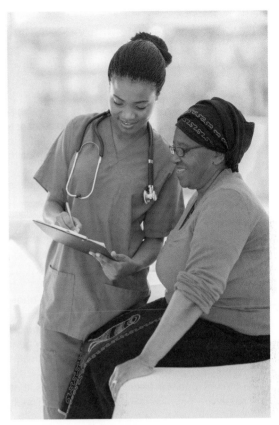

Figure 8-1. A nurse assesses an older adult client (michaeljung/Shutterstock.com).

of diabetes for American Indians/Alaska Natives is more than twice that for Whites (CDC, 2013). Similarly, Mexican-born individuals report higher rates of diabetes and related chronic illness, which directly affects higher rates of disability, than individuals in the non-Hispanic elderly population (CDC, 2013). These disparities exist for interrelated reasons, including lower-income levels, lack of insurance including supplemental insurance to Medicare, barriers in access to care, lower quality of care for some health conditions even when the individual is insured and care is received, and individual decisions to not seek care.

Both ethnicity and income level affect the older adults' health status and need for care. Older White males with the highest incomes can generally expect to live more than 3 years longer than

those in the lowest income levels. Low-income seniors are significantly more likely to encounter these health risk exposures: losing a loved one or close friend, overwhelming caregiving demands for someone else, social isolation, and poor quality housing. Elderly African Americans often suffer functional declines at earlier ages than White Americans. Older African American women have a much higher proportion of disabling conditions than older African American men and older White adults (CDC, 2013). Thus, there is no simple correlation between the need for care and increased age; care needs and health status are affected by many dimensions in an older person's life, including socioeconomic level, ethnicity, and lifestyle risk factors (e.g., dietary habits).

There are variations in disability among Hispanic or Latino subgroups. Older Puerto Rican men and women self-reported the highest levels of disability, followed by Mexican- and Dominican-born men and women. Cubans, Central Americans, and South Americans reported fewer disabling conditions, and Spanish-origin men and women reported the lowest disability among Hispanic subgroups (Markides & Gerst, 2011). While foreign-born Hispanic men had slightly lower levels of disability than US-born Hispanic men, there was no foreign-born advantage for Hispanic women (Markides & Gerst, 2011).

To serve the growing proportion of older clients and their complex demands, nurses should consider that social and economic factors, cultural variation, and available support interact and affect the **illness behavior** and related help-seeking responses of older clients. Illness behavior refers to how individuals identify that they are ill, accord symptoms significance, decide to seek care or take action to reduce their symptoms, and decide whether or not to comply with a recommended regimen or option for treatment. As nurses prepare to care for older clients, they must assess the heterogeneity of the population as ethnicity, cultural traditions, social and economic situations, living arrangements, employment status, and migration history of older adults are as varied as they are for younger adults. These background factors contribute to older adults' varied responses to the illness that brings them to the health care system.

Adults aged 65 years or older are much more likely than young and middle-aged adults to have low health literacy skills, which means they are more likely to misunderstand medical tests, end up in the emergency room, and have a harder time managing chronic diseases (CDC, 2013). A majority of older adults have trouble understanding everyday health information available in health care facilities, which indicates nurses have a role to make information and instruction understood by all patients.

Socioeconomic Status Affects Health and Illness Behavior

The United States has some of the highest expenditures for health care among developed countries, and nearly two-thirds of the health care costs are for treating chronic illnesses. National health care costs are expected to increase by 25% by 2030 with the growing numbers of older adults who have chronic illnesses (CDC, 2013). Medicare spending is projected to increase from $555 billion in 2011 to $903 billion in 2020 (Kaiser Family Foundation, 2011). The cost of caring for each adult aged 65 or older is estimated to be three to five times higher than for younger adults (CDC, 2013).

Older adults may have set aside resources for retirement, but these resources may not be sufficient to keep pace with their longer lifespans. Most older adults who retire usually live on a fixed income, but many have increased health-related expenses and may cope with the death of a spouse or life partner that also affects their personal financial resources including health care costs. Some older adults decide to continue to work part time to supplement retirement benefits or to pay for health care costs (Tang, Choi, & Goode, 2013).

Among ethnic older adults, including Hispanics and African Americans, 40% have no private savings for their retirement and will look to state

and federal reimbursement programs for health and social service needs. Poverty among some Mexican American elderly may be attributed to occupational history of low wage jobs, periods of unemployment, and lower educational levels as the proportion of Hispanic elderly with no formal education is eight times the rate for non-Hispanic White older adults (Tang et al., 2013). The reality is that many ethnic elderly of color have accumulated fewer financial assets; that is, they have a lower household income and have less income from private pensions than do elderly Whites. More ethnic elderly of color rely on Supplemental Security Income (SSI) as the primary source of income after age 65, whereas a much smaller number of elderly White clients (1 out of 20) rely on this source (Tang et al., 2013).

The majority of older adults prefer to "age in place," that is, to stay in their homes and in their neighborhoods as long as possible (Karlin, Weil, Saratapun, Pupanead, & Kgosidialwa, 2014). One of the major problems that many older adults and their families face is that limited tangible assets and lower equity in their homes may limit possible care options because families cannot afford costly community-based care of the older adult family member. Community-based services may include homemakers, adult day care, transportation, personal care, and short-term institutional care. These services may be provided to some frail elderly who meet eligibility criteria and the support services will enable more elderly to reside longer in their preferred community residences.

An example from the caseload of a nurse who provides preventive health care and assessments in a low-income housing complex for older adults illustrates that individuals have different experiences using health care services and Medicare. An 82-year-old woman working as a housekeeper did not seek health care until she had a stroke related to untreated hypertension. She had limited contributions to Social Security owing to an episodic work history, and her illness depleted any savings. She receives Medicare-funded services and continues to receive home health care through Medicaid, which is state-funded health

care coverage for individuals with low income. The home health nurse assessed that this patient and other older patients on her caseload would benefit from nursing visits and medication monitoring, but the patient's insurance and Medicare will not cover such services. Medicare pays only a small portion of home health care services, and the patient must be medically eligible to qualify. Older adults who have other insurance may have some coverage for additional home health services for a limited period of time.

This situation is representative of the experiences of many older adults who have lower socioeconomic status and are affected by the societal interventions, including Medicare, that provide health care coverage for older clients. Providing community-based care has some limitations as frail older adults in very rural areas may have to enter nursing homes as a safe housing option when there are too few community-based support services or assisted living centers to sustain the frail adult.

The care that older adults may receive will be influenced and determined by economic necessity as well as environmental situations such as resources for nursing services and homemaker resources. Older adults' needs for care, their requests for assistance, and the sources of caregivers are also dimensions that are culturally influenced. Nurses and health care professionals see numerous variations in community caregiving support resources, both formal and informal, that are provided for older adults. In addition to the demographic and economic factors that affect the older population, several theoretical assumptions underlie how people feel about aging adults and shape how resources are made available to care for older adults in communities.

Theories of Aging

There are several theories of aging that have been very popular over the years and continue to be relevant in explaining how older adults are viewed in society. Disengagement theory focuses on explaining that older adults whose status is

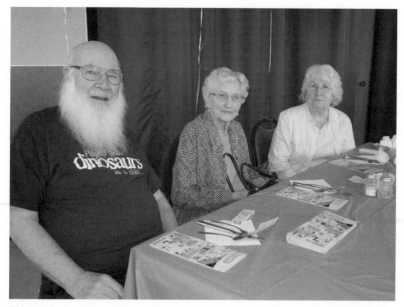

Figure 8-2. Active seniors enjoy a birthday celebration at a community center.

linked to employment perceive less self-worth in retirement when relieved of their roles and responsibilities. Activity theory describes that older adults may substitute recreational and meaningful opportunities to take the place of previous occupations and careers. Active older adults are recognized for contributing as family caregivers and as volunteers for social service organizations among other productive activities. Continuity theory focuses on supporting adults to remain engaged by adapting patterns of behavior from their younger adulthood to keep them involved into older adulthood.

Erickson's developmental theory advances that older adults may struggle with the tension between maintaining the integrity of their experience while facing the reality of declining physical and mental functions. In late older adulthood, individuals may despair with the perception that life is too short and with old age comes less authority and power (Erickson & Erickson, 1997), but they may also find joy in being a keeper of meaning and holding enduring relationships (Agronin, 2014). Cohen (2011) has described that older adults may "sum-up" their lives, which

includes a search for larger meaning in life, before having an "encore" phase of reflecting, reaffirming, and celebrating the major themes of their lives. Older adults participating in community center activities are shown in Figure 8-2.

The Older Adult in the Community: Cultural Influences

In community settings, we observe differences in how culturally and ethnically diverse older adults' life experiences will shape their **health behavior** and illness behavior. Older adults may carry out positive **health behavior,** such as not smoking, eating healthy foods, or maintaining regular exercise. Older adults could have walked daily when living in their home countries and eaten diets high in vegetables. When they are relocated into an urban setting, they may no longer feel safe to walk in unfamiliar areas and they may alter their diets to include available prepared and packaged foods. Among refugees from different regions, including

Eritrea and Ethiopia in East Africa, as well as immigrants from Eastern bloc nations, many have lived through civil wars, ethnic tensions, and political revolution, and they feel depleted in trying to cope with more changes in their lives after leaving their homelands. As aging adult immigrants, they may experience adjustment problems that warrant care in the health and mental health care system, but at the same time, they may distrust the system or have very limited experience in seeking biomedical health care.

Nurses who are providing care to clients whose background differs from their own need to be sensitive to assessing the client's culture. Individuals who have immigrated from the same country or region will differ in their needs and in the ways that their cultural background influences their health- and illness-related actions. These differences are based on a number of factors:

- Regional or religious identity
- Situation in their homeland that may have prompted them to emigrate
- Length of time they have spent in the country where they resettled or immigrated including degree of acculturation
- Proximity to immediate family or extended family members
- Network of friends and social support from their homeland
- Link with ethnic, social, and health-related institutions

To illustrate intragroup differences, we can look to the total Hispanic American population, where persons of Mexican descent are most numerous (54%), Cubans represent 14%, Puerto Ricans 9%, and other Spanish-speaking countries represent 24% (CDC, 2014). Many educated and professionally well-established Cubans immigrated to the United States in the 1960s, remained, and are now retired. In contrast, families emigrating from Mexico have been younger, some older Mexican immigrants returned to their homeland, and older Mexican Americans do not have as long a life expectancy as their Cuban American peers. The life experiences of

the individuals, including their occupations and education, and their acculturation will affect their expectations for care in their advancing years. A study of Hispanic American elders living in the community concluded that the participants who were more acculturated to mainstream culture reported better mental health, but not physical health, than less acculturated peers (Buscemi, Williams, Tappen, & Blais, 2012).

There is an incredible amount of diversity among Asian American, Native Hawaiian, and other Pacific Islanders as there are more than 40 distinct ethnic groups. Of the immigrant groups that have been represented in the United States for several generations, including Chinese, Japanese, and Filipinos, the Chinese and Filipino elderly are the most numerous. Newer immigrants include Koreans and Thais; among the refugees, the Vietnamese elderly are more numerous than Cambodians, Laotians, and Hmong. The percent of Asian Indians is growing in some regions as elder family members reunite with their adult children who relocated to North America in skills-based immigration (Sudha, 2014).

Culture influences how individuals view aging, define health, manage interpersonal crises, and face alterations in health that accompany aging. Nurses should consider that for older adults, health has multiple dimensions: physical functioning, social and emotional well-being, and quality-of-life measures, including life satisfaction and happiness. Older adults differ in their perceptions of health but generally regard their physical activity and psychological well-being as indicators of health. Poor health refers to self-reported problems with physical functioning or a need for assistance to complete daily activities.

Older adults are inclined to seek health information and to make behavioral changes to maintain their independence into old age. Older adults who use self-help strategies to maintain their health generally report better psychological well-being and physical functioning than older adults who do not use these approaches. Nurses typically provide information about the risks of not exercising as well as the benefits of increasing

activity or stopping smoking or adopting healthy eating habits. Nurses may also ask older clients about the circumstances that lead to a lack of exercise and then help clients to take small steps such as seeing how others fit exercise in their lives. Nurses who are aware of cultural variations can appreciate that older individuals will have different value orientations underlying their decisions to adopt healthy behavior over at-risk behaviors. Older adults who have peer support anticipate a possible setback in changing a behavior and plan how to get past a challenge, and use incentives through self-talk and rewards will be more likely to make positive health changes. See health promotion goals for the prevention of CVD in older adults in Table 8-1.

Practitioners should seek to understand the difficulties and different approaches that affect individual case management. Interventions should take into account older adults' cognitive ways of coping and practical strategies and support these strategies. For example, the matriarch of an extended family who has always valued the social benefits that come from sharing meals with family members may be reluctant to stop that practice and substitute exercise and low-fat meals. Older adults will also have learned responses in their help-seeking behavior to cope with chronic illness and to assess new illness symptoms. Some older African Americans have been more resourceful in their problem solving, planning, and coping that may be due in part to the lack of access to health care including mental health services that they may have experienced over time (Vinson, Crowther, Austin, & Guin, 2014).

Culture will influence the older person's expectations of what constitutes illness and will also influence whether the older adult uses traditional sources of health care, such as practices conducted by healers or actions that are known as family remedies. Older clients may preserve their traditional values that connect them to their origins and give meaning to their lives. Researchers have described the simultaneous use of Western medicine and traditional Chinese health practices that focus on restoring harmony and balance in the body and spirit among some groups of Chinese immigrants. Nurses should assess if any clients' use of traditional treatments is carried out due to a cultural preference or if a client has limited access to biomedical therapy and resorts to other sources of care (Sorkin & Ngo-Metzger, 2013). Many older clients could have grown up with limited preventive care and associate health care only with emergent conditions, so nurses should assess the older client's previous experiences in the health care system.

Table 8-1: Health Promotion Goals to Prevent Cardiovascular Disease Older Adults (Centers for Disease Control and Prevention, 2013)

Goal	Health Professionals' Actions	Indicators of Success
Reduce the number of older Americans who need cardiovascular treatment by increasing health-promoting behaviors and health protective actions to reduce disease risks	**PROMOTE** smoke-free air policies and effective tobacco packaging labels. **SUPPORT** education programs, wellness programs, and efforts to reduce sodium and eliminate trans fats in the food supply. **INCREASE** awareness of heart disease and stroke and their risk factors. **BUILD** local partnerships to enhance the effectiveness and efficiency of efforts to prevent heart attack and stroke (CDC, 2013)	Increase in the number of older adults completing health education programs offered in their communities. Reduction in numbers of older adults who smoke. Diverse groups of older adults complete wellness programs that are tailored to be culturally appropriate to encourage all individuals with different lifestyles to reduce their disease risks through increasing exercise and eating healthy. Communities respond by creating safe and accessible walking paths to increase use by older adults.

Traditional Beliefs or Practices

Older adults may have strong recollections of traditional beliefs and related remedies from their childhood. As an example, while the origins of their beliefs are very different, some Somali patients may believe illness is caused by spirit possession while some Hmong patients may believe that an illness can be caused by evil spirits if one's own spirit has left the body. Some Hindu and Sikh patients may believe that illness is due to karma, one's actions in past lives. Some older Asian Indian immigrants might follow Ayurveda, which includes the use of spices and herbs for cold, congestion, diabetes, and heart problems (Brar, Chhibber, Srinivasa, et al., 2012). Older Chinese adults experiencing chronic pain, musculoskeletal problems, and headaches might follow traditional practices including herbal medicine, massage, acupuncture, or dietary therapy. Some older Vietnamese immigrants may also use traditional remedies as well as biomedicine, but they may not disclose the use of traditional medicine to a provider, so the nurse should ask a patient what he or she does to relieve symptoms such as the ingestion of certain foods for medicinal properties.

An example of eliciting information from a patient is given in Case Study 8-1.

The patient in the case study immigrated as a young woman, but not all immigrants are young. Many immigrants who migrated after the age of 50 experience more depression, which is associated in part with their increased dependence. Depressed older adults are more likely to have lower self-rated health and may have more functional impairment. This suggests that nurses should assess the quality of the older adult's relationships, as well as their functioning status.

The older adult usually does not have an option to work, nor is public assistance an option, so the family must provide for the older adult members. Older family members may reciprocate services for younger family members. As part of a nursing assessment, the nurse should note if older adults are primary care providers for grandchildren or other family members and if an illness episode in the older adult disrupts the family.

Older adult clients may also use **traditional medicine or practices** from their family of origin as a means to prevent illness. Traditional preventive measures as well as actions to treat symptoms may combine several actions such as

CASE STUDY 8-1

Using Traditional Medicine

Sopha Danh, as a young mother in her 20s, fled with her two young children from Cambodia, settled first in the southeast United States, and then relocated to the Pacific Northwest in the late 1970s. Prior to fleeing from Cambodia, members of Sopha's extended family were tortured and died during a decade of genocide. The extended trauma resulted in patterns of posttraumatic stress disorder and depression being common among older Cambodian refugees. Older Cambodian Americans have the highest rates of disability among any of the Southeast Asians (Yang, Burr, & Mutchler,

2012). More Cambodian refugees also rate their health as poor and have poor physical functioning when compared to Pacific Islanders who were similar in age and other demographic features (Wagner, Kuoch, Tan, Scully, & Rajan, 2013).

When Sopha becomes acutely ill and her adult children bring her to a biomedical provider, she does not trust a male health care provider and is very reluctant to adhere with the biomedical care. Sopha is more familiar with traditional medicine, and her experience in help seeking is with traditional healers who took time to develop a relationship with patients. When the biomedical provider starts to elicit Sopha's history, and acknowledges how trauma affects health behavior, and when Sopha's younger family members help to interpret the cultural differences, the provider develops care recommendations that Sopha accepts.

Box 8-2 Guidelines for Communicating with Older Adult Clients

- Elicit the client's views on why the client thinks he or she has symptoms.
- Ask what home remedies or treatment the client has used and what treatment the client expects.
- Respond with information about the biomedical model using words the client can understand.
- Negotiate with the client what he or she accepts about the biomedical health care model and will likely comply with.
- Create a positive environment by being patient, inviting, and sitting close to the client so the client can hear you (avoid standing above the client). If working with an interpreter, position yourself so the client sees you. Typically, address the client in formal terms.

- Ask the client if a family member can also be present to help the client remember or participate in any client teaching.
- Have printed instructions in the client's native language, if possible. Have nonverbal methods of communication, including photographs or symbols to convey instructions, especially for clients who do not read their home language or English.
- Be aware if the client wants to make decisions or defer to family members as the decision makers about care issues.
- Demonstrate new skills that the client has to learn and discuss medications in words the client will understand. Show the client medications and help the client identify how to remember to take medications. Ask the client to repeat instructions to you.

a magical or religious element, burning a candle, offering cornmeal to the spirits, wearing an amulet, or reciting a prayer. A traditional healer is someone who is well respected for demonstrating unique abilities to relate to a person seeking help and decrease the person's discomfort. To assess the older adult's cultural beliefs and practices, the nurse can demonstrate a nonjudgmental attitude and develop culturally appropriate communication as shown in Box 8-2.

The use of traditional sources of health care concurrently with or in place of the biomedical health care system is not limited to members of recently migrated cultural groups, but is common to nearly all individuals. Several chronic conditions that often accompany age, including osteoarthritis or diabetes, increase the likelihood that older adults will use traditional sources or **self-care** to treat their symptoms. An older adult doing self-care may choose an over-the-counter medication and may use other popular remedies before, during, or after the use of prescribed sources of care. Nurses can show an interest in the client and ask them about any actions they take to

treat their conditions, in order to assess the older client's concurrent use of traditional practices, folk medicine, or popular medicine. Case Study 8-2 illustrates that assessing the client's use of alternative sources of treatment is useful in developing a care plan that the client will accept.

Understanding Culture Change

Some older adults have relocated to different regions of the country or have made a significant transition in their late adult years to be close to younger family members or for other reasons. Older clients may have the common experience of relocating or migrating, but they may vary in adjusting to new settings and to a new social environment (Keith,2014). Cultural change can contribute negatively to mental health, and this psychological stress is more intense for older refugees. For example, among some Central American immigrants living in a metropolitan area in the United States, their perceived stress was correlated with their psychological health. An example of a refugee making many social and financial adjustments is in Case Study 8-3.

CASE STUDY 8-2

How an Older Client Treats Pain

Mrs. Teadora Matthews is an 83-year-old retired seamstress who has hypertension, high cholesterol, obesity, and degenerative joint disease, which makes her joints painful and limits her mobility. She was raised in Romania, immigrated to the United States as a young woman, married a man in the mid-western United States, raised a family, and now lives in the same home as her daughter and grandchildren. She has been the primary caregiver for her grandchildren and remains active as a volunteer receptionist at her church. Her joint pain causes her to miss her planned volunteer work, and she uses over-the-counter remedies including ointments, topical applications, and pain relief patches to reduce her pain.

The nurse assesses that Mrs. Matthews tolerates a great deal of pain while carrying out her usual activities and remaining as active as possible. Her occasional use of the topical remedies does not interfere with the Mrs. Matthews' prescribed medications for her other conditions. Mrs. Matthews believes that self-medicating and using rubbing compound decreases her pain, which allows her to participate in her preferred family and volunteer activities. The nurse will continue to assess whether the use of an alternative source of treatment would interfere with a prescribed care plan.

CASE STUDY 8-3

Older Adult Adopts New Practices

Mr. Sylvestre Longo is very proud to have been born in Burundi, in central Africa. However, due to the strife, ethnic conflict, and genocide, he had to flee in his native country. He lived in refugee camps in Tanzania for almost 30 years before he was relocated by an international relief agency to Washington State. The Burundian refugees initially received financial assistance upon arrival in the United States, but after months of limited support, members of the community sought work in order to pay rent, meet their basic needs, and partially repay the costs of their relocation. Several of the Burundians learned of a social service organization that was recruiting refugees and immigrants to participate in a pilot project to develop their employment and English language skills while learning farming. The Burundians learned English vocabulary while also improving their diet by eating homegrown lettuce, beans, kale, chard, and root vegetables. The Burundians also became more physically active when they were planting and harvesting their plots and working in the fields, which also contributed to the new farmers developing peer relationships.

When Mr. Longo experiences shortness of breath and he seeks treatment through a neighborhood health clinic, a nurse elicits basic information about his health history, his social network, and his life transitions. Although he is only 50 years old, he is regarded as an elder among the other Burundians, who are in their 30s, some of whom lived their entire lives in refugee camps. Mr. Longo often attends monthly get-togethers of the local Burundians in which the younger, more acculturated members help to explain the cultural practices of their adopted country, such as completing applications to get entry-level jobs, buying food in large markets, and making appointments to request financial assistance.

Mr. Longo's nurse identifies several of his health-promoting behaviors. His informal social network could offer him some informational support to comply with his prescribed medications. She also assesses that he eats a diet high in fresh vegetables. This is in contrast to many immigrants and older adults who have income only from public benefits; typically, they have very limited access to fresh food when they live in neighborhoods without grocery stores (Yamashita & Kunkle, 2012). The nurse also assesses that Mr. Longo walks daily because he cannot afford other transportation, and this regular exercise contributes to his overall health and decreased risk factors for chronic conditions.

Box 8-3 Assessing Older Adults' Social Roles

- Family relationships and social interaction of the older client within the family—that is, the role the older adult has with a spouse, partner, adult children, and grandchildren as well as the role of the elder with peers and others in a social network
- Environment to which the older client will return
- Adherence of the client and the family to traditional values including the preferences of the patient to prepare, cook, or eat traditional foods. Adoption of new nutritional patterns

- of eating prepared and packaged foods in place of traditional foods
- Linguistic or social isolation of the older client
- Desire to maintain a moderate level of activity
- Ability to take personal responsibility for one's health
- Access to services and amenities including a safe place to exercise, senior center, and transportation
- Significance of spirituality and religious practices to health

The nurse in this case study assesses several areas that are relevant to assess for any older adult client to maintain good health; these are listed in Box 8-3. For many Burundian refugees and other refugees and immigrants, low socioeconomic status could be a barrier to health care, especially for early diagnosis and treatment of chronic conditions. Access to affordable health insurance is increasing for many low-income individuals, but paying insurance premiums often remains a challenge. Some of the older immigrants from East Africa experience mild declines in their health when they gradually become less active and modify their diets to eat more of the prepared high carbohydrate foods that are abundant in their new country. Supplemental nutrition programs including community lunches high in fresh vegetables and a protein serve several purposes of supporting positive mental health through peer interaction and stimulating healthy eating practices to promote health. These communal meals often increase the participants' intake of healthy foods and decrease their risks for poor nutritional status, which are associated with some older adults' functional limitations, cognitive dysfunction, decreased physical activity level, social isolation, alcohol or substance abuse, or other factors.

Caregiving of Older Adults

Older family members are part of the **informal social support** in their families, so they may be the caregivers for grandchildren or younger family members and they may receive assistance and support from other family members (see Figure 8-3) (Khan, 2014). If the older adult becomes ill, then families may have to adapt to find an alternate caregiver. Older adults in their family social support networks may also be in need of assistance and nurturing. Consider the preferences of the older person and his or her family members, as well as the capacities of the older adult for self-care and the willingness and capabilities of the families to offer support and assistance with care. The type and duration of support that can be provided by family members must be considered in relation to sources of **formal support** from home health workers, hospice care, and visiting nurses and therapists that could be used to sustain the family care.

There are many contexts for formal support and health care for the older adults. The image of care for older adults in skilled nursing facilities has given way to a continuum of services that includes self-care, supported self-care, assisted living communities, and skilled care. The roles

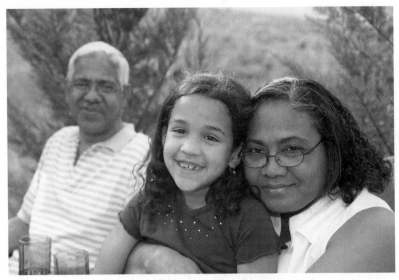

Figure 8-3. Grandparents are often the primary caregivers for grandchildren or younger family members (Rob Marmion/Shutterstock.com).

that family members take in each of these levels of care vary according to cultural, socioeconomic, and demographic characteristics. Although intergenerational caregiving is becoming increasingly common for some families across the United States, families in other countries have values more consistent with caring for aging parents in extended families. All families have culturally influenced patterns of responsibility to care for older family members, but these patterns vary across cultures.

Culture influences the role that the family members will take in the care of older family members. Nurses and health care professionals must be increasingly aware of how social and economic factors may alter families' retention of traditional values that affect caring for older family members. Nurses working with older adults should be sensitive to the evolving needs of family caregivers that will be influenced by the caregivers' acculturation and their time since immigration, factors that place the caregiver between value systems.

The economic necessity that two adults in many households must work to provide adequate household income has contributed to a decline in the availability of adult female children as

caregivers to parents and grandparents. Adult children and other family members may be available to provide episodic assistance, emotional support through short visits, or some financial assistance to purchase in-home services. Because it is not possible to talk about older adults or their families as if they were a homogeneous group, it is necessary to consider that cultural diversity and lifestyle choices may determine the options for care of the older adult. Several examples of community care options for older adults are highlighted in Table 8-2.

In caring for older adults, community nurses may have to coordinate how families caring for older adult members can access and use formal support services (visiting nurse services, chore services, adult day care) and **informal support** services (family members, neighborhood volunteers, meal delivery). Nurses are giving increasing attention to assessing the caregiver's capacities, needs, and resources in planning for extended care of an older adult at home. A nurse needs to assess the caregiver's health and well-being as well as that of the older adult client, considering a caregiver may be a working mother sandwiched in the care of an older parent and adolescent

Table 8-2: Highlights of Selected Health Care Studies of Caregiving and Older Adults

Study Author (Date) Topic or Group Studied	Cultural Concepts Relevant in Care of Older Adult Client	Implications for Nursing Care
Friedemann, M., Buckwalter, K. C., Newman, F. L., & Mauro, A.C. (2013) Four groups in South Florida: Cubans, other Hispanic, Caribbean Black, and White elders who were being cared for in the community.	Four groups of caregiver respondents had similar feelings of obligation, emotional attachment, use of family or community help for older family members. They also similarly acknowledged the role of spirituality.	Families' cultural values and emotional reactions to caring for a family member determined how they balanced their caregiving with available formal or community sources. Intergroup and intragroup differences should be assessed to plan appropriate care.
Sudha, S. (2014) Asian Indians from Tamil or Telugu ethnic groups who resided in North Carolina. Older adults and their midlife adult family members were interviewed. Some older South Asians have a pattern of moving between India and North America as their health and financial circumstances change.	Coresidence of elder family members with adult children, called joint families, was a social norm in South Asian populations. Older family members sometimes spent time to live in the households of their different children to increase interaction and decrease interpersonal tensions.	A major concern of the midlife and older adults has been affording health care. Many immigrant seniors have not been able to afford insurance and only sought health care with emergent needs. Some relief is likely with certain provisions of the Affordable Care Act.
Wang-Letzkus, M., Washington, G., Calvillo, E. R., & Anderson, N. L. R. (2012) Older diabetic Chinese Americans living in southern California.	Two adult day care centers serving community-based Chinese elders were the sites of a study using a community-based participatory research approach. The nurse researchers emphasized a colearning atmosphere and included community advisors at each site to promote information exchange with the participants.	Elder participants considered diabetes to be a social stigma, and they did not wish to speak of their illness. Chinese elders did desire to pass along their wisdom to younger generations, so bilingual research assistants, who were students, encouraged the elders to discuss their life experiences.

children, or a caregiver may be a retired worker in her 60s with a chronic illness.

Not only are clients more diverse, but their potential family caregivers vary widely in socioeconomic status, educational levels, and acculturation patterns. These factors will influence whether the caregivers, who are often wives, daughters, or other close relatives, will be expected to care for older family members.

Dimensions of Social Support

Social support has been delineated in three ways: affective support, or expressions of respect, and love; affirmational support, or having endorsement for one's behavior and perceptions; and tangible

support, or receiving some kind of aid or physical assistance, such as accompanying a person to an appointment. Many older adults are deprived of the informal social supports due to losses:

- Separation from immediate family members because of geographic mobility
- Age-related segregation caused by increased nuclear families in neighborhoods
- Loss of spouse or partner because of death or illness
- Loss of leisure pursuits or entertainment due to illness, loss of income, or declining physical abilities

It is especially important for many older adults to have social, emotional, and physical sources of

support to assist them to remain as independent as possible. We know that social support may mitigate the negative effects of social stress, but the exact mechanisms are unclear. We do understand variations in these patterns of support, which helps to prepare nurses who work in acute, extended-care, or community settings. Some minority older adult clients may have more connections to kin in their support networks, but they may also be more vulnerable to conflicts in tight-knit networks; this is less common for older adults who have multiplex networks of family, friends, neighbors, and coworkers (Lincoln, 2014).

Having sufficient social support has been associated with positive health-related quality of life. Mobilizing social support along with spiritual dimensions was related to decreasing depression and improving health-related quality of life for some Korean American older adults (Lee, Kim, & Han, 2013). In a different study, remaining self-reliant, having strong social support, having adequate income, and being in good health all contributed to positive quality of life in a study of health care implications of aging lesbians (Averett & Jenkins, 2012).

Culture may influence the types of social support family members offer to older clients, and nurses may assess that families' size and structure affect how informal support is provided. Some families, including German Americans, and families of English heritage often have a linear structure. The expectation is that adult children will assume care responsibilities for aging parents, and grandchildren will assume caregiving for aging parents and grandparents when needed. Another family structure is collateral when the perceived bonds are more diffuse. Parents, aunts, uncles, grandparents, and family friends may be part of the collateral bonds of families. Among families with a collateral structure are some Irish, Polish, and African American families, who expect to receive and to provide informal support among all collateral contacts. The expectation for care among many Irish families is that relatives must assist each other when needed. Many Irish and Irish American families would agree

that their relatives are obliged to enter into generalized reciprocity. Being a member of a large extended family does not ensure being a recipient of informal support, but brings an expectation of providing social support to older family members (Gallant et al., 2010).

Socially isolated older adults may have more self-reported health problems but may "do without" health care services due to their income status and lack of social support. When these older adults do seek care, they tend to be sicker and need more extensive care. Access to needed services in a timely manner could help older adults address health conditions and promote well-being in the short term.

In addition to cultural variation in patterns of giving help and support, socioeconomic status will influence the amount and level of assistance that family members provide to older adult family members. Demographic factors, such as family size, migration patterns, rural/urban residence, and socioeconomic factors, including income level and educational level, affect patterns of family support to their older members. These factors may determine the availability of family members to offer assistance and may influence the type of support that is offered. Thus, nurses must assess the influence of these factors on the older adult's social support network and identify that demographic and socioeconomic factors may be blended with culturally influenced patterns of behavior.

There are elders of American Indian nations who have lived in urban areas and have developed cultural resilience through bridging their native and dominant cultures, while also maintaining a strong sense of identity (Grandbois & Sanders, 2012). Many elder Native Americans tend to socialize less outside of their extended families and expect that the needs of extended family members will come before those of the individual (see Figure 8-4). Native American values support the care of older family members in the home, but the pool of available caregivers is diminishing because of some of the same patterns observed for other families that includes

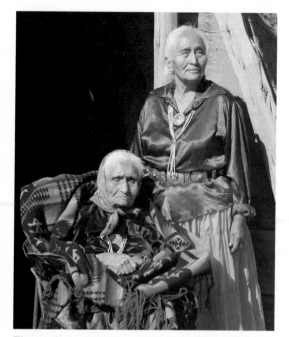

Figure 8-4. Elderly Navajo women on the reservation.

employment mobility. Elder Native Americans living in multigenerational households are more likely than White peers to have significant disabilities (CDC, 2013). A pattern that has been seen in some Native American families is that each adult child, in birth order, assumes the burden of responsibility and cost of care for the aging parent, which may exhaust the son's or daughter's personal financial resources.

Variations Among Members of Cultural Groups

The large older Hispanic population includes very diverse individuals who not only represent different countries, traditions, and acculturation status but who also have many variations in their patterns of social support from friends and family. While there are intragroup and intergroup differences, some patterns have been observed in studies of Hispanic elders. Older Cuban Americans are more likely than Mexican Americans and older Puerto Ricans to get together often with friends. Older Mexican Americans are more likely than either Cuban Americans or Puerto Ricans to attend church and to have daily contact with their children (Friedemann, Buckwalter, Newman, & Mauro, 2013).

There are also significant variations in groups of older Asian Americans and Pacific Islanders. Older Korean Americans may have immigrated with their highly educated adult children, but a higher proportion of the older clients wish to live independently from the adult children. The Korean American elderly may socialize with their peers through Korean churches but some are more likely to be lonely and isolated than Chinese, Japanese, and Filipino elderly (Park, Roh, & Yeo, 2011).

The nurse may look for ways to support an older adult immigrant in making ties to his or her home country to enhance self-esteem and feelings of belonging. Nurses may ask if an older adult can talk to a group of children at an ethnic community center, such as the Ukrainian Community Center, El Centro de la Raza, or the Polish Association. The older adult can also tell the history of his or her immigration to adolescents who may be tracing their cultural heritage for an oral history project. Senior adults may also be connected to school-age children by walking them to and from school or tutoring them through an after-school project. Nurses who are working with ethnic elderly clients may want to look for resources in the local community to do outreach to these community members and to involve them in their care.

The Older Adult: Caring for Individual Clients

At an individual level, older adults continue to meet developmental tasks similar to the way young adults and middle-aged adults also fulfill developmental tasks. The developmental tasks that older adults achieve include the satisfaction of basic needs, such as safety, security, and dignity, and the fulfillment of integrity and self-actualization. For the majority of older adults,

meeting these needs is intertwined with the lifestyle and the residence of the older adult. The older adult also usually prefers to maintain self-esteem through exercising self-determination in planning where he or she will live. Older adults may confer with their family members in discussing what housing option provides a safe environment where risks for injury or falls are reduced and social and health supports are available for the older adult. Depending on whether older adults reside in a community setting or an institutional residence, the individual may find an outlet for individual or group activity, volunteer efforts, artistic activity, or socialization that are sources of self-esteem. For most older adult clients, participating in some meaningful activity contributes to the positive fulfillment of the developmental tasks of aging (see Figure 8-5).

Across different cultural groups, aging is a developmental experience for individuals who are in a stage of reflecting on life experiences and finding meaning in their lives. Older adults may have many transitions that are chosen or are inevitable with growing older. These often include retirement, grandchildren, changed living arrangements, family mobility, declining health, and deaths of family members including a spouse, siblings, or children. Older adults may assume new roles, and nurses who work with older adults in community settings can reinforce changing roles as opportunities for positive growth. Nurses often view the strengths and residual abilities that older clients possess rather than dwelling on the losses, and in doing so, the nurse promotes optimal functioning when the older adult may be experiencing unavoidable dependency.

Cultural factors, including the cultural group history, and life experiences, including immigration, will interact and determine the older client's efforts to achieve security, autonomy, and integrity. In achieving integrity, the older client has a need to bring closure to life and acceptance of eventual death. A nurse may assess this need in a client's family and be a sensitive listener when the client works through the steps of achieving integrity. Older clients need time for a purposeful life review. The older adult may relinquish some aspects of their typical responsibilities, such as paying bills, to an adult child, so they can be free to spend time on other activities or have more time to reflect.

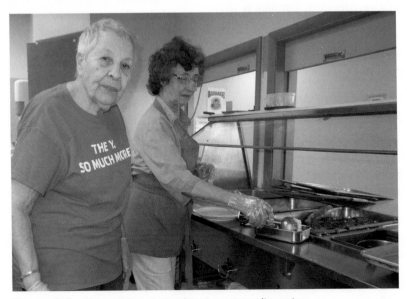

Figure 8-5. Older adults volunteering at a community center.

Faith and Spirituality

Many older adults experience an increase in religion or spirituality, which is evident in showing increased humanistic concern for future generations, changing relationships with others, and spending time coming to terms with one's mortality. Older adults respond differently to these spiritual development tasks as influenced by their culture, life experiences, and individual qualities. Religion and spirituality may be a source of emotional support, a psychosocial resource, or a coping mechanism for older adults who experience challenging health conditions, losses in personal relationships and fulfilling roles, and stress.

Previous studies have found that older adults' immigration status and countries of origin influence different religious and spiritual participation and devotion behavior. Some African American female elders have reported higher importance of religion and spirituality in their lives when compared to younger adults, and church-based social support was related to positive well-being and life satisfaction (Krause, 2010). Another example of spirituality is evident in older black Caribbean elders with higher education who were more likely to attend church services, while the younger and less educated black Caribbeans reported more devotional nonorganized behaviors (Chatters, Nguyen, & Taylor, 2014).

There are examples of older adults perceiving benefits of religiosity and spirituality. Some elder Japanese Americans reported that religion brings them peace while some Thai elderly, who were studied, reported attending temple helps them find meaning in life, which is a way to maintain health in later life (Iwamasa & Iwasaki, 2011). In a study of some elderly Koreans, religiosity was related with greater life satisfaction (Park et al., 2011) and with improved health status (Lee & Hwang, 2014).

Decisions on a Continuum of Care

Many older adults will require three types of care: (1) intensive personal health service, depending on the presence of acute and chronic conditions; (2) health maintenance and restorative care, depending on chronic conditions; and (3) coordinated nursing, social services, and ancillary services that may be provided on an episodic basis for older clients in the community. Many older adults will require care and assistance to manage chronic conditions; a public health goal is to encourage adults to adopt and follow health-promoting actions in their earlier years to minimize the occurrence of chronic conditions.

Depending on their level of ability or disability, older adult clients may choose to continue to live in their own home with assistance, with family members, in an assisted living residence, or in a skilled nursing facility. Nurses will observe that older clients express different attitudes that range from resignation to acceptance when they must change residences. The nurse can assess that the older client's attitudes about community or facility residence have been influenced by social and peer groups, and the nurse can be sensitive to the older client's reactions.

Families have often developed culturally influenced patterns of caregiving and social support. The nurse may assess the following: Does the family modify the environment and assist in home care so that the older adult remains at home? Do children and grandchildren share tasks, provide meals, and run errands so the grandparents can live alone? Do family members have a plan to have relatives share responsibility to provide support and supervision for an older family member? Does the older family member have caregivers and alternates who can provide care as needed if the older adult wishes to remain at home?

Some differences have been noted in the patterns of living arrangements according to ethnic background. When family assistance and informal as well as formal sources of health care and social support are coordinated in a plan of care, some older adults may remain in a community setting longer before being cared for in long-term care facilities. The proximity of the older adult to younger family members who are willing and prepared to provide assistance with activities of daily living, transportation, nutrition, respite care, and

social support may defer or delay nursing home placement for older family members (Kolb, 2013). Nurses must also assess that the values of independence and self-reliance may be very strong for some older clients, and they may refuse any assistance from family members, so the nurse should evaluate clients' behaviors relative to underlying values.

The adult children of older parents may feel obliged to respect their elders and provide home care when possible. As an example, some older Koreans have felt that their children should care for them, which is consistent with the value of filial responsibility (Kolb, 2013). However, these families, much like many other families of different cultural backgrounds, often face employment and financial challenges that limit their availability to care for aging parents, so the options for community care or nursing home placement should be considered. The interaction of factors including the availability, acceptability, and affordability of a skilled nursing facility that is in proximity to the ethnic populations also definitely impacts the overall residence patterns by members of cultural and ethnic groups (Khan, 2014).

Older adults who for the majority, if not all, of their lifetime have spoken their native language and surrounded themselves with friends who also shared their customs might find it enormously difficult to enter a skilled nursing facility that would appear quite different in its practices. Nurses and other health care professionals are not always aware that certain behaviors, such as an insistence on schedules, order, and cleanliness, might not be valued equally by all older adults. Older adults may feel especially uncomfortable if they do not understand why they are awakened at a certain time, required to be dressed, and asked to participate in group socialization and may find the skilled nursing facility to be hostile and unfriendly (Kolb, 2013).

Nurses can do much to ease the entry of adults into health care facilities when they assess each resident's cultural background, food preferences, choices for daily care and personal schedule, and interaction with family members. A nurse may ask questions on topics that were meaningful to the older client, for example, what was most important for them to maintain in their daily routines and what would they like to do so they could be as independent as possible. Older clients in long-term care facilities have expressed their desires to maintain their quality of life by controlling personal care and making decisions about their personal affairs whenever possible.

Some older adults, coping with terminal illnesses and debilitating and painful conditions, may choose to be cared for in hospice care in facilities or in their homes with professional, formal, and informal sources of care. Nurses preparing to care for and support hospice patients who experience chronic pain may refer to evidence-based practices in pain management as shown in Evidence-Based Practice 8-1.

Clinical guidelines have been evolving that are based on evidence-based practices for care of the older adult client with acute and chronic conditions who reside in community and institutional settings. Several sources in print and visual media help guide the nurse in assessing the older client; see Table 8-3.

Community-Based Services for Older Adults

The skilled nursing facility represents only one option for extended care of the older adult. The current nursing facility resident is typically an individual who has exhausted the opportunities for care in the community after implementing home care and assisted living. Long-term care nursing consultants and nurses working in ambulatory care settings often are asked to assess older clients to help determine the best care option. Criteria that the nurse often considers when recommending the level of care or residential placement include mental orientation, physical mobility restrictions (use of assistive devices and ability to walk unaided), degree of assistance needed to complete activities of daily living, frequency of incontinence, and level of risk for accident or injury if living independently.

Pain Management in Older Adults: Accommodating for Cultural Variation

A panel of researchers for the British Pain Society and British Geriatrics Society has published reviews on the assessment of pain and the management of chronic pain in older adults (Abdulla et al., 2013). The majority of cited studies were of community-based adults, but also included adults in residential care. Cited studies had been done on older adults in Australia, the United Kingdom, and North America. The review was designed to identify best practices for clinical providers to implement in managing pain for older adults, including sectors of the old and very old. A study finding was that older adults' attitudes and beliefs play an important role in mediating the way in which patients engage with treatment and the pain experience in general (pain intensity, psychological distress, functional impairment, and coping strategies used). Another finding based on small-scale studies found that several of the complementary therapies, including acupuncture, transcutaneous electrical nerve stimulation (TENS), and massage, had some efficacy among the older population. These approaches affect pain and anxiety, but require more investigation including research on older adults of different ages. Another finding was that some psychological approaches, including guided imagery and biofeedback training, were useful with subgroups of the older population. Limited evidence also supported the use of cognitive–behavioral therapy among some nursing home populations, but additional evidence would be needed to extend the findings.

Clinical Implications

Nurses working in acute care settings, extended care settings, and in the community interact with patients and their caregivers to negotiate an acceptable pain management plan. Nurses should assess for the patient's tolerance for pain, past and present experience with pain, effect of pain on quality of life, and the meaning attached to pain; these are all factors that can be influenced by the patient's cultural background and the patient's life experiences. The nurse who is striving to be culturally competent will assess the patient's culturally influenced explanatory model about the cause of the pain and the patient's expectations of treatments to relieve the pain. Behavioral therapies, which may include meditation, music, imagery, and aromatherapy, were not widely supported in the review but have been reported by groups of older patients to be effective. The nurse may assist in integrating the patient's preferences to use traditional and popular remedies including cold packs, herbal remedies, heat applications, or other therapies along with the Western prescribed medicines when the traditional or alternative sources would not harm the patient, give comfort to the patient, and do not interact with prescribed medications.

Nurses can assess social and cultural factors that influence the care that older adults will need, the resources to meet those needs, and the locations for residence and care that are most acceptable to the client. Nurses must assess the physiologic status of the older adult and consider the safety of the client in a residential setting, including medication management. The nurse should assess for the older clients' understanding of medication directions, as the client's eyesight may be failing, and should clarify directions, which may be open to multiple interpretations. The cultural values held by the older client and his or her family will influence the available resources, including informal sources of support such as children and grandchildren who are called upon to provide personal care, assistance with activities of daily living, and financial support.

Nurses and health care professionals who are aware of the older adult client's preferences for in-home care or for residence in skilled nursing facilities realize that the client's economic resources

Table 8-3: Clinical Guidelines for Caring for Older Adult Clients

Reference for Practice	Source	Evidence Base or Focus for Clinical Practice
Gerontological nurses are held to standards of Gerontological Nursing, which describe required nursing knowledge and specific nursing skills and abilities. Assessment is identified as a key skill for working with older adult clients.	Hartford Institute for Gerontological Nursing at New York College of Nursing and the American Journal of Nursing developed a visual and print series on assessment of the older adult client, which can be accessed online (http://www.nursingcenter.com).	The *How To Try This* evidence-based geriatric assessment tools were translated into nursing approaches and guidelines on 30 topics including pain assessment, pain rating scale, nutrition assessment, working with families, predicting pressure sore risk, assessing caregiver strain, and activities of daily living scale.
The Stanford Geriatric Education Center set goals to increase knowledge of evidence-based interventions for diabetes and depression in the elderly and to infuse ethnogeriatrics in the practice of health care professionals.	Stanford Geriatric Education Center, Ethnogeriatric Resources. Publications on diverse older adult populations, as well as webinars and handouts from the Ethnogeriatric webinar series, can be accessed online (http://sgec.stanford.edu).	The 2012 Ethnogeriatric webinar series on Applying Best Practices to Diverse Older Adults and Tackling the Tough Topics in Ethnogeriatrics include why culture matters in elder mistreatment, HIV and aging, pain management, behavioral issues, and elders at risk.
The module series on Meeting the Health Care Needs of Older Adults was developed for social workers and has relevant topics for nurses and other health professionals.	University of Minnesota School of Social Work developed modules on Meeting the Health Care Needs of Older Adults. The modules can be accessed online (http://www.cehd.umn.edu/ssw).	The Health Literacy and Cultural Competency module topics include demographics of older adults, health literacy, cultural competency, health communication, working with interpreters, chronic disease, and pain management.

may affect preferred care options. For the low-income elderly person, purchasing part-time personal health care services or attendant care that would enable him or her to remain at home may not be an option, so the older adult manages in less-than-desirable or potentially unsafe living situations. Nurses who are working with individual clients and those who are assigned a caseload of groups of older adults in community settings, such as apartment complexes and assisted living centers, will assess the client's needs, available sources of support from the family, and formal sources of support that are affordable to the client in a total plan of care for each client. Community-based care typically includes a broad spectrum of services, often using formal and informal networks of caregivers, as well as resources such as home-delivered meals or older adult day care. Local programs through the Division of Aging,

Aging Services, or a comparable agency may leverage available state or federal funds in innovative programs to reduce rental costs to assist elderly clients so they can remain in the community.

Local or church-affiliated agencies that recruit and train volunteer visitors and caregivers to the elderly may be used in conjunction with the aging agency programs to enable the fragile older adult to function at home with formal sources of support. These organized sources of support that may include a weekly visitor or a person to do chores for the elderly client may supplement the care and support that family members may provide. For many older adults, the long-held value of independence is so strong that the person would rather live alone, even in poor health, than be a burden to his or her family.

Older individuals who are independent or self-sufficient are the most likely candidates for

what are termed continuing care or assisted living retirement communities. There is a wide variety of assisted living programs in terms of size, structure, sponsorship, amenities, cost, and service availability. These are common residential locations that offer the older adult a comfortable apartment, a range of levels of assistance with activities of daily living, meals, social activities, and supervised exercise programs. Some residential communities have an attached facility for the skilled nursing care to move the client to higher levels of care based on the older client's needs, which may change over time due to acute illness, postsurgical care, and declines in functional abilities associated with falls or accidents.

Some older adults choose to relocate to these smaller, safer residences late in their lives to maintain their independence, but those decisions can lead to increased unfamiliarity in new neighborhoods (Lofqvist et al., 2013). The opportunity to interact with peers, and the option to participate in community resources, including cultural events, or shopping trips is fulfilling for some older adults (see Figure 8-6). But other older adults would feel stigmatized by residence in such a facility and would prefer to live in an independent location in the community. Other prospective residents might prefer the stimulation of intergenerational contact outside of an age-related residence and would prefer living on their own. Older adults deciding on any of these options are typically working through developmental tasks of finding where they will feel satisfied and fulfilled and find meaning in their lives.

The challenge that the majority of older individuals will face is the high cost of paying for levels of care in residential communities or in skilled nursing facilities. Many older clients and their families assume that Medicare will be the means for paying for such care. However, Medicare has limitations for hospital care and posthospital rehabilitation and does not cover what is termed custodial care of the older client. Older individuals and their families may exhaust their personal resources to cover extended care needs.

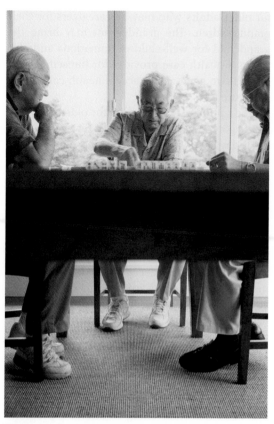

Figure 8-6. Retirees enjoy an activity in their residential community.

There has been an increase in the development of day programs in communities that provide nursing assessment, physical or occupational therapy, group socialization, and nutrition to older adults. These programs may supplement the affective support and tangible assistance that families give, and the programs provide settings that affirm the older clients' dignity. The range of these services provided at each site varies according to the support of the local community, including volunteers and professional staff. Some sites provide group socialization and nutrition for a lunchtime meal. The older adults are usually ambulatory or able to be independent with assistive devices, so they may be transported to the sites by public or private transportation. Some adult day centers offer programs and services

for older adults who may be caregivers for their grandchildren. The grandparent may bring the grandchild for well-child examinations and also access a health care provider for himself or herself, so two generations access health care at the same site.

The options are expanding for older clients to participate in community-based services such as adult day care, which may follow a social model, a health support model, or a combined service delivery approach (Wang-Letzkus, Washington, Calvillo, & Anderson, 2012). Adult day health programs were endorsed in the 2010 Affordable Care Act as a possible means to extend older adults' residence in their communities. The number of adult day programs has more than doubled in the last two decades, but the increase is not keeping pace, nor are services being funded at an adequate level to meet the needs of ethnically diverse older adults trying to remain in their familiar settings as they grow older (Brown, Friedemann, & Mauro, 2014). Nurses working in health care facilities or in community settings may want to assess the availability of local health and social enrichment programs and encourage the older adult client to attend a program. Many mutual assistance associations or cultural affiliations may provide programs for older adults to interact with young people and to share cultural traditions. These cultural center programs and similar church-affiliated programs provide a means for older clients to receive affirmational peer support and to reinforce their cultural identity in a way that restores self-esteem and dignity.

Other intergenerational programs support older adults becoming involved within the community and the educational system. These types of programs include the Older American Volunteer Program, the Retired and Senior Volunteer Program, and the Foster Grandparents Program. There are also intergenerational child care centers that are demonstrating that older volunteers are resources in the community, and the children and older adults benefit. Evaluations of multigenerational programs found that the older volunteers had a high level of life satisfaction,

including psychosocial adjustment, positive social exchanges, and self-esteem (Pilkington, Windsor, & Crisp, 2012).

Summary

A cultural approach to the older client recognizes that individuals are the products of, as well as the participants in, an encompassing societal framework. Within the societal framework, the cultural backgrounds of the older clients will influence their variations in their perceptions, behavior, and practices. Culture serves as a guide to the older client to determine what health-related choices and actions are appropriate and acceptable. Within cultural groups, individual variation is evident in responses to the physiologic signs and the psychosocial demands of increasing age. Examples of older immigrant clients demonstrate that the clients' views and perceptions may differ from those of family members and from the views of the nurse. The different attitudes, practices, and behaviors among older clients result from their heritage, experiences, education, acculturation, and socioeconomic status.

Nurses who are providing care in acute care settings or in the community often ask several questions as part of the nursing assessment:

1. Is the older adult isolated from culturally relevant supportive people, or is the older client enmeshed in a caring network of relatives and friends?
2. Has a culturally appropriate network replaced family members in performing some tasks for the older adult client?
3. Does the older adult expect family members to provide care, including nurturance and emotional support, which family members are unable to provide?
4. Does language create a barrier in the older client's receipt of services from formal resources?

Older adult clients have often developed their own informal support systems for coping with illness and with changes associated with age. Formal

resources may be used to sustain the informal support systems to promote the lifestyle preferred by the older client. Nurses caring for older adult clients should give attention to the client's family and social roles and develop care plans that maintain and restore the individual to his or her usual roles and patterns of activity. In the future, nurses will assess and work with more older clients as they progress along a continuum of services and through more than one type of residence in the community.

Clients may be reluctant to use services for various reasons that include cultural and linguistic differences or prior negative experiences in health care settings. To overcome any of the barriers that are perceived by older clients, nurses can assume several approaches to interact effectively with older adults from diverse groups:

- Be sensitive to the life experiences and previous health care experiences of the older clients.
- Listen attentively to the older client's complaints, recollections, and strengths.
- Listen to related conversations to assess for underlying depression.
- Elicit information about the older client's preferences for care, including diet and use of self-care remedies, and include them when appropriate.
- Identify available sources of informal support and confirm availability.

REVIEW QUESTIONS

1. What resources, needs, and limitations should the nurse assess to develop a care plan for a recently discharged 82-year-old chronically ill man who is returning to a single-room occupancy hotel in a crowded inner city location?
2. As the nurse who does health assessments for frail older adults who attend a community comprehensive day program, what information should the nurse assess to identify culturally appropriate care plans or service delivery plans for older Filipino and Chinese American clients?
3. The short-term subacute unit where you are the nurse manager serves a multinational group

of older clients who are admitted for orthopedic surgery. What cultural assessments do you teach the staff to use in identifying the needs of clients and their families?

CRITICAL THINKING ACTIVITIES

1. Many local communities offer adult day care for older adults with chronic health care problems who are residing alone or with family members. Services usually include health screening by a nurse as well as occupational health and/or physical activity sessions for these community-based older adults. Request permission to attend an activity as an observer and attentive listener. Through observation and, if possible, conversation with a participant, try to assess the levels of self-care that session participants possess and identify the types of assistance that these clients require to remain in the community.

2. If you are a case manager for a managed care organization, you receive many authorization requests for in-home nursing services to assist older adults who have been discharged home following hospitalization for acute illnesses or surgery. List the factors that you will consider and the types of data that you need to make an informed decision about the nursing and health-related services and the duration of services that the older client should receive while at home.

3. In many communities, nurses provide hospice services to residents in long-term care facilities or to older adults living in other settings. Contact a community-based hospice nurse to request information about how the services meet older adults' needs for love and belongingness, as well as reflection and recollection that are expressed late in life.

4. With your awareness that cultural traditions and life experiences influence many older adults to prefer independent living, prepare a letter as a home health nurse to the appropriate official to request government-funded home health services for older adults.

REFERENCES

Abdulla, A., Adams, N., Bone, M., Elliott, A. M., Gaffin, J., Jones, D., …, British Geriatric Society. (2013). Guidance on the management of pain in older adults. *Age and Ageing, 42*(Suppl. 1), i1–i57.

Agronin, M. E. (2014). From Cicero to Cohen: developmental theories of aging, from antiquity to the present. *The Gerontologist, 54*(1), 30–39.

Averett, P., & Jenkins, C., (2012) Review of the Literature on Older Lesbians: Implications for Education, Practice, and Research. *Journal of Applied Gerontology, 31*(4):537–561.

Brar, B. S., Chhibber, R., Srinivasa, V. M., Dearing, B. A., McGowan, R., & Katz, R. V. (2012). Use of Ayurvedic diagnostic criteria in Ayurvedic clinical trials: A literature review focused on research methods. *Journal of Alternative and Complementary Medicine, 18*(1), 20–28.

Brown, E. L., Friedemann, M., & Mauro, A. C. (2014). Use of adult day care service centers in an ethnically diverse sample of older adults. *Journal of Applied Gerontology, 33*(2), 189–206.

Buscemi, C. P., Williams, C., Tappen, R. M., & Blais, K. (2012). Acculturation and health status among Hispanic American elders. *Journal of Transcultural Nursing, 23*(3), 229–236.

Centers for Disease Control and Prevention. (2013). *The state of aging and health in America 2013.* Atlanta, GA: Centers for Disease Control and Prevention, US Department of Health and Human Services.

Centers for Disease Control and Prevention. (2014). Minority health Hispanic or Latino populations. Retrieved December 30, 2014 from http://www.cdc.gov/minorityhealth/populations/REMP/hispanic.html

Chale, A., Unanski, A. G., & Liang, R. Y. (2012). Nutrition initiatives in the context of population aging: Where does the United Stated stand? *Journal of Nutrition in Gerontology and Geriatrics, 31*(1), 1–15.

Chatters, L. M., Nguyen, A. W., & Taylor, R. J. (2014). Religion and spirituality among older African Americans, Asians, and Hispanics. In K. E. Whitfield & T. A. Baker (Eds.), *Handbook of minority aging* (pp. 47–64). New York, NY: Springer Publishing Company.

Cohen, G. D. (2011). The geriatric patient. In M. E. Agronin & G. J. Maletta (Eds.), *Principles and practice of geriatric psychiatry* (2nd ed., pp. 15–30). Philadelphia, PA: Lippincott Williams & Wilkins.

Erickson, E. H., & Erickson, J. M. (1997). *The life cycle completed.* New York, NY: W.W. Norton & Company.

Federal Interagency Forum on Aging-related Statistics. (2012). *Older Americans 2012: Key indicators of well-being.* Retrieved March 15, 2014 from http://www.agingstats.gov

Fredriksen-Goldsen, K., & Muraco, A. (2012). Aging and sexual orientation: A 25-year review of the literature. *Research on Aging, 32*(3), 372–413.

Friedemann, M., Buckwalter, K. C., Newman, F. L., & Mauro, A. C. (2013). Patterns of caregiving of Cuban, other Hispanic, Caribbean black, and white elders in South Florida. *Journal of Cross-Cultural Gerontology, 28*, 137–152.

Gallant, M. P., Spitze, G., & Grove, J. G. (2010). Chronic illness self-care and the family lives of older adults: A synthetic review across four ethnic groups. *Journal of Cross-Cultural Gerontology, 25*(1), 21–43.

Grandbois, D. M., & Sanders, G. F. (2012) Resilience and stereotyping: The experience of native american elders. *Journal of Transcultural Nursing, 23*(4), 389–396.

Iwamasa, G. Y., & Iwasaki, M. (2011). A new multidimensional model of successful aging: Perceptions of Japanese american older adults. *Journal of Cross-Cultural Gerontology, 26*(3), 261–278.

Kaiser Family Foundation. (2011). Medicare spending and financing fact sheet. Kaiser Family Foundation Web site. Retrieved March 15, 2014 from http://www.kff.org/medicare/upload/7305-06.pdf

Karlin, N., Weil, J., Saratapun, N., Pupanead, S., & Kgosidialwa, K. (2014). Etic and emic perspectives on aging across four countries: Italy, Thailand, Botswana, and the United States. *Ageing International, 39*(4), 348–368.

Keith, V. M. (2014). Stress, discrimination, and coping in late life. In K. E. Whitfield & T. A. Baker (Eds.), *Handbook of minority aging* (pp. 65–84). New York, NY: Springer Publishing Company.

Khan, H. (2014). Factors associated with intergenerational social support among older adults across the world. *Ageing International, 39*(4), 289–326.

Kolb, P. K. (2013). *Social work practice with ethnically and racially diverse nursing home residents and their families* (p. 177). New York, NY: Columbia University Press.

Krause, N. (2010). The social milieu of the church and religious coping responses: A longitudinal investigation of older whites and older blacks. *International Journal for the Psychology of Religion, 20*(2), 109–129.

Lee, K. H., & Hwang, M. J. (2014). Private religious practice, spiritual coping, social support, and health status among older Korean adult immigrants. *Social Work in Public Health, 29*(5), 428–443.

Lee, J., Kim, M. T., & Han, J. (2013). Correlates of health-related quality of life among Korean immigrant elders. *Journal of Applied Gerontology, 33*(1), 1–14.

Lincoln, K. (2014). Social relationships and health among minority older adults. In K. E. Whitfield & T. A. Baker (Eds.), *Handbook of minority aging* (pp. 25–46). New York, NY: Springer Publishing Company.

Lofqvist, C., Granbom, M., Himmelsbach, I., Iwarsson, S., Oswald, F., & Haak, M. (2013). Voices on relocation and aging in place in very old age—a complex and ambivalent matter. *The Gerontologist, 53*(6), 919–929.

Markides, K. S., & Gerst, K. (2011). Immigration, aging, and health in the United States. In R. A. Settersten Jr & J. L. Angels (Eds.), *Handbook of sociology of aging* (pp. 103–116). New York, NY: Springer Science and Business Media.

Ortman, J. M., Velkoff, V. A., & Hogan, H. (2014). An aging nation: The older population in the United States population estimates and projections. U. S. Department of Commerce., US Census, Current Population Reports Issued May 2014.

Park, J., Roh, S., & Yeo, Y. (2011). Religiosity, social support, and life satisfaction among elderly Korean immigrants. *The Gerontologist, 52*(5), 641–649.

Pew Research Center. (2014). Baby boomers retire. Pew research center web site. Retrieved March 15, 2014 from http://pewresearch.org/databank/dailynumber/?NumberID=1150

Pilkington, P. D., Windsor, T. D., & Crisp, D. A. (2012). Volunteering and subjective well-being in midlife and older adults: The role of supportive social networks. *Journals of Gerontology. Series B, Psychological Sciences and Social Sciences, 67B*(2), 249–260.

Sorkin, D. H., & Ngo-Metzger, Q. (2013). The unique health status and health care experiences of older Asian americans: Research findings and treatment recommendations. *Clinical Gerontologist, 37*, 18–32.

Sudha, S. (2014). Intergenerational relations and elder care preferences of Asian Indians in North Carolina. *Journal of Cross-Cultural Gerontology, 29*, 87–107.

Tang, F., Choi, E., & Goode, R. (2013). Older americans employment and retirement. *Ageing International, 38*, 82–94.

U.S. Department of Health and Human Services. (2010). *Multiple chronic conditions: A strategic framework—Optimum health and quality of life for individuals with multiple chronic conditions.* Washington, DC: US Dept of Health and Human Services. http://www.hhs.gov/ash/initiatives/mcc/mcc_framework.pdf

Vinson, L. D., Crowther, M. R., Austin, A. D., & Guin, S. M. (2014). African americans, mental health and aging. *Clinical Gerontologist, 34*(1), 4–17.

Wagner, J., Kuoch, T., Tan, H. K., Scully, M., & Rajan, T. V. (2013). Health beliefs about chronic disease and its treatment among aging Cambodian Americans. *Journal of Cross-Cultural Gerontology, 28*, 481–489.

Waites, C. (2012). Examining the perceptions, preferences, and practices that influence healthy aging for African American older adults: An ecological perspective. *Journal of Applied Gerontology, 32*(7), 855–875.

Wang-Letzkus, M. F., Washington, G., Calvillo, E. R., & Anderson, N. L. R. (2012). Using culturally competent community-based participatory research with older diabetic Chinese Americans: Lessons learned. *Journal of Transcultural Nursing, 23*(3), 255–261.

Yamashita, T., & Kunkle, S. (2012). Geographic access to healthy and unhealthy foods for the older population in a US metropolitan area. *Journal of Applied Gerontology, 31*, 287–313.

Yang, M. S., Burr, J. A., & Mutchler, J. E. (2012). The prevalence of sensory deficits, functional limitations, and disability among older southeast Asians in the united States. *Journal of Aging and Health, 24*, 1252–1274.

Part Three

Nursing in Multicultural Health Care Settings

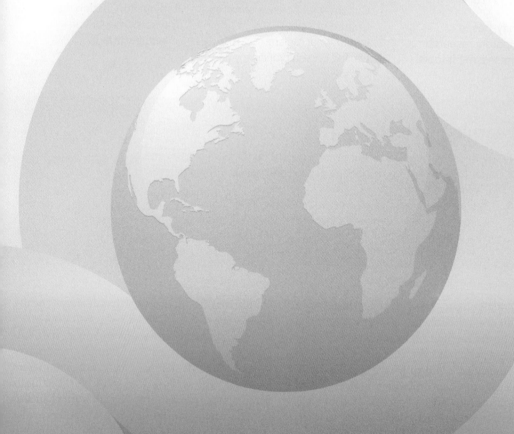

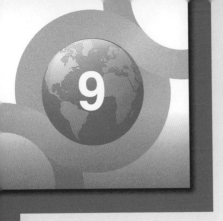

9

Creating Culturally Competent Health Care Organizations

● Patti Ludwig-Beymer

Key Terms

Community-based
  participatory research
Cultural assessment tools

Culturally congruent services
Culturally responsive services
Culture of safety
Institutional racism
Limited English proficiency (LEP)

Magnet designation
Participatory action research
Transcultural nursing
  administration

Learning Objectives

1. Assess the need for culturally competent health care organizations.
2. Identify how health disparities can be decreased or eliminated.
3. Evaluate organizational cultures.
4. Describe how organizations can develop cultural competency.
5. Assess culturally competent initiatives designed and implemented by health care organizations.

An individual's culture affects access to health care and health-seeking behaviors, as well as perceived quality of care. In addition to understanding the culture of clients, however, it is also essential to examine the culture of health care organizations. The interplay of client, provider, and organizational cultures may create barriers, lead to a client's lack of trust or reluctance to access services, cause cultural conflicts, and ultimately result in health care inequities. Conversely, organizational culture may facilitate access that decreases health disparities.

This chapter serves to augment the current dialogue on creating culturally competent organizations. It defines a culturally competent organization, explains the need for culturally competent organizations, describes mechanisms for assessing organizational culture, and provides strategies for developing culturally competent organizations.

Defining a Culturally Competent Health Care Organization

Cultural competence refers to the ability of health care providers and organizations to understand and respond effectively to the cultural and linguistic needs of clients (Office of Minority Health, 2011). Cultural competence encompasses a variety of diversities, including age, culture, ethnicity, gender, language, race, religion, sexual preference, and socioeconomic status. Cultural competence encompasses a wide range of activities and considerations and includes providing respectful care that is consistent with cultural health beliefs of the clients and family members. A **culturally competent organization** is broadly defined as an organization that provides services that are respectful of and responsive to the cultural and linguistic needs of the clients they serve.

The Need for Culturally Competent Health Care Organizations: External Motivations

Nursing has been at the forefront of cultural competence in individuals and organizations. The Transcultural Nursing Society was established in 1975 to advance cultural competence for nurses worldwide, advance scholarship of the discipline, and develop strategies for advocating social change for culturally competent care (Transcultural Nursing Society, 2014). An expert panel identified ten standards of practice for culturally competent nursing care. Salient to this chapter is Standard 6, Cultural Competence in Health Care Systems and Organizations. The standard holds that "Healthcare organizations should provide structures and resources necessary to evaluate and meet the cultural and language needs of their diverse clients" (Douglas et al., 2014, p. 113).

The American Nurses Association (1998) has also been proactive in addressing discrimination and racism in health care and promoting justice in access and delivery of health care to all people. The organization supported affirmative action programs in 1972 and passed a resolution on cultural diversity in 1991. ANA (2010) developed a position statement on ethics and human rights in an effort to address institutional racism, environmental disparities, class discrimination, sexism, ageism, heterosexism, homophobia, and discrimination based on physical or mental disabilities. Box 9-1 contains a partial listing of their recommendations. Sigma Theta Tau (Wilson, Sanner, & McAllister, 2003) and the American Organization of Nurse Executives (2011) include publications on diversity and the need for cultural competence in health care.

Regulatory agencies address the need for culturally competent organizations. For example, The Joint Commission has set standards, outlined in Box 9-2, to ensure that clients receive care that respects their cultural, psychosocial, and spiritual values (Joint Commission Resources, 2014).

The US government has also addressed culturally appropriate health care systems. For example, the Institute of Medicine (IOM) report "Health Professions Education: A Bridge to Quality" (Greiner & Knebel, 2003) identifies five core competencies for all health professionals: provide patient-centered care, work in interdisciplinary teams, employ evidence-based practice, apply quality improvement, and utilize informatics. Providing patient-centered care includes sharing power and responsibility with clients and caregivers; communicating with clients in a shared and fully open manner; taking into account clients' individuality, emotional needs, values, and life issues; implementing strategies for reaching those who do not present for care on their own, including care strategies that support the broader community; and enhancing prevention and health promotion. In order to accomplish the goal of meeting clients' individuality, emotional needs, values, and life issues, the IOM report further indicates that clinicians must provide care in the context of the culture, heath status, and health needs of the client.

In addition, National Standards for Culturally and Linguistically Appropriate Services in Health Care (CLAS Standards), outlined in Box 9-3, were

Box 9-1 American Nurses Association Recommendations Related to Cultural Competence

- All nurses advocate for human rights of patients, colleagues, and communities.
- Health care agencies pay close attention to potential for human rights violation as they relate to patients, nurses, health care workers, and others within their institutions.
- Nurses work collaboratively within the profession and with other health care professionals to create moral communities that promote, protect, and sustain ethical practice and the human rights of all patients and professional constituents.
- Nurse researchers conduct research that is relevant to communities of interest and guided by participation of these communities in

identifying research problems and that strives to benefit patients, society, and professional practice.
- Nurse administrators assess policy and practice and identify risks for reduced quality of care that may occur as a result of unacknowledged violations of human rights.
- Nurse administrators actively promote a caring, just, inclusive, and collaborative environment.
- Nurse administrators look beyond the immediate environment to the wider community for opportunities to contribute or participate in efforts to promote health and human rights.

Source: American Nurses Association. (2010). *The nurse's role in ethics and human rights: Protecting and promoting individual worth, dignity, and human rights in practice settings.* Washington, DC: American Nurses Association.

Box 9-2 2014 Joint Commission Standards That Address Culture

Leadership Standards

LD.03.01.01 Leaders create and maintain a culture of safety and quality throughout the hospital.
LD.04.01.01 The hospital provides services that meet patient needs.
LD.04.07.07 Patients with comparable needs receive the same standard of care, treatment, and services throughout the hospital.

Human Resource Standards

HR.01.06.01 Staff are competent to perform their responsibilities.

Rights and Responsibilities of the Individual

RI.01.01.01 The hospital respects, protects, and promotes patient rights.

RI.01.01.03 The hospital respects the patient's right to receive information in a manner he or she understands.
RI.01.02.01 The hospital respects the patient's right to participate in decisions about his or her care, treatment, and services.
RI.01.03.01 The hospital honors the patient's right to give or withhold informed consent.
RI.01.03.05 The hospital honors the patient's right to give or withhold informed consent to produce or use recordings, films, or other images of the patient for purposes other than his or her care.
RI.01.03.05 The hospital protects the patient and respects his or her rights during research, investigation, and clinical trials.
RI.01.05.01 The hospital addresses patient decisions about care, treatment, and services received at the end of life.

RI.01.06.05 The patient has the right to an environment that preserves dignity and contributes to a positive self-image.

RI.01.07.03 The patient has the right to access protective and advocacy services.

Provision of Care, Treatment, and Services

PC.01.01.01 The hospital accepts the patient for care, treatment, and services based on its ability to meet the patient's needs.

PC.01.03.01 The hospital plans the patient's care.

PC.02.01.01 The hospital provides care, treatment, and services for each patient.

PC.02.01.21 The hospital effectively communicates with patients when providing care, treatment, and services.

PC.02.02.01 The hospital coordinates the patient's care, treatment, and services based on the patient's needs.

PC.02.02.13 The patient's comfort and dignity receive priority during end-of-life care.

PC.02.03.01 The hospital provides patient education and training based on each patient's needs and abilities.

PC.04.01.01 The hospital has a process that addresses the patient's need for continuing care, treatment, and services after discharge or transfer.

PC.04.01.05 Before the hospital discharges or transfers a patient, it informs and educates the patient about his or her follow-up care, treatment, and services.

Source: Joint Commission Resources. (2014). The Joint Commission Edition. Accessed March 16, 2014 at: http://edition.jcrinc.com

---

Box 9-3 National Standards for Culturally and Linguistically Appropriate Services (CLAS) in Health Care

Standards

1. Provide effective, equitable, understandable, and respectful quality care and services that are responsive to diverse cultural health beliefs and practices, preferred languages, health literacy, and other communication needs.

Governance, Leadership, and Workforce

2. Advance and sustain organizational governance and leadership that promotes CLAS and health equity through policy, practices, and allocated resources.

3. Recruit, promote, and support a culturally and linguistically diverse governance, leadership, and workforce that are responsive to the population in the service area.

4. Educate and train governance, leadership, and workforce in culturally and linguistically appropriate policies and practices on an ongoing basis.

Communication and Language Assistance

5. Offer language assistance to individuals who have limited English proficiency (LEP) and/or other communication needs, at no cost to them, to facilitate timely access to all health care and services.

6. Inform all individuals of the availability of language assistance services clearly and in their preferred language, verbally and in writing.

7. Ensure the competence of individuals providing language assistance, recognizing that the use of untrained individuals and/or minors as interpreters should be avoided.

8. Provide easy-to-understand print and multimedia materials and signage in the languages commonly used by the populations in the service area.

(continued)

Engagement, Continuous Improvement, and Accountability

9. Establish culturally and linguistically appropriate goals, policies, and management accountability, and infuse them throughout the organizations' planning and operations.

10. Conduct ongoing assessments of the organization's CLAS-related activities, and integrate CLAS-related measures into assessment measurement and continuous quality improvement activities.

11. Collect and maintain accurate and reliable demographic data to monitor and evaluate the impact of CLAS on health equity and outcomes and to inform service delivery.

12. Conduct regular assessments of community health assets and needs, and use the results to plan and implement services that respond to the cultural and linguistic diversity of populations in the service area.

13. Partner with the community to design, implement, and evaluate policies, practices, and services to ensure cultural and linguistic appropriateness.

14. Create conflict and grievance resolution processes that are culturally and linguistically appropriate to identify, prevent, and resolve conflicts or complaints.

15. Communicate the organization's progress in implementing and sustaining CLAS to all stakeholders, constituents, and the general public.

Source: Office of Minority Health, Department of Health and Human Services. (2011). The National CLAS standards. Accessed February 23, 2014 at http://minorityhealth.hhs.gov/templates/browse.aspx?lvl=2&lvlID=15

developed by the U.S. Department of Health and Human Services' Office of Minority Health in 2001 and updated in 2011 to advance health equity, improve quality, and help eliminate health care disparities. All people entering the health care system should receive equitable and effective care in a culturally and linguistically appropriate manner. The CLAS standards are inclusive of all cultures and are especially designed to address the needs of racial, ethnic, and linguistic populations that experience unequal access to health services. Ultimately, the aim of the standards is to contribute to the elimination of racial and ethnic health disparities and to improve the health of all Americans.

The Need for Culturally Competent Organizations: Eliminating Health Disparities

Disparities in health have long been acknowledged; these racial and ethnic disparities document the reality of unequal health care treatment. The National Institutes of Health (2010) defines disparities in health as "differences in the incidence, prevalence, mortality, and burden of diseases and other adverse health conditions that exist among specific population groups in the United States." At the most basic level, disparities are evident in life expectancies. For example, the Centers for Disease Control and Prevention National Vital Statistics System (Hoyert & Xu, 2012) reports that the overall US life expectancy is 78.7 years. However, life expectancy varies by race, with White males (76.6 years) and White females (81.3 years) higher than African American males (72.1 years) and African American females (78.2 years).

Annually, the Agency for Healthcare Research and Quality (AHRQ) tracks disparities in health care delivery as it relates to racial and socioeconomic factors. Three themes emerged from the 2012 National Healthcare Disparities Report (AHRQ, 2012):

1. Health care quality and access are suboptimal, especially for minority and low-income groups.
2. Overall quality is improving, access is getting worse, and disparities are not changing.

3. Urgent attention is warranted to ensure continued improvements in:
   a. Quality of diabetes care, maternal and child health, and adverse events
   b. Disparities in cancer care
   c. Quality of care among states in the south

Access (getting into the health care system) and quality care (receiving appropriate, safe, and effective health care in a timely manner) are key factors in achieving good health outcomes. While many believe that access to high-quality care is a fundamental human right, the poor and racial and ethnic minorities often face more barriers to care and receive poorer quality of care when they access care.

The U.S. Department of Health and Human Services (HHS) uses a variety of measures to evaluate access to health care. Based on the 2012 National Healthcare Disparities Report (AHRQ, June 2013), blacks experienced better access to care compared to whites for 14% of measures and worse access for 33% of measures. When comparing Hispanics and Whites, Hispanics experienced better access to care for 14% of the measures and worse access for 71% of the measures. When comparing those below the poverty level to those with high incomes, those with low incomes experienced worse access for all measures. Both Blacks and Hispanics were more likely than were Whites to be unable to receive care or to delay care.

HHS also uses a variety of measures to evaluate the quality of health care. Blacks experienced better quality of care compared to whites for 15% of the measures and worse quality of care for 43% of the measures. Hispanics experienced better quality of care for 21% of measures and worse quality of care for 42% of measures. Those with low incomes experienced better quality of care for 5% of measures and worse quality of care for 60% of measures. Between 2000 to 2002 and 2008 to 2010, access measures showed no improvement, and quality of care measures improved more slowly in racial and ethnic minorities than for the total population. Disparities that are worsening over time are summarized in Box 9-4 (AHRQ, June 2013).

Box 9-4 Increasing Health Care Disparities for Select Groups

Group	Measures
African American or Black compared to White	• Advanced stage invasive breast cancer incidence per 100,000 women age 40+ • Maternal deaths per 100,000 live births
American Indian/Alaskan Native compared to White	• Hospital patients with heart failure and left ventricular dysfunction who were prescribed ACE inhibitor or ARB at discharge • Adults age 50+ who ever received a colonoscopy, sigmoidoscopy, or proctoscopy
Asian compared to White	• Adjusted incidence of end-stage renal disease due to diabetes per million population • Hospice patients who received the right amount of help for feelings of anxiety of sadness • Adults ages 18–64 at high risk (e.g., COPD) who ever received pneumococcal vaccination
Hispanic compared to non-Hispanic White	• Home health care patients who have less shortness of breath • Adults age 40+ with diagnosed diabetes who received 2 or more hemoglobin A1c measurements in the calendar year • Hospital patients with heart attack who received fibrinolytic medication within 30 minutes of arrival

(continued)

Low income compared with high income[a]	• People without a usual source of care who indicated a financial or insurance reason for not having a source of care • Adults age 50 and over who ever received a colonoscopy, sigmoidoscopy, or proctoscopy • Adults with diabetes with short-term complications per 100,000 population, age 18+

[a]Low income is defined as people whose individual or family income falls below specific poverty thresholds, established annually by the U.S. Bureau of the Census based on family size and composition. Poverty rates vary by race and ethnicity, with 14.3% of individuals and 11.1% of families below the poverty level in 2009. Individual rates vary as follows: 25.8% of Black, 25.3% of Hispanic, 12.5% of Asian and Pacific Islander, and 12.3% of White individuals classified as poor in 2009.

Sources: AHRQ (June 2013). 2012 National Healthcare Disparities Report. Agency for Healthcare Research and Quality, Rockville, MD. http://www.ahrq.gov/research/findings/nhqrdr/nhdr12/index.html; United States Census Bureau (2012).

Canada's experience with universal access to care suggests that access may help to reduce health disparities between groups but does not eliminate them (Alter, Stukel, Chong, & Henry, 2011). Their longitudinal study followed nearly 15,000 people for over a decade and found that clients with lower incomes used more health care resources than did those with a higher socioeconomic status. Regardless, individuals with lower incomes had poorer health, including depression, hypertension, diabetes, cancer, and cataracts, and were more likely to die during the follow-up. These findings imply that factors in addition to access may account for some health disparities. Potential barriers that contribute to the disparities may be related to demographics, culture, and the health care system itself. Potential barriers are summarized in Box 9-5.

Box 9-5 Potential Demographic, Cultural, and Health System Barriers

Demographic Barriers

Age
Gender
Ethnicity
Primary language
Religion
Educational level and literacy level
Occupation, income, and health insurance
Area of residence
Transportation
Time and/or generation in the United States

Cultural Barriers

Age
Gender, class, and family dynamics
Worldview/perceptions of life
Time orientation
Primary language spoken
Religious beliefs and practices
Social customs, values, and norms

Traditional health beliefs and practices
Dietary preferences and practices
Communication patterns and customs

Health System Barriers

Differential access to high-quality care
Insurance and other financial resources
Orientation to preventive health services
Perception of need for health care services
Lack of knowledge and/or distrust of Western medical practices and procedures
Cultural insensitivity and incompetence in providers, including bias, stereotyping, and prejudice
Lack of diversity in providers
Western versus folk health beliefs and practices
Poor provider–client communication
Lack of bilingual and bicultural staff
Unfriendly and cold environment
Fragmentation of care
Physical barriers (such as excessive distances)
Information barriers

Although identifying disparities in care is important, it is not sufficient. To reduce health disparities, individuals must deliver culturally competent health care that focuses on risk reduction, vulnerability reduction, and promotion and protection of human rights (Flaskerud, 2007). Organizational culture is one area that may influence both cultural competence and health disparities. A culturally competent organization is extremely complex. Within the health care setting, practitioners must be aware of the effects of culture on individual behaviors.

Assessing Organizational Culture

Organizational culture has emerged as an important variable for behavior, performance, and outcome in the workplace. Organizations are complex, with multiple and competing subcultures. The subcultural systems have inherent values and beliefs, folklore, and language; these systems are organized in a hierarchy of authority, responsibilities, obligations, and functional tasks that are understood by members of the organization. Leininger (1996) defines organizational culture as the goals, norms, values, and practices of an organization in which people have goals and try to achieve them in beneficial ways.

Organizational culture has been studied as it relates to accountability, change, emotional intelligence, effectiveness, implementation of best practices and research, leadership and management, Magnet recognition status, mentoring, and patient safety. Organizational culture affects not only people working in the institution, such as employees, physicians, and volunteers, but also those who access the institution's services, such as clients, families, and community members. The social organization of hospitals and other health care facilities has a profound effect on clients, both directly through the care provided and indirectly through organizational policies and philosophy. However, no current studies have linked organizational culture to client or provider outcomes or to the provision of culturally competent care.

Theories of Organizational Culture

A variety of definitions, methods of measurement, and theories for organizational culture exist. There is reasonable consensus on the following (Strasser, Smits, Falconer, Herrin, & Bowen, 2002):

- An organization's culture consists of shared beliefs, assumptions, perceptions, and norms leading to specific patterns of behaviors.
- An organization's culture results from an interaction among many variables, including mission, strategy, structure, leadership, and human resource practices.
- Culture is self-reinforcing; once in place, it provides stability, and changes are resisted by organizational members.

Bolman and Deal's Organizational Culture Perspective

Bolman and Deal (1997) describe four organizational culture perspectives or "frames" that affect the way in which an organization resolves conflicts: human resource, political, structural, and symbolic. The human resource frame strives to facilitate the fit between person and organization. When conflict arises, the solution considers the needs of the individual or group as well as the needs of the organization. The political frame emphasizes power and politics. Problems are viewed as "turf" issues and are resolved by developing networks to increase the power base. The structural frame focuses on following an organization's rules or protocols. This culture relies on its policies and procedures to resolve conflict. The symbolic frame relies on rituals, ceremony, and myths in determining appropriate behaviors.

To understand how these four perspectives will result in different outcomes, consider typical responses to the following situation. Hospital A is located on the border of two communities. One community is primarily African American. The other community is primarily Hispanic.

The hospital has traditionally provided care to African Americans and is well regarded by that community. The hospital has noted, however, that few members of the Hispanic community use its services. The hospital's board of directors realizes that, to survive, the hospital must expand its client base. The approach to this challenge will vary based on the organization's culture.

Hospital leaders with a human resource perspective are likely to approach the situation by assessing the needs of both communities and the staff. For example, the hospital may convene focus groups with members of the Hispanic community to identify why the hospital's services are not used by that community. At the same time, the hospital will assess the African American community's perspective on the hospital's plan to expand its services and become a more inclusive organization. The hospital will also provide opportunities for staff members to provide input and to express their feelings about the goals of the organization. In the end, the hospital with a human resource perspective will reach a decision that balances the needs of all of these groups while enhancing the goal of expanding the client base.

Hospital leaders in a political culture will take a different approach. They will identify key "power" leaders in the Hispanic community. Perhaps they will invite a Hispanic leader to join their board of directors or serve in another advisory capacity, or ask a priest from a Hispanic congregation to serve as a hospital chaplain. In addition, they will actively recruit Hispanic physicians and other clinician leaders. They will build a Hispanic power base within the hospital and use it to reach out to the larger Hispanic community and expand the client base.

Hospital leaders in a structural culture will develop policies and procedures to attract more Hispanic clients. For example, they may make certain that all signage appears in both English and Spanish or develop a policy that requires all client educational materials to be available in both Spanish and English. They may require all staff to attend a session on Hispanic culture, and

may strongly encourage or mandate Spanish-language training for key personnel.

Hospital leaders in a symbolic culture will use ceremony to meet their goal. They will make physical changes to the environment to attract more Hispanics. For example, they may create or alter a chapel, inviting a priest from a Hispanic congregation to say mass. They may display other religious symbols, such as a crucifix or a statue of Our Lady of Guadalupe, or alter their artwork to be more culturally inclusive. They may also include Hispanic stories and rituals in their internal communications. These leaders will draw on symbols and rituals that will make persons of Hispanic culture more comfortable in the hospital environment and that will attract a larger Hispanic client base.

None of these organizational cultures are inherently good or bad, just different. Each presents both strengths and weaknesses, and more than one culture may exist in an organization. For example, an organization may be guided primarily by both human resource and symbolic perspectives.

Schein's Organizational Culture

Schein (2004) describes organizational culture at three levels: (1) observable artifacts, (2) values, and (3) basic underlying assumptions. Artifacts are visible manifestations of values. Artifacts may include signage, statues and other decorations, pictures, décor, dress code, traffic flow, medical equipment, and visible interactions. Values are explicitly stated norms and social principles and are manifestations of assumptions. Underlying assumptions are shared beliefs and expectations that influence perceptions, thoughts, and feelings about the organization; they are the core of the organization's culture. Assumptions define the culture of the organization, but because they are invisible, they may not be recognized. At times, the assumptions of an institution are ambiguous and self-contradictory, especially when an institutional merger or acquisition has occurred.

Organizational Culture, Employees, and the Community

Many organizations are aware of the impact of organizational culture on its employees. When filling positions, recruiters consider the "fit" between the organization and the potential employee, because a good "fit" results in better retention and satisfied employees. Nurses and other health care professionals also learn how to determine whether an organization will match their personal values. For example, a nurse who wants to provide care in a culturally competent manner to lesbian, gay, bisexual, and transgender (LGBT) individuals will not be happy in a critical care unit that restricts visitors to nuclear family members.

Humans need care to survive, thrive, and grow. According to Leininger (1996), organizations need to incorporate universal care constructs, including respect and genuine concern for clients and staff. These caring organizations are needed for nurses and other staff members. Historically, however, organizations have made few attempts to nurture and nourish the human spirit.

An inclusive workplace is characteristic of a caring organization. Such a workplace, however, is not satisfied simply by a diverse workforce. Instead, such an organization focuses on capitalizing on the unique perspectives of a diverse workforce, in essence "managing for diversity" rather than "managing diversity" (Chavez & Weisinger, 2008). An inclusive workplace also reaches out beyond the organization by encouraging members of the workforce to become active in the community and participate in state and federal programs, working with the poor and with diverse cultural groups. Rather than espousing the golden rule (treat others as you wish to be treated), an inclusive workplace treats others as they wish to be treated, in what is sometimes called the platinum rule (Alessandra, 2010). Organizations with inclusive workplaces draw staff members who are committed to cultural competence and who value diversity and mutual respect for differences.

Although the impact of organizational culture on employees has been acknowledged, the impact of organizational culture on the community being served has received less attention. For years, hospitals and other health care organizations have espoused the view that "If we build it, they will come" (i.e., all that is needed is to offer the services). Now, there is a growing recognition that health care services should be structured in ways to appeal to and meet the needs of various members of the community. Health care leaders recognize that cultural competence in organizations is essential if organizations are to survive, grow, satisfy customers, and achieve their goals. Image is critically important for an organization's survival. A variety of factors are needed to move an organization toward cultural competence.

Assessment Tools

Organizational culture may be assessed in numerous ways. The Magnet Hospital Recognition Program for Excellence in Nursing Services evaluates organizational climate or culture (American Nurses Credentialing Center, 2013) and is used by many organizations as a blueprint for achieving excellence (Schaffner & Ludwig-Beymer, 2003). Evidence-Based Practice 9-1 outlines the original research that resulted in the creation of Magnet designation. Evaluating the five key components of the Magnet model may be helpful in assessing the culture of an organization. These five key components are transformational leadership; structural empowerment; exemplary professional practice; new knowledge, innovations, and improvements; and empirical outcomes.

Leininger's (1991) theory of culture care diversity and universality is also helpful in assessing the culture of an institution. Leininger's culture care model may be used to conduct a cultural assessment of the organization, with dominant segments of the sunrise model identified. An example of such an assessment is provided in Box 9-6. Other cultural care assessment tools are available to assess the culture of an institution. This assessment is then compared with the values

Magnet Research and the Forces of Magnetism

The Magnet Recognition Program for Excellence in Nursing Services grew out of a 1982 descriptive study conducted by the American Academy of Nursing's Task Force on Nursing Practice (McClure, Poulin, Sovie, & Wandelt, 1983). The study began by asking Fellows from the American Academy of Nursing to identify hospitals that attracted and retained professional nurses who experienced professional and personal satisfaction in their practice. The Fellows nominated 165 institutions. These institutions were viewed as "Magnets." The task force then began narrowing the list based on specific criteria and the hospitals' willingness and availability to participate in the study.

Data were then collected from staff nurses and nursing directors in 41 hospitals. Nurses identified and described variables that created an environment that attracted and retained well-qualified nurses and promoted quality patient care. Nurses were asked nine questions, which remain valuable for structuring nursing input even today:

1. What makes your hospital a good place to work?
2. Can you describe particular programs that you see leading to professional/personal satisfaction?
3. How is nursing viewed in your hospital, and why?
4. Can you describe nurse involvement in various ongoing programs/projects whose goals are quality of patient care?
5. Can you identify activities and programs calculated to enhance, both directly and indirectly, recruitment/retention of professional nurses in your hospital?
6. Could you tell us about nurse–physician relationships in your hospital?
7. Describe staff nurse–supervisor relationships in your hospital.
8. Are some areas in your hospital more successful than others in recruitment/retention? Why?
9. What single piece of advice would you give to a director of nursing who wishes to do something about high RN vacancy and turnover rates in his or her hospital?

Staff nurses identified a variety of conditions that made a hospital a good place for nurses to work, specifically related to administration, professional practice, and professional development. Clustered together, a very clear culture of nursing emerged from this descriptive study.

Based on findings from the original Magnet study, the Magnet Recognition Program was developed in 1990. The program was created to advance three goals:

- Promote quality in a milieu that supports professional practice
- Identify excellence in the delivery of nursing services to patients/residents
- Provide a mechanism for the dissemination of "best practices" in nursing services

Clinical Implications

As they rotate to different facilities for their clinical experiences, nursing students are in an ideal position to evaluate organizational climate. Nurses and nursing students are encouraged to use the Magnet framework to assess nursing subcultures and determine organizational fit.

Reference: McClure, M. L., Poulin, M. A., Sovie, M. D., & Wandelt, M. A.; for the American Academy Task Force on Nursing Practice in Hospitals. (1983). *Magnet hospitals. Attraction and retention of professional nurses.* Kansas City, MO: American Nurses Association.

BOX 9-6 Example of Leininger's (1991) Culture Care Model Used to Conduct an Organizational Assessment in a Hypothetical Hospital

Factor: Environmental Context

Types of Questions: What is the general environment of the community that surrounds the organization? Socioeconomic status? Race/ethnicity? Emphasis on health? Living arrangements? Access to social services? Employment? Proximity to other health facilities?

Sample Findings: Hospital A is in a low-income urban setting. The majority of residents in the area are African Americans, with a few Asians and Whites. A public housing complex is located within a few blocks of the hospital. The economy is depressed, and many are out of jobs. Drug abuse and alcoholism are rampant. Families are challenged to survive, and they tend to view disease prevention as unimportant. There is a short-term perspective on health, which is defined as being able to do normal activities. Several social agencies nearby provide assistance with food pantries. There are no other hospitals within a 5-mile radius.

Factor: Language and Ethnohistory

Types of Questions: What languages are spoken within the institution? By employees? By patients and clients? How formal or informal are the lines of communication? How hierarchical? What communication strategies are used within the institution? Written? Poster? Electronic? Oral? "Grapevine"? How did the institution come to be? What was the original mission? How has it changed over the years?

Sample Findings: Clients primarily speak English. Employees typically speak English, although Polish and Russian are heard, particularly among the housekeepers. The grapevine is alive and well at Hospital A. Although memos and e-mails are circulated, verbal communication is prized throughout the institution. The president/chief executive officer, chief nursing officer, and chief medical officer all maintain an open-door policy in their offices. Posters are also used to communicate, especially in the elevators. Electronic communication to direct care staff via e-mail has not been successful because computer workstations are in short supply throughout the institution. Hospital A was founded by a Roman Catholic religious order of nuns in 1885. The original mission was to provide care to immigrants and the poor. Immigrants from many nations, including Ireland, Poland, Hungary, and Russia, originally inhabited the area. The mission is still to provide the highest quality of care to the poor and underserved, although that is becoming increasingly difficult financially.

Factor: Technology

Types of Questions: How is technology used in the institution? Who uses it? Is client documentation electronic? Is electronic order entry in place? Is cutting-edge technology in place in the emergency department (ED), critical care units, labor and delivery, radiology, surgical suites, and similar units? Are instant messaging, text messaging, and tweets used? Is Web-based technology embraced?

Sample Findings: There are a few computer workstations on each nursing unit, which are primarily used by the clinical secretaries. Nurses do not document electronically, and physicians do not use electronic order entry. Hospital A received external funding several years ago to renovate their old ED. The new ED has state-of-the art equipment, as do the critical care units. The labor and delivery area is cramped and overcrowded. Equipment is well worn. Similarly, the surgical suites are dated. The radiology department is scheduled for a major capital investment next year.

Factor: Religious/Philosophical

Types of Questions: Does the institution have a religious affiliation? Are religious symbols displayed within the facility? By clients? By staff? Is the institution private or public? For-profit or not-for-profit?

(continued)

Sample Findings: Founded by a religious order, Hospital A is very clearly viewed as Roman Catholic. Outside, the hospital is marked with a large cross on its roof. Inside, a crucifix hangs in each client room. A large chapel is used for daily mass. A chaplain distributes communion to clients and staff every evening. Nurses demonstrate a variety of religious symbols. One nurse is seen wearing a cross; another wears a Star of David. Clients adhere to a variety of faith traditions, including Southern Baptist and Black Muslim. Chaplains come from a variety of faith traditions and attempt to meet the needs of diverse groups.

Factor: Kinship and Social Factors

Types of Questions: What are the working relationships within nursing? Between nursing and ancillary services? Between nursing and medicine? How closely are staff members aligned? Is the environment emotionally "warm" and close or "cold" and distant? How do employees relate to one another? Do they celebrate together? Rely on each other for support? Do employees get together outside of work?

Sample Findings: RNs at Hospital A tend to be white and are often the children of immigrants. They are most often educated in associate degree or diploma programs. Aides tend to be African American. There is tension between the two groups especially as the role of the aide has expanded. Nurses tend to be somewhat in awe of physicians. Physicians' attitudes toward nurses range from respect to disrespect. Many physicians are angry about the erosion of their autonomy and economic security. Most units tend to be tight knit, with celebrations of monthly birthdays and recognition provided when staff members "go the extra mile." Nurses rarely socialize with one another outside of work. Staff nurses are middle aged (mean age 45). Most of them commute from the suburbs to the hospital and return home after their shift. In contrast, many of the aides are from the immediate community, know each other, and socialize outside of work.

Factor: Cultural Values

Types of Questions: Are values explicitly stated? What is valued within the institution?

What is viewed as good? What is viewed as right? What is seen as truth?

Sample Findings: The institution clearly identifies its mission and strives to fulfill it in economically difficult times. Its stated values are collaboration and diversity. Although diversity training has been provided to managers, tensions still exist between work groups, particularly because the workforce tends to be racially divided.

Factor: Political/Legal

Types of Questions: How politically charged is the institution? Where does the power rest within the institution? With medicine? With finance? With nursing? With information technology? Is power shared? What types of legal actions have been taken against the institution? On behalf of the institution?

Sample Findings: Historically, Hospital A has been politically naive. It has gone about its mission without regard to the external environment. Recently, the hospital has begun to lobby for better reimbursement for care provided under Medicaid. Institutional power rests with the strong medical staff and department chairs.

Factor: Economic

Types of Questions: What is the financial viability of the institution? Who makes the financial decisions? How do the salaries and benefits compare with those of competitors in the immediate environment?

Sample Findings: Hospital A has a very low profit margin, 0.5%, compared with an industry standard of more than 3%. This means that little money is available for capital improvements, which results in less technology and some units being cramped. Community needs are considered, along with all financial decisions. People are valued, and efforts are made to keep salaries competitive. Starting salaries are increasing for new graduates, and experienced nurses are complaining of salary compression.

Factor: Educational

Types of Questions: How is education valued within the institution? What type of assistance (financial, scheduling, flexibility) is

provided for staff seeking advanced degrees? Does the institution provide education for medicine, nursing, and other professions? Are advanced practice nurses utilized? What is the educational background of staff nurses? Nurse managers? Nursing leaders? How does this compare with education of other professional groups? With competing organizations?

Sample Findings: With an in-house diploma school, nurses are most often educated at the diploma level. Although flexible scheduling and limited tuition reimbursement are provided, many nurses do not take advantage of the benefits because of the need to work extra shifts to ensure staffing and competing personal and family priorities. All new nurse managers and directors are required to have a BSN; however, most existing managers are educated at the diploma level. Nursing students from five different programs rotate through the institution, with first priority given to the hospital's diploma program. Hospital A provides a summer preceptor program to students from one baccalaureate degree program, and some faculty members are employed during summers and holidays. Medical education is provided at Hospital A, with 150 residents and many 3rd year and 4th year medical students rotating through the facility. The residents, while learning, also provide important service to the community, particularly through their clinic rotations. Students in respiratory, social work, dietitian, physical therapy, occupational therapy, speech therapy, and pastoral care also have clinical rotations at Hospital A.

and beliefs of the groups who use the health care organization. Andrews (1998) provides an assessment tool for cultural change that examines demographic/descriptive data; strengths; community resources; continued growth; perspectives of clients, families, and visitors; institutional perspective; and readiness for change. This tool allows organizational leaders to assess the needs of the community they serve and to use their findings to guide strategic planning for the future.

Building Culturally Competent Organizations

Cultural competence has been identified as a key strategy for eliminating racial and ethnic health disparities. However, the competence must extend beyond the provider, into the system of health care. It would be naive to assume that building culturally competent organizations will resolve all health disparities. However, when health care is delivered within a culturally competent organization, diverse health care consumers may be more likely to access the services, return for services, adhere to the plan of care, and make necessary lifestyle changes.

Weech-Maldonado, Elliott, Pradhan, Schiller, Hall, et al. (2012) conducted research to examine the relationship between hospital cultural competence and satisfaction with inpatient care. They found that inpatients reported higher satisfaction with hospitals that had greater cultural competency. The findings were particularly striking among minority patients, who reported higher satisfaction with nurse communication, physician communication, staff responsiveness, pain control, and environmental factors in hospitals with greater cultural competency.

Guerrero (2012) examined the extent to which internal and external organizational pressures contributed to the degree of adoption of culturally and linguistically responsive practices in outpatient substance abuse treatment systems. Higher adoption of culturally competent practices was found in programs with more external funding and regulation and with managers who had higher levels of cultural sensitivity. Organizations with a large number of professional staff had lower adoption of culturally competent practices when compared to organizations with fewer professional staff members.

As with cultural competence in individuals, cultural competency in organizations develops over time as part of a journey. The process involves all aspects of the organization. Malone (1997) describes several strategies for improving organizational cultural competence. Strategies include training that helps the organization to value and manage cultural diversity; rewarding practice that values differences and is culturally appropriate and collaborative; recruiting nurses who are culturally competent; and hiring nurses who are culturally diverse. Purnell, Davidhizar, Giger, Strickland, Fishman, and Allison (2011) provide a guide to developing culturally competent organizations that address four key areas: administration and governance, orientation and education, language, and staff competence. Marrone (2010, 2012) provides a comprehensive assessment of organizational cultural competency. Douglas et al. (2014) recommend ten practices by leaders to build cultural competence in health care organizations, summarized in Box 9-7. Fung, Srivastava,

and Andermann (2012) present a framework, consisting of eight domains, to plan for organizational cultural competence in mental health care service settings. Delphin-Rittmen (2013) describes seven essential strategies for promoting and sustaining cultural competence.

For the purpose of this chapter, the concepts identified above have been combined and consolidated. Seven specific areas critical to fostering culturally competent health care organizations are discussed in the sections below: governance and administration, internal evaluation of adherence to cultural competence standards, staff competence, the physical environment of care, linguistic competence, community involvement, and culturally congruent services and programs.

Governance and Administration

For the purposes of this chapter, governance is defined as members of the board of directors and any subboards, such as Board Finance or Board

Box 9-7 The Role of Health Care Organization Leaders in Developing Culturally Competent Health Care Systems and Organizations

1. Develop systems to promote culturally competent care delivery.
2. Ensure that mission and organizational policies reflect respect and values related to diversity and inclusivity.
3. Assign a managerial-level task force to oversee and take responsibility for diversity-related issues within the organization.
4. Establish an internal budget for the provision of culturally appropriate care, such as for the hiring of interpreters, producing multi-language client education materials, adding signage in different languages, and so on.
5. Include cultural competence requirements in job descriptions, performance measures, and promotion criteria.

6. Develop a data collection system to monitor demographic trends for the geographic area served by the agency.
7. Obtain patient satisfaction data to determine the appropriateness and effectiveness of services.
8. Collaborate with other health agencies to share ideas and resources for meeting the needs of culturally diverse populations.
9. Bring health care directly to the local ethnic populations.
10. Enlist community members to participate in the agency's program planning committees, for example, for smoking cessation or infant care programs.

Source: Douglas, M. K., Rosenkoetter, M., Pacquiao, D., Callister, L. C., Hattar-Pollara, M., Lauderdale, J., ..., Purnell, L. (2014). Guidelines for implementing culturally competent nursing care. *Journal of Transcultural Nursing*, 25(2), 109–121.

Box 9-8 Strategies and Tools for Reducing Health Disparities

Local research and analysis of disparities

Primary health care practices and resources
   Location of Services
   Appropriate care

Partnerships
   Poverty reduction collaborations
   Early childhood development
   School-based strategies

Public education and policy advocacy

Community development and participation

Source: Kouri, D. (2012, March). Reducing health disparities: How can the structure of the health system contribute? *Wellesley Institute.* Accessed March 16, 2014 at http://www.wellesleyinstitute.com/wp-content/uploads/2012/09/Reducing-Health-Disparities-how-can-health-system-structure-contribute.pdf

Quality. Administration is defined as those individuals who serve as department heads. Together, governance and administration are responsible for ensuring that the organization is continually developing cultural competence. The Wellesley Institute in Ontario (Kouri, 2012) identifies key strategies and tools helpful for reducing health disparities; several strategies helpful for governance and administration to consider are summarized in Box 9-8.

Ideally, both board members and administrators reflect the ethnic and racial diversity of the community served. The board and administration set the strategic plan for the organization. The strategic plan sets the direction for an organization and is used to communicate organizational goals and the actions needed to achieve those goals. The strategic planning process should begin with an assessment of community strengths and needs. In a study designed to determine factors related to organizational cultural competence, Guerrero (2013) found that leadership skills and strategic climate in addiction health service settings resulted in a better understanding and responsiveness to community needs.

Board members and administration also establish the mission, vision, and values for the organization. The mission statement describes the purpose of the organization, its reason for existing. The mission statement should be inclusive, and the strategic plan should include tactics for developing culturally congruent services and programs to meet community needs, partnering with key community organizations, and developing the organization's cultural competence. The basic premises of an organization, reflected in its mission statement, provide insight into the presence or absence of a commitment to providing culturally competent care. Many organizations also establish a vision and values to guide their culture. The vision projects the future status of an organization and inspires and generates a shared purpose among organization members. Whether or not they are explicitly stated, all organizations have values. Values are the standards that guide the perspective and action of the organization and help to define an organization's culture and beliefs. As seen in Box 9-9 the mission, vision, and values may also include specific behaviors demonstrated toward both customers and colleagues.

Administration also develops the organization's budget, which is then approved by the board of directors. Financial resources, including funding for capital, staff, and programs for the delivery of care, must be allocated appropriately to foster organizational cultural competence. For example, the environment should be welcoming, with the space and décor appropriate for the cultural groups served. Funding for staff recruitment, orientation, and training is also essential. Funding for the delivery of care must always consider cultural components. For example, funding is needed to advertise new and existing programs, using the venues and languages appropriate to the community. Pictures on the advertising materials must reflect the client population.

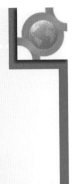

Box 9-9 Edward Hospital Mission, Vision, and Values

Mission

To support health and strengthen communities by providing outstanding health care services

Vision

Locally preferred, regionally referred, nationally recognized

Values

Patients first
Integrity

Compassion
Responsibility
Collaboration
Passion

Behaviors

We will always…

    Communicate openly
    Care for you
    Provide quality

Courtesy of Edward Hospital and Health Services. (2013). Naperville, IL.

Nurse executives can take the lead in developing culturally competent health care organizations. Leininger (1996) defined transcultural nursing administration as "a creative and knowledgeable process of assessing, planning, and making decisions and policies that will facilitate the provision of educational and clinical services that take into account the cultural caring values, beliefs, symbols, references and lifeways of people of diverse and similar cultures for beneficial or satisfying outcomes" (1996, p. 30). Nurse administrators must ensure that organizational policies are culturally sensitive and appropriate and that they recognize the rights of individuals and families. Such policies should incorporate Leininger's (1991) decisions and actions of culture care preservation/maintenance, culture care accommodation/negotiation, and culture care repatterning/restructuring.

Nurse leaders who recognize the importance of transculturally based administration are essential for culturally competent health care organizations. The American Organization of Nurse Executives (AONE, 2011) identifies five nurse executive competencies: communication, knowledge, leadership, professionalism, and business skills. Nurse executive competencies related to diversity are summarized in Box 9-10. Nurse administrators must foster a climate in which

nurses and other health care providers realize that provider–client encounters include the interaction of three cultural systems: the organization, the providers, and the client (American Nurses Association Council on Cultural Diversity in Nursing Practice, 1991).

In culturally competent health care organizations, nurse leaders also recognize the relationship between a culturally diverse nursing workforce and the ability to provide culturally competent patient care. The need to attract students from underrepresented groups is gaining importance (American Association of Colleges of Nursing, 2014) and calls for new partnerships between practice, community, and academic settings.

Administration and the board of directors must work together to ensure that the health care organization continues the journey toward cultural competence. This includes setting strategic priorities and funding appropriate programs for staff and clients.

Internal Evaluation of Adherence to Cultural Competence Standards

In addition to recognizing and acknowledging the overall culture of a health care organization, organizations must also evaluate how they are adhering to cultural competence standards as an

Box 9-10 American Organization of Nurse Executives (AONE) Nurse Executive Communication and Relationship-Building Competencies Related to Diversity

- Create an environment that recognizes and values differences in staff, physicians, patients, and communities.
- Assess current environment and establish indicators of progress toward cultural competency.
- Define diversity in terms of gender, race, religion, ethnicity, sexual orientation, age, etc.

- Analyze population data to identify cultural clusters.
- Define cultural competency and permeate principles throughout the organization.
- Confront inappropriate behaviors and attitudes toward diverse groups.
- Develop processes to incorporate cultural beliefs into care.

Source: American Organization of Nurse Executives. (2011). The AONE nurse executive competencies. Accessed February 22, 2014 at www.aone.org/resources/leadership%20tools/PDFs/AONE_NEC.pdf

organization and determine how effectively the organization is meeting the needs of the populations they serve. The evaluation may be conducted in a variety of ways.

Roizner (1996) identifies a checklist for culturally responsive health care services. Health care services are evaluated based on their availability, accessibility, affordability, acceptability, and appropriateness. When the organization is evaluated by this model, it is important to consider these "five A's":

- Are the health services that are needed by the community readily available? In a community with rampant illicit drug use, for example, one should expect to find a variety of types of drug abuse prevention and treatment programs offered that are readily available to the local population.
- Are health care resources accessible? A pediatrician's office, for example, might need to expand its hours of operation to accommodate the schedules of working parents. Geographic location should be considered in terms of proximity to public transportation, traffic patterns, and available parking. Structural changes may also be needed to accommodate specific types of clients, such as those who use wheelchairs.
- Are the services affordable? Partnerships between public and private organizations may be needed to ensure that services are afford-

able. A sliding scale might be developed to accommodate the needs of people with limited financial resources.
- Are the services acceptable? Providers need to carefully consider this question. Do community members who use the services perceive the services to be of high quality? Do community members value the services? Are the waiting rooms stark, dimly lit, or untidy? Is the furniture worn or the reading material frayed and outdated? Providers need to understand what makes services acceptable to the community they seek to serve. Community members may avoid a particular agency or institution because services are delivered in a noncaring and patronizing fashion.
- Are the services appropriate? Community members may not use services if they do not perceive that these services meet their needs. For example, community members who struggle with day-to-day survival with limited financial and social resources may not use fitness classes. Programs that are disconnected from the daily life of community members constitute a recipe for failure.

Fung et al. (2012) present a methodology for evaluating cultural competence in health care organizations involving mixed qualitative and quantitative methods. An organization may also compare their performance to standards provided by regulatory bodies, government agencies,

and professional organizations. Annually, members of the Language, Culture and Religion Committee at some organizations critically compare current practice with Joint Commission and CLAS standards. The committee members determine where there are gaps and develop a strategic plan to address the gaps.

The Cultural Competency Assessment Tool for Hospitals (CCATH) allows an organization to assess adherence to the CLAS standards (Hays et al., 2006). The instrument measures 12 composites: leadership and strategic planning, data collection on inpatient population, data collection on service area, performance management systems and quality improvement, human resource practices, diversity training, community representation, availability of interpreter

services, interpreter services policies, quality of interpreter services, translation of written materials, and clinical cultural competency practices (Weech-Maldonado, Dreachslin, et al., 2012). Weech-Maldonado, Elliott, Pradhan, Schiller, Dreachslin, et al. (2012) found that hospitals that were not-for-profit, served a more diverse inpatient population, and were located in more competitive and affluent markets exhibited a higher degree of cultural competency.

To evaluate how effectively the health care organization is meeting community needs, a variety of data elements may be considered, including clinical data and patient satisfaction. Health care organizations should assess their own practices to determine if there are unknown disparities in care. As an example, Figure 9-1 presents

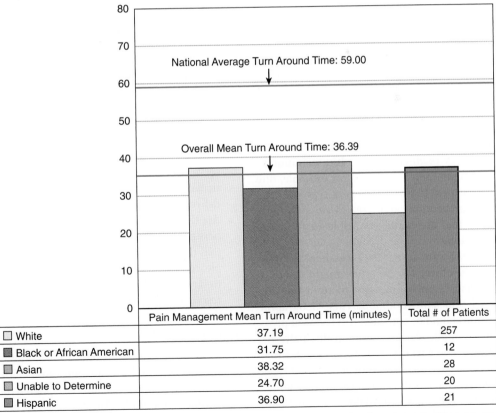

	Pain Management Mean Turn Around Time (minutes)	Total # of Patients
☐ White	37.19	257
▨ Black or African American	31.75	12
▨ Asian	38.32	28
▨ Unable to Determine	24.70	20
▨ Hispanic	36.90	21

Figure 9-1. Example of emergency department information for turnaround time for pain medication in clients with long bone fracture by race/ethnicity, FY2013 (Data from Edward Hospital at Edward-Elmhurst Healthcare).

data for long bone fracture pain management from an emergency department. The mean and median turnaround time for pain medication is shorter than the national average for all groups, but is slightly longer for the Asians compared to all other populations at the author's hospital. Examination of the data helps the organization to determine the causes of the variations.

Staff Competence

Individual health care providers are essential for building culturally competent organizations. All staff members must be competent; this is especially critical for direct care nurses and other staff members. Many times, nurses and other care providers interact based on their own cultural values, experience, and preferences. They need to be taught how to interact with patients from diverse cultures to provide patient-centered care and serve as patient advocates (Sherrod, 2013). Key processes, including organizational support, orientation, and ongoing education, are needed to enhance staff competence.

The human resource department typically provides organizational support for staff. The department plays a key role in ensuring that recruitment and hiring activities reflect the diversity of the community they serve. The department can also prioritize recruitment of bilingual staff members and ensure appropriate compensation. Policies, position descriptions, and performance reviews, typically overseen by human resources, must reflect cultural competence.

Orientation and ongoing education are needed for employees at all levels to develop and foster cultural sensitivity and competence. Diversity in its broadest terms should be discussed in orientation. This should include race, ethnicity, religion, age, gender, sexual orientation, socioeconomics, and educational backgrounds of both clients and staff members. Volunteers and medical staff members also need to be oriented to the organization's culture, strategy, and expectations.

Beyond orientation, ongoing education is needed to reinforce the learning. While staff cannot learn about all diversity, they should be equipped with a general cultural framework and have specific knowledge about the cultural groups for whom they most often provide care. A first step to learning about culture is to identify the values and worldview of one's own culture. This may be facilitated through reflection and discussion. By acknowledging one's own beliefs, staff members may be helped to avoid stereotyping and cultural imposition. A variety of formats may be used to educate staff, including live education sessions, electronic learning, journal clubs, and discussion groups. Inviting members of a particular culture or religion to discuss their beliefs and practices is often engaging for both the community and staff. To help hold staff members accountable for their actions, performance reviews must reflect the organization's commitment to cultural competence.

Nurses and other health care staff members need training to ensure appropriate care and accurate data. Gomez, Le, West, Santariano, and O'Connor (2003) found that while 85% of hospitals reported collecting data on race, approximately half of them obtained the data by observing a client's physical appearance. In addition, only 12% of the hospitals reported having a procedure for recording the race and/or ethnicity of a client with mixed ancestry, and 55% reported never collecting ethnicity data. Regenstein and Sickler (2006) found that 78.4% of hospitals collect race information, 50.4% collect data on client ethnicity, and 50.2% collect data on language preference. However, only 20% have formal data collection policies, and fewer than 20% use the data to assess and compare care quality, health services utilization, health outcomes, or patient satisfaction.

According to a report from the Commonwealth Fund and the American Hospital Association's Health and Research Educational Trust (Hasnain-Wynia, Pierce, & Pittman, 2004), fewer than 80% of hospitals collect data on race and ethnicity. Most often, data are collected because of a law or regulatory requirement. However, the information that is collected may not be accurate or valid.

The report recommends that hospitals standardize who provides the information, when it is collected, which racial and ethnic categories should be used, and how the data are stored. Staff members need to be taught why this is important and how to collect the information.

Culturally competent staff is essential for building culturally competent health care organizations. Staff members who lack the competency may fail to take the client's culture seriously, misinterpret the client's value system, and elevate their own value systems. This posture is culturally destructive because it minimizes the other person's culture. Culturally competent staff members will take time to ask questions about what the client prefers and listen attentively. In the end, this will increase understanding, trust, collaboration, adherence, and satisfaction.

Nurses and other health care providers can help the organization grow in cultural understanding. If they listen and attend carefully, health care providers have a valuable window directly into the world of their clients. They can take what they learn and share it with the administration to improve the cultural responsiveness of their organization. Individuals and groups of clinicians can also develop special programs to meet the needs of the specific populations they serve. Speaking the language is a definite advantage.

The Physical Environment of Care

The physical environment should always be assessed. Approaching this assessment as a potential client is helpful, and a variety of factors should be considered. What message does the organization send through its physical surroundings? How is the facility organized physically? How does the entryway present the culture of the organization to the public? Is the entrance warm and inviting? Is the signage prominent? What languages are included on the signs? Is information presented clearly and unambiguously? Are amenities available to clients and their family members? Are the doors open or closed? Do people talk with one another, and what languages are

spoken? What is the traffic pattern, and what is the general flow of traffic? Does the environment appear calm or turbulent? Are the staff members attentive and courteous?

A physical environment may send unintentional messages. For example, consider the birthing center at a city hospital. The hospital's service area is undergoing tremendous changes, with a large influx of African American, Hispanic, Indian, and Polish American populations. The birthing unit is beautifully and tastefully decorated with oak furniture and pastel prints. Every picture on the walls, however, shows a Caucasian family. This clearly sends a message of exclusivity rather than inclusiveness. When this is brought to the attention of the nurse manager, she is completely dumbfounded and quickly takes steps to rectify the situation. Ethnocentrism and stereotyping are in play here, and it takes a degree of cultural competence to identify this and bring it to recognition and resolution.

Organizational leaders must also assess the physical environment of care to identify potential barriers. A flow chart is a helpful tool for determining such barriers. For example, in an effort to provide comprehensive women's health programs in a caring fashion, organizational leaders may examine the steps for admission to the hospital for the delivery of a baby. To determine this, staff members walk through the care process and create a flow chart that outlines the steps. Staff members must be alert, in particular, for possible sources of confusion for parents at this highly stressful time. The flow chart can then be used to design changes in the environment that can be implemented to decrease barriers and improve services.

Linguistic Competence

Language is a major barrier to quality health care (Office of Minority Health, 2013). The Institute of Medicine (2002) reports that 51% of providers believe that clients do not adhere to treatment because of culture or language. At the same time, nurses and other health care providers report

having received no language or cultural competency training (Baldonado et al., 1998; Park et al., 2005). Twenty-two percent of medical residents feel unprepared to treat patients who have LEP (Weissman et al., 2005). Similarly, while both nurses and baccalaureate nursing students perceive an overwhelming need for transcultural nursing, only 61% report confidence in their ability to provide care to culturally diverse patients (Baldonado et al., 1998). Providing care to non–English-speaking patients presents a special challenge.

Addressing this challenge begins when the nurse determines the preferred language for health care discussions from the patient. This information must be recorded and shared with all health care providers. Patients must be informed that an interpreter will be provided for them at no cost. Interpreter services may be provided in person, by videoconferencing, or by telephone.

Competent interpreter services are necessary when providing care and services. Because communication is a cornerstone of patient safety and quality care, every patient has the right to receive information in a manner he or she understands. Effective communication allows patients to participate more fully in their care, is critical to the informed consent process, and helps practitioners and health care organizations give the best possible care. For communication to be effective, the information provided must be complete, accurate, timely, unambiguous, and understood by the patient. Many patients of varying circumstances require alternative communication methods, including patients who speak and/or read languages other than English, patients who have limited literacy in any language, patients who have visual or hearing impairments, patients on ventilators, patients with cognitive impairments, and children.

Health care organizations have many options to assist in communication with these individuals, such as interpreters, translated written materials, pen and paper, and communication boards. It is up to the hospital to determine which method is the best for each patient. Various laws and regulations and guidelines are relevant to the use of interpreters. These include Title VI of the Civil Rights Act, 1964; Executive Order 13166; policy guidance from the Office of Civil Rights regarding compliance with Title VI, 2004; Title III of the Americans with Disabilities Act, 1990; state laws; and the American Medical Association's Office guide to communicating with LEP patients (AMA, 2007).

Policies addressing interpreter services should be in place, and staff members should be educated on them. Signage, consent forms, patient education, and other written materials should be translated and available in the most commonly spoken languages. Written materials should augment, not substitute for, discussion in the patient's language. The organization should evaluate written documents for cultural sensitivity. When collecting data, such as patient satisfaction or quality of life surveys, the organization should provide the surveys in the patient's preferred language. The organization should also work with the community to address health literacy and provide and encourage attendance at English as a Second Language classes.

Large health care organizations may have resources to secure trained professional interpreters and bilingual providers. Regardless of setting, however, Youdelman and Perkins (2005) suggest the following eight-step process for developing appropriate language services:

1. Designate responsibility
2. Conduct an analysis of language needs
3. Identify resources in the community
4. Determine what language services will be provided
5. Determine how to respond to LEP patients
6. Train staff
7. Notify LEP patients of available language services
8. Update activities after periodic review

Community Involvement

Understanding what culturally competent health care means from the standpoint of patients is an important step in building culturally competent

organizations. Napoles-Springer, Santoyo, Houston, Perez-Stable, and Stewart (2005) conducted 19 community focus groups to determine the meaning of culture and what cultural factors influenced the quality of their medical visits. Culture was defined in terms of value systems, customs, self-identified ethnicity, and nationality. African Americans, Latinos, and non-Latino Whites all agreed that the quality of health care encounter was influenced by clinicians' sensitivity to complementary/alternative medicine, health insurance discrimination, social class discrimination, ethnic concordance between patient and provider, and age-based discrimination. Ethnicity-based discrimination was identified as a factor for Latinos and African Americans. Latinos also described language issues and immigration status factors. Overall, participants indicated greater satisfaction with clinicians who demonstrated cultural flexibility, defined as the ability to elicit, adapt, and respond to patients' cultural characteristics.

Health care institutions exist to provide care. A variety of factors, such as tobacco and alcohol use, poor diet, and physical inactivity, contribute to mortality in the United States and Canada. Addressing these factors requires individual behavioral change, community change, social change, and economic change. Health care organizations cannot confront these complex factors in isolation; they must partner with their communities to build trust in their institutions and meet the needs of their local communities.

Community partnerships may be configured in a variety of ways. Hospitals and health care systems usually articulate their desire to improve the health of the communities they serve. Historically, hospitals have fulfilled this mission through charity care, health care provider education, health care research, community education programming, and community outreach (Pelfrey & Theisen, 1993). However, true improvements in the health of a community require the focused efforts of the entire community. Such improvement may occur only in partnerships with community members and community organizations.

An ethnographic study of community (Davis, 1997) revealed five themes related to the experience of community caring. Three of these themes are of particular significance to this discussion: (1) Reciprocal relationships and teams working together are central to building healthy communities, (2) education with a focus on prevention is key to enhancing health, and (3) understanding community needs is a primary catalyst for health care reform and change.

Health care professionals in culturally competent organizations collaborate with surrounding communities to conduct community health assessments. In community mapping, staff collect a variety of data, including demographics, health status, community resources, barriers, and enablers. Both strengths and needs are identified from the perspective of the community. All of the data are then used collaboratively with communities to set priorities. An example of such a community assessment is provided in Box 9-11. Data from these assessments are used to set priorities and guide the planning and implementation of key initiatives. These initiatives are most well accepted when they are sponsored by a variety of community organizations rather than by a single health care organization such as a hospital.

Focus groups may assist an organization in assessing how well they are meeting the needs of the populations they serve. For example, the Boston Pain Education Program worked collaboratively with community representatives to develop a culturally sensitive, linguistically appropriate cancer pain education booklet in 11 languages and for 11 ethnic groups. Focus groups were used to develop materials that would empower patients and families to more effectively partner with health care professionals and manage pain in culturally competent ways (Lasch et al., 2000).

Community-based participatory research or participatory action research may be helpful in understanding a community and developing health improvement initiatives with community members. The method uses collaborative,

Box 9-11 Community Assessment Example

The Advocate Lutheran General Hospital completed an assessment of the communities it serves. By analyzing data from clinical practice, staff members realized that Hispanics made up an increasing proportion of the population and were the most frequently underserved population. As a result, a family practice physician initiated the idea for a community center for health and empowerment. A coalition composed of individuals from social services, health care agencies, schools, police, churches, businesses, city government, and other community services also identified the Hispanic community as underserved. This group provided an etic, or outsider, view of the Hispanic community.

To provide a local, or emic (insider), view, community members worked with health care personnel to design and conduct a door-to-door community assessment. Leininger's theory of cultural diversity and universality served to guide the assessment. The assessment process involved 2 focus groups, 15 community interviewers, and 220 door-to-door interviews. In addition, 5 meetings, attended by 180 community members, were held to report the findings to community members and solicit their input on how to maintain strengths and address needs. As a result, numerous task forces were formed to preserve strengths or mediate needs.

The major strengths identified were access to friends and families to socialize and get support,

prenatal and postnatal care, and pediatric care. The major needs identified were affordable housing, programs to help immigrants, Spanish-speaking dentists, and activities for youth.

The community was involved in key decision making from the beginning, including selecting the site for the center, choosing the name for the center, and establishing a sliding scale for fees. The bilingual center provides primary health care services, a Women–Infant–Children program run by the county health department, and a community empowerment program. A salaried community outreach worker coordinates the community empowerment program. In collaboration with businesses, churches, and city services, community members have undergone training in group work and priority setting. Monthly dental services through a dental van were added at the center.

Activities for youth were identified as concerns in the community assessment. As a result, community members and center personnel have actively partnered with the park district, schools, churches, and the police to provide recreational activities for the youth. The community also uses this as an opportunity to celebrate their cultural heritage. Health promotion materials and activities are also provided through collaboration.

participatory approaches to develop sustainable services (Koch & Kralik, 2006). An example is a participatory action research project that is addressing organizational barriers to cultural competence in hospice care through a university–community–hospice partnership (Reese, 2011). In addition, the National Center on Minority Health and Health Disparities (NCMHD), located within the National Institutes of Health, has funded disease intervention research in reducing and eliminating health disparities using community-based participation research that is jointly conducted

by health disparity communities and researchers (NIH, 2010).

Conducting community assessments requires cultural awareness and sensitivity. Interpreting the data requires knowledge of the cultural dimensions of health and illness. Using the data to develop and implement programs in conjunction with the community requires the ability to plan and implement culturally competent care. The skill of a transcultural nurse or other culturally competent health care professional is invaluable in these situations.

Culturally Congruent Services and Programs

Culturally competent nurses and other health care providers are able to develop and evaluate culturally competent initiatives. Many important factors must be considered in planning programs across cultural groups. In many cases, cultural competence must be demonstrated with multiple cultures simultaneously. For example, one hospital in the Chicago area provides care for individuals who speak 64 different languages. This calls for much effort and creativity on the part of patients, health care providers, and interpreters. Case Study 9-1 describes the development and implementation of a culturally competent initiative. This case study focuses on one culturally

Case Study 9-1

Caring Hospital, a not-for-profit hospital, serves clients who differ in multiple ways, including socioeconomic status, education, race, ethnicity, religion, language, and culture. Organizational leaders embrace Leininger's theory of culture care. In particular, nursing leaders believe that nursing care must be congruent with the client's culture in order to promote the client's health and satisfaction.

Through a healthy community program, the hospital remains grounded in the reality of their clients. The healthy community program, developed and staffed by two nurses with community health backgrounds, is responsible for broadly defining community-based health promotion initiatives that address individual, social, and community factors. Their goal is to establish partnerships with community members and governmental and community organizations to ensure that everyone has access to the basics needed for health; that the physical environment supports healthy living; and that communities control, define, and direct action for health.

The nurses in the healthy community program bring together resources from settings both within and outside their hospital. For example, they work closely with other community-focused staff members, such as home care and parish nurses. They also work with multiple external organizations, such as local health departments and other government agencies, religious institutions, community businesses, schools, and other health care entities. These nurses work specifically with the communities

surrounding their facility. In this way, they acknowledge the specific needs of diverse groups.

The healthy community nurses use Leininger's culture care diversity and universality model in their practice. They use data gathered from cultural assessments to assist them in understanding the communities they serve. They consider environmental context, ethnohistory, language, kinship, cultural values and lifeways, the political and legal system, and technologic, economic, religious, philosophic, and educational factors. They understand the interactions among the folk system, nursing care, and the professional systems. They also understand the importance of using the three culture care modalities: preservation/maintenance, accommodation/negotiation, and repatterning/restructuring.

Because of their community health backgrounds, the nurses are knowledgeable about disparities in health. The nurses use data from a variety of sources, including hospital-specific data, census tract data, and health department data, to help them understand health and access disparities in their area. They also talk to community members and to health care providers to identify competing priorities. Using these processes, they discover that their communities have not achieved the Healthy People 2020 immunization goals for children by the age of 2 years.

To address the lack of immunizations, the nurses acknowledge that the issues that affect immunizations are multifaceted. The immunization schedule changes frequently and is quite complex. Even health care providers have difficulty interpreting it. Communication with parents has been sketchy and has been complicated by controversy. Immunizations are sometimes seen by parents as nonessential for young children until they enter elementary school.

Immunizations may not be easily accessible, available, and affordable. Parents may make decisions based on misinformation, rumor, or hearsay. The nurses know, however, that community members want to keep their children healthy and that immunizations have contributed greatly to reduced illness in individuals and better overall health for the community. They also know that community members prefer to have their children immunized in a consistent place, as part of an overall medical home.

Because the childhood immunization levels are suboptimal in the communities served by the hospital, childhood immunization is selected as a quality initiative. A group of consumers and clinicians is convened to implement a program with the goal of increasing immunization to the Healthy People 2020 goals. There is much discussion on the best way for increasing immunization rates, using a broad-based program. The group considers mailed, telephoned, e-mailed, and texted reminders and opts to combine texted reminders with follow-up by mailed reminders.

Various materials are developed in both English and Spanish, and incentives are put into place to assist parents. Babies are automatically enrolled in the program when they are born in the hospital. Mailings occur at regular intervals and include a personalized letter indicating what vaccines are due, a vaccine record, vaccine information statements, and a growth and development newsletter. Additionally, incentives are mailed to help keep the parents motivated to use preventive services. Materials are written at a sixth-grade level. All materials are reviewed for cultural congruity, and the illustrations include babies from various ethnic groups.

New materials are developed as needed, based on a continuous assessment of the needs of the parents. For example, reproducing all the materials in all the languages used by clients is too expensive, so a multiple-language brochure is developed in the 11 most common languages. The brochure explains the program and asks that non–English-speaking and non–Spanish-speaking families obtain help in translating the materials. In addition, after families express a major concern about the multiple injections required to keep their babies fully immunized and their babies' resultant distress and crying, a "calming strategies" flyer is developed.

Because financial barriers still exist among parents seeking immunizations for their children, the healthy community nurses implement several additional strategies. First, they work with physicians and help them enroll in the Vaccines for Children program, making vaccines available at no cost or low cost right in their offices. They also work with the staff in physicians' offices to enhance their role in fostering childhood immunizations. In addition, they work with the health department to provide monthly immunizations on-site at the hospital.

competent program provided to a community; however, additional programs, targeting the needs of other groups, may also be envisioned. For example, adult immunizations are a challenge for many communities, so a program might be developed that focuses specifically on older adults and their immunization needs. Similarly, programs might be instituted to deal with other health issues of concern to community members. The case study demonstrates the importance of incorporating an understanding of culture in every aspect of an initiative. To design and implement an effective program, the cultural values of patients must be understood and addressed.

Overcoming the Barrier of Institutional Racism in Health Care

Prejudice, racism, stereotyping, and ethnocentrism are present in health care settings. Institutional racism, sometimes referred to as institutionalized racism, is defined as differential access to goods, services, and opportunities based on race (Peek et al., 2010); this includes differential access to health insurance. The dominant subgroup is often ignorant of its own privilege. For example, services may be organized for the

convenience of providers, and providers may be unaware that inconvenient hours or locations are affecting the community members who seek services. In contrast to individual behaviors, institutional racism occurs when systematic policies and practices disadvantage certain racial or ethnic groups. Institutions may be overtly racist, as when they specifically exclude certain groups from service. More often, however, institutions are unintentionally racist. For example, a dress code that requires everyone to wear the same hat would institutionally discriminate against Sikh men, who are expected to wear turbans, and Muslim women, who wear the hijab or veil. Institutions don't necessarily adopt such policies with the intention of discriminating and often revise their practice once the discrimination is identified.

Institutional racism is an international concern. In England, institutional racism is defined as "the collective failure of an organisation to provide an appropriate and professional service to people because of their colour, culture, or ethnic origin" (McKenzie & Bhui, 2007, p. 649). Henry, Houston, and Mooney (2004) suggest that health care in Australia is institutionally racist and that such racism represents one of the greatest barriers to improving the health of Aboriginal and Torres Strait Islander people. Examples include funding inequities, differences in performance criteria, and differences in treatment regimens. Reports in Sweden and the United Kingdom suggest continued concerns about discrimination and inequity in services (Bhopal, 2007). Differences in the treatment of mental illness have been documented in England and Wales (McKenzie & Bhui, 2007). Contributing factors include the actions of individual staff members and policies that are based on the needs of the ethnic majority population rather than considering the needs of minority populations (Bhopal, 2007).

Cultural differences and lack of knowledge create institutional racism, and indifference nurtures it. Cultural differences must be acknowledged and celebrated rather than denigrated (Henry et al., 2004). Health care organizations must be built upon the cultural values of the people they serve. The strategies outlined in this chapter and throughout this book are needed to overcome institutional racism and build culturally competent health care organizations.

Summary

As with individuals, the quest for organizational cultural competence is a continuous journey. There is always room for improvement. To be truly effective in improving patient care for all, health care services and social services that take cultural diversity into account must make an organizational commitment to cultural competence. Cultural competence cannot live in one or two nurses; it must be systemic. It must involve individuals at all levels of the organization: governance members, administrators, managers, providers, and support staff. In addition, an organization must have a mutually beneficial relationship with the community it serves to achieve cultural competence and must involve community members in its quest for cultural competence.

REVIEW QUESTIONS

1. What types of access, health care, and health outcome disparities exist nationally? In your community?
2. How does the culture of an organization affect the quality of care provided?
3. What tools or models are helpful for assessing organizational culture?
4. How does an organization's culture influence or affect its employees?
5. What specific areas must receive attention in order to build culturally competent health care organizations?

CRITICAL THINKING ACTIVITIES

1. An excellent way to understand a culturally competent organization is to assess the organizational culture using the "five A's"

described in this chapter. With some of your classmates, compare and contrast the availability, accessibility, affordability, acceptability, and appropriateness of one health care organization. Discuss what actions could be taken by the organization to increase its cultural competency.

2. Use Leininger's (1991) theory of culture care diversity and universality to assess the culture of the same organization. Box 9-6 in this chapter provides an example of how Leininger's culture care model can be used. Compare and contrast the values and beliefs of the organization with the values and beliefs of the groups using the

health care organization's services. What areas would be most problematic, and why?

3. Many members of ethnic or minority communities lack adequate access to care because they do not have adequate health insurance. Often, these individuals use the emergency departments (EDs) of city hospitals for episodic care. Visit a busy ED. What languages do you hear? Assess the physical environment to determine potential barriers to culturally competent care. Develop a flow chart that outlines the steps a client takes when he or she seeks care in an emergency room. Identify changes that would decrease barriers and improve services if they were implemented.

REFERENCES

Agency for Healthcare Research and Quality. (2012). *National healthcare disparities report, 2021.* Rockville, MD: U.S. Department of Health and Human Services, Agency for Healthcare Research and Quality. Accessed February 22, 2014 at www.ahrq.gov/research/findings/nhqrdr/nhdr11/nhdr11.pdf

Agency for Healthcare Research and Quality. (2013). *2012 National Healthcare Disparities Report.* Agency for Healthcare Research and Quality, Rockville, MD. http://www.ahrq.gov/research/findings/nhqrdr/nhdr12/index.html

Alessandra, T. (2010). *The platinum rule.* Accessed February 21, 2010 at http://www.alessandra.com

Alter, D. A., Stukel, T., Chong, A., & Henry, D. (2011). Lessons from Canada's Universal Care: Socially disadvantaged patients use more health services, still have poorer health. *Health Affairs, 30*(2), 274–283.

American Association of Colleges of Nursing. (2014). Enhancing diversity in the nursing workforce. Accessed March 1, 2014 at http://www.aacn.nche.edu/media-relations/fact-sheets/enhancing-diversity

American Medical Association. (2007). Office guide to communicating with limited English proficient patients. Accessed February 23, 2014 at http://www.ama-assn.org/ama1/pub/upload/mm/433/lep_booklet.pdf

American Nurses Association. (1998). *Discrimination and racism in health care.* Washington DC: American Nurses Association.

American Nurses Association. (2010). *The nurse's role in ethics and human rights: Protecting and promoting individual worth, dignity, and human rights in practice settings.* Washington, DC: American Nurses Association.

American Nurses Association Council on Cultural Diversity in Nursing Practice. (1991). *Cultural diversity in nursing practice [position statement].* Washington DC: Author.

American Nurses Credentialing Center. (2013). *2014 Magnet application manual.* Silver Spring, MD: American Nurses Credentialing Center.

American Organization of Nurse Executives. (2011). *The AONE nurse executive competencies.* Accessed February 22, 2014 at www.aone.org/resources/leadership%20tools/PDFs/AONE_NEC.pdf

Andrews, M. M. (1998, October). A model for cultural change. *Nursing Management, 66,* 62–64.

Baldonado, A., Ludwig-Beymer, P., Barnes, K., Starsiak, D., Nemivant, E. B., & Anonas-Ternate, A. (1998). Transcultural nursing practice described by registered nurses and baccalaureate nursing students. *Journal of Transcultural Nursing, 9*(2), 15–25.

Bhopal, R. S. (2007). Racism in health and health care in Europe: Reality of mirage? *European Journal of Public Health, 17*(3), 238–241.

Bolman, L. G., & Deal, T. E. (1997). *Reframing organizations: Artistry, choice, and leadership* (2nd ed.). San Francisco, CA: Jossey-Bass.

Chavez, C. I., & Weisinger, J. Y. (2008). Beyond diversity training: A social infusion for cultural inclusion. *Human Resource Management, 47*(2), 331–350.

Davis, R. N. (1997). Community caring: An ethnographic study within an organizational culture. *Public Health Nursing, 14*(2), 92–100.

Delphin-Rittmen, M. E. (2013). Seven essential strategies for promoting and sustaining systemic cultural competence. *Psychiatric Quarterly, 84*(1), 53–64.

Douglas, M. K., Rosenkoetter, M., Pacquiao, D., Callister, L. C., Hattar-Pollara, M., Lauderdale, J., ..., Purnell, L. (2014). Guidelines for implementing culturally competent nursing care. *Journal of Transcultural Nursing*, *25*(2), 109–121.

Flaskerud, J. H. (2007). Cultural competence: What effect on reducing health disparities? *Issues in Mental Health Nursing*, *28*, 431–434.

Fung, K., Srivastava, R., & Andermann, L. (2012). Organizational cultural competence consultation to a mental health institution. *Transcultural Psychiatry*, *49*(2), 165–184.

Gomez, S. L., Le, G. M., West, D. W., Santariano, W. A., & O'Connor, L. (2003). Hospital policy and practice regarding the collection of data on race, ethnicity, and birthplace. *Journal of Public Health*, *93*(10), 1685–1688.

Greiner, A. C., & Knebel, E. (Eds.), Institute of Medicine. (2003). *Health professionals education: A bridge to quality*. Washington, DC: The National Academies Press.

Guerrero, E. (2012). Organizational characteristics that foster early adoption of cultural and linguistic competence in outpatient substance abuse treatment in the United States. *Evaluation and Program Planning*, *35*(1), 9–15.

Guerrero, E. G. (2013). Organizational structure, leadership and readiness for change and the implementation of organizational cultural competence in addiction services. *Evaluation and Program Planning*, *40*, 74–81.

Hasnain-Wynia, R., Pierce, D., & Pittman, M. A. (2004, May). Who, when, and how: The current state of race, ethnicity, and primary language data collection in hospitals. *The Commonwealth Fund and the American Hospital Association's Health Research and Educational Trust*. Accessed February 20, 2006 at http://www.cmwf.org

Hays, R., Weech-Maldonado, R., Brown, J., Sand, K., Dreachslin, J., & Dansky, K. (2006). *Cultural Competency Assessment Tool for Hospitals (CCATH). Final Report for Contract Number 282-00-0005, Task Order # 7*. Washington, DC: Department of Health and Human Services; Office of Minority Health.

Henry, B. R., Houston, S., & Mooney, G. H. (2004). Institutional racism in Australian healthcare: A plea for decency. *Medical Journal of Australia*, *180*(10), 517–520.

Hoyert, D., & Xu, J. (2012, October 10). Deaths: Preliminary data for 2011. *National Vital Statistics Report, U.S. Department of Health and Human Services, Centers for Disease Control and Prevention, National Center for Health Statistics, National Vital Statistics System*. Accessed March 16, 2014 at http://www.cdc.gov/nchs/data/nvsr/nvsr61/nvsr61_06.pdf

Institute of Medicine. (2002). *Unequal treatment: Confronting racial and ethnic disparities in health care*. Washington, DC: National Academies Press.

Joint Commission Resources. (2014). The Joint Commission Edition. Accessed March 16, 2014 at http://e-dition.jcrinc.com

Koch, T., & Kralik, D. (2006). *Participatory action research in health care*. Oxford: Wiley-Blackwell.

Kouri, D. (2012, March). Reducing health disparities: How can the structure of the health system contribute? *Wellesley Institute*. Accessed March 16, 2014 at http://www.wellesleyinstitute.com/wp-content/uploads/2012/09/Reducing-Health-Disparities-how-can-health-system-structure-contribute.pdf

Lasch, K. E., Wilkes, G., Montuori, L. M., Chew, P., Leonard, C., & Hilton, S. (2000). Using focus group methods to develop multicultural cancer pain education materials. *Pain Management Nursing*, *1*(4), 129–138.

Leininger, M. (1991). *Culture care diversity and universality: A theory of nursing care*. New York, NY: National League for Nursing Press.

Leininger, M. (1996). Founder's focus: Transcultural nursing administration: An imperative worldwide. *Journal of Transcultural Nursing*, *8*(1), 28–33.

Malone, B. L. (1997). Improving organizational cultural competence. In J. A. Dienemann (Ed.). *Cultural diversity in nursing: Issues, strategies, and outcomes*. Washington, DC: American Academy of Nursing.

Marrone, S. R. (2010). Organizational cultural competency. In M. Douglas & D. Pacquiao (Eds.), *Core curriculum in transcultural nursing and health care*. Thousand Oaks, CA: Sage.

Marrone, S. R. (2012). Organizational cultural competency. In L. Purnell (Ed.). *Transcultural health care: A culturally competent approach* (4th ed.). Philadelphia, PA: F.A. Davis.

McClure, M. L., Poulin, M. A., Sovie, M. D., & Wandelt, M. A.; for the American Academy Task Force on Nursing Practice in Hospitals. (1983). *Magnet hospitals. Attraction and retention of professional nurses*. Kansas City, MO: American Nurses Association.

McKenzie, K., & Bhui, K. (2007). Institutional racism in mental health care. *BMJ*, *334*(7595), 649–650.

Napoles-Springer, A. M., Santoyo, J., Houston, K., Perez-Stable, E. J., & Stewart, A. L. (2005). Patients' perceptions of cultural factors affecting the quality of their medical encounters. *Health Expectations*, *8*, 4–17.

National Institutes of Health. (2010). Accessed February 21, 2010 at http://www.nih.gov

Office of Minority Health, Department of Health and Human Services. (2011). National CLAS standards. Accessed February 23, 2014 at http://minorityhealth.hhs.gov/templates/browse.aspx?lvl=2&lvlID=15

Office of Minority Health, Department of Health and Human Services. (2013, April). Accessed February 23, 2014 at http://minorityhealth.hhs.gov/templates/browse.aspx?lvl=2&lvlID=16

Park, E. R., Betancourts, J. R., Kim, M. K., Maina, A. W., Blumenthal, D., & Weissman, J. S. (2005). Mixed messages: Residents' experiences learning cross-cultural care. *Academic Medicine*, *80*(9), 874–880.

Peek, M. S., Odoms-Young, A., Quinn, M. T., Gorawara-Bhat, R., Wilson, S. C., & Chin, M. H. (2010). Racism in healthcare: Its relationship to shared decision-making

and health disparities. *Social Science and Medicine, 71*(1), 13–17.

Pelfrey, S., & Theisen, B. A. (1993). Valuing the community benefits provided by nonprofit hospitals. *Journal of Nursing Administration, 23*(6), 16–21.

Purnell, L., Davidhizar, R. E., Giger, J. N., Strickland, O. L., Fishman, D. & Allison, D. M. (2011). A guide to developing a culturally competent organization. *Journal of Transcultural Nursing, 22*(1), 7–14.

Reese, D. J. (2011). Proposal for a university-community-hospice partnership to address organizational barriers to cultural competence. *American Journal of Hospital & Palliative Care, 28*(1), 22–26.

Regenstein, M., & Sickler, D. (2006). Race, ethnicity, and language of patients. *National Public Health and Hospital Institute.* Accessed February 21, 2010 at http://www.naph.org

Roizner, M. (1996). *A practical guide for the assessment of cultural competence in children's mental health organizations.* Boston, MA: Judge Baker's Children's Center.

Schaffner, J. W., & Ludwig-Beymer, P. (2003). *Rx for the nursing shortage.* Chicago, IL: Health Administration Press.

Schein, E. H. (2004). *Organizational culture and leadership* (3rd ed.). San Francisco, CA: Jossey-Bass.

Sherrod, D. (2013). Ask, listen, respect. *Nursing Management, 44*(11), 6.

Strasser, D. C., Smits, S. J., Falconer, J. A., Herrin, J. S., & Bowen, S. E. (2002). The influence of hospital culture on rehabilitation team functioning in VA hospitals. *Journal of Rehabilitation Research and Development, 39*(1), 115–125.

Transcultural Nursing Society. (2014). Accessed March 2, 2014 at http.www.tcns.org

United States Census Bureau. (2012). Income, Expenditures, Poverty, & Wealth. *The National Data Book 2012 Statistical Abstract.* Accessed March 16, 2014 at http://www.census.gov/compendia/statab/2012/tables/12s0710.pdf

Weech-Maldonado, R., Dreachslin, J. L., Brown, J., Pradhan, R., Rubin, K. L., Schiller, C., & Hays, R. D. (2012a). Cultural competency assessment tool for hospitals: Evaluating hospitals' adherence to the culturally and linguistically appropriate services standards. *Health Care Management Review, 37*(1), 54–66.

Weech-Maldonado, R., Elliott, M. N., Pradhan, R., Schiller, C., Dreachslin, J., & Hays, R. D. (2012b). Moving toward culturally competent health systems: Organizational and market factors. *Social Science and Medicine, 75*(5), 815–822.

Weech-Maldonado, R., Elliott, M., Pradhan, R., Schiller, C., Hall, A., & Hays, R. D. (2012c). Can hospital cultural competency reduce disparities in patient experiences with care? *Medical Care, 50,* S48–55.

Weissman, J. S., Betancourt, J. R., Campbell, E. G., Park, E. R., Kim, M., Clarridge, B., & Maina, A. W. (2005). Resident physicians' preparedness to provide cross-cultural care. *Journal of the American Medical Association, 294*(9), 1058–1067.

Wilson, A. H., Sanner, S. J., & Mcallister, L. E. (2003) The Honor Society of Nursing, Sigma Theta Tau International Diversity Paper. Accessed February 23, 2014 at http://www.nursingsociety.org/aboutus/PositionPapers/Documents/Diversity_paper.pdf

Youdelman, M., & Perkins, J. (2005). Providing language services in small health care provider settings: Examples from the field. *The Commonwealth Fund.* Accessed October 17, 2005 at http://www.cmwf.org

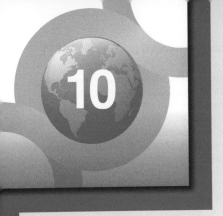

Transcultural Perspectives in Mental Health Nursing

● Joanne T. Ehrmin

Key Terms

Cultural blindness
Cultural blind spot
Cultural norms

Cultural pain
Culture shock
Disenfranchised grieving
Historical unresolved grief
Historical trauma

Interpersonal communication
Mental health
Shared decision making

Learning Objectives

1. Recognize the importance of cultural values, beliefs, and practices when planning and implementing mental health nursing care.
2. Examine best practice treatment options in caring for culturally diverse mental health clients.
3. Understand the influence of culture on decisions about mental health care.
4. Evaluate strategies to provide competent transcultural mental health nursing care.
5. Recognize the importance of evidence-based transcultural mental health nursing research in caring for clients seeking mental health care in a culturally congruent and competent manner.

Mental health and mental illness are described as two extreme end positions on a continuum, with many varying degrees between mental health and mental illness. Dealing with the loss of a job, the emotional pain of grieving the loss of a loved one, and having a severe mental illness, such as schizophrenia or bipolar disorder, all fall along this continuum. A landmark *Supplement to Mental Health: A Report of the Surgeon General: Culture, Race, and Ethnicity* (2001) brought a focus to mental health and culture, race, and ethnicity for the first time in such a clear and distinct manner (Manson, 2003). According to Galson (2009), interim Surgeon General, mental disorders are frequently "untreated, underdiagnosed, misdiagnosed, ignored, stigmatized, and dismissed" (p. 190).

In this chapter, we discuss mental illnesses within a transcultural nursing perspective, exploring how culture influences the way in which we interpret and behave with mental illnesses. The goal of this chapter is to help nurses gain the necessary knowledge and skills to improve the mental health and well-being of clients from all cultural backgrounds. As culture strongly influences how clients experience illness, and culture is the framework for the interpretation of that experience, transcultural mental health nursing knowledge is integral for culturally competent mental health care. According to the American Psychiatric Association (2013), mental disorders are defined according to "cultural, social and familial norms and values" (p. 14). Furthermore, culture provides the framework that is used to interpret "the experience and expression of the symptoms, signs and behaviors that are criteria for diagnosis" (p. 14).

The concept of **cultural norms** is relevant to transcultural mental health nursing, as one's culture shapes what is considered normal and, by default, what is considered abnormal. Cultural norms are patterns, values, meanings, expressions, beliefs, practices, and experiences that are typical of specific cultural groups. Such norms are learned and passed down by family, friends, communities, and other members of the cultural group (Figure 10-1 shows students learning to make drums, a tradition that is passed down from one generation to the next). Given the broad influence of culture, culture and mental health care are described as intricately related and dependent on one another. In fact, there is growing evidence that culture influences perceptions and attitudes with respect to mental illness (Mellor, Carne, Shen, McCabe, & Wang, 2013).

Many people think of wellness in terms of illness, concluding the absence of illness indicates wellness. The distinction between *disease* and *illness* is relevant to mental health nursing care. Disease comes out of the medical model, is objective, is physiologically based, and requires a "cure," whereas illness is subjective, comes from the perspective of the client, is culturally based, and requires "care." According to Eisenberg (1977), "patients suffer 'illnesses'; doctors 'diagnose' and treat diseases" (p. 2). Illnesses are perceived by

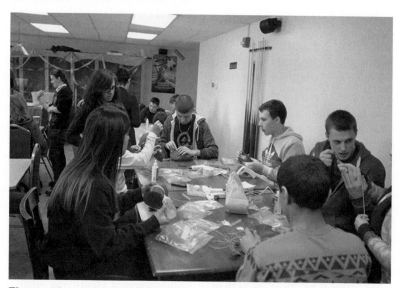

Figure 10-1. Drum making is taught to students to help them learn about traditional Native American culture. These classes help to keep the Native American cultural values, beliefs, and practices alive with youth in the community and demonstrate a sense of pride in traditional customs and lifeways (Ruffino, 2013, p. 28).

the client as a disruption in their daily activities. Diseases, on the other hand, are abnormalities in the anatomy and/or physiology of the body. For example, an individual may feel ill-health as tired, fatigued, anxious, or irritated, and the diagnosis out of the medical model may be posttraumatic stress disorder. Traditional healers are often more open "to the psychosocial context of illness" (p. 2). Interestingly, disease can occur without illness and illness can also occur without disease. An individual who feels ill may first self-medicate and then consult with family, friends, local healer, pharmacist, and so on. Numerous sociocultural factors are considered prior to reaching out to the traditional health care system and providers. What may be perceived as illness or disease in one culture may not have the same meaning in another culture. Since culture determines how clients experience illness, and culture is the framework for the interpretation of that experience, transcultural mental health nursing knowledge is necessary for culturally competent and congruent mental health care.

Defining Mental Health Within a Transcultural Nursing Perspective

The World Health Organization (WHO) (2014a) indicated that "over 450 million people suffer from mental disorders." WHO further postulated: "Mental health is an integral part of health; indeed, there is no health without mental health" (WHO, retrieved 2-14). Interestingly, the definition of mental health, by WHO, has not been changed since 1948. WHO included mental well-being in their definition of health: "Health is a state of complete physical, mental and social well-being and not merely the absence of disease or infirmity." Included in this definition is the implication that "mental health is more than the absence of mental disorders or disabilities" (WHO, 2014). WHO (2014b) further specified that **mental health** is "a state of well-being

in which the individual realizes his or her own abilities, can cope with the normal stresses of life, can work productively and fruitfully, and is able to make a contribution to his or her community" and that this understanding of mental health can be interpreted "across cultures" (p. 1). WHO further elaborated that "mental well-being, historically has frequently been misunderstood and forgotten." In the Rural Healthy People 2020 Report, survey results of state and local rural leaders indicated that mental health and mental disorders are the third most often identified rural health priority (Bolin & Bellamy, 2013).

Furthermore, WHO (2013) identified a comprehensive mental health action plan for 2013 to 2020. The plan encourages community-based mental health care and focuses on recovery, moving away from a strictly medical model and deals with income, education, and "other social determinants of mental health in order to ensure a comprehensive response to mental health." WHO (2013) identified there are numerous determinants of mental health at any given point in time for an individual, including "social, psychological and biological factors." Some of the social/psychological factors include persistent poverty, risks of violence and human rights violations, gender discrimination, and social exclusion. There are also biological factors including chemical imbalances.

According to the National Alliance on Mental Illness (NAMI) (2014), mental illness is a condition that "disrupts a person's thinking, feeling, mood, ability to relate to others and daily functioning." NAMI identified some of the most serious mental illnesses include "major depression, schizophrenia, bipolar disorder, obsessive compulsive disorder (OCD), panic disorder, posttraumatic stress disorder (PTSD), and borderline personality disorder."

Leininger (Leininger, 1991a; Leininger & McFarland, 2002), in Culture Care Diversity and Universality: A Theory of Nursing, theorized the importance of identifying what is common and universal among cultures, while at the same time understanding there is individual diversity within cultures. Diversity for transcultural mental health

nurses encompasses not only culture and ethnicity but also gender, sexual orientation, socioeconomic status, age, physical abilities or disabilities, religious beliefs, and political beliefs or other ideologies (Figure 10-2).

Gaining a better understanding and more in-depth knowledge base of patterns of values, beliefs, and practices for mental health care can be used as one "tool" in caring for clients, families, and communities from diverse cultural groups. This is different from simplistic overgeneralizations that can lead to stereotyping a particular culture. Stereotyping is a "fixed, overgeneralized belief about a particular group or class of people" (Cardwell, 1996). Stereotypes can lead to erroneous misrepresentations of diverse cultural groups, age groups, gender identity, etc.

Stereotypes can be used as an underlying rationale to distort mental illness symptoms and misdiagnose culturally diverse individuals, families, and communities. Stereotypes can also serve to exploit culturally diverse clients, particularly in the area of mental health care, where differences in group norms can sometimes be used to inappropriately label clients with a mental health diagnosis. Dow (2011) identified the dangers of racism and stereotyping, particularly for migrants, which can increase an already high level of stress, thereby adding to the psychological burdens migrants experience, possibly even threatening their survival. She further identified racism and stereotyping as being more prevalent in communities with minimal cultural diversity.

Transcultural nurses do not promote stereotyping of clients, families, and communities because of unique characteristics. Stereotyping labels people and is a form of prejudice that is damaging and harmful to any recipient, let alone a client with a mental illness! Furthermore, stereotyping is generally inaccurate and is often based more on the individual expressing the stereotypical view than the cultural group being targeted. Stereotyping identifies a cultural group or members of that culture as identical and indistinguishable from each other. Some examples of common stereotyping are beliefs that African Americans are "better at sports" and "dancing" than are other cultural groups. Other examples of stereotypes are that Irish Americans are "quick tempered," or Turkish women are "belly dancers."

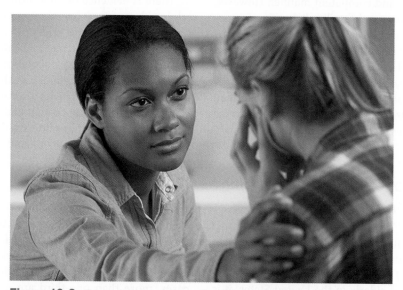

Figure 10-2. Transcultural nurses practice within a framework of sensitivity, knowledge, and skill to promote health and care for individuals diagnosed with a mental illness in culturally congruent ways (Monkey Business Images/Shutterstock.com).

Identifying people as all looking the same or thinking the same is stereotyping. Transcultural mental health nursing does not promote applying a stereotypical "cookbook" approach to mental health care.

Another concept that is important to consider in transcultural mental health nursing is ethnocentrism. "In its mildest form, ethnocentrism presents as subconscious disregard for cultural differences; in its most severe form, it presents as authoritarian" (Sutherland, 2002, p. 280). Ethnocentrism can manifest as feelings of superiority or discrimination with respect to one's own group or culture over another group or culture. For example, ethnocentrism can manifest as a belief that one's own religious beliefs are superior to another group or culture's religious beliefs and that one's own health care beliefs and practices are superior to another culture's health care beliefs and practices. US-trained health care professionals are frequently guilty of the latter ethnocentric assumption.

Many cultural groups have distinct patterns of values, beliefs, and practices that can be used as a basis for providing mental health care in a culturally congruent and competent manner. However, many individuals and families belonging to specific cultural groups may have more diverse mental health care needs than do those of the cultural group norm. The term "norm" is used to identify patterns of values, beliefs, and practices specific to mental health that have been identified through research and caring for culturally diverse clients, families, and communities.

Population Trends and Mental Health

The US population is projected to increase in age and cultural diversity as we move toward the middle of the century. Given the increasing numbers of elderly in the United States, it is important to understand trends in utilization of mental health care services for older populations

of all cultures. According to the 2010 U.S. Census, the United States is projected to become a more diverse nation. In fact, the United States is expected to become a "majority–minority" nation by 2043. Currently, minorities (Hispanic, African American, Asian, American Indians, Alaska Natives, etc.) represent 37% of the US population and are expected to represent 57% of the population in the United States by 2060. The implications and need for educated transcultural mental health nurses are immense (United States Census Bureau, 2012).

According to National Institute of Mental Health (NIMH) (2012), mental illnesses are identified as "common" in the United States. Approximately 43.7 million adults (approximately 19% of all adults in the United States), aged 18 or older, were currently, or within the past year, diagnosed with a mental, behavioral, or emotional disorder and excluding substance use disorders. When broken down by culture, Asians had the lowest percentage of adults diagnosed with mental illness (13.9%) and American Indian/Alaska Natives had the highest percentage of adults diagnosed with mental illness (28.3%).

There is evidence of underutilization of mental health services by many minority groups. Community education and outreach programs are needed to increase mental health service use in older ethnic minority populations (Jang, Kim, Hansen, & Chiriboga, 2007). Although mental health nurses care for clients of all age groups and all cultural groups, the current and future trends in population projections do have major implications for transcultural nursing and mental health services in the United States.

According to Kessler, Chiu, Demler, and Walters (2005), approximately 26.2% of Americans 18 years old and older, or 1 in 4 adults, suffer each year from a mental disorder that is defined in the Diagnostic and Statistical Manual, 4th edition (DSM-IV), of the American Psychiatric Association (APA) mental disorders. Of those cases, more than one-third are mild. However, approximately 6%, or 1 in 17 individuals, suffer from a "serious mental illness," including suicide,

mental or substance abuse, nonaffective psychosis, bipolar I or II disorder, or acts of violence.

The institutionalized view of mental health care as portrayed in the movie "One Flew Over the Cuckoo's Nest" (1975) is no longer the norm for care today. Increasingly, mental health care is moving from state and general "mental" hospitals to community-based service centers. The U.S. Department of Health and Human Services' Center for Mental Health Services (CMHS) is the Federal agency within the U.S. Substance Abuse and Mental Health Services Administration (SAMHSA) charged with improving prevention and mental health treatment services in the United States. For 2008, CMHS statistics for utilization of community-based mental health treatment was 19.15%, as compared to treatment in state hospitals and other psychiatric inpatient settings just over 2%. The cultural diversity of mental health clients is increasing, as is the use of community-based mental health treatment centers. These statistics can help to guide the direction nursing will take in meeting the needs of mental health clients.

Decision Making and Mental Health Care

Consumers of mental health care (clients, families and significant others, and communities) are more knowledgeable now than they have ever been in the past. With the advent of the Internet, mental health care information is more widely available to those seeking knowledge. Continuous news broadcasts offer health care information to both consumers and professionals alike. National and international news and research breakthroughs are increasingly available to consumers, almost as soon as they are available to professionals. In addition, our society is more open to talking about mental health conditions, such as depression and bipolar disorder, in ways that would have been unthinkable just two decades ago.

Clients, families, and significant others want an active role in decision making about their mental health care, and they use numerous resources to make those decisions. Mental health clients, particularly, can become agitated when their voice is not heard or taken into consideration with regard to treatment decisions. For culturally diverse clients with mental health care needs, and diverse values, beliefs, and practices that may not be understood by health care providers, this can be even more frustrating and can lead to misunderstandings on both sides. Clients may feel misunderstood and isolated in a health care system that can seem cold, frightening, rigid, and controlling. Offering support and clear communication can be key to bringing about favorable outcomes for all clients, but it can be particularly challenging with clients, families, and significant others from diverse cultural groups seeking mental health care.

The U.S. Department of Health and Human Services (2010) propose **shared decision making (SDM)** as a practice to advance mental health care. SDM encourages providers and consumers to collaborate on mental health care for the consumer. Mental health care providers can offer suggestions for treatment options depending on the needs of the consumer. In addition, by making the consumer an integral part of the mental health plan of treatment, it demonstrates a commitment to the autonomy and decision-making role of the consumer (Schauer et al., 2006).

It has become important for mental health care professionals to attempt to include clients and family members in care decisions. At times, this can be problematic for mental health care providers, particularly if the mental health status of the client is considered to be questionable in making critical personal decisions regarding his or her own care. Consumer treatment input can also seem a daunting task for those care providers who have based practice decisions on a strictly authoritarian framework. Understanding and taking into account the client's values, beliefs, and practices is crucial to ensuring favorable outcomes. Evidence-based or "best" practice options

can be discussed with clients and family members who are able to participate in care decisions. However, the ultimate decision lies with the client and his or her family or relatives. It is important for nurses to assess the knowledge level of their clients, family members, and/or significant others regarding the client's status and care the client is receiving. Try to include the client in decisions affecting his or her care whenever possible.

Disparities in Mental Health Care

Reducing and eliminating disparities in health care has been a focus of numerous initiatives in recent years. Healthy People 2020 (2015) identified mental disorders are one of the most common causes of disability and further identified one of the main goals was to "improve mental health through prevention and by ensuring access to appropriate, quality mental health services." The American Psychological Association (APA) (2015) called for reform in disparities in mental health status and care. APA identified that mental health is frequently lacking for diverse minority communities. In addition, concerns were raised about mental health symptoms that are "undiagnosed, underdiagnosed, or misdiagnosed for cultural, linguistic, or historical reasons." The National Institute of Nursing Research (NINR) identified strategies to reduce and eventually move toward elimination of health disparities among a number of underrepresented cultural groups. The Federal Collaborative for Health Disparities Research selected mental health disparities as one of four areas that merited immediate national research attention (Safran et al., 2009).

When asking the question "What can nursing do about health disparities?" Smith (2007) suggested that nursing has lost its vision and capacity for caring, which qualifies the profession to address disparities. Caring is essential to the theory and practice of nursing. Nursing "has been seduced by the scientific model" (p. 285),

and Smith asked the question about where that leaves nursing with respect to human suffering. She further identified nursing is more alienated with respect to the needs of oppressed groups. It is imperative that all health care providers, including mental health nurses, care about and reach out to those individuals and families suffering from mental health care disparities.

Disparities in mental health treatment have existed from the earliest historical recordings. Those with behavior that was considered to be "abnormal" were thought to be "deranged" or "mad," and in many cases, they were sent to asylums, under the harshest of conditions, to live out the remainder of their lives. Psychiatric mental health nurses have been at the forefront in paving the way for the humane care and treatment of mental health clients and, yet, mental health still remains wrought with disparities and stigma that do not exist for many other health conditions (see Evidence-Based Practice 10-1). Gluck (2014) defined stigma as "a perceived negative attribute that causes someone to devalue or think less of the whole person." Individuals with mental illness have been identified as one of the most highly stigmatized groups in the American culture. Gluck further identified that many individuals with a mental health disorder may define stigma with such phrases and terms as feeling discriminated against, hurtful, and humiliating.

The first Surgeon General's report on mental health identified disparities among diverse cultural groups in seeking and being treated for mental illness: "Even more than other areas of health and medicine, the mental health field is plagued by disparities in the availability of and access to its services. A major factor in mental health disparities, particularly for underrepresented and underserved cultural groups was the deinstitutionalization of mental health care in the mid 20th Century. Moving mental health clients from psychiatric state hospitals to community-based settings never fully materialized. Instead, individuals with mental health problems frequently ended up in emergency rooms for short-term treatment. Eventually jails and prisons became the long-term placement

Overcoming Stigma for Those Seeking Mental Health Treatment

Unfortunately, mentally ill people have evoked adverse responses across various cultures, frequently leading to living with the mental illness, rather than seeking treatment, for fear of being labeled and rejected by society. Stigma is a word with Greek origins, which referred to a symbol cut or burnt into the body, and was used to signify something negative about the moral status of the individual. It was further identified that stigma could lead to a "spoiled identity" and "damaged sense of self" (Goffman, 1964, p. 116). According to the Surgeon General's report on mental health, mental illness stigma is "the most formidable obstacle to future progress in the arena of mental illness and health" (Hinshaw, 2007, p. x). The pain of mental illness is difficult enough, "but the devastation of being invisible, shameful and toxic, can make the situation practically unlivable" (Hinshaw, 2007, p. xi). Mental illness "affects personal well being, economic productivity, and public health, fueling a vicious cycle of lowered expectations, deep shame, and hopelessness" (p. x).

Untoward consequences of mental illness, stigma, and discrimination can impact nearly every aspect of an individual's life, as well as the lives of their family and significant others. Rao, Feinglass, and Corrigan (2007) theorized that "diagnoses of mental illness are given based on deviations from sociocultural, or behavioral norms. Therefore, mental illness is a concept deeply tied to culture, and accordingly, mental illness stigma is likely to vary across cultures" (p. 1020).

Given the importance of understanding stigma associated with mental illness, it is concerning that limited research has been conducted on this phenomenon. Cheon and Chiao (2012) identified that "cultural variations in automatic affective reactions toward mental illness suggest that cultural differences in the meanings or assumptions associated with mental illness may underlie cultural variations in stigma. For example, for the Asian culture, danger and mistrust are associated with mental illness (Abdullah & Brown, 2011).

Hansson, Jormfeldt, Svedberg, and Svensson (2013) conducted a study with mental health care staff and mental health care patients themselves about attitudes and beliefs about mental illness. Mental health care staff caring for patients with a psychosis and staff working with inpatients held the most negative attitudes. Overall, patient attitudes were in keeping with those of the staff. The researchers expressed concerns about staff holding negative attitudes and beliefs about their patients with mental illness, and the impact on treatment and development and implementing evidence-based services. The researchers also identified the importance of developing interventions that would focus on both patient and staff beliefs about mental illness, in order to facilitate a more recovery-oriented outcome.

Clinical Implications

It is important for nurses and other health care providers caring for individuals, family members, and significant others to understand the impact of mental health stigma on the patient diagnosed with a mental illness. Understanding the stigma of mental illness can even influence the patient, family, and significant others' willingness to contact health care providers for treatment and can help caregivers help patients, families, and significant others understand mental illness within the context of health care. If nurses are to help the patient deal with the untoward effects of stigma associated with mental illness, it is crucial that nurses get in touch with their own biases and negative attitudes about mental illness. It is also important for nurses to understand that the patient, family, and significant others may resist a mental illness diagnosis, based on the societal and specific cultural values, beliefs, and practices associated with mental illness. Peer discussions among nurses about personal and professional values, beliefs, and practices associated with mental illness could facilitate getting in touch with negative attitudes and beliefs about mental illness. Nurses can also participate in workshops and other educational experiences to improve their understanding of cultural values, beliefs, and

(continued)

Overcoming Stigma for Those Seeking Mental Health Treatment (continued)

practices related to mental illness in general and to specific mental illness diagnoses.

References

Abdullah, T., & Brown, T. L., (2011). Mental illness stigma and ethnocultural beliefs, values, and norms: An integrative review, *Clinical Psychology Review*, *31*, 934–938.

Cheon, B., & Chiao J. Y. (2012). Cultural variations in implicit mental illness stigma. *Journal of Cross-Cultural Psychology*, *43*(7), 1058–1062.

Goffman, E. (1964). Stigma. London, UK: Penguin.

Hansson, L., Jormfeldt, H., Svedberg, P. & Svensson, B. (2013). Mental health professionals' attitudes towards people with mental illness: Do they differ from attitudes held by people with mental illness? *International Journal of Social Psychology*, *59*(1), 48–54.

Hinshaw, S. P. (2007). *The mark of shame: Stigma of mental illness and an agenda for change*. New York, NY: Oxford University Press.

Rao, D., Feinglass, J., & Corrigan, P. (2007). Racial and ethnic disparities in mental illness stigma. *The Journal of Nervous and Mental Disease, 195*(12), 1020–1023.

for many individuals with mental health diagnoses (Safran et al., 2009). These disparities are viewed readily through the lenses of racial and cultural diversity, age, and gender" (U.S. Department of Health and Human Services, 1999, p. vi).

Historically, racism in America has led to difficulties in acknowledging and/or discussing differences in cultural values and lifeways for diverse cultural groups. Bell and Peterson (1992) indicated that slavery, segregation, and institutionalized racism have resulted in numerous problems faced by African Americans, resulting in what the authors labeled as *cultural pain*. **Cultural pain** is defined as feeling "insecure, embarrassed, angry, confused, torn, apologetic, uncertain, or inadequate because of conflicting expectations of and pressures from being a minority" (Bell & Peterson, 1992, p. 8). Leininger (1995) identified cultural pain as "the suffering, discomfort, or unfavorable responses of an individual group towards an individual who has different beliefs or lifeways, usually reflecting the insensitivity of those inflicting the discomfort" (p. 67).

A number of diverse cultural groups have experienced what is called **historical trauma** (also referred to as **Historical Unresolved Grief** or **Disenfranchised Grieving**; see Evidence-Based Practice 10-2). Evans-Campbell (2008) discussed historical trauma in Native American and Alaska Native communities and defined historical trauma as: "a collective complex trauma inflicted on a group of people who share a specific group identify or affiliation-ethnicity, nationality, and religious affiliation. It is the legacy of numerous traumatic events a community experiences over generations" (p. 320). In contrast to personal traumatic experiences, "the concept of historical trauma calls attention to the complex, collective, cumulative, and intergenerational psychosocial impacts that resulted from the depredations of past colonial subjugation" (Gone, 2013).

Yellow Horse Brave Heart and DeBruyn (1998, p. 60) observed that "American Indians experienced massive losses of lives, land, and culture from European contact and colonization resulting in a long legacy of chronic trauma and unresolved grief across generations." Past emotional harm done to people of a diverse culture includes such examples as the Jewish holocaust, slavery of African American people in the United States, internment of Japanese Americans in America during World War II, and treatment of American Indians. In order to help individuals heal from historical unresolved grief or historical trauma, nurses need to understand how experiences of the past shape the present and future (Struthers & Lowe, 2003; Yellow Horse Brave Heart & DeBruyn, 1998). Helping clients to move through

"Historical Unresolved Grief" or "Historical Trauma"

Certain cultural groups, including First Nations such as American Indian, Native Alaska, and Canadian Aboriginal, have experienced what is called "historical unresolved grief" or "historical trauma." They have experienced loss of people, land, and culture as a result of European colonization. This phenomenon "contributes to the current social pathology of high rates of suicide, homicide, DV, child abuse, alcoholism, and other social problems among American Indians" (p. 60). Other cultural groups experience the phenomenon of historical unresolved grief or historical trauma as well, as a result of, for example, the Jewish holocaust, slavery of African Americans, and the internment of Japanese Americans during World War II. Nurses can help specific cultural groups grieve the past traumatic event(s) and allow them to acknowledge the events that occurred. It is important to help individuals, groups, and communities identify methods and solutions to move forward in the healing process.

Gone (2013) identified First Nations' communities have repeatedly linked their high rates of mental health distress with historical traumatic experiences of European colonization. Gone differentiates historical trauma from posttraumatic stress disorder in three different aspects: First, historical trauma is more complex in what preceded it, how it evolved, and the outcome. Second, historical trauma is a collective phenomenon shared by communities following deliberate conquest, colonization, or genocide. Finally, historical trauma is cumulative in its effect over time. Gone further stipulated various

traditional cultural practices to help First Nations suffering from historical trauma, such as talking circles, pipe ceremonies, sweat lodges, and other cultural practices for therapeutic healing purposes. (See Figures 10-1, 10-4, and 10-5 for other examples of healing tribal ceremonies and activities.)

Clinical Implications

As individuals, families, and communities continue to grieve the emotional pain associated with historical trauma, it is important for transcultural mental health nurses to acknowledge the emotional feelings (insecurity, embarrassed, angry, confused, torn, apologetic, uncertain, or inadequate) associated with such grief and the conflicting expectations of and pressures from being a minority. It is important for transcultural mental health nurses to facilitate a safe and healing environment for individuals, families, and communities to work through the feelings associated with historical unresolved grief or historical trauma.

References

Bell, P., & Peterson, D. (1992). Cultural pain and African Americans: Unspoken issues in early recovery. Hazelden Publishing Center City, MN.

Gone, J. P. (2013). Redressing First Nations historical trauma: theorizing mechanisms for indigenous culture as mental health treatment, *Transcultural Psychiatry*, *50*(5), 683–706.

Yellow Horse Brave Heart, M., & DeBruyn, L. M. (1998). The American Indian holocaust: Healing historical unresolved grief. *American Indian & Alaska Native Mental Health Research*, 8(2), 60–82.

the process of unresolved grief is an important care measure nurses and other health care providers must consider when caring for individuals and families from cultures who have experienced horrific events or trauma in the past. Often, interventions are directed toward the community at large rather than focused on specific individuals. Working *with* clients, families, and communities and encouraging their voices to be heard is key to

helping those who have experienced pain associated with racial, social, and economic disparities and oppression.

Johnston and Boyle (2013) conducted an ethnographic study with Northern British Columbian Aboriginal mothers with adolescents diagnosed with fetal alcohol spectrum disorder and observed that the mothers who participated in the study lived within a marginalized

and poverty-stricken context. Intergenerational alcohol abuse had played a major role in all of the women's lives. "Mothering from the Margins" was a major theme discovered in the study. The women's lives were "framed within a post colonial context of racial prejudice and stereotypical notions of Aboriginal motherhood" (p. 65). The researchers suggested that nurses need to take a leadership role to reduce health disparities with marginalized and poverty-stricken populations, particularly when there is evidence of prejudice, including stereotyping. It is important for nurses to advocate on behalf of such individuals and communities.

Zayas, Torres, and Cabassa (2009) compared mental health diagnostic agreement in an outpatient unit with Hispanic and non-Hispanic health care providers. The non-Hispanic care providers rated client's functional ability and the severity of symptoms significantly worse than do the Hispanic care providers. The authors noted that because the mental health labor force is primarily non-Hispanic, Hispanic individuals are likely to be assigned a non-Hispanic care provider. The authors questioned the possibility of the care provider's cultural and social biases, and wondered if those factors were responsible for the discrepancy in diagnoses. It is important for mental health professionals not only to identify but also to understand racism and the role it plays in mental health, at both a conscious and unconscious level, in order to eradicate racial inequalities in mental health care.

Mental Health Care for Immigrants

There has been extensive debate about immigration policy during the past several years in the United States as well as internationally. In the United States, the debate has become heated politically with political parties arguing the implications, from their standpoint, of immigration policies. Health care for those immigrants who are not in this country legally has also been extensively debated, again with both sides stating the merits of their views on whether such immigrants, or undocumented individuals, have a right to health care in this country. At the same time, however, there has been minimal understanding of these issues from the perspective of the undocumented immigrants and the impact immigration has on their mental health (see Evidence-Based Practice 10-3).

Use of the terms "illegal alien," and "illegal immigrant," is increasingly identified as "racially charged" and offensive terminology to describe "undocumented workers," or "undocumented immigrants." In fact, according to the PEW Research Center (2013), a nonpartisan think tank located in Washington, D.C., use of the term "illegal alien" reached its low point in 2013, dropping to 5% of terms used. It had consistently been in double digits in the other periods studied, peaking at 21% in 2007. According to the Central Broadcasting System (CBS) (2014), Supreme Court Justice Sonia Sotomayor, the first Hispanic Supreme Court Justice, uses the term "undocumented immigrants" rather than the term "illegal alien." Justice Sotomayor identified that "labeling immigrants criminals seemed insulting to her." She further stated: "I think people then paint those individuals as something less than worthy human beings and it changes the conversation." The undocumented worker's voice is generally absent in policy debates and implementation. In fact, undocumented immigrants are "often forced to live in the shadows of society for fear of deportation," which further alienates and silences the voice of the undocumented immigrant (Summers-Sandoval, 2008, p. 581).

Setting aside the political debate, transcultural mental health nurses have cared for both documented and undocumented immigrants for many years and are increasingly caring for those immigrants who are feeling the emotional pressures of such a political climate. The term **culture shock** was coined by the anthropologist Kalervo Oberg (1960) to describe individuals, such as immigrants, who enter a new culture. Culture shock

Mental Health Needs of the Immigrant Population

Based on the 2009 American Community Survey (ACS), approximately 38.5 million or 12.5% of the population in the United States are foreign born (U.S. Census Bureau, 2010). Schock-Giordano (2013) found that assimilation into the American culture may have a negative impact on mental health. The mental health needs of the immigrant population increase with the stresses encountered in learning the values, beliefs, and practices of a new culture. In addition, language and financial needs can limit the immigrant population from seeking adequate health care services, particularly mental health services. The immigrant population faces numerous challenges in seeking professional mental health care, including a lack of understanding of the mental health care system and how to go about accessing mental health services (Dow, 2011).

A major barrier that can impede an immigrant from seeking mental health care services is language. Immigrants may delay seeking mental health care based on fear of not being able to communicate or a fear of embarrassment about their language difficulties. Misdiagnoses may result from difficulties with communication and may impede appropriate mental health treatment (Dow, 2011). In order to provide optimal care to immigrants seeking mental health services, it is important for nurses to facilitate, to the best of their ability, a willingness to understand the client's perspective and help the client with language difficulties, to communicate their symptoms and perceptions about their mental health state. It is important for nurses to let the immigrant client know they are willing to listen, help interpret, and understand the client's perspective about their symptoms within a nonjudgmental setting. Particularly for the immigrant client with financial and insurance difficulties, it is most important for the nurse to work with the client and the health care system to facilitate the client's care or their ability to access available and appropriate care, including a certified translator if needed.

Immigrants from diverse cultures have unique patterns of beliefs and values as to the meaning of health or illness. These patterns of beliefs and values, interpreted within a distinct cultural context, then influence how symptoms are identified and interpreted and determine when to seek mental health services and appropriate treatment (Dow, 2011). It is important for mental health care providers to interpret symptoms and perceptions within a cultural context, in order to determine appropriate care. To provide culturally congruent mental health care, it is important for nurses to assess for the client's understanding of symptoms; their migration story and potential trauma associated with their immigrant status; spiritual and religious values, beliefs, and practices; stressors associated with acculturation; and available support system, all of which can influence the patient receiving appropriate diagnosis and treatment for their symptoms (Caplan et al., 2013).

References

Caplan, S. Caplan, S., Escobar, J., Paris, M., Alvidrez, J., Dixon, J. K., … Whittemore, R. (2013). Cultural influences on causal beliefs about depression among Latino immigrants, *Journal of Transcultural Nursing, 24(1),* 68–77.

Dow, H. D. (2011). An overview of stressors faced by Immigrants and Refugees: A guide for mental health practitioners, *Home Health Care Management and Practice, 23(3),* 210–217.

Schock-Giordano, A. (2013). Ethnic families and mental health: Application of the ABC-X model of family stress, *Sage Open, 1,* 1–7.

U. S. Census Bureau. (2010). *Place of birth of the foreign-born population: 2009.*

is "precipitated by the anxiety that results from losing all our familiar signs and symbols of social intercourse" (p. 177). Oberg suggested that the "signs" or "cues" that people use within a culture—such as the words people speak—customs people follow, and even nonverbal communication such as gestures and facial expressions are not recognized by those who are new to the culture.

This leads to feelings of frustration and anxiety even in those persons who would be considered "mentally healthy." Imagine how these negative feelings would be confounded for an individual who has entered the country as an undocumented immigrant and fears arrest, detention, and deportation.

The concept of **acculturation** was initially defined by Redfield, Linton, and Herskovits (1936) as "those phenomena which result when groups of individuals having different cultures come into continuous first-hand contact, with subsequent changes in the original cultural patterns of either or both groups" (p. 149). Acculturation can be a stressful and complex process, particularly for immigrants who experience difficulty adjusting to the new culture. Ho (2014) conducted a systematic review of research on implications of acculturation on Chinese immigrants. Acculturation discrepancy between immigrant Chinese parents and their children, specifically in the American orientation, was indirectly related to a higher level of adolescent delinquency. In other words, "the parents' acculturation in the host orientation may be more saliently related to children's conduct or delinquent behaviors" (p. 155). Some individuals

may find themselves unable to work through the stress of acculturation and have great difficulty in modifying their **cultural values, beliefs, or practices** and feel isolated from their new culture or even from their culture of origin. Depression (see Evidence-Based Practice 10-4) is the most common mental health problem among immigrants in the United States and has been associated with the process of acculturation (Al-Omari & Pallikkathayil, 2008; Choi, Miller, & Wilbur 2009). Immigrants and refugees may be fleeing war and other traumatic political environments and may exhibit symptoms of posttraumatic stress disorder as well as depression (Figure 10-3).

Walsh, Shulman, and Maurer (2008) studied immigration distress in young adults immigrating to Israel from Eastern Europe and found young immigrants experienced immigration distress, including feelings of guilt and shame, failure, and incompetence and not feeling wanted, understood, or a sense of belonging. Immigration distress can be a result of economic adversity, language difficulties, loss of support networks, even loss of family members, as well as prejudice and discrimination. Because of the difficulties faced by immigrant

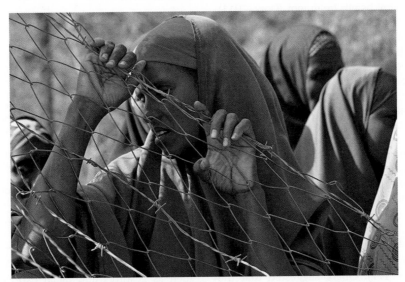

Figure 10-3. In addition to being uprooted or fleeing war-torn and impoverished living conditions in their home countries, many immigrants from diverse cultural groups suffer from mental health issues (hikrcn/Shutterstock.com).

Depressive Disorders Interpreted Within a Cultural Context

According to WHO, depression is one of the most common mental disorders and leading cause of disability worldwide (World Health Organization, 2012). "Globally, more than 350 million people of all ages suffer from depression" (2012). Similarly, the U.S. Department of Health and Human services, in the Healthy People 2010 report, identified depressive disorders have been categorized as major, persistent, premenstrual, substance/medication-induced, depressive disorder R/T another health condition, other specified and unspecified (DSM-V, 2013). Common symptoms among the depressive disorders are "presence of sad, empty, or irritable mood, accompanied by somatic and cognitive changes" (p. 155) that significantly affect the individual's ability to carry out functions of daily living. What varies among the depressive disorders are "duration, timing, or presumed etiology" (p. 155).

How depression is identified, treated, and talked about is frequently connected to one's cultural values, beliefs, and practices. In a study about the influences and causal beliefs about depression among Latino immigrants, Caplan et al. (2013) identified disparities in depressive mental health care for Latinos are not completely explained by difficulties with insurance and language but may be more a reflection of the patient's cultural values, including religious values, and a lack of understanding of these values by health care providers. The researchers found that "the perceived importance of supernatural and religious causation beliefs, which might contribute to a reluctance to fully accept medical interventions" (p. 75). Therefore, it is important for nurses to explore these sensitive areas with their patient's and/or family/significant others. Patients may be reluctant to discuss deeply held cultural beliefs such as supernatural, voodoo, and various rituals little understood by health care providers, unless an open, accepting discovery mode is provided.

Brintnell, Sommer, Kuncoro, Setiawan, and Bailey (2013) conducted a concept mapping study on the expression of depression among Java, Indonesia, participants from local mental health hospitals, aged 15 to 55 years old. Investigators held individual meetings rather than group meetings, related to a cultural norm of not wanting to share private health information in public. Participants had received a clinical diagnosis of recurrent major depressive disorder depending on severity (2013, p.162). Participants were asked, "How do you experience your illness/sickness?" Six underlying themes were identified: interpersonal relationships, hopelessness, physical/somatic, poverty of thought, discouragement, and defeat. Researchers concluded the findings indicated common features with Western populations with the disorder.

Clinical Implications

When health care providers lack an understanding of the diverse cultural groups for whom they provide care, failure to accurately diagnose an individual with the correct diagnosis increases. For example, with depression, Brintnell et al. (2013) concluded that there is a discrepancy in current diagnostic tools to address depressive experiences/illnesses when compared to how individuals actually experience their illness/sickness. The authors concluded the discrepancy could ultimately influence diagnosing depression in diverse non-Western cultural groups. Gwynn et al. (2008) reported that immigrants in the United States who suffered from depression were 60% less likely to be diagnosed than were individuals born in the United States, even if those individuals born in the United States were of the same culture as the immigrants (Gwynn et al., 2008). For example, Asian immigrants who suffered from depression were often inadequately diagnosed and treated, which ultimately led to serious psychosocial and functional impairments (Gwynn et al., 2008).

Based on the findings in the Brintnell et al. (2013) study, "religion or spiritual interconnectedness acts as a common coping mechanism and screening tools might benefit by including these aspects" (p. 593). The researchers also suggested the need to place more emphasis on somatic complaints and problems with concentration.

It is important for nurses to understand both past and present life experiences are interpreted through the lens of deeply held cultural, religious, and spiritual

(continued)

Depressive Disorders Interpreted Within a Cultural Context (continued)

beliefs. It is important for nurses to try to understand beliefs, values, practices, and expectations grounded in one's culture, to more fully understand a patient's symptoms, their perspective about their illness, and expected outcomes of treatment for depression.

References

American Psychiatric Association. (2013). *Diagnostic and Statistical Manual of Mental Disorders, DSM-5* (5th ed.). Washington, DC: American Psychiatric Association.

Brintnell, S. E., Sommer, R. W., Kuncoro, B., Setiawan, P. G., & Bailey, P. (2013). The expression of depression among Javanese patients with major depressive disorder: A concept mapping study. *Transcultural Psychiatry, 50*, 579–598.

Caplan, S., Escobar, J., Paris, M., Alvidrez, J., Dixon, J. K., Desai, M. M., ... Whittemore, R. (2013). Cultural influences on causal beliefs about depression among Latino immigrants. *Journal of Transcultural Nursing, 24*(1), 68–77.

Gwynn, R. C., McQuistion, H. L., McVeigh, K. H., Garg, R. K., Frieden, T. R., & Thorpe, L. E. (2008). Prevalence, diagnosis, and treatment of depression and generalized anxiety disorder in a diverse urban community. *Psychiatric Services, 59*, 641–647.

World Health Organization. (2012). Fact Sheet N369. Retrieved 4-17-14 http://www.who.int/mediacentre/factsheets/fs369/en/

families, their children are at higher risk for depression, anxiety disorders, substance abuse, and other mental health problems. Mental health nurses working with immigrants and their families need to be aware of the risk for mental health problems.

Ho (2014) identified nurses are uniquely qualified to identify acculturation discrepancy problems with immigrant parents and children at the clinical and mental health community levels. Based on their holistic perspective and skills, nurses are able to develop links among the individual, family, and social environment, thereby helping to prevent negative child outcomes associated with acculturation in immigrant families. Many immigrants may express their anxiety as somatic complaints, so nurses working with immigrant populations need to be aware of the linkages between somatic complaints, such as headaches, backaches, and the like, and mental health problems (Lamberg, 2009).

Bridges, Andrews, and Deen (2012) studied 84 adult Hispanic immigrants in the Mid-Southern United States, their mental health needs, and their use of services; they found 36% of participants met the criteria for at least one mental disorder. Forty-two percent of the sample saw a physician in the previous year, primarily because of somatic complaints; however, religious leaders were providing mental health services to the participants. Findings indicated that many of the Hispanic immigrants participating in the study recognized mental health services would be beneficial; however, systemic barriers existed, including economic and linguistic. The authors recommended recruiting bilingual medical and nursing students into the health care professions and offering incentives to retain the students. The authors also identified a need to work closely with religious leaders to recognize mental health problems and help to form a beneficial referral system.

Cultural Criteria Changes in Diagnostic Statistical Manual-V

In the newest DSM-V, the culture-bound syndromes that have routinely been used by mental health professionals have now been replaced with three cultural concepts. An overview of the three concepts follows, along with the reasons identified for the change in the DSM-V. In addition, several key mental health organizations have come out against the DSM-V, and those organizations and reasons for their views on the DSM-V will be discussed.

A Cultural Formulation Interview (CFI) has been identified in the DSM-V and is a set of 16 questions clinicians can use in a mental health assessment. The questions are geared to the impact of culture on the individual's current clinical picture.

The three cultural concepts in the DSM-V (American Psychiatric Association, 2013) are cultural syndrome, cultural idiom, and cultural explanation. Cultural syndrome is identified as a cluster or co-occurring group of symptoms found in a specific cultural group or community (e.g., *ataque de nervios*). The syndrome may not be identified as an illness by the cultural group, yet would be identified as an illness by an outside observer. Cultural idiom of distress is a means of identifying suffering among a cultural group with shared ethnicity and religion (e.g., *kufungisisa*). Kufungisisa is associated with "a range of psychopathology," including "anxiety, excessive worry, panic attacks, depressive symptoms and irritability" (p. 834). The cultural idioms of distress may not be associated with specific symptoms and may be used to demonstrate discomfort in a variety of situations, including social circumstances versus mental health issues, and cultural explanation or perceived cause is a label that provides a cultural etiology (e.g., *maladi moun*). "Interpersonal envy and malice cause people to harm their enemies by sending illnesses such as psychosis, depression. A related condition is the 'evil eye' (p. 835)." Explanations about the cause may be features or folk classifications used by cultural healers or lay individuals (see Table 10-1).

Table 10-1: DSM-V (2013) Cultural Concepts of Distress

Cultural Concept of Distress	Culture	Symptoms
Ataque de nervios	Latino	Intense emotional upset; acute anxiety, anger, or grief; screaming and shouting uncontrollably; attacks of crying; trembling; heat in the chest rising into the head; verbal and physical aggression Dissociative experiences; seizure-like and fainting; suicidal gestures
Dhat syndrome	India Pakistan	Associated with semen loss in young males Anxiety, fatigue, weight loss, impotence
Khyal cap	Cambodians in United States and Cambodia	Panic attacks; anxiety, tinnitus, and neck soreness
Kufungisisa	Shona of Zimbabwe	Anxiety, depression Somatic problems (Indicative of interpersonal and social difficulties)
Maladi moun Sent sickness	Haiti	Humanly caused illness (envy of other's success, hatred) Attractive, intelligent, and wealthy are at risk
Nervios	Latinos in the United States	Emotional distress Somatic disturbance Inability to function Headaches and brain aches
Shenjing shuairuo	Chinese	Weakness, emotions, excitement, nervous pain, sleep disturbances, 3:5 required
Susto	Some Latinos in United States, Central America, South America	Frightening event causing soul to leave body Unhappiness and sickness Difficulty in key social roles
Taijin kyofusho	Japanese	Interpersonal fear disorder Anxiety and avoidance of interpersonal situations Fear of inadequacy and offensiveness to others

The NIMH, the world's largest and most influential funding agency for mental health research, and a key supporter and funding agency for research for the previous editions of the DSM, withdrew support for the DSM-V. In fact, the NIMH stated that the agency would no longer fund research based strictly on the DSM criteria. The DSM criteria have been used for many years to diagnose and treat clients with mental health illness, as well as serving as the basis for insurance reimbursement payments. Thomas R. Insel, M.D., the Director of the NIMH, identified that a major weakness of the DSM was "its lack of validity." He further identified the DSM diagnoses "are based on a consensus about clusters of clinical symptoms, not any objective laboratory measure" (Lane, 2013).

Culture-Bound Syndromes

Although culture-bound syndromes have been removed from the DSM-V, they are presented here as still existent within the cultures identified and in the mental health system. Various mental health symptoms are experienced by people all over the world. Cultural meanings, beliefs, and practices regarding specific symptoms may vary depending on one's culture and socioeconomic status within the culture. Although specific identifying terms, manifestations, and meanings within

different cultures may vary, a diagnosis such as depression is similar around the world. However, cultural values, beliefs, and practices shape how various groups interpret symptoms, identify causality, and determine appropriate treatment.

In contrast, **culture-bound syndromes**, also called folk illnesses, culture-specific illnesses, or culture-specific syndromes, often are localized to a particular cultural group. According to American Psychiatric Association (2000), culture-bound syndromes are described as recurrent, locality specific patterns of aberrant behavior and troubling experiences that may or may not be linked to a particular DSM-IV diagnostic category. Many of these patterns are indigenously considered to be "illnesses," or at least afflictions, and most have local names. Culture-bound syndromes are generally limited to specific societies or culture areas and are localized, diagnostic categories that frame coherent meanings for certain repetitive, patterned, and troubling sets of experience and observations (p. 898).

As mental health care is changing to meet the increasing multicultural diversity of the client population, it is important for mental health nurses to recognize the culture-bound syndromes. Table 10-2 lists the most frequently cited culture-bound syndromes. Since values, beliefs, and practices of people are culturally constructed, the syndromes can only be interpreted within the context of the specific culture in which they exist.

Table 10-2: Culture-Bound Syndromes

Syndrome	Culture	Symptoms
Amok	Malaysia	Period of brooding with subsequent aggressive behavior followed by amnesia or exhaustion
Cafard, cathard	Polynesia	
Mal de pelea	Puerto Rico	Typically occurs in young to middle-aged males who have experienced recent loss
Iich'aa	Navajo	
Ataque de nervios	Latino Puerto Rico	Uncontrollable shouting, crying, trembling, and aggressive behavior Sensation of heat in the chest Possible fainting or seizure-like activity Triggered by stressful familial event and buildup of anger Typically occurs in women 45 years and older

Table 10-2: Culture-Bound Syndromes (continued)

Syndrome	Culture	Symptoms
Bilis, colera, muina	Latino	Acute nervous tension, trembling, screaming, gastrointestinal disturbances Cause is thought to be unexpressed anger or rage
Bouffee delirante	West Africa, Haiti	Abrupt outburst of agitation, aggression, and confusion May be associated with hallucinations (visual and auditory) and paranoia
Brain fag, brain fog	West Africa	Brain "fatigue," difficulty concentrating or sleeping, weakness Crawling sensation under skin Feelings of depression Most often afflicts high school or college students
Dhat, Jiryan Sukra Prameha Shen k'uei	India Sri Lanka China, Taiwan	Somatic complaints of dizziness, fatigue, weakness, loss of appetite, guilt, and sexual dysfunction associated with semen-loss anxiety
Falling out, blacking out	Southern United States, Caribbean	Spinning sensation and dizziness prior to collapse Visual impairment Difficulty interacting with environment
Ghost sickness	Navajo	Weakness, pending sense of "doom," loss of appetite, feeling of suffocation, fainting, dizziness, and hallucinations Preoccupation with death
Hwa-byung	Korea	Insomnia, chest discomfort, dizziness, headaches, fearful, sadness, suicidal ideation, and guilt Typically occurs in middle-aged or elderly women
Koro Shuk yang, Shook yong, Suo yang Jinjinia bemar Rok joo	Malaysia China Assam Thailand	Fear of penis in men and vulva and nipples in women retracting into the body and possibly causing death
Latah Amurakh, irkunii, olan, myriachit, menkeiti Bah tschi, bah tsi, baah ji Imu Mali-mali, silok Locura	Malaysia Siberia Thailand Ainu, Sakhalin, Japan Philippines Latin America and Latinos in United States	Exaggerated startle response, screaming, cursing, laughing, echopraxia, echolalia Typically occurs in women

continued

Table 10-2: Culture-Bound Syndromes (continued)

Syndrome	Culture	Symptoms
Mal de ojo, evil eye	Mediterranean	Typically occurs with children and can also affect women Sleep disturbances, crying, diarrhea, vomiting, and fever
Nervios	Latino	Feeling of vulnerability and emotional distress to stressful life experiences Irritability, sleep disturbances, nervous, difficulty concentrating, tearfulness, and dizziness
Pibloktoq, Arctic hysteria	Inuit	Fatigue, depressive silences, confusion Typically follows a major loss
Qigong psychotic reaction	Chinese	Dissociation and paranoia Headache, dizziness, disorientation Can occur following Qigong meditation
Rootwork	Southern United States Caribbean	Witchcraft, voodoo, hexing, or evil influence are responsible for illnesses.
Mal puesto, brujeria	Latino	GI disturbances, anxiety, fear of being poisoned or killed ("voodoo death")
Sangue dormido	Portuguese Cape Verde Islanders	Pain, numbness, paralysis, convulsions, stroke, heart attack, infection, and miscarriage
Shenjing	Chinese	Depression, anxiety, dizziness, headaches, GI and sleep disturbances, and sexual dysfunction
Shin-byung	Korean	Anxiety, weakness, dizziness, fear, sleep and GI disturbances Somatic complaints are followed by dissociation and feeling possessed by ancestral spirits.
Spell	Southern United States	Trancelike state, communication with deceased spirits May be misdiagnosed as psychosis
Susto, fright, soul loss (espantro, pasmo, perdida del alma chibih)	Latinos in United States Mexico Central America South America	Actual "fright" Sleep and appetite disturbances, tripa ida, sadness, lack of motivation, low self-esteem, muscle aches, headache, and GI disturbances Typically follows a frightening event resulting in the soul leaving the body Symptoms can occur immediately following event or years later
Taijin kyofusho	Japan	Intense fear that one's body (appearance, odor, nonverbal communication) embarrasses or offends others
Zar	North Africa Middle East	Feeling possessed by a spirit Dissociation (laughing, hurting self, singing, crying), withdrawal, difficulty caring for self May develop relationship with spirit

Data from (2000). *American Psychological Association: Diagnostic and Statistical Manual of Mental Disorders* (4th ed.); and Hales, Yudofsky & Gabbard (Eds.). (2008). *The American Psychiatric Publishing Textbook of Psychiatry* (5th ed.)

Cultural Values, Beliefs, and Practices of Specific Cultural Groups as They Relate to Mental Health

Nurses have always cared for diverse populations of clients, and community-based nurses have focused in particular on newly arrived immigrant populations. A century ago, nurses and other health professionals were concerned about contagious diseases and malnutrition in caring for immigrant populations. Currently, there is a great deal of research being conducted to better understand nursing care for culturally diverse immigrant clients and their family members who are seeking care. Many of these studies focus specifically on mental health care, particularly helping immigrant clients, families, and communities adjust to life in their new country. In addition, health care services for immigrant communities also place an emphasis on mental health, particularly since many recent immigrants have experienced war, displacement, and other associated traumas.

Transcultural mental health nurses and other mental health care providers want to help clients of all cultures achieve their optimal level of human functioning. However, an individual's optimal level of human functioning can be specifically tied to the meanings and expressions of care of one's culture. Historically, the majority of research on psychological functioning with immigrants from diverse cultures has relied on the deficit model. According to the deficit model, hostile environmental factors such as prejudice and inequality in social conditions lead to increased rates of stress among minority populations, which ultimately lead to inferior or self-destructive methods of coping (Kaplan & Sue, 1997). Although the deficit model drew attention to the effects of prejudice and inequality in social conditions, there was a tendency to equate one's psychological functioning with negative rather than positive forces. Researchers now seek more positive frameworks

to describe diverse experiences, beliefs, and transitions, emphasizing the strengths of immigrant and minority populations.

According to Constantine and Sue (2006a, 2006b), an individual's optimal level of human functioning is dependent upon the cultural context in which it is being defined. In fact, Western goals associated with optimal human functioning, such as happiness and self-determination, which are grounded in a Eurocentric cultural value system, may differ greatly with individuals from diverse cultures. Optimal human functioning of culturally diverse persons may be better understood by studying the values, beliefs, and practices of the cultural group. For example, in the United States, optimal level of human functioning for African Americans and Native Americans may include such concepts as collectivism, racial and ethnic pride, spirituality, religion, holistic health, and family and community or tribal importance. In addition, overcoming such adversity as racism may serve as a strength and helps mental health care providers better understand optimal human functioning for diverse cultural groups (Constantine & Sue, 2006a, 2006b).

Modern medical care may not be viewed the same as traditional health care in reservation or immigrant communities. Native Americans, as well as newly arrived immigrants, may experience some difficulty in trusting modern-day (allopathic) mental health care providers. For example, some Native Americans may be reluctant to consult professionally educated mental health care providers, particularly if they perceive that the mental health care professionals are attempting to "brainwash" them into accepting the cultural values, beliefs, and practices of the Western health care system (Gone & Alcantara, 2007, p. 356).

Nurse researchers and other health-related disciplines have continued to explore the health beliefs and practices of culturally diverse clients specific to mental health. An overview of mental health beliefs and practices of selected cultural groups follows. The overviews are not intended

to stereotype or generalize the specific cultures. They are only intended as a resource for transcultural nurses and others to increase the awareness of patterns of values, beliefs, and practices related to mental health of the selected cultural groups. However, the transcultural nurse is also encouraged to understand the diversity within cultural groups with respect to mental health beliefs and practices. Many clients and families of specific cultural groups may not exhibit traditional patterns of values, beliefs, and practices of any specific cultural group. Transcultural nurses should conduct a thorough history and cultural assessment to ensure competent cultural care for each client.

African American Culture: An Overview of Mental Health Concerns

Individuals of African descent comprise 14.7% of the total US population by 2060 (United States Census Bureau, 2012). The concept of African Americans as a distinct group in the United States is grounded historically in their shared social and environmental contexts, historical events, as well as family and kin memories of those experiences. Bell and Peterson (1992) noted that slavery, segregation, and institutionalized racism created a climate that resulted in health disparities, structural inequalities, marginalization, and cultural pain for African Americans. Acknowledging and understanding this cultural context is an important first step prior to providing transcultural mental health care to African American individuals, families, and communities.

According to the Mental Health Screening Organization (2014), even though many African Americans have endured discrimination, and may have ancestors who have endured slavery, they have led productive lives and built dynamic communities. Historically, African Americans were forced to deal with inequities with education, employment, and health care and thereby learned to turn to each other and community leaders for help. Currently, African Americans frequently turn to family, friends, neighbors,

community, church, and religious leaders for help and to cope and deal with mental health issues.

Numerous health disparities are of great concern in the African American population, and mental health issues have often gone unnoticed, taking a back seat to other health concerns. Many in the Black community, especially young Black males, may believe that depression is not really an illness or that it is a sign of weakness, so they tend not to seek help. There is a notion that is prevalent among young Black men (as well as others) that because of machismo, being macho or tough, Black men cannot be suicidal. It is one of the most pervasive and damaging falsehoods within and outside of the African American community. Some studies have shown that some African Americans believe that depression is a personal weakness and the result of improper lifestyles (e.g., too much worry, working too hard, not being religious enough) (Shellman & Mokel, 2010).

African American men, as in other diverse cultural groups, often express their depression through bodily symptoms like headaches, stomach aches, pains, and so on. Within the Black community, there can be considerable stigma about mental illnesses. Prevention of depression and suicide is extremely important, and education is the key to early prevention. Although the African American church has traditionally viewed suicide as a sin, many religious organizations are now starting to create mental health programs. The Black church is a major institution in the community and pastors can be trained to recognize signs of depression among parishioners and to refer troubled individuals to the proper professionals (Taliaferro, 2006). Depression in African American individuals can be overlooked; unfortunately, it is sometimes cultural insensitivity that leads health care providers to overlook symptoms of depression.

There are other mental health issues within the African American community that lead to premature mortality or morbidity. The societal costs of substance abuse can be calculated in terms of violence, disease, and death. There is a close relationship between substance abuse and

HIV/AIDS and other sexually transmitted diseases. In a grounded theory study focused on understanding the use of street drugs among older African Americans, Pope, Wallhagen, and Davis (2010) found that a close relationship with family members was often the precipitating factor for entrance into rehabilitation. Close relationships and the context of those relationships are sometimes a precipitating factor for beginning substance abuse, also. Respondents in this study also identified several media images that negatively portrayed African American culture and influenced the use of illegal substances. The negative images portrayed by "harmful one-dimensional characterizations surrounding criminal culture/drug culture, negative characterizations and comedic renderings" were profoundly described by the sample (p. 251). These images have two major effects: they glamorize a drug lifestyle and they perpetuate the stereotype of African American involvement in crime, violence, and deviant behavior (see Evidence-Based Practice 10-5.)

Although major health disparities affect the African American community, mental health issues need immediate attention as these issues are complex and require creative and substantive interventions. There is clearly a need for concerted action as the core issues of substance abuse and suicide cannot be addressed by just one discipline alone; the environmental and larger societal forces must be attended to by multidisciplinary actions on numerous fronts. There are several important factors to keep in mind when providing transcultural mental health care to African Americans. First, family and kin networks, while perhaps not as strong as in the past, are still extremely important in assisting the recovery process. Outreach and education to family members about depression, suicide, and substance abuse are extremely important. For many African Americans who have experienced difficulty with mental health issues of substance and drug abuse and serious and persistent mental illnesses, such as depression, family and community are very important components in the recovery process.

Maintaining a connection with family members and others in the community assists clients to feel accepted and demonstrates to themselves and others that they are responsible and can move forward in the recovery process (Armour, Bradshaw, & Roseborough, 2009; Ehrmin, 2005). Secondly, the African American church is a key player in changing community perceptions about depression and suicide as well as a leading player in substance abuse programs. The Black church is a major institution and where many African Americans choose to go for help. Spirituality has been a traditional cultural norm in African cultures and the modern African American church has incorporated the spiritual component into healing and care.

Native American Culture: An Overview of Mental Health Concerns

According to the 2010 U.S. Census Bureau, 5.2 million people in the United States identified as Native Americans (American Indians and Alaska Natives) either alone or in combination with 1 or more other cultures. In the United States, there are 566 Federally Recognized Native American Tribes (Bureau of Indian Affairs, 2012) and Nations. In Canada, as documented in the Indian Register (2011), maintained by the Aboriginal Affairs and Northern Development Canada, there are 617 First Nation communities.

There is a need to improve mental health care for Native Americans. The Indian Health Service (IHS), U.S. Department of Health and Human Services (2015) Mental Health Program, a part of the Federal Program for American Indians and Alaska Natives, offers culturally sensitive, comprehensive mental health services. For example, the Winnebago Counseling Center (WCC) in South Dakota offers counseling for "grief, anxiety, sleep problems, depression, anger management, stress, posttrauma reactions, family problems, interpersonal problems, and many other life situations." According to Walker (2014), the annual budget for IHS was $4.6 billion, of which only $266 million is allocated to mental health and

The Challenge of Recovery for African American Women

Alcohol and substance abuse is a national and transcultural phenomenon of epidemic proportions in many cultures. Substance abuse within the African American culture and communities has been a significant challenge for health care providers who care for the patients, families, and communities wrought with this debilitating epidemic. Hunte and Barry (2012) identified African Americans who feel unfairly treated, including being treated with less respect and courtesy, were more likely to treat their emotional pain with alcohol and drugs. The researchers found this finding troubling, as African Americans are more likely to live in neighborhoods advertising alcoholic beverages through billboards, signs, and local markets.

Reverend Williams (1992), at Glide Memorial Church in San Francisco's Tenderloin neighborhood, identified an epidemic of drug abuse in inner cities, what he identified as today's new form of slavery, "a slavery of addiction" (p. 3). Reverend Williams began a recovery program based on what he called a "smell of death" (p. 2). The "smell of death" came from many people, especially young mothers, strung out on crack cocaine, and the Reverend declared a "war on addiction" (p. 3). Since most of the individuals attending services at Glide memorial were African Americans, Williams developed a recovery program in conjunction with the church and community members. The recovery program was "culturally based" (p. 7) and included acts of recognition, self-definition, rebirth, and community and eventually formed the basis of the recovery program. Williams stressed that recovery was a process in which everyone needed to participate. He was able to help a community begin to deal with their cultural pain and move through the process of recovery from their drug and alcohol abuse.

In a transcultural ethnonursing research study conducted using Leininger's Culture Care Diversity and Universality: Theory of Nursing, Ehrmin (2000, 2001, 2005) entered the African American women's emic world to study the women living in an inner city transitional home for substance abuse. Transcultural nursing concepts and principles were valuable to gain insight about the women and their cultural experiences, with respect to their values, beliefs, meanings, and practices that influenced their use and abuse of substances and their cultural care needs in recovery. In order for substance-dependent African American women to successfully move through treatment and recovery for their substance abuse, they needed to feel respected, cared for, listened to, and treated in a nonjudgmental manner. The women wanted to be guided and directed in their treatment to learn to be productive members of society. The women also needed to resolve past cultural pain experiences. The predominant reason that women sought treatment and recovery for their addiction was their children. For many of the women, their children either had been taken away from them by Children's Services Board (CSB) or were currently living with family or other relatives. The women expressed unresolved maternal feelings of guilt and shame for their use of alcohol and drugs. Dealing with those feelings was key to women moving successfully through the process of recovery for substance abuse.

Clinical Implications

African American families are generally matriarchal families, and women have strong gender roles within the family. To facilitate the success of women in recovery, transcultural mental health nurses can help women learn to trust and develop positive supportive relationships with female care providers, other recovering women, and female members of their families. Substance-dependent women need to be supported in a nonjudgmental manner as they resolve past painful life experiences, particularly those having to do with perceived maternal failures during their active addiction. It is important to assess substance-dependent women for comorbid depression, which can increase a woman's risk for relapse.

References

Hunte, H., & Barry, A. (2012). Perceived discrimination and DSM-IV–based alcohol and illicit drug use disorders. *American Journal of Public Health, 102*(12), 111–117.

Ehrmin, J. T. (2000). Cultural implications of the 12-approach in addictions treatment and recovery. *Journal of Addictions Nursing, 12*, 37–41.

Ehrmin, J. T. (2001). Unresolved feelings of guilt and shame in the maternal role with substance-dependent African-American women. *Journal of Nursing Scholarship, 33*, 53–58.

Ehrmin, J. T. (2002). Family violence and culture care with African and Euro-American cultures in the United States. In M. Leininger & M. R. McFarland (Eds.), *Transcultural nursing: Concepts, theories, research & practice* (3rd ed., pp. 333–346). New York, NY: McGraw-Hill.

Ehrmin, J. T. (2005). Dimensions of culture care for substance-dependent African American women. *Journal of Transcultural Nursing, 16*, 117–125.

Williams, C. (1992). *No hiding place, empowerment and recovery for our troubled communities*. San Francisco, CA: Harper San Francisco.

substance abuse programs. Much work remains to be accomplished in overall mental health care for American Indians and Alaska Natives.

The Native American culture believes in holistic health care and generally has a holistic outlook in all aspects of their lives. Holism is a belief that the physical, mental, emotional, and spiritual dimensions of an individual are perceived as one. Native Americans, as a cultural group, are also perceived as one, although each tribe may have unique characteristics. The mind–body separation of Western health care is not present in the Native American culture (Yurkovich & Lattergrass, 2008). Traditional peoples bring cultures together in contemporary life in many ways. Ideally, individuals with more than one cultural affiliation can bring parts of each culture together without conflict. Figure 10-4 shows Native American

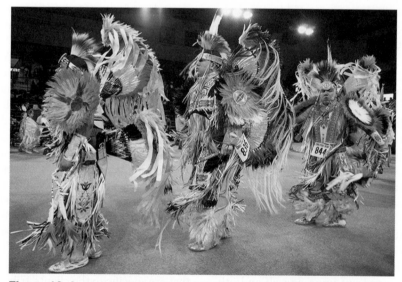

Figure 10-4. Native American Fancy Dancers (e-miizinigaajig) embrace their culture. Youth from the Saginaw Chippewa Tribe participate in a "powwow" where youth learn long-held traditions of their Native American culture. The theme of the powwow is "Celebrating Life," which refers to actively and energetically living your life to the fullest with your family (Wright, 2013).

Fancy Dancers (*e-miizinigaajig*) in a powwow at a Saginaw Chippewa Festival.

For Native Americans, acknowledging positive cultural strengths such as spirituality in all aspects of their lives, resiliency, and positive identity are necessary for healing within a cultural care perspective (Yurkovich & Lattergrass, 2008). It is important for nurses working with Native American clients to focus on such strengths as spirituality, resiliency, and positive identity to help clients in the healing process. In order to provide culturally competent care, health care professionals should work closely with native healers to integrate spirituality and other indigenous beliefs into treatment processes (Yurkovich & Lattergrass, 2008).

Gone (2009) conducted a study on the legacy of Native American historical trauma with staff and clients in a Native American Healing Lodge. Findings suggested connecting evidence-based and culturally sensitive treatment options with indigenous programs to create culturally sensitive interventions congruent with community values and norms. Program staff identified the importance of embracing the Native American indigenous heritage, identity, and spirituality in order to begin healing the detrimental effects of historical trauma and colonization. Nurses can help specific cultural groups grieve the past traumatic event(s) and resolve some of the past pain associated with such grief and trauma.

Alcohol has had an overwhelming impact on the mental health of Native Americans. Forced into a harsh reservation system, Native Americans were forced to give up their native lands and ways of life. Yellow Horse Brave Heart and DeBruyn (1998) utilized the literature on Jewish Holocaust survivors to develop the construct of historical trauma. The authors suggested that, for many individuals, the resulting anger and oppression are acted out upon oneself and others like the self, such as members of one's group. Native Americans have repeatedly suffered losses of family and community members to alcohol-related accidents, homicides, and suicide. Abuse, such as domestic violence (DV) and child abuse,

is a leading mental health concern among Native American communities throughout the country. "These layers of present losses in addition to the major traumas of the past fuel the anguish, psychologic numbing, and destructive coping mechanisms related to disenfranchised grief and historical trauma" suffered by Native Americans (Yellow Horse Brave Heart, & DeBruyn, 1998, pp. 68–69). The initial groundbreaking work of Yellow Horse Brave Heart and DeBruyn (1998) developing the theory of historical trauma provides mental health care professionals currently treating Native American clients for mental health illnesses, "an understanding of how the historical losses suffered generations ago have resulted in historical loss symptoms being transferred to subsequent and current generations of Native Americans" (Brown-Rice, 2014).

Kasl (1992) observed an anniversary celebration of a Native American healing center. He suggested that the Native Americans in attendance drew from several belief systems and referred to this phenomena as an "integrated faith." Other examples of integrated faith may be an informal Catholic mass integrating Native American wisdom and then followed by an Alcoholic Anonymous (AA) meeting. Many Native American tribes have developed their own mental health treatment centers that incorporate the concept of integrated faith, including those that specifically treat chemical dependencies (alcohol and drugs). These treatment centers (both inpatient and outpatient) are fully accredited by appropriate accreditation agencies and employ certified and licensed counselors, who are often Native Americans themselves. The services combine traditional beliefs with professional treatment. The services focus on wellness and healing; they may include spiritual retreats, talking circles, sweats, burning sage, smudge, and other practices that are specific to the clients' tribes.

For the Anishinabe people of the Michigan, Great Lakes region, a smudging ceremony or purification ceremony can take place anytime and is frequently used during times of stress at work or in the home. Some people perform a smudging

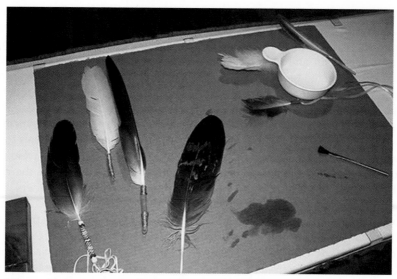

Figure 10-5. The eagle feather cleansing and honoring and feast of the Saginaw Chippewa Tribe promote cultural awareness and demonstrate honoring the life of the Anishinabe people (Great Lakes region) and the spirit of the eagle. This "gives blessings and strength to our people" (Sowmick, 2013).

ceremony when they hear bad news such as illness or death of a loved one. Four sacred medicines are used: sema, kiishig, mshkwadewashk (sage), and wiingash. The smoke from the medicines is used to cleanse the mind, body, and spirit. Eagle feathers are used to fan the smoke from burning the sacred medicine. Feathers, particularly eagle feathers (see Figure 10-5), symbolize trust, honor, and wisdom for Native Americans and are held as part of the Native American ethnohistory. Eagle feathers are also used in what is known as a talking circle ceremony in the Native American culture. Individuals sit in a circle and can talk about a specific topic or anything they want, depending on the circle. An eagle feather is passed around the circle and gives participants an opportunity to talk when they hold the feather (Anishinaabemdaa, 2014). Many of these ceremonies serve similar purposes as group therapy that is used in traditional mental health counseling treatment centers. Group therapy is generally facilitated by a group leader, commonly a mental health professional, to work with a group on individual mental health–focused issues within a group setting.

Native Americans frequently communicate through storytelling. So, allowing Native American clients to tell their story is an important and useful way to get information. Use of broad, open-ended questions facilitates obtaining a health history and other information in a culturally competent manner. As there is a focus on tribal and family viewpoints, how one views himself or herself is frequently based on how others in their tribe or family view them. So, rather than discourage tribal and family inclusion in treatment approaches, it may be important to help the client form an "interdependent" view of themselves, acknowledging the impact of treatment on the tribe and family is important to the client (DeCoteau, Anderson, & Hope, 2006).

Asian/Pacific Islander Culture: An Overview of Mental Health Concerns

For the United States 2010 to 2060 period, Asian Americans and Pacific Islanders are one of the fastest growing minority groups in the United States, second only to the Hispanic or Latino cultural groups. The Asian population is projected

to more than double, from 15.9 million in 2012 to 34.4 million in 2060, with its share of nation's total population climbing from 5.1% to 8.2% in the same period. The Native Hawaiian and Other Pacific Islander population is expected to nearly double, from 706,000 to 1.4 million (United States Census Bureau, 2012). Asian Americans and Pacific Islanders of Asian ancestry represent 43 diverse cultural groups from Korea, Japan, China, India, Cambodia, Vietnam, Indonesia, Philippines, and Papua New Guinea, to name only a few (United States Census Bureau, 2012).

For some Asian Americans and newly arrived immigrants from China and Japan, stigma related to mental health problems can be a stumbling block in seeking appropriate care. For example, a study by Gilbert et al. (2007) focused on Asian and non-Asian young women's shame related to mental health care and identified three components of shame: external, internal, and reflected. External shame is a belief that an individual will be viewed negatively for mental health problems; internal shame is evaluating oneself negatively; and reflected shame is a belief that having mental

health problems could bring shame to an individual's family or community. Results of this study suggest that Asian women had higher external and reflected shame beliefs than did non-Asian women. Asians also expressed concerns about confidentiality when talking about personal feelings/anxieties. This study suggests that stigma may play a role in seeking mental health care and may encourage individuals to seek care only among friends and family, avoiding professional mental health services and the risk of bringing shame to themselves and others.

Asian Americans' core cultural values of honor and pride and patriarchal obligations, particularly with elders, are important to understanding Asian American culture. Collective group harmony, including family and kin, rather than individual concerns, are significant cultural values (Leininger, 1995). Understanding core cultural values of the Asian American culture, particularly the importance of maintaining harmony, will help transcultural nurses plan care for clients with mental health problems in a culturally competent manner (see Figure 10-6).

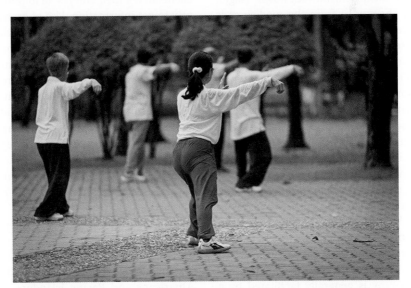

Figure 10-6. Tai chi, a low-impact Chinese martial art, is practiced to facilitate the relief of stress and a sense of mental well-being. Transcultural mental health nurses can explore the use of alternative techniques becoming more popular with diverse cultural groups (vanHurck/Shutterstock.com).

In a study of older Korean Americans exploring cultural attitudes toward mental health services, Jang et al. (2007) found that individuals who had been in the United States for a shorter time frame and had more severe levels of depression were more likely to have negative attitudes about mental health services. Cultural values and beliefs of older Korean Americans seemed to have a major influence on whether or not they viewed mental health services in a negative manner. Those individuals who identified mental illness with personal weakness or shame held more negative attitudes about using mental health services. However, if the individual associated depression as a health condition, then he or she had a more positive attitude about mental health services. Cultural values and beliefs about mental illness, including stigma associated with mental illness, were also found to be influential in individual's attitudes toward mental health services.

Community agencies have often provided mental health services specifically to Asian Americans. The National Alliance on Mental Illness (2011) reported deep cuts to state health care dollar allocations for mental health treatment for children and adults living with a serious mental illness. Many of these community agencies have suffered a severe cutback in services and are unable to provide the level and kinds of care that they have provided in the past. Recognition of cultural barriers, such as language, that have a direct effect on communication between nurses and other health care providers and clients and their family/significant other(s) can be preemptive and lead to more positive client outcomes.

Hispanic/Latino Culture: An Overview of Mental Health Concerns

Individuals of Hispanic or Latino descent are the fastest growing cultural group in the United States (United States Census Bureau, 2012). By 2060, approximately 128 million people, nearly one in three US residents, will self-identify as Hispanic Americans (United States Census Bureau, 2012). Hispanic countries include such diverse places as

Mexico, Puerto Rico, Cuba, Spain, and the United States; there is tremendous cultural diversity among the Hispanic/Latino groups.

In general, Mexican Americans (American citizens identifying as having Mexican ancestry) tend to rely on their family and extended family networks. Family and the extended family members are viewed as a whole and are highly valued. Family members rely on each other for socialization, support (emotional and monetary), and childcare, and, often, they expect loyalty from other family members. "Familismo (loyalty, reciprocity, and solidarity within the immediate and extended family)" is an important cultural value indicating the importance of the family in the Hispanic culture (Galanti, 2003). Nurses and other health care providers need to consider the importance of the family when making health care decisions for a client who has entered the American health care system, where individuality is valued. Mexican Americans have a lower incidence of mental illness when compared to other diverse cultural groups, possibly due to strong extended family connections and the role family networks play in dealing with anxiety and stresses, as well as the role of religion.

For many Hispanic immigrants, use of mental health services in the United States is low when compared to use of health care services for general health concerns. According to a report by the U.S. Department of Health and Human Services (2009), less than 1 in 11 Hispanic Americans with a mental health illness contacts a mental health care provider while less than 1 in 5 contacts a health care provider for a general health concern. For Hispanic immigrants with a mental health illness, less than 1 in 20 contacts a mental health care provider while 1 in 10 contacts a health care provider for general health concerns. According to the American Psychiatric Association (2015), many Hispanic individuals rely on their extended family, the community, traditional folk healers known as *curanderos* or *herbalistas*, and churches for help during a health crisis. Consequently, many Hispanic individuals with mental illness often go without seeking professional help for

mental health treatment. One of the main reasons for failure to seek professional mental health care services is Hispanics are the largest uninsured population in the United States. Cultural barriers, including language and fear of being stigmatized with a mental health illness, also serve to obstruct access to seeking professional mental health care.

In providing mental health care for Mexican Americans, nurses need to understand the values, beliefs, and practices of the culture that impact the mental health needs of their clients. The bonds in the traditional Mexican American family are often very strong, and the father is the authority figure. *Machismo* is a term used in the Latino culture to describe the traditional male gender role. Machismo has both positive (strength, courage, responsibility) and negative (aggression, dominance over women and the family) connotations (Dietrich & Schuett, 2013; Torres, Solberg, & Carlstrom, 2002). Dietrich and Schuett (2013) described machismo as the traditional male gender role in the Latino culture. Machismo is often viewed by outsiders as "exaggerated male pride." However, in the Latino culture, it is a respected position of honor vital to one's self-esteem and manhood. The father or oldest male relative is the power figure in most families and may make health decisions for other family members. While in private, some women may hold more power, in public, women show respect for their husbands. The authors also talked about the importance of what is called "Culture of Honor," which encourages women and family members to consider the reputation of the family. If the woman is abused for violating the honor of the male, then the abuse may be considered culturally acceptable. For example, if a married woman flirted with another man, the woman's husband would be justified in abusing his wife to maintain the honor of his family. Many of these deep-seated cultural practices and values are difficult for mental health care providers to influence and help to modify unhealthy behaviors.

Although intimate partner violence (IPV) and family violence associated with male dominance in the Mexican American culture may be prevalent, as in other cultural groups, it is frequently underreported (Kemp, 2005) (see Evidence-Based Practice 10-6). Dietrich and Schuett (2013) identified that using even the most conservative prevalence estimates about IPV in the Latino culture calls for immediate attention to this serious problem.

The Latino culture also holds strong expectations for women, with an emphasis on submissiveness and reverence toward men. The female role has its roots with the Virgin Mary and is referred to as *marianismo*, indicating women should be pure and self-sacrificing and devote their lives to their family. The traditional Hispanic cultural values for females may lead to a higher incidence of IPV, where women are encouraged to be submissive and "obey" their husbands. Nurses and other health care providers need to be aware of the importance of modesty for Hispanic women, particularly older women, and should try to keep them covered during physical exams (Galanti, 2003).

Religion is very influential in Hispanic communities and may play a major role in the mental health illnesses of Hispanic Americans. Many Hispanic Americans are Roman Catholics, and faith and church activities are an influential part of their daily life activities (Kemp, 2005). Some studies have identified religious and cultural barriers to professional mental health care as some Hispanic Americans report that they trust in God, and "if I am sick, it is his will" (Carter-Pokras et al., 2008). These attitudes often delay appropriate preventative care as well as treatment of mental health illnesses.

The hot and cold system is one of the most prevalent folk systems found in Mexican American cultural groups. The hot and cold system is based on balancing substances in the body and the outside environment. Various substances including food, water, and different herbs and medications are considered hot or cold. Lack of balance is thought to be the cause for illness: the mind and body are viewed as intertwined, and balance is sought in all aspects of life (Berry, 2002). Various diseases are identified as either hot or cold and treated with the corresponding therapy. Hot diseases are treated with cold and cold diseases are

Violence Against Women

DV or IPV is of epidemic proportions and affects individuals, primarily women, in virtually all cultures, nationally and internationally. According to the National Coalition Against Domestic Violence (NCADV), domestic violence "is the willful intimidation, physical assault, battery, sexual assault, and/or other abusive behavior perpetrated by an intimate partner against another" (National Coalition Against Domestic Violence, 2014, downloaded 4-13-14). WHO identified recent prevalence figures of "35% of women worldwide have experienced either intimate partner violence or non-partner sexual violence in their lifetime" (2013). Risk factors for being a victim of intimate partner and sexual violence include "low education, witnessing violence between parents, exposure to abuse during childhood and attitudes accepting violence and gender inequality" (World Health Organization, 2014c).

Approximately 30% of women in a relationship have experienced physical or sexual violence by their partner. The subheading of "victim" is identified rather than "survivor," because not all women survive the violence. According to WHO, approximately "38% of murders of women are committed by an intimate partner" (2013). The statistics identified are staggering and indicate how widespread this epidemic has become. However, equally alarming, according to the NCADV, is the fact that most cases of DV/IPV go unreported.

According to Gonzalez-Guarda, Cummings, Becerra, Fernandez, and Mesa (2013), given that Hispanics are disproportionately affected by IPV, limited IPV prevention interventions have been identified for this population. The Partnership for Domestic Violence Prevention (PDVP) conducted a 1-year participatory action research study at the level of the community to identify IPV prevention interventions. Immigrants, particularly undocumented immigrant Hispanic women, were identified as most vulnerable because of perceived obstacles to leaving an abusive relationship. It was identified that prevention programs should target some of the most vulnerable Hispanic subgroups including Hispanic youth, undocumented Hispanic immigrants, and pregnant women. Interventions should address the cultural context of IPV within the Hispanic community. Cultural factors included family, faith, traditional gender roles that promote male dominance, the acculturation process, community ties, and various barriers to access appropriate services. School-based teen dating prevention programs were identified by community members as important in stopping the IPV cycle. It was identified the Center for Disease Control at the Federal level is working on "Safe Dates" programs specific to family, school, and neighborhood environments to address the issues of dating violence (Centers for Disease Control and Prevention [CDC], 2014).

Risk factors for being a perpetrator include "low education, exposure to child maltreatment or witnessing violence in the family, harmful use of alcohol, attitudes accepting of violence and gender inequality" (World Health Organization, 2014c).

Clinical Implications

It is important to talk to women about DV/IPV when they come in for health care services. Mexican American women are generally open to disclosing and discussing their experiences of DV and IPV if they believe the health care provider is willing to listen and facilitate breaking the silence surrounding the abuse; it is important to help the women find resources available to them in their respective communities (Gonzalez-Guarda, et al., 2011). It is important for nurses and other health care providers to understand the devastating lifelong implications of sexual violence. Care should be taken to understand abuse nationally and internationally, and "future policies and programs should focus on abuse within families and eliminate the acceptance of and impunity surrounding sexual violence" (Peterman, Palermo, & Bredenkamp, 2011, p. 1060).

References

Centers for Disease Control and Prevention (CDC). (2014). Dating matters TM initiative. Retrieved August 19, 2014 from http://www.cdc.gov/violenceprevention/datingmatters/index.html

(continued)

Violence Against Women (continued)

Gonzalez-Guarda, R., Cummings, A., Becerra, M., Fernandez, M., & Mesa, I. (2013). Needs and preferences for the prevention of intimate partner violence among Hispanics: A Community's perspective. *Journal of Primary Prevention*, 34,221–235.

National coalition against domestic violence. (2014). Downloaded on 4-13-14, http://www.ncadv.org/files/DomesticViolenceFactSheet(National).pdf

Peterman, A., Palermo, T., & Bredenkamp, C. (2011). Estimates and Determinants of Sexual Violence Against Women in the Democratic Republic of Congo. *American Journal of Public Health, 101*(6), 1060–1067.

World Health Organization. (2014c). Violence against women: Intimate partner and sexual violence against women. Fact sheet N°239 http://www.who.int/mediacentre/factsheets/fs239/en/

treated with hot (Spector, 2013). It is imperative that mental health nurses understand the importance of these cultural practices when caring for their Hispanic and Latino clients; seemingly "bizarre" behavior or practices can be common and culturally acceptable treatment options.

Arab Muslim Culture: An Overview of Mental Health Concerns

There are over 48 countries with at least half of the population identified as Muslim, or people who practice the Islamic faith, including Pakistan, Turkey, Egypt, Iran, Afghanistan, Iraq, Saudi Arabia, Syria, Libya, and Jordan. The Arabic language is spoken in Arab Muslim countries, and Islam is the main religion of the people. Islam is growing more rapidly than any other religion in the world. There are two major religious orthodoxies of Muslims: the Sunni and the Shi'a (Luna, 2002). More than a billion Muslims follow the Islamic fundamental beliefs that are described as "Articles of Faith." Worship in the Islamic faith is known as the "five pillars of Islam" and consists of the "declaration of faith, prayer, fasting, charity, and pilgrimage" (Mofty, 2013). Ramadan is the 9th month of the Islamic calendar and was the month in which the Koran was revealed to the Prophet Muhammad. During the month of Ramadan, Muslims are required to abstain from food and drink from dawn until dusk. Devout Muslims pray five times each day. Prior to prayer,

each person must perform a cleansing of the body, which signifies a pure soul.

There are a number of Islamic religious requirements specific to men and women such as an unrelated male should not touch females, including shaking hands; make direct eye contact with each other; or be alone in a room with one another (Simpson & Carter, 2008). In the Arab Muslim culture, women are required to avoid raising their voices so they will not be overheard by strangers (Abushaikha & Oweis, 2005). Talking in a manner in which other clients and observers can overhear what is being communicated would then seem to be incongruent with the women's needs of privacy. In a study conducted by Simpson and Carter (2008) on Muslim women's experiences with health care in the rural United States, one participant described writing a letter to her physician prior to her health care appointment to identify her religious needs. She stated: "I don't shake hands and I would prefer not to be examined by a male. I don't speak with a male unnecessarily either, and conversations with males will be succinct and to the point" (p. 19). When Arab Muslim women believed their religious beliefs were violated, they experienced feelings of guilt and viewed the health care experience as negative; when no religious beliefs were violated, they viewed their experience as more positive. However, the women also expressed an understanding that it is difficult for health care providers outside of their culture to understand all of their cultural beliefs and

practices. Several women identified being treated differently by health care providers because they wore the Islamic head covering (hijab) (Simpson & Carter, 2008).

There are a limited number of psychiatric beds in Arab countries, ranging from 30 to less than five per 100,000 population. Psychiatric nurses range from 23 in Bahrain to 0.03 in Somalia per 100,000 population. A number of countries have agreed to integrate mental health into their current health care delivery system, yet few have actually integrated the services. Cultural beliefs about being possessed and sorcery or the "evil eye" affect interpretation of mental health symptoms. Prior to seeing health care professionals, Arab Muslims may seek traditional healers for mental health problems. Traditional healers hold special importance to Arab Muslim people because of their affiliation and connection to the community. Traditional healers also deal with mystical and unknown (Okasha, 2012).

Seventy to 80% of mental health clients in Arab countries tend to present with somatic symptoms for psychological issues. There is a stigma about mental health problems, and the client who presents with somatic complaints is protected from the stigma of being diagnosed with a mental health illness. However, this creates difficulties for the client as he or she is treated for physical rather than psychological problems (Okasha, 2003). Nurses and other health care providers in emergency departments need to be aware of this phenomenon and assess the client for any mental health concerns. The subordinate position of Arab women places them at risk for developing mental health disorders such as depression, anxiety, and suicidal behaviors (Douki, Ben Xineb, Nacef, & Halbreich, 2007). For individuals from Arab communities, stigma associated with mental illness is considered a major barrier to accessing mental health services related to the shame associated with disclosing personal and family issues to outsiders (Ciftci, Jones, & Corrigan, 2013).

Jadalla and Lee (2012) conducted a study on the relationship between acculturation and health status for Arab Americans living in southern California to assess the physical and mental health of the participants. The researchers found that acculturation was an important factor when assessing the well-being of Arab Americans, particularly their mental health. The results indicated that the Arab American participants who had a higher assimilation into the American culture were associated with significantly better mental health.

While acculturation has been shown to be beneficial, Arab Americans moving to the United States can experience great stress associated with acculturation difficulties. There is evidence to suggest that the experience of prejudice, intolerance, and hostility toward Arab Americans has increased in the United States following the terrorist attacks on 9/11. Arab Americans have been victims of racism, aggression, insulting speech, and discrimination on the basis of their cultural religious beliefs and practices and national origin (Kulwicki, Khalifa, & Moore, 2008). Arab American nurses in Detroit participated in a study to explore the influence of the terrorist attacks on 9/11 on their profession as nurses. Overall, the Arab American nurses had not experienced hate crimes or major work-related retaliation, such as termination. The discrimination the nurses did experience was in the form of verbal insults about their cultural and religious practices such as wearing a hijab, the traditional head covering worn by Muslim women. One in seven of the nurse participants had experienced a situation wherein clients and their families refused their care (Kulwicki, Khalifa, & Moore, 2008).

Culturally Competent Mental Health Care

The interpretation of behavior generally transpires within the context of the specific culture in which it occurs. However, when clients and families from diverse cultural groups come to institutions of the dominant culture, the behavior is identified and interpreted by the

dominant culture. Frequently, behavior can be misinterpreted and/or distorted if health care providers are not knowledgeable about caring for clients from diverse cultural groups. Particularly with mental health, diagnoses applied to clients based on certain behaviors may be inaccurate; if the same behavior were understood and interpreted within the context of the client's culture, a different diagnosis might be made, with different treatment, or no diagnosis at all. Inaccurate mental health labels can have a negative impact on an individual and family for years. Communication and cultural knowledge, leading to cultural competency, can have a positive impact on the mental health care that is provided to clients of diverse cultural groups and lead to positive experiences for both clients and the nurses providing the care.

Developing Cultural Competence

Developing a mutually trusting relationship with clients improves plans of care and increases the likelihood of more optimal health outcomes; this is particularly important in mental health nursing care. Because of difficult experiences with past family and other relationships, it may be difficult for some clients with mental health needs to trust others, including mental health care providers. Early on, Leininger (1991b) recognized the importance of developing a trusting relationship with participants in a research study and developed "Leininger's Stranger to Trusted Friend Enabler Guide" (p. 82). Leininger also identified the guide would be helpful for clinicians. The purpose of the enabler was to facilitate the researcher, or clinician, to "move from mainly a distrusted stranger to a trusted friend" (p. 82) in order to establish a trusting relationship as a clinician. According to Egan (2014), helpers need to have an understanding that some clients have a fear of betrayal and, therefore, have a more difficult time in developing trust with the helper. Clients who have difficulty in trusting others may reveal themselves in a much more guarded manner, particularly in a mental health care setting. Particularly for mental health nurses, patience

and encouragement are needed when helping clients with a fear of trust. An understanding of the client's culture increases the likelihood of improved health outcomes.

Nurses are increasingly caring for clients from diverse cultures and are expected to have a broad understanding of culture in order to provide culturally competent mental health care. Culturally competent nursing care for clients from diverse cultures becomes crucial in caring for clients with mental health needs. Some questions that nurses may be asking are what exactly does *culturally congruent care* mean? How can a transcultural mental health nurse understand the cultural values, beliefs, and practices of all the culturally diverse clients a nurse will care for over the lifetime of his or her career? Well, one answer may be that, of course, you cannot understand the values, beliefs, and practices of all of the clients you will care for in your career. However, nurses can become familiar with the values, beliefs, and practices of the culturally diverse groups to whom they do provide care.

Nurses have identified the importance of culturally sensitive care. Although learning to be sensitive to client's cultural values, beliefs, and practices is important, it has became obvious that transcultural nurses need to move beyond being "sensitive" to competency-based cultural care. *Cultural competence* is defined as a process in which nurses strive to work successfully within the cultural context of individuals, families, and communities (Andrews & Boyle, 1997; Campinha-Bacote, 2002). Campinha-Bacote (2009) identified that cultural competency "requires nurses to see themselves as becoming culturally competent rather than being culturally competent" (p. 49).

Buchwald et al. (1994) used the term "**cultural blind spot**," sometimes referred to as **cultural blindness**, to describe the assumption that if a person is similar in appearance and behaviors as the care provider, then there are no perceived cultural differences or potential barriers to giving appropriate care. The cultural blind spot supports people's beliefs that they understand the culture

and have had similar cultural encounters. Thus, a person could conclude he or she has culturally competent skills. However, it is this lack of awareness of differences that creates the cultural blind spot. Transcultural mental health nurses need to be aware of the phenomenon of cultural blind spot/cultural blindness because of the unintended influence it can have on care of diverse populations of mental health clients.

Intrapersonal Reflection

Several transcultural nursing leaders identified the importance of conducting a personal inventory of one's own cultural values, beliefs, and practices to begin to identify, understand, and remove personal cultural bias, ethnocentrism, and prejudice (Andrews & Boyle, 1997; Leininger, 2000). It is important for nurses to explore and reflect on their own cultural values, beliefs, practices, expressions, meanings, and own cultural norms in order to identify and begin to understand personal biases, prejudices, and other barriers to caring for clients in a culturally congruent and competent manner. Although tolerance may be the opposite of prejudice, it is an inadequate benchmark in caring for clients in a culturally competent manner. Nurses and other health care providers need to celebrate diversity and recognize the challenge to continually explore areas within themselves or others that may block or serve as barriers to caring for clients in a culturally competent manner. Each nurse needs to explore his or her own personal values, beliefs, and practices in order to recognize areas of prejudice, bias, stereotyping, and ethnocentrism of culturally diverse individuals, families, and communities.

Gordijn, Koomen, and Stapel (2001) studied whether an individual's level of knowledge of cultural stereotypes about minority groups was universal or whether that knowledge was influenced by that individual's level of prejudice. Findings indicated that an individual's level of prejudice was related to that individual's level of knowledge about cultural stereotypes with minorities. Findings such as these should encourage transcultural mental health nurses to explore their personal prejudices and biases toward people from diverse cultures and peel away and expose stereotypes that impede caring for culturally diverse clients.

Important Factors to Consider in Transcultural Mental Health Nursing

Three important factors that need to be considered when discussing transcultural mental health nursing are communication and language, spirituality, and experiences of pain. Mental health care is dependent on initiating a dialogue with the client. It is even more important for transcultural mental health care providers to effectively communicate with clients who may have some difficulty with meanings and expressions of the dominant English language in the United States. Spirituality is an integral part of mental well-being and has become a focus for mental health care providers. Transcultural mental health care providers are increasingly exploring diverse cultural expressions, meanings, and practices of spirituality. Chronic pain is generally thought of as a physical, bodily pain; however, there is an emotional and mental health component to experiences of pain that may vary widely depending on one's cultural values, beliefs, and practices.

Communication and Language

Communication, both verbal and nonverbal, is one of the most important skills for mental health nurses. Communication is even more important with culturally diverse mental health clients, where language may serve as a barrier and make the process of communication more difficult. **Interpersonal communication** helps mental health nurses assess each client's values, beliefs, and practices about their mental health care. Communicating with each client is important in caring for clients in a culturally congruent and competent manner.

Communication between the mental health nurse and the client and family generally brings together the exchange of two diverse cultures, that of the nurse and that of the client. Therefore, it is also important for nurses to have an understanding of their own cultural values, beliefs, and practices, so they can better understand the diversity between their own cultural values, beliefs, and practices and those of the client and family, particularly as these phenomena relate to mental health care.

Culture influences each interaction nurses have with clients. Since an important part of mental health care is communicating and providing counseling for clients with mental health illnesses, if nurses are not knowledgeable about the cultural context in which their communication is being interpreted, there is a possibility that the message can be misunderstood. Rosenberg (2003) described how cultural conditioning, a socialization process that influences how we think and behave, has a major impact on each of us. Becoming consciously aware of our individual cultural conditioning is a key to lessening the effect it has on us. Communication is crucial when nurses are caring for culturally diverse clients with such mental health problems as schizophrenia, bipolar disorder, or major depression, where clients and their family or kin may be confused or even fear a health care system in which they have no previous experience. Effective cross-cultural communication skills are particularly important when caring for mental health clients. Developing lasting meaningful relationships across potential social barriers such as ethnicity and culture contributes to improved communication.

Mental health nurses understand the importance of developing trust with clients and their family/kin networks. Taking time to develop trust with clients who do not speak English or speak minimal English can be very challenging, particularly given the increasingly culturally diverse population seeking mental health care. Sometimes, health care providers can become irritated that clients and family members do not speak the dominant English language. When there is a possibility

to have a certified translator/interpreter serve as an interpreter, that is the ideal choice rather than using family members or other staff who may not understand complex health situations. Family members should be encouraged to offer family support rather than serve as an interpreter.

People who do not speak English identify care as less supportive and more rushed than do those individuals who do speak English (Simpson & Carter, 2008). Whenever possible, a translator is preferred for barriers in communicating the language between care provider and clients seeking treatment, particularly for mental health care. Caregivers are more confident when a translator is present and interprets the client's words verbatim whenever possible, in order to maintain accuracy and reduce translation bias (Olivares & Altarriba, 2009). However, Bowes and Domokos (1995) found that speaking the same language, while important, is not the most important element in communicating with clients from diverse cultural backgrounds. The attitude of the care provider is instrumental in helping the client be open to treatment options. Communicating an understanding of cultural diversity helps facilitate the client–nurse relationship. On the other hand, authoritarian care providers have a negative impact on treatment compliance.

Bowes and Domokos (1995) make a distinction between language and communication, suggesting that language has more to do with the technical aspect of speech, while communication consists of both verbal and nonverbal elements, including the provider's attitude. For a number of culturally diverse clients and their families/kin, there are cultural values that influence what subjects are appropriate to discuss with health care providers. Some topics (e.g., sexual activities) may be considered inappropriate to discuss with health care providers. Other topics that most of us consider appropriate to discuss with a health care provider in the United States are not necessarily viewed that way by persons from different cultures. For example, in Asian and Latino cultures, individuals would not communicate dissatisfaction with services. In a study on Latino health disparities, one

nurse participant in the study stated, "If someone does not like the doctor or does not agree, they will not speak up or say anything because they are taught that it is rude to do this" (Carter-Pokras et al., 2008, p. 163). Even in conducting a health history and assessment, what are culturally acceptable questions to ask in the United States may not be acceptable in other countries and cultures. There are other factors that may have a profound influence on the communication between clients and health care providers. Undocumented migrants may fear that health care providers would turn them in to the authorities if providers learned that their clients were in the United States illegally (Carter-Pokras et al., 2008).

Empathy is one of the most important communication skills that transcultural mental health nurses and other health care providers can use with clients from diverse cultural backgrounds. In using empathy in communicating with clients, health care providers are attempting to understand what a client is experiencing or has experienced—trying to put themselves in the client's place and feel and experience what the client is feeling and experiencing—and then communicating that understanding back to the individual client (Egan, 2014). Empathic communication helps the health care provider to better understand the situation or context of the client as well as the cultural norms and values that structure that context and influence the client. For example, if a client was sitting in his or her hospital room crying, the nurse would know to further explore that client's feelings. According to Rasoal, Jungert, Hau, Stwine, and Andersson (2009), the ability to use "ethnocultural empathy" (p. 300) has become crucial for health care providers in their interactions with clients. It is important to communicate back to the client and family your understanding of their experience so they may clarify whether you have accurately identified the client's perception of a particular experience (Egan, 2014).

Empathy becomes very important in trying to understand the experience and feelings of mental health clients and their families. Attempting to understand the experience of abuse, schizophrenia, depression, bipolar disorders, and other mental health issues is crucial to understand the perspectives of the client and family (Figure 10-7).

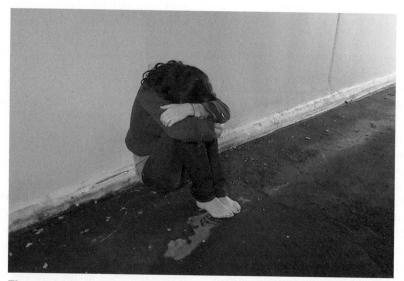

Figure 10-7. A rape victim covers her face. Numerous feelings haunt rape survivors for years. Fear, shame, humiliation, and emotional pain are areas transcultural mental health nurses can facilitate healing through therapeutic empathy and counseling (ChameleonsEye/Shutterstock.com).

For transcultural mental health care providers, empathy needs to be communicated, taking into consideration the beliefs, values, and practices, or in other words the "norms," of a culture. When communicating with clients from other cultures, particularly for those who do not speak English or for whom English is a second language, there is an increased risk of miscommunication.

Mental health nurses need to practice culturally competent communication skills to improve care for an ever-increasing population of culturally diverse mental health clients. Becoming aware of the importance of communication is key to providing culturally competent mental health care. Taking into account the cultural values, beliefs, meanings, practices, expressions, and cultural norms of specific cultures takes knowledge, experience, and patience in acquiring these skills. In addition, basic verbal and nonverbal communication skills such as tone of voice, use of probes and clarification, listening, empathy, facial expressions and body gestures, for both the nurses themselves and for the clients and family members, will help to improve overall communication and culturally competent mental health care.

Spirituality

Although the terms spirituality and religion are sometimes used interchangeably, *spirituality* refers to a broad sense of the inner experience of the self and a search for meaning while *religion* generally involves an institution with a given set of rules and observances involving devotion and ritual. There are many spiritual and religious themes to mental health disorders such as schizophrenia, bipolar disorder, psychosis, hallucinations, and delusions. Transcultural mental health nurses care for clients who have diverse cultural values, beliefs, meanings, and practices, many of which are grounded in spiritual and religious beliefs. This applies to clients and families from all of the world's major religious systems, Jewish, Christian, Islamic, and others.

A phenomenological research study attempted to answer the question with Australian mental health clients from a community mental health center: "What does spirituality mean for people with a mental illness?" (Wilding, Muir-Cochrane, & May, 2006, p. 144). Clients were not recruited to the study if they were experiencing psychosis or exacerbation of symptoms. Findings indicated that spirituality became increasingly important in client's lives after being diagnosed with a mental illness. Spiritual experiences of the clients could be interpreted as signs and symptoms of mental illness, depending on who was interpreting the experiences. Clients expressed a fear that mental health nurses would label them as mentally ill when their spiritual beliefs and experiences were similar to symptoms of mental illness. As previously discussed, the interpretation of one's cultural values, beliefs, and practices takes place within the dominant culture or power structure in which the situation or event occurs. Therefore, it is quite likely that within a mental health setting, values, beliefs, and practices would be interpreted according to the mental health professional's views rather than those of the client.

Spirituality and religious practices can play an influential role in enhancing mental health and emotional stability. For example, many African Americans view their church as the focal point of their lives. Within the African American church, emotions can be released that cannot be expressed in many other social situations and friendships. The African American church functions in promoting a high level of self-esteem, particularly for those individuals and communities in poverty-stricken environments. The role of the African American church "as a cornerstone for optimal health care cannot be emphasized enough" (Geiger, Appel, Davidhizar, & Davis, 2008, p. 382). Given this important role the African American church plays in the lives of parishioners, the churches may be uniquely positioned to overcome barriers such as stigma, distrust, and limited access that contribute to racial disparities in professional mental health care and service utilization (Hankerson & Weissman, 2012). In addition, health care providers could partner with churches and develop culturally congruent interventions

to improve care African Americans connected to various churches. Church leaders could also begin to develop relationships with professional mental health care providers to refer parishioners needing more acute mental health care services.

Bonifield (2009), in a report for CNN about African American churches fighting mental health "demons," described how African American church leaders were taking a lead in reaching out to those who need mental health services. In an effort to change attitudes about mental illness, concerned Black clergy of Atlanta established a connection with the National Alliance on Mental Illness to educate their church members about the signs and symptoms of mental illness. The church leaders suggested that it may be helpful for an individual to go to a church pastor if he or she was experiencing minor depression. Pastors were trained to recognize early signs and symptoms of depression and how to refer parishioners with major depression to mental health facilities. In another example, the Tennessee Department of Mental Health and Magellan Health Services, in collaboration with African American churches in various Tennessee communities, initiated "Emotional Fitness Centers" to screen for signs and symptoms of mental illness with parishioners seeking emotional support. Listening was stressed as the most important skill a pastor can use with someone seeking emotional support.

Experiences of Pain

In mental health nursing, the client's experience of pain can be manifested in many different ways. Unlike other somatic symptoms frequently associated with mental health issues, pain has a component that includes emotional elements. Psychosocial factors have been found to influence pain. In a study by Palmer et al. (2008) on somatic complaints, mood, and self-rated health as predictors of arm pain, mental health was found to be a strong predictor of complaints of arm pain in adults from a British community. Beliefs about causation and prognosis of arm pain were also associated with persistence of symptoms.

There is increasing evidence to suggest that pain can be a physical symptom of depression and that pain and depression are common comorbidities. According to Hall-Flavin (2013), depression can lead to pain and vice versa. In fact, pain and depression may create a "vicious cycle in which pain worsens symptoms of depression, and then the resulting depression worsens feelings of pain." It seems to be extremely difficult to separate the somatic, physical component of pain from the psychological component of pain. In a study conducted by Bonnewyn et al. (2009), researchers found that chronic pain and mood disorders were common in elderly populations. Elderly individuals with a 12-month major depressive episode were more likely to have painful physical symptoms than were those persons without major depression.

There is the concept of psychosomatic pain, or pain with psychological components, and this pain is expressed differently by cultural groups. One of the distinct types of depression with Haitian women is "douluer de corps (pain in the body)" (Nicholas et al., 2007, p. 87). Barkwell (2005) studied Native Americans (Ojibwa) with cancer pain. They described their pain as "all that was most painful in life" and included the following properties in their description of cancer pain: "physical sensation, threatening cognitions, emotional, social and spiritual anguish, and intuitive sensing" (p. 454). In a study to differentiate somatic versus psychological symptoms as a cultural expression of depression, Chinese outpatients reported more somatic symptoms compared to Euro-Canadians, who reported more psychological symptoms specific to the diagnosis of depression (Ryder et al., 2008).

Lee, Kleinman, and Kleinman (2007) have suggested that knowledge about depression and other mental illnesses is based on research conducted with Western populations. In a study with Chinese clients in Guangzhou (Canton), China, in an outpatient mental health service, clients experiencing symptoms of depression identified numerous affective symptoms, including sadness, preverbal pain, social disharmony,

and sleeplessness. The authors emphasized how important it is to study depression cross-culturally, in order to be more sensitive and appropriate with culturally diverse populations.

Summary

This chapter explored perspectives on transcultural mental health nursing care. The goal is to help nurses provide culturally competent care that improves the health and well-being of culturally diverse mental health clients. Nurses can increase their competency by understanding cultural values, beliefs, practices, meanings, expressions, and cultural norms of diverse cultures specific to the mental health and well-being of individuals, families/kin, and communities. Competency-based transcultural knowledge is essential in today's complex mental health environment.

REVIEW QUESTIONS

1. Describe the influence of culture on mental health care values, beliefs, and practices.
2. Identify specific cultural values, beliefs, and practices of three diverse cultural groups and how transcultural mental health nurses might facilitate culturally congruent care in a mental health care system.
3. Compare and contrast your cultural values, beliefs, and practices about mental health care with that of another cultural group.
4. Critically explore and reflect on any personal or familial biases, prejudices, and other culturally specific barriers that would impact your ability to provide culturally congruent care.
5. Identify five communication skills that facilitate culturally competent mental health care.

CRITICAL THINKING ACTIVITIES

1. Describe a personal clinical experience you have had or observed where a cultural

misunderstanding occurred. How did you feel either as a participant or as an observer? How do you believe the other individual(s) involved in the situation felt? How might the situation have been resolved in a culturally congruent manner?

2. Role-play several clinical situations in which cultural misunderstandings occurred. Then, role-play how you would resolve the cultural misunderstandings in a culturally congruent manner.

3. Discuss the impact an incorrect mental health diagnosis and label might have on individuals' lives.

4. Collect data on knowledge and skills for culturally congruent transcultural mental health nursing by interviewing someone from a culture that is very different from your own. Practice some basic interpersonal communication skills to get to know the person and establish some basic trust; ask the individual about their values, beliefs, and practices related to mental health and mental illness. Then, search the literature for information to read about that individual's cultural group. Regardless of whether your interviewee is from Haiti, Japan, or another cultural group and is gay, young, or elderly, consider if what you have read either represents or does not represent the individual you have interviewed.

5. Think about various times in your life that you have been involved with a group of people with whom you have felt comfortable, connected to, and shared similar values, beliefs, and practices. Think about the times in your life that you have been involved with a group of people with whom you did not feel comfortable and connected to and did not share similar values, beliefs, and practices. Compare and contrast those different experiences in your life. How might it feel for an individual from a different culture to come

into the group you felt comfortable with, connected to, and shared similar values, beliefs, and practices?

6. Imagine you are working with several nurses who imitate clients and their families who have difficulty speaking English and make fun of some of the cultural values, beliefs, and practices of culturally diverse individuals and families who are different from their own. How might you deal with this situation? Try role-playing the situation from different perspectives and using different communication skills not only to challenge the actions of your coworkers but also to help them begin to understand the impact of their behavior on others.

7. Imagine you are working with a client and his or her extended family who do not speak English. What are some ways you might communicate with your client and the family? Role-play some options you might try to communicate with your client and family.

8. You are caring for a patient from an Arab Muslim culture in a clinical setting, and the patient is exhibiting behaviors that you believe may be signs and symptoms of mental illness. Describe some of the signs and symptoms you might be observing. Describe some of the techniques you might use to differentiate whether the behavior is a manifestation of cultural values, beliefs, and practices you are not familiar with or are a result of a mental illness?

REFERENCES

Abdullah, T., & Brown, T. L. (2011). Mental illness stigma and ethnocultural beliefs, values, and norms: An integrative review, *Clinical Psychology Review, 31*, 934–938.

Abushaikha, L., & Oweis, A. (2005). Labor pain experience and intensity: A Jordanian perspective. *International Journal of Nursing Practice, 11*(1), 33–38.

Al-Omari, H., & Pallikkathayil, L. (2008). Psychological acculturation: A concept analysis with implications for nursing practice. *Journal of Transcultural Nursing, 19,* 126–133.

American Psychiatric Association. (2000). *Diagnostic and statistical manual of mental disorders* (4th ed.—text revision). Washington, DC: American Psychiatric Association.

American Psychiatric Association. (2013). *Diagnostic and Statistical Manual of Mental Disorders, DSM-5* (5th ed.). Washington, DC: American Psychiatric Association.

American Psychiatric Association. (2015). Hispanic-latino mental health. Retrieved January 10, 2015. http://www.psychiatry.org/mental-health/people/hispanics-latinos

Andrews, M. M., & Boyle, J. S. (1997). Competence in transcultural nursing care. *American Journal of Nursing, 98*(8), 16AAA–16DDD.

Anishinaabemdaa. (2014). Ceremonies, Manidokewinan. Retrieved 5, 2014. http://www.anishinaabemdaa.com/ceremonies.htm

Armour, M. P., Bradshaw, W., & Roseborough, D. (2009). African Americans and recovery from severe mental illness. *Social Work in Mental Health, 7*(6), 602–622.

Barkwell, D. (2005). Cancer pain: Voices of the Ojibway people. *Journal of Pain and Symptom Management, 30*(5), 454–464.

Bell, P., & Peterson, D. (1992). *Cultural pain and African Americans: Unspoken issues in early recovery.* Hazelden Publishing Center City, MN.

Berry, A. (2002). Culture care of the Mexican American family, In M. Leininger & M. R. McFarland (Eds.), *Transcultural nursing: Concepts, theories, research & practice* (3rd ed., pp. 363–373). New York, NY: McGraw-Hill.

Bolin, J. N., & Bellamy, G. (2013). Rural Healthy People 2020. Available online http://www.srph.tamhsc.edu/centers/srhrc/images/rhp2020#rhp2020

Bonifield, J. (2009). African-American churches fighting mental health 'demons.' CNN: Paging Dr. Gupta, July 17, 1–6. URL: http://pagingdrgupta.blogs.cnn.com/2009/07/17/African-American-churches-fighting-mental-healthdemons

Bonnewyn, A., Katona, C., Bruffaerts, R., Haro, J. M., de Graaf, R., Alonso, J., & Demyttenaere, K. (2009). Pain and depression in older people: Comorbidity and patterns of help seeking. *Journal of Affective Disorders, 117*(3), 193–196.

Bowes, A., & Domokos, T. (1995). South Asian women and their GPs: Some issues of communication. *Social Sciences in Health: International Journal of Research & Practice, 1*(1), 22–33.

Bridges, A. J., Andrews III, A. R., & Deen, T. L. (2012). Mental health needs and service utilization by Hispanic

immigrants residing in Mid-southern United States, *Journal of Transcultural Nursing, 23*(4), 359–368.

Brintnell, S. E., Sommer, R. W., Kuncoro, B., Setiawan, P. G., & Bailey, P. (2013). The expression of depression among Javanese patients with major depressive disorder: A concept mapping study. *Transcultural Psychiatry, 50,* 579–598.

Brown-Rice, K. (2014). Examining the theory of historical trauma among Native Americans. (2014). *The Professional Counselor.* Retrieved January 10, 2015. http://tpcjournal.nbcc.org/examining-the-theory-of-historical-trauma-among-native-americans/

Buchwald, D., Caralis, P. V., Gany, F., Hardt, E. J., Johnson, T. M., Muecke, M. A., & Putsch, R. W. (1994). Caring for patients in a multicultural society. *Patient Care, 28,* 105–123.

Bureau of Indian Affairs. (2012). Indian entities recognized and eligible to receive services from the Bureau of Indian Affairs. Retrieved August 24, 2014. http://www.bia.gov/cs/groups/public/documents/text/idc-020700.pdf

Campinha-Bacote, J. (2002). The process of cultural competence in the delivery of healthcare services: A model of care. *Journal of Transcultural Nursing, 13*(3), 181–184.

Campinha-Bacote, J. (2009). A culturally competent model of care for African Americans. *Urologic Nursing, 29*(1), 49–54.

Caplan, S., Caplan, S., Escobar, J., Paris, M., Alvidrez, J., Dixon, J. K., Desai, M. M.,..., Whittemore, R. (2013). Cultural influences on causal beliefs about depression among Latino immigrants. *Journal of Transcultural Nursing, 24*(1), 68–77.

Cardwell, M. (1996). *Dictionary of psychology.* Chicago, IL: Fitzroy Dearborn.

Carter-Pokras, O., Brown, P., Martinez, I., Solano, H., Rivera, M., & Pierpont, Y. (2008). Latin American–trained nurse perspective on Latino health disparities. *Journal of Transcultural Nursing, 19*(2), 161–166.

Centers for Disease Control and Prevention (CDC). (2014). Dating matters initiative. Retrieved August 19, 2014 from http://www.cdc.gov/violenceprevention/datingmatters/index.html

Central Broadcasting System. (2014). Sotomayor: Labeling illegal immigrants criminals is insulting. Retrieved May 12, 2014. http://washington.cbslocal.com/2014/02/04/sotomayor-labeling-illegal-immigrants-criminals-is-insulting

Cheon, B., & Chiao J. Y. (2012). Cultural variations in implicit mental illness stigma. *Journal of Cross-Cultural Psychology, 43*(7), 1058–1062.

Choi, J., Miller, A., & Wilbur, J. (2009). Acculturation and depressive symptoms in Korean immigrant women. *Journal of Immigrant Minority Health, 11,* 13–19.

Ciftci, A., Jones, N., & Corrigan, P. (2013). Mental health stigma in the Muslim community, *Journal of Muslim Mental Health, 7*(1), 17–32.

Constantine, M. G., & Sue, D. W. (2006a). Factors contributing to optimal human functioning in people of color in the United States. *Counseling Psychologist, 34,* 228–244.

Constantine, M. G., & Sue, D. W. (Eds.) (2006b). *Addressing racism: Facilitating cultural competence in mental health and educational settings.* Hoboken, NJ: John Wiley & Sons.

DeCoteau, ., Anderson, J., & Hope, D. (2006). Adapting manualized treatments: Treating anxiety disorders among Native Americans. *Cognitive and Behavioral Practice, 13,* 304–309.

Dietrich, D. M., & Schuett, J. M. (2013). Culture of honor and attitudes toward intimate partner violence in Latinos, *Journal of Transcultural Nursing, 3*(2), 1–11.

Douki, S., Ben Xineb, S., Nacef, F., & Halbreich, U. (2007). Women's mental health in the Muslim world: Cultural, religious, and social issues. *Journal of Affective Disorders, 102*(1–3), 177–189.

Dow, H. D. (2011). An overview of stressors faced by Immigrants and Refugees: A guide for mental health practitioners, *Home Health Care Management and Practice, 23*(3), 210–217.

Egan, G. (2014). *The skilled helper: A problem management and opportunity development approach to helping* (10th ed.). Belmont, CA: Thomson Brooks/Cole.

Ehrmin, J. T. (2000). Cultural implications of the 12-approach in addictions treatment and recovery. *Journal of Addictions Nursing, 12,* 37–41.

Ehrmin, J. T. (2001). Unresolved feelings of guilt and shame in the maternal role with substance-dependent African-American women. *Journal of Nursing Scholarship, 33,* 53–58.

Ehrmin, J. T. (2005). Dimensions of culture care for substance-dependent African American women. *Journal of Transcultural Nursing, 16,* 117–125.

Eisenberg, L. (1977). Disease and illness: Distinctions between professional and popular ideas of sickness. *Culture, Medicine and Psychiatry, 1*(1), 9–23.

Evans-Campbell, T. (2008). Historical trauma in American Indian/Native Alaska Communities: A multilevel framework for exploring impacts on individuals, families and communities. *Journal of Interpersonal Violence, 23*(3), 316–338.

Galanti, G. A. (2003). The Hispanic family and male-female relationships: An overview. *Journal of Transcultural Nursing, 14*(3), 180–185.

Galson, S. K. (2009). Surgeon general perspectives: Mental health matters. *Public Health Reports, 124,* 189–191.

Geiger, J. N., Appel, S. J., Davidhizar, R., & Davis, C. (2008). Church and spirituality in the lives of the African American community. *Journal of Transcultural Nursing, 19*(4), 375–383.

Gilbert, P., Bhundia, R., Mitra, R., Mcewan, K., Irons, C., & Sanghera, J. (2007, March). Cultural differences in shame-focused attitudes towards mental health problems in Asian and Non-Asian student women. *Mental Health, Religion & Culture, 10*(2), 127–141.

Gluck, S. (2014). What is stigma?. Retrieved January 4, 2015. http://www.healthyplace.com/stigma/stand-up-for-mental-health/what-is-stigma/

Goffman, E. (1964). *Stigma*. London, UK: Penguin.

Gone, J. P. (2009). A community-based treatment for Native American historical trauma: Prospects for evidence-based practice. *Journal of Consulting and Clinical Psychology, 77*(4), 751–762.

Gone, J. P. (2013). Redressing First Nations historical trauma: Theorizing mechanisms for indigenous culture as mental health treatment. *Transcultural Psychiatry, 50*(5), 683–706.

Gone, J. P., & Alcantara, C. (2007). Identifying effective mental health interventions for American Indians and Alaska Natives: A review of the literature. *Cultural Diversity & Ethnic Minority Psychology, 13*(4), 356–363.

Gonzalez-Guarda, R. M., Vasquez, E. P., Urrutia, M. T., Villarruel, A. M., and Peragallo, N., (2011). Hispanic Women's Experiences With Substance Abuse, Intimate Partner Violence, and Risk for HIV, *Journal of Transcult Nursing, 22*(1) 46–54.

Gonzalez-Guarda, R. M., Cummings, A. M., Becerra, M., Fernandez, M. C. & Mesa, I. (2013). Needs and preferences for the prevention of intimate partner violence among Hispanics: a community's perspective, *Journal of Primary Prevention, 34*(4), 221–235.

Gordijn, E. H., Koomen, W., & Stapel, D. A. (2001). Level of prejudice in relation to knowledge of cultural stereotypes. *Journal of Experimental Social Psychology, 37*, 150–157.

Gwynn, R. C., McQuistion, H. L., McVeigh, K. H., Garg, R. K., Frieden, T. R., & Thorpe, L. E. (2008). Prevalence, diagnosis, and treatment of depression and generalized anxiety disorder in a diverse urban community. *Psychiatric Services, 59*, 641–647.

Hall-Flavin, D. K. (2013). Is there a link between pain and depression? Can depression cause physical pain? Disease and Conditions (Major Depressive Disorder). Retrieved January10, 2015. http://www.mayoclinic.org/diseases-conditions/depression/expert-answers/pain-and-depression/faq-20057823

Hankerson, S. H., & Weissman, M. M. (2012). Church-based health programs for mental disorders among African Americans: A review, *Psychiatric Services, 63*(3), 243–249.

Hansson, L., Jormfeldt, H., Svedberg, P., Svensson, B. (2013). Health professionals' attitudes towards people with mental illness: Do they differ by attitudes held by people with mental illness ? *International Journal of Social Psychiatry, 59*(1), 48–54.

Healthy People 2020. (2015). Mental health and mental disorders. Retrieved January 14, 2015. https://www.healthypeople.gov/2020/topics-objectives/topic/mental-health-and-mental-disorders

Ho, G. (2014). Acculturation and its implications on parenting for Chinese Immigrants: A systematic Review. *Journal of Transcultural Nursing, 25*(2), 145–158.

Hunte, H. E., & Barry, A. E. (2012). Perceived discrimination and DSM-IV-based alcohol and illicit drug use disorders, *American Journal of Public Health, 102*(12), 111–117.

Indian Health Service, U.S. Department of Health and Human Services. (2015). Mental Health Winnebago counseling Center. Retrieved January 5, 2015. http://www.ihs.gov/winnebago/services/mentalhealth/

Indian Register. Aboriginal Affairs and Northern Development Canada. (2011). Retrieved January 5, 2015. https://www.aadnc-aandc.gc.ca/eng/1100100032475/1100100032476

Jadalla, A., & Lee, J. (2012). The relationship between acculturation and general health of Arab Americans. *Journal of Transcultural Nursing, 23*(2), 159–165.

Jang, Y., Kim, G., Hansen, L., & Chiriboga, D. A. (2007). Attitudes of older Korean Americans toward mental health services. *Journal of the American Geriatric Society, 55*, 616–620.

Johnston S., & Boyle, J. (2013). Northern British Columbian Aboriginal mothers: Raising adolescents with fetal alcohol spectrum disorder, *Journal of Transcultural Nursing, 24*(1), 60–67.

Kaplan, J. S., & Sue, S. (1997). Ethnic psychology in the United States. In D. F. Halpern & A. E. Voiskounsky (Eds.) *States of mind: American and post-Soviet perspectives on contemporary issues in psychotherapy* (pp. 349–369). New York, NY: Oxford University Press.

Kasl, C. D. (1992). *Many roads one journey: Moving beyond the 12 steps*. New York, NY: Harper Collins.

Kemp, C. (2005). Mexican and Mexican-Americans: Health beliefs & practices. http://bearspace.baylor.edu/Charles_Kemp/www/hispanic_health.htm

Kessler, R. C., Chiu, W. T., Demler, O., & Walters, E. E. (2005). Prevalence, severity, and comorbidity of twelve month DSM IV disorders in the National Comorbidity survey replication (NCS-R). *Archives of General Psychiatry, 62*, 617–627.

Kulwicki, A., Khalifa, R., & Moore, G. (2008). The effects of September 11 on Arab American nurses in metropolitan Detroit. *Journal of Transcultural Nursing, 19*(2), 134–139.

Lamberg, L. (2009). Children of Immigrants may face stresses, challenges that affect mental health. *Journal of the American Medical Association, 300*(7), 780–781.

Lane, C. (2013). The NIMH withdraws support for DSM-5, Psychology Today. Retrieved June 10, 2014. http://www.psychologytoday.com/blog/side-effects/201305/the-nimh-withdraws-support-dsm-5

Lee, D. T. S., Kleinman, J., & Kleinman, A. (2007). Rethinking depression: An ethnographic study of the experiences of depression among Chinese. *Harvard Review of Psychiatry*, *15*, 1–8.

Leininger, M. M. (1991a). The theory of culture care diversity and universality. In M. M. Leininger (Ed.). *Culture care diversity and universality: A theory of nursing* (pp. 5–68). New York, NY: National League for Nursing Press.

Leininger, M. M. (1991b). Ethnonursing: A research method with enablers to study the theory of culture care. In M. M. Leininger (Ed.) *Culture care diversity and universality: A theory of nursing* (pp. 73–117). New York, NY: National League for Nursing Press.

Leininger, M. M. (1995). *Transcultural nursing: concepts, theories, research and practice.* New York, NY: McGraw-Hill.

Leininger, M. M. (2000). Founders focus: Transcultural nursing is discovery of self and the world of others. *Journal of Transcultural Nursing*, *11*, 312–313.

Leininger, M. M., & McFarland, M. R. (2002). *Transcultural nursing: Concepts, theories, research and practice* (3rd ed.). New York: McGraw Hill.

Luna, L. J. (2002). Arab Muslims and culture care. In M. Leininger, & M. R. McFarland (Eds.) *Transcultural nursing: Concepts, theories, research and practice* (3rd ed., pp. 301–332). New York, NY: McGraw-Hill.

Manson, S. M. (2003). Extending the boundaries, bridging the gaps: Crafting mental health: culture, race, and ethnicity, a supplement to the Surgeon General's Report on Mental Health. *Culture, Medicine and Psychiatry*, *27*, 395–408.

Mellor, D., Carne, L., Shen Y., McCabe, M., & Wang, L. (2013). Stigma toward mental illness: A cross-cultural comparison of Taiwanese, Chinese immigrants to Australia and Anglo-Australians. *Journal of Cross Cultural Psychology*, *44*(3), 352–364.

Mental Health Screening Organization. (2014). Mental health in the African American community. Retrieved 8-24-14 https://www.mentalhealthscreening.org/screening/resources/mental-health-in-the-african-american-community.aspx

Mofty, C. (2013). Core Values of Islam. (Retrieved 8-21-14) http://www.islamreligion.com/articles/10256/

National Alliance on Mental Illness. (2011). State mental health cuts: The continuing crisis. Retrieved 1-10-15, http://www.nami.org/Content/NavigationMenu/State_Advocacy/State_Budget_Cuts_Report/State_Mental_Health_Cuts_The_Continuing_Crisis.htm

National Alliance on Mental Illness. (2014). On the homepage or website of NAMI. http://www.nami.org/Template.cfm?Section=By_Illness

National Coalition Against Domestic Violence. (2014). Downloaded 4-13-14, http://www.ncadv.org/files/DomesticViolenceFactSheet(National).pdf

National Institute of Mental Health. (2012). Transforming the understanding and treatment of mental illnesses. Retrieved 1-5-15, http://www.nimh.nih.gov/health/statistics/prevalence/any-mental-illness-ami-among-adults.shtml

Nicholas, G., Desilva, A. M., Subrebost, K., Breland-Noble, A., Gonzalez-Eastep, D., Manning, N., Prosper, V., & Prater, K. (2007). Expression and treatment of depression among Haitian immigrant women in the United States: Clinical observations, *American Journal of Psychotherapy*, *61*(1), 83–98.

Oberg, K. (1960). Cultural shock: Adjustment to new cultural environments. *Practical Anthropology*, 177–182.

Okasha, A. (2003). Arab Studies Quarterly. http://findarticles.com/p/articles/mi_m2501/is_4_25/ai_n6129825

Okasha, A. (2012). Mental health services in the Arab world. *World Psychiatry*, *11*(1), 52–54.

Olivares, I. & Altarriba, J. (2009). Mental health considerations for speech-language services with bilingual Spanish-English speakers, *Seminars in Speech and Language*, *30*(3), 153–161.

Palmer, K. T., Reading, I., Linaker, C., Calnan, M., & Coggon, D. (2008). Population-based cohort study of incident and persistent arm pain: Role of mental health, self-rated health and health beliefs. *Pain*, *136*, 30–37.

Peterman, A., Palermo, T., & Bredenkamp, C. (2011). Estimates and Determinants of Sexual Violence Against Women in the Democratic Republic of Congo. *American Journal of Public Health*, *101*(6), 1060–1067.

Pew Research Center. (2013). 'Illegal,' 'undocumented,' 'unauthorized': News media shift language on immigration. Retrieved 5-12-14, http://www.pewresearch.org/fact-tank/2013/06/17/illegal-undocumented-unauthorized-news-media-shift-language-on-immigration

Pope, R. C., Wallhagen, M., & Davis, H. (2010). The social determinants of substance abuse in African American baby boomers: Effects of family, media images, and environment. *Journal of Transcultural Nursing*, *21*, 246–256.

Rao, D., Feinglass, J., & Corrigan, P. (2007). Racial and ethnic disparities in mental illness stigma. *The Journal of Nervous and Mental Disease*, *195*(12), 1020–1023.

Rasoal, C., Jungert, T., Hau, S., Stwine, E. E., & Andersson, G. (2009). Ethnocultural empathy among students in health care education. *Evaluation & the Health Professions*, *32*(3), 300–313.

Redfield, R., Linton, R., & Herskovits, M. (1936). Memorandum on the study of acculturation. *American Anthropologist*, *38*, 149–152.

Rosenberg, M. B. (2003). *Nonviolent communication: A language of life.* Encinitas, CA: PuddleDance Press.

Ruffino, L. (2013). Drum making with students, The Saginaw Chippewa Indian Tribe of Michigan, Bonus Coverage, (10-16-2013). *Tribal Observer, The Saginaw Chippewa*

Indian Tribe of Michigan, 24(5), 28. http://www.sagchip.org/tribalobserver/archive/2013-pdf/050113-v24i05.pdf

Ryder, G., Yang, J., Zhu, X., Yao, S., Yi, J., Heine, S. J., & Bagby, M. R. (2008). The Cultural shaping of depression: Somatic symptoms in china, psychological symptoms in North America? *Journal of Abnormal Psychology, 117*(2), 300–313.

Safran, M. A., Mays, R. A., Huang, N. L., McCuan, R., Pham, P. K., Fisher, S. K., …, Trachtenberg, A. (2009). Mental Health Disparities. *American Journal of Public Health, 99*(11), 1962–1966.

Schock-Giordano, A. (2013). Ethnic families and mental health: Application of the ABC-X model of family stress. *Sage Open, 1*, 1–7.

Shellman, J., & Mokel, M. (2010). Overcoming barriers to conducting an intervention study of depression in an older African American population. *Journal of Transcultural Nursing, 21*(4), 361–369.

Simpson, J. L., & Carter, K. (2008). Muslim women's experiences with health care providers in a rural area of the United States. *Journal of Transcultural Nursing, 19*(1), 16–23.

Smith, G. R. (2007). Health disparities: what can nursing do? *Policy, Politics & Nursing Practice, 8*, 285–291.

Sowmick, J. V. (2013). Eagle Feather Cleansing, Tribal Observer, The Saginaw Chippewa Indian Tribe of Michigan, Bonus Coverage, (Retrieved 10-16-2013). http://www.sagchip.org/tribalobserver/article.aspx?article=2014#.U34Z3l7cjca

Spector, R. (2013). *Cultural Diversity in Health and Illness* (8th ed.). Boston, MA: Pearson.

Struthers, R., & Lowe, J. (2003). Nursing in the Native American culture and historical trauma. *Issues in Mental Health Nursing, 24*(3), 257–272.

Summers-Sandoval, T. F. (2008). Disobedient bodies: Racialization, resistance, and the mass (Re) articulation of the Mexican immigrant body, *American Behavioral Scientist, 52*(4), 580–597.

Sutherland, L. L. (2002). Ethnocentrism in a pluralistic society: A concept analysis. *Journal of Transcultural Nursing, 13*(4), 274–281.

Taliaferro, P. (2006). The myth about black men and suicide. Retrieved October 2, 2010, from http://www.blackvoices.com/blacklifestyle/health_headlines_featuresadvice/canvas/feat

The American Psychological Association. (2015). Health care reform: disparities in mental health status and mental health care. Retrieved January 4, 2015. http://www.apa.org/about/gr/issues/health-care/disparities.aspx

Torres, J. B., Solberg, V. S., & Carlstrom A. H. (2002). The myth of sameness among Latino men and their machismo. *American Journal of Orthopsychiatry, 72*(2), 163–181.

U. S. Department of Health and Human Services. (1999). *Mental health: A report of the surgeon general.* Rockville,

MD: Center for Mental Health Services, National Institutes of Health, National Institute of Mental Health. Retrieved January 5, 2015. http://www.surgeongeneral.gov/library/mentalhealth/home.html

U.S. Department of Health and Human Services. (2009). Office of the Surgeon General, SAMHSA, Fact sheet: Latino/Hispanic Americans. Retrieved October 25, 2009, from http://mentalhealth.samhsa.gov/cre/fact3.asp

U.S. Department of Health and Human Services. (2010). *Shared Decision-Making in Mental Health Care: Practice, Research and Future Directions.* HHS Publication No. SMA-09-4371. Rockville, MD: Center for Mental Health Services, Substance Abuse and Mental Health Services Administration. http://store.samhsa.gov/shin/content/SMA09-4371/SMA09-4371.pdf

United States Census Bureau (2010). Place of Birth of the Foreign-Born Population: 2009. https://www.census.gov/prod/2010pubs/acsbr09-15.pdf

United States Census Bureau. (2012). U.S. Census Bureau projections show a slower growing, older, more diverse nation a half century from now. Retrieved January 10, 2015. https://www.census.gov/newsroom/releases/archives/population/cb12-243.html

Walker, D. (2014). Detecting the True "Culture" of Indian Health Service Mental Health Programs, Mad in America, science, Psychiatry and community. Retrieved January 5, 2015. http://www.madinamerica.com/2014/09/detecting-true-culture-indian-health-service-mental-health-programs-counting-words/

Walsh, S., Shulman, S., & Maurer, O. (2008). Immigration distress, mental health status and coping among young immigrants: A 1-year follow up study. *International Journal of Intercultural Relations, 32*, 371–384.

Wilding, C., Muir-Cochrane, E., & May, E. (2006). Treading lightly: Spirituality issues in mental health nursing. *International Journal of Mental Health Nursing, 15*, 144–152.

Williams, C. (1992). *No hiding place, empowerment and recovery for our troubled communities.* San Francisco, CA: Harper San Francisco.

World Health Organization. (2012). Fact Sheet N369. Retrieved April 17, 2014. http://www.who.int/mediacentre/factsheets/fs369/en/

World Health Organization. (2014a). Mental health: Strengthening our response. http://www.who.int/mediacentre/factsheets/fs220/en/

World Health Organization. (2014b). Mental health: a state of well-being. http://www.who.int/features/factfiles/mental_health/en/

World Health Organization. (2014c). Violence against women: Intimate partner and sexual violence against women. Fact sheet N°239. http://www.who.int/mediacentre/factsheets/fs239/en/

Wright, M. (2013). Native American Fancy Dancers (e-miizinigaajig) embrace their culture at the CMU

Powwow, Tribal Observer, The Saginaw Chippewa Indian Tribe of Michigan, 24(5), 14. http://www.sagchip.org/tribalobserver/archive/2013-pdf/050113-v24i05.pdf

Yellow Horse Brave Heart, M., & DeBruyn, L. M. (1998). The American Indian holocaust: Healing historical unresolved grief. *American Indian & Alaska Native Mental Health Research, 8*(2), 56–78.

Yurkovich, E. E., & Lattergrass, I. (2008). Defining health and unhealthiness: Perceptions held by Native American Indians with persistent mental illness. *Mental Health, Religion & Culture, 11*(5), 437–459.

Zayas, L. H., Torres, L. R., & Cabassa, L. J. (2009). Diagnostic, symptom, and functional assessments of Hispanic outpatients in community mental health practice. *Community Mental Health Journal, 45*, 97–105.

Culture, Family, and Community

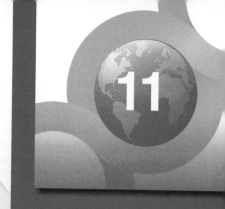

11

Joyceen S. Boyle and Martha B. Baird

Key Terms

Aggregates
Alternative therapies
Assimilation
Asylee
Community-based nursing
Community-based
  collaborative action
  research (CBCAR)
Community-based setting
Community health nursing

Community nursing
Community settings
Cultural assessment
Cultural health systems
Cultural knowledge
Cultural sensitivity
Culturally competent care
Cultural integration
Dinka culture
Immigrants
Kinship
Levels of prevention

Medically underserved areas
Primary prevention
Public health nursing
Secondary prevention
Specialized community
  interventions
Subcultures
Sudanese culture
Tertiary prevention
Traditional health beliefs and
  practices
Worldview

Learning Objectives

1. Use cultural concepts to provide nursing care to families, communities, and aggregates.
2. Understand the necessary components of a cultural assessment of an aggregate group.
3. Explore interactions of community and culture as they relate to concepts of community-based nursing practice and specialized community interventions.
4. Analyze how cultural factors influence health and illness of groups.
5. Assess factors that influence the health of diverse groups within the community.
6. Evaluate potential health problems and solutions in refugee and immigrant populations.
7. Identify interventions that are culturally sensitive and relevant to address health concerns of a refugee population.

An understanding of culture and cultural concepts contributes to the nurse's knowledge and facilitates culturally competent nursing care in **community-based settings**. Currently, many nurses practice in community settings with clients from a wide variety of cultural backgrounds; this trend is expected to increase with more nurses moving from acute care institutions to

community settings. The care of clients in the community can be extremely complex, calling for a high level of nursing skill. Cultural diversity is also expected to increase in the United States; "by 2050 nearly one-half of the U.S. population will be composed of racial minorities" (McKenzie, Pinger, & Kotecki, 2012, p. 272). Significant changes in the health care system, as well as an increased emphasis on health promotion and disease prevention, have influenced nurses to make changes in their practice as well as the setting in which care is delivered. Concepts such as health equality, diversity, partnership, empowerment, and facilitation now form the basis for community-based nursing practice with individuals, families, and **aggregates** in the community. An aggregate is a collection of people who can be thought of as a whole simply because they happen to be in the same place at the same time. For some time, national nursing associations, including the National Institute of Nursing Research (NINR), have urged a community and population focus in both nursing research and practice. Involving clients in planning for and providing community nursing services is the foundation of culturally competent care.

Specialized community interventions that are culturally relevant to the people served are built on collaboration and partnerships between community leaders, health consumers, and health care providers. When community residents or health consumers are involved as partners, community-based services are more likely to be responsive to locally defined needs, are better used, and are sustained through local actions. **Community-based collaborative action research (CBCAR)** is an approach for nurses to partner with communities to address health issues (Pavlish & Pharris, 2011). Specialized community interventions are complex and often very time consuming. They require a high level of nursing knowledge and skill in working with and relating to different individuals and groups. In many instances, the complexity is increased when clients and their families come from diverse cultures. Nurses must understand how to help persons from various cultures work with community leaders and health care providers to form partnerships that are responsive and can structure nursing and health care in ways that are culturally sensitive and appropriate. It is often the cultural factors that determine whether a particular population or group will choose to participate in community-based health services. There is always a need for continuing communication among health care providers and community residents that is characterized by mutual understanding and respect. It is this understanding and respect that forms the basis for culturally relevant and competent nursing care.

In this chapter, the terms **community nursing, community-based nursing, community health nursing,** and **public health nursing** are used interchangeably, even though they have different meanings in some settings and in different contexts (Canales & Drevdahl, 2014; Williams, 2012). Whether the nurse is employed as a public health nurse or a community health nurse in a health department or practices in a community-based setting, he or she needs the knowledge and skills to provide culturally competent care. The practice of nursing in a community setting requires that nurses be comfortable with clients from diverse cultures and the broader socioeconomic context in which they live. As the population continues to grow in diversity, health disparities have become more apparent in diverse populations and are now a vital area of focus for researchers and practitioners. Care that is not congruent with the client's value system is likely to increase the cost of care because it compromises quality and inhibits access to services. Furthermore, members of diverse cultural groups, such as the officially designated minority groups in the United States, tend to experience greater health inequalities than do members of the general population. This was the impetus for targeting the four ethnic minority groups in *Healthy People 2000* (U.S. Department of Health and Human Services, 1990) and *Healthy People 2010* (U.S. Department of Health and Human Services, 2000) because

Box 11-1 What's New in Healthy People 2020?

- Emphasizing ideas of health equity that address social determinants of health and promote health across all stages of life
- Replacing the traditional print publication with an interactive website as the main vehicle for dissemination

- Maintaining a website that allows users to tailor information to their needs and explore evidence-based resources for implementation

Source: http://www.healthypeople2020.gov

cultural diversity must be respected and taken into account by health care professionals. Equally important, we must address the stark inequalities that exist in health status between minority groups and the wider American society. *Healthy People 2020* is a set of goals and objectives with 10-year targets designed to guide national health promotion and disease prevention efforts to improve the health of all people in the United States (U.S. Department of Health and Human Services, 2010). Box 11-1 shows what is new in *Healthy People 2020.*

Overview of Culturally Competent Nursing Care in Community Settings

Nurses practice in many settings within the community, including worksites, schools, physicians' offices, health care program sites, clinics, churches, and public health departments. The use of **cultural knowledge** in community-based nursing practice begins with a careful assessment of clients and families in their own environments. Cultural data that have implications for nursing care are selected from clients, families, and the environment during the assessment phase and are discussed with the client and family to develop mutually shared goals. The Andrews/Boyle Transcultural Nursing Assessment Guide for Individuals and Families (Appendix A) and the Andrews/Boyle Transcultural Nursing

Assessment Guide for Groups and Communities (Appendix B) are helpful when assessing clients, families, groups, and communities.

Cultural data are important in the care of all clients; however, in community nursing, they are a prerequisite to successful nursing interventions. Community nursing is practiced in a community setting, often in the home of the client, and frequently requires more active participation by the client and family. Often, the client and family must make basic changes in lifestyle, such as changes in diet and exercise patterns. Cultural competence requires that the nurse understand the family lifestyle and value system, as well as those cultural forces that are powerful determinants of health-related behaviors. Nurses often work closely with clients with chronic diseases or those who have other health problems, and nursing interventions must include aspects of counseling and education as well as anticipatory guidance directed toward helping clients and families adjust to what may be lifelong conditions. Nurses must take into account the diverse cultural factors that will motivate clients to make successful changes in behavior because improvement in health status requires lifestyle and behavioral modifications.

Transcultural nursing practice has the potential to improve the health of the community as well as the health of individual clients and families. An additional consideration of the nurse who is involved in community-focused planning is the health needs of populations at risk. Special at-risk groups can be found in all communities: the homeless, the poor,

persons with HIV/AIDS and/or tuberculosis, refugees, prison populations, and the elderly are groups at risk for decreased health status.

Consider what problems might arise if one were to design a health program for a community composed primarily of Somali refugees who recently arrived in the United States. They may have spent years in refugee camps in other countries and lost many family members, or their family members may be still in Somalia and the refugees are now making a life for themselves in a strange country. Certainly, language would be a major problem, but so could many other cultural differences, from nuances in communication to differences in beliefs of what constitutes health and illness as well as treatment and cure. A failure to understand and deal with these differences would have serious implications for the success of any health or nursing intervention. Nurses who have knowledge of, and an ability to work with, diverse cultures are able to devise effective community interventions to reduce risks in a manner that is consistent with the community and group, as well as individual values and beliefs of community members.

A Transcultural Framework

A distinguishing and important aspect of community-based nursing practice is the nursing focus on the community as the client (Stanhope & Lancaster, 2012). Effective community nursing practice must reflect accurate knowledge of the causes and distribution of health problems and of effective interventions that are congruent with the values and goals of the community. A social–ecological approach can be used by the community nurse to collect, organize, and analyze information about high-risk groups that are encountered in community practice. The underlying foundation of the social–ecological approach is that behavior has multiple levels of influences. This approach focuses on the interaction between and the interdependence of factors within and across all levels of a health problem (McKenzie, Pinger, & Kotecki, 2012). Using a cultural overlay with a social–ecological approach enhances nurse–community interactions in numerous ways.

Identifying Subcultures and Devising Specialized Community-Based Interventions

A transcultural framework for nursing care helps the nurse to identify subcultures within the larger community and to devise community-based interventions that are specific to community health and nursing goals. For example, in the multicultural society of the United States, it is common to speak of "the Black community," "the Hispanic community," or "the Francophone community." We might also speak more broadly of "the immigrant community," or the "refugee community," or of other unique groups within or near a local community. A cultural focus allows this variety and facilitates data collection about specific groups based on their health risks. A cultural/social/ecological framework facilitates a view of the community as a complex collective yet allows for diversity within the whole. Interventions that are successful in one subgroup may fail with another subgroup of the same community, and often, the failure can be attributed to cultural differences or barriers that arise because of these differences. Often, the community location of a diverse subculture reflects distinctive aspects of the cultural group. Figure 11-1 shows murals on the wall of a library in El Rio, a Mexican American barrio in Tucson, AZ.

Identifying the Values and Cultural Norms of a Community

A transcultural framework is essential for the community health nurse to identify the values and cultural norms of a community. Although values are universal features of all cultures, their types and expressions vary widely, even within the same community. Values often serve as the foundation for a community's acceptance and use of health resources or a group's participation in community-based intervention programs to

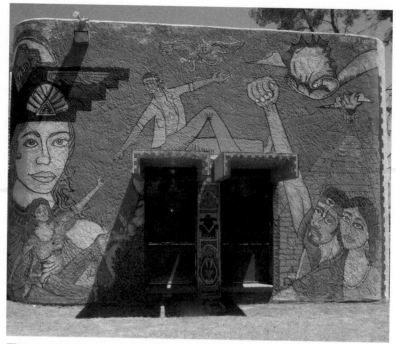

Figure 11-1. These murals reflect the Mexican American culture of the El Rio barrio. They were painted by community residents.

promote health and wellness. Just as nurses share data and collaborate with clients and families to establish mutually acceptable goals for nursing care, the community-based nurse works with the community or aggregates within the community to plan community-focused health programs. In addition to forming partnerships with communities, the community nurse considers the influences of social, economic, ecological, and political issues. Larger policy issues directly and profoundly affect many, if not all, community health issues. These larger policy issues are, in turn, influenced by the wider national and/or international culture.

Cultural Issues in Community Nursing Practice

The need for nurses to be sensitive to clients who are culturally different is increasing as we become more aware of the complex interactions between health care providers and clients and how these interactions might affect the client's health. Diverse client groups who have limited access to health services, along with barriers resulting from language and cultural differences, often suffer from a variety of health inequalities (Dreachslin, Gilbert, & Malone, 2013). The information in this chapter will assist nurses to become aware of cultural factors that affect health, illness, and the practice of nursing in community settings.

Purnell (2013) and Giger and Davidhizar (1991) have provided models or frameworks to guide the nurse in the assessment of cultural factors in patient care. The Andrews/Boyle Transcultural Nursing Assessment Guide (see Appendices A and B) provides outlines for the nurse to collect and assess cultural data relevant to individuals, families, and communities. Most cultural assessment guides are oriented to individual client and occasionally to families. The Andrews/Boyle assessment guides have the comprehensive view necessary for assessing cultural

factors for intervention at the individual, family, and community levels. Because individual clients and their families constitute larger communities, nurses who work in community settings must understand cultural issues as they relate to individuals and families and the context in which they live—communities.

Cultural Influences on Individuals and Families

Cultural influences—values, norms, beliefs, and behaviors—have a profound effect on health. When assessing individuals and families, the community health nurse should carefully examine the following:

1. Family roles, typical family households and structure, and dynamics in the family, particularly communication patterns and decision making
2. Health beliefs and practices related to disease causation, treatment of illness, and the use of indigenous healers or folk practitioners and other alternative/complementary therapies
3. Patterns of daily living, including work, school, and leisure activities
4. Social networks, including friends, neighbors, kin, and significant others, and how they influence health and illness
5. Ethnic, cultural, or national identity of client and family, for example, identification with a particular group, including language
6. Nutritional practices and how they relate to cultural factors and health
7. Religious preferences and influences on well-being, health maintenance, and illness, as well as the impact religion might have on daily living and taboos or restrictions arising from religious beliefs that might influence health status or care
8. Culturally appropriate behavior styles, including what is manifested during anger, competition, and cooperation, as well as relationships with health care professionals, relationships between genders, and relations with other groups in the community

A cultural assessment of individuals and families includes all of the preceding factors. This list is a starting point for community nurses to use when assessing individuals and families in everyday practice. Cultural values shape human health behaviors and determine what individuals and families will do to maintain their health status, how they will care for themselves and others who become ill, and where and from whom they will seek health care. Most importantly, family members are often the ones who decide on the course of treatment. Families have an important role in the transmission of cultural values and learned behaviors that relate to both health and illness. It is within the family context that individuals learn basic ways to stay healthy and to ensure their own well-being and that of their family members.

One commonality shared by members of functioning families is a concern for the health and wellness of each individual within the family because the family has the primary responsibility for meeting the health needs of its members. The nurse must not only assess the health of each family member but must also determine how well the family can meet family health needs. Just how well families can meet the needs of each family member will determine how, when, and where interventions will take place. A cultural orientation assists the nurse in understanding cultural values and interactions, the roles that family members assume, and the support system available to the family to help them when health problems are identified.

The family is usually an individual's most important social unit and provides the social context within which illness occurs and is resolved. Health promotion and maintenance also occur within the family group. Most **traditional health beliefs and practices** promote the health of the family because they are generally family and socially oriented. Frequently, traditional beliefs and practices reinforce family cohesion. Some values are more central and influential than others; given a competing set of demands, these central values will typically determine a family's priorities. In families that adhere to traditional

cultural values, the families' (or tribe's and/or community's) needs and goals often will take precedence over an individual's needs and goals. The culturally competent nurse can recognize and use the family's role in promoting and maintaining health. This requires an appreciation of the family context in health and illness and how this varies among diverse cultures.

Cultural Factors Within Communities

In addition to identifying and meeting the cultural needs of clients and families, the community health nurse must consider social and cultural factors on a community level to respect cultural values, mobilize local resources, and develop culturally appropriate health programs and services. Important factors to consider include the influence of demographics on health care, subcultures in the United States, refugee and immigrant populations (special consideration is given here to the Dinka refugees from South Sudan), maintenance of traditional cultural values and practices, and access to health and nursing care for diverse cultural groups.

Demographics and Health Care

During the 21st century, the United States and many other countries will face enormous demographic, social, and cultural changes. The United States is becoming more diverse, and it is incumbent on nurses to be prepared to respond appropriately as the health status of individuals differs dramatically across cultural/ethnic groups and social classes. Certain groups in the United States face greater challenges than does the general population in accessing timely and needed health care services. Major indicators such as morbidity and mortality rates for adults and infants show that the health status of minority Americans in the United States is substantially worse than that of White Americans. Health status is worse among those who are medically underserved—populations who have inadequate access to quality health care. Community nurses must assess groups within the community in a very sensitive

manner; often those characteristics that we assume are related to the group's culture may be influenced by other factors instead.

Subcultures or Diversity Within Communities

Caring for diverse groups within the community has been a focus of public health nursing since the days of Lillian Wald, an early nurse leader. Home care was provided to inner city residents, particularly recently arrived immigrants. Because nurses were not from the same cultural background as their clients, they had to deal with cultural differences between themselves and the persons in their care (Degazon, 2012). The need for nurses to provide culturally relevant care is greater than ever. Currently, the focus of community nursing is on diversity in the United States across and within **subcultures**. Subcultures are aggregates of people that establish certain rules of behavior, values, and living patterns that are different from mainstream culture. Leininger described subcultures as having "distinctive patterns of living with sets of rules, special values and practices that are different from the dominant culture" (Leininger, 1995, p. 60). There can also be diversity within each subculture. Hispanic culture as a group is very broad and includes Mexican Americans, Puerto Ricans, Dominicans, Cubans, and Central and South Americans. There is diversity within each of these groups as well.

Certain geographic areas of the country, such as Appalachia, can be singled out as containing subcultures. Persons born and reared in the southern states or in New York City can often be identified by their dialect and mannerisms as members of a distinct subculture. The United States used to be described as a "melting pot" culture, indicating that new arrivals gave up their former languages, customs, and values to become Americans. This concept may not be appropriate, however. A more accurate metaphor for the American population is a rich and complex tapestry of colors, backgrounds, and interests. One subculture that has retained many aspects

of their traditional culture is the Hmong people from Southeast Asia. They came to the United States in the 1970s as refugees after the Vietnam War. The large Hmong community in Fresno, CA, sponsors a New Year's Day Celebration that is attended by as many as 100,000 Hmong from all over the United States (Figure 11-2).

Refugee and Immigrant Populations

Immigrants are persons who voluntarily and legally immigrate to the United States to live. Immigrants come of their own choice, and most plan to eventually become citizens of their new host country. Currently, immigration of undocumented individuals, or those who do not have the appropriate documentation to immigrate, can be a contentious issue in the industrialized nations of the world. Many of the key issues in the debate about immigration policies in the United States are based on economic and political issues (Ayón, 2009).

Many persons do come to the United States, Canada, and Western Europe without the proper documentation. Although terms differ for these persons, in the United States, they usually are referred to as "undocumented" migrants, "illegal immigrants," or "illegal aliens." McGuire (2014)

states that these latter terms originate in nativism, an anti-immigrant attitude rooted in self-interest and maintenance of the status quo. The terms "illegal" and "alien" should be avoided in nursing discourse and the professional literature to show respect for the undocumented immigrant as a human being (McGuire, 2014).

Under international law, **refugee** is a special term that describes a person who is outside of his or her country of nationality or habitual residence and who has a well-founded fear of persecution if he or she returns to his or her own country. By definition then, refugees are persons escaping persecution based on race, religion, nationality, or political stance (The UN Refugee Agency, UNHCR, 1966). Evidence-Based Practice 11-1 presents a study about the barriers to human rights that women encountered in southern Sudan. Violence against women is considered the most pervasive human rights violation in the world. Violence against women is exacerbated in war-torn countries, with a high incidence of rape and other physical/sexual abuse during armed conflicts. Women and girls, often unaccompanied by family members, are particularly at high risk. Many refugee women who come to the United States have experienced these human

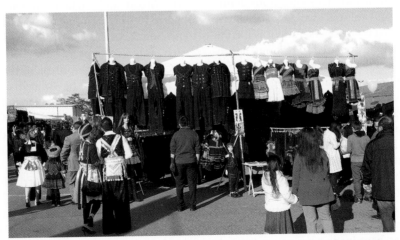

Figure 11-2. The Hmong New Year's Celebration in Fresno, CA, is attended by 100,000 Hmong. In this photo, several Hmong admire the merchandise in a booth selling traditional clothes.

Human Rights Barriers for Displaced Persons in Southern Sudan

This is a community-based research study that explores community perspectives on barriers to human rights that women encounter in a postconflict setting of southern Sudan. Violence against women is considered the most pervasive human rights violation in the world and is exacerbated in war-torn countries with high incidence of rape and other physical/sexual abuse during armed conflicts; women and girls are at particularly high risk. Violence against women is often rooted in social values and mores and potential success of change depends on learning more about local priorities regarding gender relationships, practices, and rights.

The region of southern Sudan is the site of a 40-year civil war that has had a horrific effect on the population as well as the social, economic, and physical infrastructures and health care services. Focus groups and key informant interviews provided the data for this ethnographic study. Themes found in human rights structures and subsequent barriers to human rights are described. Most human rights situations are dealt with by the traditional clan system and then go on to the more formal court and police system. Customary behavior often prevails and often women are disadvantaged because of their social positions and power differentials. Although some police officials receive procedural training in law enforcement and occasionally informal training in human rights, key informants reported that the police might actually perpetuate human rights abuses. The formal court system is still "developing" and does not always offer protection to women. Numerous barriers exist to extending human rights and protection to women. These barriers include (1) shifting legal frameworks that create a lack of knowledge about what constitutes a human rights violation, (2) mistrust and doubt about human rights, (3) weak government infrastructure, and (4) poverty.

Clinical Implications

- Nurses should be aware of the everyday struggle for justice and human dignity that refugees from the Sudan have experienced. Similarly, nurses must consider the broader historical and cultural factors that contribute to human rights abuses when working with displaced or refugee communities.
- Given their advocacy role and direct contact with communities, nurses can help educate community members regarding the health effects of human rights violations. Furthermore, by questioning social practices that violate women's rights (e.g., domestic violence), nurses can create opportunities for social change.
- Research results also indicated that enacting human rights was frequently associated with a sense of connectedness and community responsibility, suggesting that nurses can work with local residents and service providers in addressing violence against women and promoting human rights.
- Nurses are in a key position to help refugee communities analyze and address human rights barriers, thus advancing women's health and well-being.

Reference: Pavlish, C., & Ho, A. (2009). Human rights as barriers for displaced persons in southern Sudan. Journal of Nursing Scholarship, 41, 284–292.

rights violations (Ashford & Huet-Vaughn, 1997; Vickers, 1993).

Barnes, Harrison, and Heneghan (2004) suggested that there is a need for research about refugees that is distinct from other categories of immigrants. The circumstances that lead to forced migration of refugees are very different from those that influence an immigrant to relocate, and these differences can have distinct health implications. In recent times, refugees have come to the United

States from countries in Africa, including Sudan and Somalia, Eastern Europe, Afghanistan, Iraq, Syria, and other countries undergoing violent conflicts; refugees are fleeing war, famine, and other social upheavals. They are fleeing for their lives and safety rather than personally choosing to leave their homeland. The term refugee and the status of an individual who is a refugee have legal meanings and designations that differ from those of immigrants.

Another classification of newcomers is asylees—persons who come to a particular country seeking political asylum from some sort of persecution in their home country. These various types of classification—immigrant, undocumented immigrant, refugee, and asylee—often determine the rights of individuals. The individual's status will determine eligibility for work permits, residency status, and the types of social and health services he or she may be entitled to. In addition, those who are undocumented, or without appropriate residency status, may face arrest and deportation to their country of origin. Table 11-1 shows terms used for individuals residing in a country who are not citizens.

Many recent immigrants and refugees are not acculturated to prevailing Western norms related to health beliefs or behaviors. Furthermore, they do not understand the complex US health care system. Many arrive with scant economic resources and must learn English and become economically self-sufficient as quickly as possible. Certain factors, such as settlement patterns or living near friends or family, communication networks, social class, and education, have helped many immigrants maintain their cultural traditions. Immigrant or refugee communities provide support for newcomers and opportunities for cultural continuity because these ethnic communities reflect the identities of the home countries. At the same time, belonging to such a community tends to set immigrants and refugees apart and isolate them from the larger community. For example, newcomers from Mexico realize that they need to learn English to get better jobs, but they often join expanding Latino communities where most residents speak Spanish. Learning English well enough to obtain employment in the English-speaking world is difficult and takes time. It is to their credit that most immigrants and refugees do learn English and make significant contributions to their new country.

In addition to the legal entrance of immigrants and refugees, other persons seeking political asylum have entered the United States from all over the world. Often, those seeking asylum or those who enter the country both legally and illegally are at considerable risk for health and

Table 11-1: Terms Used for Individuals Residing in a Country Who Are Not Citizens

Term	Description
Illegal immigrant	A person who is in a country without the appropriate documentation and permission
Immigrant	A person who comes to a country to take up permanent residence
Refugee	A person who is escaping persecution based on race, religion, nationality, or political persuasion
Emigrant	A person departing from a country to settle elsewhere
Émigré	A person forced to emigrate for political reasons
Asylee	A person seeking political asylum from persecution in his or her home country
Temporary stay migrant	A person who moves to another country with the intention of staying there for only a limited time, usually for occupational reasons
Undocumented	A person without the required documents that provide evidence of status or qualification, such as nationality or specified length of time a person may legally reside within a country

social problems. In particular, health care along the US–Mexico border, where many individuals are undocumented, poses special problems and challenges for health care providers (Ayón, 2009; McEwen & Boyle, 2007). Immigrants, refugees, and asylees face language and employment barriers and usually have scant economic resources. Some have experienced rapid change and traumatic life events, their coping abilities have been overwhelmed, and few resources are available to assist them. Refugees, asylees, and immigrants in general, whether they are here legally or undocumented, have special health risks.

The next section in this chapter highlights a special refugee community, known as the Dinka, from the African nation of Sudan. A prolonged civil war and famine in the Sudan has displaced millions over the last two decades, and many of them have been women and children. Many Dinka refugees have been resettled in the United States and have had to make profound adjustments to learn to live in the American society and culture.

A Refugee Community: The Dinka of South Sudan

The prolonged civil war in the African country of Sudan has resulted in large numbers of refugees. It is estimated that 2 million people died and 4 million others were displaced as a result of this war Al-Tohami, K. (2011). The war was the result of religious and ethnic conflict between the predominantly Muslim north and the minority indigenous and Christian south. South Sudan officially ceded from North Sudan on July 9, 2011, and became a separate nation (Gettleman, 2011). However, civil war resumed in South Sudan in December 2013 between two of the largest ethnic tribes, the Nuer and Dinka, as each vies for control of the new country (The UN Refugee Agency [UNHCR], 2014). The United Nation estimates that 6.9 million people were in need of humanitarian assistance at the end of January 2014, as a result of the continued conflict in Sudan (The UN Refugee Agency [UNHCR], 2015).

Sudan received worldwide attention for documentation of human rights violations, including genocide and slave trade (The UN Refugee Agency [UNHCR], 2015). The story of "The Lost Boys of Sudan" gained worldwide attention through books Bixler, 2006; Eggers, 2006), documentaries for television (Mihalovich, 2014), and a Hollywood film (Luckinbill et al., 2014). This story of the Lost Boys chronicles the plight of 20,000 South Sudanese children, mostly young boys, who walked across Sudan to escape the genocide. They sought refuge in neighboring African countries, and many have been resettled to Western countries such as the United States, Australia, and Canada.

Sudanese refugees have undergone stressful, traumatic, and even catastrophic experiences such as war, torture, refugee camps, death of family members, and loss of homeland. Many of the health problems experienced by the Sudanese refugees are the result of prolonged civil war and a lack of nutrition and basic health care. Refugees from Sudan may have a variety of health problems including severe malnutrition and diseases endemic to Sudan, such as gastrointestinal diseases, tuberculosis, schistosomiasis, sleeping sickness, and HIV/AIDS (Brown, 2004; Pinto et al., 2005). Because of the human rights atrocities that Sudanese refugees have experienced, many also experience extreme mental distress.

The World Health Organization reports that more than 50% of refugees suffer from mental health problems (World Health organization [WHO], 2012). Studies indicate that many refugees experience posttraumatic stress disorder (PTSD), which follows a psychologically traumatic event outside of the range of usual human experiences. The symptoms may include nightmares, depression, withdrawal, hopelessness, sleep disorders, and other somatic complaints (American Psychiatric Association, 2013). Despite the high incidence of mental disorders, many refugees are reluctant to seek care in mainstream mental health facilities (Jaranson et al., 2004), preferring instead to seek traditional methods to deal with mental stress and psychological disorders.

The Sudanese refugees were forced out of their communities and often traveled many miles, some on foot, adapting to temporary environments and harsh conditions. Many have lost close family members in the conflicts as well as all that is familiar to them, thus losing a sense of identity and community. Many others have witnessed and/or experienced the worst kind of human atrocities, including forced slavery, rape, and genocide. Refugee Sudanese women were especially vulnerable during migration when they did not have the protection and support of their families and communities. However, trying to make a new life in a new host country has also been very stressful for Sudanese refugees. Factors such as unemployment, decreased family income, changes in lifestyle, lack of ability to speak English, cultural conflict, and separation from family and loved ones continue to add to stress and decrease the quality of life for many Sudanese refugees.

The Dinka tribe is one of the largest tribes in South Sudan, and its members were some of the most persecuted. Their Christian faith and practices made them a target of ethnic persecution by the Islamic northern militia. Many Dinka have come to Western countries as refugees. This section highlights traditional Dinka culture, including characteristics of a Dinka community, family, and the roles of women. Although the focus of this section is on Dinka refugees, many of the issues, challenges, and topics identified here have relevance to other refugee and immigrant groups as well.

Traditional Dinka Culture. The traditional **Dinka culture** is community oriented with kinship and family ties that extend beyond blood relatives. The Dinka are a patriarchal society who revere and respect their elders. As a tribal society, the Dinka are a social group with a territorial affiliation and a strong cultural and ethnic identity. They are very proud of their traditional tribal culture and their identity as "Dinka." They refer to themselves as *Monyjang*, which means "The lord of all people" (Deng, 1984, p. 2). Cattle hold special significance in Dinka culture and traditions

and also provide a livelihood for the tribe. Cattle are considered an important aspect of Dinka marriage rituals; bridewealth (or a bride's value) depends on the amount of cattle her union will bring to her family (Deng, 1984).

The Dinka are considered very religious, and their Christian practices are an integral part of their traditions. In keeping with a common practice among the Dinka, both men and women are given a "Christian" or "Biblical" name at birth, as well as a traditional Dinka name. They have a belief in an inseparable connection between the natural and supernatural world. Even in resettlement, the Dinka have established strong Christian practices within their new communities. Health and illness are closely linked to spirituality and supernatural forces. Illness is considered a community affair, and family and friends often gather at the bedside of a sick member to pray or to sit in watchful silence.

Characteristics of a Dinka Refugee Community. There is no "one" Dinka refugee community. Dinka refugees have been resettled in cities all over the world. The experiences of men, women, and children who have grown up outside of Sudan may be strikingly different from their elders. Many Dinka adults, as well as their children, have spent years in refugee camps or countries of transit before arriving in countries of resettlement. It is also quite possible that they have experienced traumatic events prior to relocation, and such factors may have a profound effect on transition to life in the new country. In essence, any attempt to bring health care services to the community or to address the community's health problems must take into account the tremendous diversity within the whole community. This requires flexibility and ingenuity on the part of health care professionals.

Further complicating this situation is language. Some Dinka may have learned English in their homeland due to postcolonial British occupation. Most Dinka speak the tribal language (also called Dinka), and many speak Arabic, although few are literate in either. As Dinka are resettled, they are

learning a new language, seeking employment, and sending their children to school. Many Dinka families live in close proximity to each other, as well as other African refugees. Although this practice may isolate newly arrived refugees from those in the dominant society, close association with persons from their own culture and tribe can form a supportive network for new arrivals. Refugee communities that facilitate healthy transitions include support from family, friends, and health care professionals. Social support has been identified in the resettlement process as one of the most critical factors that promotes health and well-being (Simich, Beiser, & Mawani, 2003). The cultural values and traditions that refugees maintain after resettlement, such as a sense of communality, hope, and religious practices, are resources that enable them to develop healthy strategies to cope with resettlement experiences (Baird & Boyle, 2012).

The Dinka Family. Family life is at the core of Dinka culture. Men in Dinka society are expected to provide for their family and to make most of the important decisions concerning family affairs. Once a woman is married, she and her children are considered to belong to her husband's family. In fact, in the case of a divorce, the children are expected to remain with the husband or his family members. In addition, if the husband dies, his wife or wives will often be taken in by one of his brothers to support. Married Dinka couples do not share the same last name, and it is common for their children to be given a family name.

Polygamy is not uncommon in the Dinka tribal culture of South Sudan. A husband may have more than one wife, and he and his cowives, along with their children, may exist as one extended family within the family compound. Resettlement may lead to dissolution and separation of families as husbands may have to choose only one wife. This can pose difficulties for those wives and their children who are left without a father and no one to support the family in resettlement. Husbands are sometimes threatened by their wives'

newfound sense of equality and independence, and this often leads to marital discord and sometimes to domestic violence. Domestic violence is not well tolerated in Western cultures, and refugee women learn that they do not have to tolerate beatings from their husbands. Women who pursue a divorce because of domestic violence or polygamy are often discouraged by their families back in Sudan as well as the Dinka community in the United States. When a woman seeks a divorce, her family may be expected to return the bridewealth that was paid to her husband's family as part of the marital contract. The loss of the bridewealth can lead to serious financial problems for the woman's family back in Sudan. If a Dinka woman should seek a divorce, she will likely face considerable stigma and be censored by friends and her community.

The Dinka tend to socialize almost exclusively with family members and members of their own tribe. This can create challenges for refugee families in the diaspora who may live a considerable geographic distance from each other, thus making frequent visits very difficult. The Dinka go to considerable efforts to maintain ties with family members back in the Sudan through technology such as cell phones and Skype.

This group communality provides an important buffer for the refugees, especially new arrivals. Dinka communities usually have a Sudanese community church, which serves as the religious and social center for the members (Figure 11-3). During weekly services, traditional cultural practices include chanting Christian hymns in the Dinka language accompanied by tribal drums. Social events held at the church might include birthday celebrations, baby showers, and memorial services for those family members who have died in Sudan. In addition, the church provides updates on the current political and social situations in their home country. Women are able to continue their traditions of language, dress, food, and music through their association with the church. The weekly events at the church allow the refugees to stay connected with each other and give them a sense of belonging and familiarity.

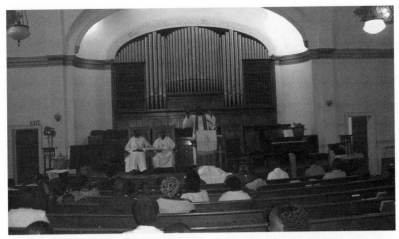

Figure 11-3. This Sudanese church serves as a religious and social center for the highly devout Christian Dinka in Kansas City, KS, and has served as a site for health fairs for members of the congregation.

Many social concerns that are relevant to the Dinka community are addressed through the Sudanese church. Sermons might include lessons about issues that face Dinka families such as the importance of continuing education or methods to resolve domestic disputes. Often, there is a women's group at the church that provides help to Dinka families when there is illness or financial difficulty; they collect money or cook food for a family in need. It is through attendance at the Sudanese church that the Dinka value of respect for the elderly is reinforced in the socialization of Dinka children.

Dinka women are at the center of family life and responsible for the transmission of the cultural values, beliefs, and practices to the children. There is still tremendous social pressure from family members and the Dinka community to continue these cultural traditions after resettlement. This may cause problems for refugee women who are also coping with tremendous role changes in countries of resettlement.

Dinka Women's Roles. In the traditional patriarchal culture of the Dinka, women are dependent on and subservient to men. Marriage and childbearing have traditionally been the only acceptable roles for Dinka women. The family clan

system in the Dinka culture continues to subjugate women, even after resettlement. Women in Sudan typically do not work outside the home and do not make important decisions within the family. If difficulties arise between a husband and wife, the husband is likely to communicate with his family back in Sudan who may then apply pressure on her to maintain traditional ways. For example, the Dinka culture values large families and encourages women to have many children, as children are a sign of prosperity. However, refugee women soon learn that large families are not affordable or practical in countries of resettlement. Baird (2009) described an interaction that occurred between a husband and wife at a hospital after the birth of their fourth child. The physician broached the subject of a tubal ligation. The woman was interested, but the husband said "No." When the physician persisted, saying that the woman should have input into the decision, the husband again replied, "No. We will talk with her at home." If a Dinka woman is reluctant to have another child or refuses outright, the family back in Sudan might arrange for a second wife for the husband.

Raising children in the American culture has proved challenging for Dinka mothers. As children are exposed to American culture at

school and on television, sex, violence, and other controversial aspects of American life prove pervasive and difficult to avoid. Children tend to acculturate more rapidly than do their parents, learning English more quickly and, in general, adapting to new social roles and gender identities, as well as establishing roots in American culture. Mothers struggle to help their children with their homework: often, the mothers' English reading skills and educational background are very limited. Mothers can experience pressure from their children to cook certain foods and participate in cultural celebrations and activities in the new culture, such as Halloween, which may be foreign to Dinka parents. Disciplining children by using corporal punishment is not acceptable in the United States, and mothers may be afraid of being reported to authorities who would then take their children away. Dinka parents soon learn that in the United States, children are expected to express their feelings and opinions openly and to question rules and authority. This is rather shocking to Dinka parents. Many mothers are concerned that their children will identify with the antisocial behaviors they see in their neighborhood or on television—smoking cigarettes, drinking alcohol, and sexual promiscuity. These conflicts can create cultural clashes between generations of refugees.

In summary, Dinka women, like other women refugees, have experienced profound role changes. In many cultures, a woman's proper place is in the home. The freedoms and opportunities refugee women gain when they come to countries of resettlement may create conflict and power imbalances in their marriages and family relationships, thus adding to their stress. The following section addresses health care interventions nurses can implement to help refugees adapt to the stress of the cultural transition.

Planning Nursing Care for Refugee Families and Communities

Careful assessment of cultural backgrounds and individual factors can help nurses anticipate and work with difficulties that are experienced by refugees and immigrants who seek health care. The Boyle/Baird Assessment Guide for Refugees (Appendix E) is recommended for use with refugee clients and their families. In response to the large numbers of refugees admitted to the United States after the Vietnam War, Lipson & Meleis (1983) identified important factors to assess when working with refugees. This outline provides minimum information for the nurse to plan culturally competent care:

- Length of time since the client and family left their country of origin
- The different locations (countries or refugee camps) and number of years spent prior to resettlement. Not only is the country important, but rural and urban differentiation may also be important, as well as social, political, and economic levels.
- Language spoken in the home and language skill in English
- Nonverbal communication style
- Religious practices
- Ethnic affiliation or identity
- Family roles and how they are influenced by the resettlement experience
- Social support or networks, especially relatives or family members in the new country

Assessment of these factors will assist the nurse in planning health care for refugee and/or immigrant families. Health services, preventive care, and health education have been identified over the years as important needs in health surveys that have been conducted in refugee communities.

The stress of resettlement is often a significant problem for members of refugee communities. Stress is related to the refugee experience and also to inadequate income, work-related problems, and loss of culture and traditions. The lack of mental health services is a real concern in refugee and immigrant communities and requires creative and innovative solutions. In refugee communities, a church, synagogue, or mosque can play a positive and important role—religion is often identified as a protective factor by refugees

in facilitating wellness and increasing quality of life. Refugee men and women may be reluctant to seek mental health services because of the stigma of mental illness as well as their traditional male/female roles. Postmigration stress may be exacerbated by unemployment or underemployment and may contribute to depression, PTSD, alcohol abuse, and poor general health status.

Many refugees come from underdeveloped countries with limited health care services, and the idea of preventive care is foreign to them. Preventive health practices such as dental care, breast self-examination, mammography, and Papanicolaou (Pap) smears are important for refugee women (see Evidence-Based Practice 11-2). Refugee men need preventive health care as well including regular prostate and testicular exams. Many barriers to good preventive care are environmental and social rather than cultural. Constraints are based on the refugee's individual situations as well as language, economic, occupational, and transportation problems. Cultural groups differ in regard to the priority given to individual goals versus those of the larger group. For example, many refugee communities, such as those of the Dinka, are a collectivist society that values the good of the group, traditional values, and group loyalty. This often conflicts with the individualistic American society. Many African refugees may suffer from racism and discrimination when they resettle in the United States, and this too impacts mental health and successful resettlement.

Many refugee women may have experienced gender-based violence (GBV) including torture, rape, and human rights abuses, and nurses and other health professionals must learn sensitive ways of broaching these subjects and helping refugee women access culturally appropriate care. Health care professionals, especially women physicians and nurses, can design programs that consider problems in access and appropriate language as well as culturally sensitive health care for women who have experienced GBV.

Health education, including information about access to care, is always important in planning services for refugee and immigrant communities.

Many refugees and immigrants do not use health education services, not necessarily because of cultural barriers but because of difficulties with language and access, the need for translation and transportation, the desire for women health care providers, and other barriers such as child care.

Health care institutions and agencies, from the beginning, should include bicultural health care providers on their staff. Community health workers could be trained to serve as interpreters and translators. It is always problematic for health care providers to use various family members as interpreters because of divisions along age and gender lines. Children do learn English more quickly than do their parents, but it would be inappropriate to expect a young boy to interpret a conversation about results of his mother's Pap smear. The health care provider's gender is important, as many refugee women are not comfortable with male doctors or nurses and might avoid health care altogether if female care providers are not available. Health care providers must be knowledgeable about the refugees' or immigrants' experiences and background, cultural and social factors, and other unique aspects of the population they serve. Refugees and new immigrants need access to language-appropriate and culturally relevant health care. Many refugees from community-oriented societies prefer to receive such information in a group or social setting rather than a one-to-one basis that is common in many US health care settings. For many refugee and/or immigrant communities, churches, mosques, and synagogues are appropriate settings for health education (Figure 11-4). Health fairs sponsored by community nurses and held within the refugee or immigrant communities have been very successful (Figure 11-5). Often, health fairs have been cosponsored by churches that serve immigrant or refugee communities.

The classic definition of community uses a geographic boundary, such as a village, town, or an urban settlement such as a city. This sense may be conveyed somewhat in terms such as Little Havana, Little Kabul, and Little Saigon, but such designations do not really convey the nature or

A Community-Based Collaborative Action Research (CBCAR) Intervention with Sudanese Refugee Women

This project was a partnership between students and faculty from a Midwestern school of nursing and a group of refugee women from South Sudan to address some of the health concerns in their community. This CBCAR intervention provided informational support, social support, and job skills to empower the women to help themselves, their families, and their community.

The intervention was a series of five educational seminars held at the Sudanese Community Church on a Saturday to accommodate the women's work schedules. Transportation and child care were provided. The students and faculty presented information to the women on the following topics:

- Well-woman health
- Parenting children in the United States
- Prevention of sexually transmitted diseases (STDs)
- Managing childhood illnesses
- Women's stress (depression, anxiety, and PTSD)

After each seminar, the students, faculty, and women shared social time and ate lunch together. Then a focus group was held to get the women's perspectives about the information presented in the seminars. A final focus group was held at the end of the project so participants could evaluate the project and discuss plans for future partnerships. A young refugee woman from South Sudan, who was trained as a professional interpreter, interpreted for each of the seminars and focus groups in both Dinka and Arabic, the primary languages spoken by the Sudanese women, and back into English.

The women responded very positively to the health information. Five of the thirteen women who attended the seminar on well-woman health followed up and scheduled their first mammogram. The students and faculty reported they learned as much from the experience as the refugee women. For instance, the women explained that the concept of preventive health care did not exist in South Sudan and people only went to clinics or hospitals when they were seriously ill. Some of the refugee women experienced discrimination during their visits with US health providers in settings such as the emergency department and health clinics. The women explained that it was difficult to communicate their concerns to health providers using an interpreter in the brief, 15-minute time-limited visits typical in these settings. Overall, the faculty, students, and refugee women learned valuable lessons about the differences in cultural perspectives that will influence future health encounters.

Clinical Implications

- Involve clients in a partnership to address health concerns that are important to them.
- Use trained, professional interpreters.
- Understand that many clients are most comfortable in a place that is familiar to them, such as a community church.
- Encourage clients/participants to discuss traditional health care behaviors and to describe their encounters with the US health care system.

Reference: Baird, M. B., Domian, E. W., Mulcahy, E. R., Mabior, R., Jemutai-Tanui, G., & Filippi, M. K. (2015, January 9). Creating a bridge of understanding between two worlds: Community-based collaborative-action research with Sudanese refugee women [Epub ahead of print]. *Public Health Nursing.* doi: 10.1111/phn.12172

quality of the refugee or immigrant experience, which tends to cross geographic boundaries. Although refugees from certain geographical areas such as Sudan tend to be resettled in common locations when they arrive in the United States, they may later move to be closer to relatives or families who came from the same village back home. The sense of shared displacement or "uprootedness" that serves to unite and distinguish immigrant or refugee communities from

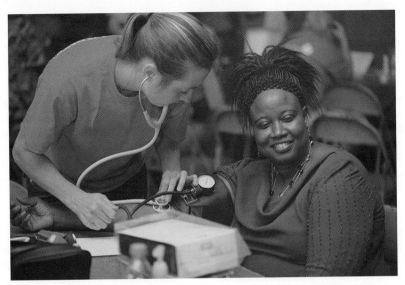

Figure 11-4. A Dinka refugee woman getting her blood pressure taken at a health fair conducted in the Sudanese Community Church by a volunteer from Heart to Heart International.

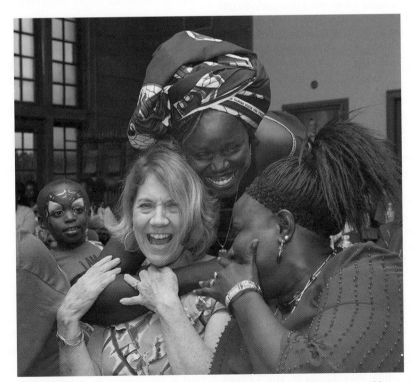

Figure 11-5. Two Dinka women celebrate a successful health fair partnership with American community health nurse, Martha Baird PhD, APRN, CTN.

other groups or communities is quite profound and cannot be ignored when planning for community-based health services.

Immigrants and refugees are often seen by health professionals as dominated by psychoemotional experiences and consequences of relocation. In other words, we focus on the effects of stress, relocation, and human rights violations. Indeed, much of the literature on immigrants and refugees focuses on PTSD. Although many immigrants and refugees have endured horrific experiences, this focus alone is not holistic. This view, according to DeSantis (1997), focuses on the primacy of the individual (an American value) rather than the community and thus prescribes psychiatric treatment instead of addressing the sociocultural and economic barriers at the macro level. It is at the macro level that transcultural health care providers must be engaged if they are to be effective participants in building healthy refugee and immigrant communities. This does not mean that individual health concerns should be ignored; it simply acknowledges that health care can be more effective when incorporated within a community focus, especially when dealing with immigrant or refugee communities.

Maintenance of Traditional Cultural Values and Practices

An important aspect of transcultural nursing is the collection of cultural data and the assessment of traditional values and practices and how they are maintained over time. The terms **assimilation** and **acculturation** are often used to describe how immigrants and refugees adapt and change over time in a new country. Both of these terms imply that newcomers give up their traditional lifestyle to adapt to the dominant culture. **Integration** may be a better term to describe the experience: it implies that an immigrant or refugee incorporates certain aspects of the new culture into his or her lifestyle, such as language and food, while still maintaining his or her cultural traditions and values. Both individuals and groups may be resistant to some changes and retain many traditional

cultural traits. Hispanics are the largest cultural/ethnic group in the United States, and in several large American cities, they constitute large percentages of the population. In these ethnic communities, it is easier to speak Spanish and to maintain other traditional cultural practices. Because traditional health beliefs and practices influence health and wellness, it is important for the nurse to understand the degree to which clients, families, and communities adhere to traditional health values and how nursing practice should reflect those values. Spector (2012) suggests that a person's health care and behavior during illness may well have roots in that person's traditional belief system. Unless community health nurses understand the traditional health beliefs and practices of their clients and communities, they may intervene at the wrong time or in an inappropriate way. Evidence-Based Practice 11-3 describes the hypertension prevention beliefs of a group of Hispanics and how they might influence barriers to preventive behaviors.

Many factors influence the likelihood that clients, families, and communities will maintain traditional health beliefs and practices. For example, the length of time a person lives in the new host country will influence factors such as language and the use of media (e.g., radio, television, and computers). Teenagers may quickly adjust to American culture and use a smartphone or an Ipad. The ability to speak English and to communicate with members of the majority culture is crucial to learning about the new host culture and beginning to feel comfortable. The size of the ethnic or cultural group is also important; if the group is small, individuals from that group are more likely to be exposed to outsiders and will not spend all their time within their own group or community. Although this may hasten integration in the new culture, not being around individuals from their own cultural group may deprive members of an immigrant or refugee community of the social support and presence of a large ethnic community.

Generally, children acculturate more quickly because they are exposed to their peer group

Hypertension Prevention Beliefs of Hispanics

This qualitative study used focus group methodology to explore attitudes and beliefs of Hispanics regarding hypertension prevention behaviors. The investigators found that participants were knowledgeable about hypertension and had a positive attitude about prevention. However, they identified numerous barriers to preventive behaviors.

The participants believed that hypertension is strongly influenced by unhealthy diets, lack of exercise, and being overweight. Certain emotions such as "worry" and "upset" were also identified as causes of hypertension. Participants agreed that the consequences of hypertension were serious, such as stroke or kidney disease. They believed that lifestyle modification (diet and managing stress) would be best to control hypertension, although medication was helpful too.

The participants described three subcategories of limitations—health insurance for hypertension screening, money for purchasing healthy food, and lack of time. Lack of time was the greatest barrier to preventing hypertension as time constraints interfered with a healthy lifestyle and engaging in activities to reduce stress.

Every participant described Hispanic food as "a link to the past" and saw Hispanic food as a symbol of love, affection, and hospitality. Hispanic food was generally described as "unhealthy" because it was fried, salty, and contained large portions of lard, meat, and carbohydrates. While healthy adaptations of Hispanic food were acknowledged, traditional foods were the choice for social occasions as they are symbolic of hospitality and affection.

The participants described cultural norms that valued spending time with family and friends rather than regularly scheduled exercise or "working out." Dancing (with Latin music) was suggested as more appropriate than going to a yoga class. Another deterrent to hypertension prevention was not seeking health care unless symptomatic—"I'd better be pretty darn sick before I step into a doctor's office." Participants described a cultural norm that defined overweight as normative. Many Hispanics think being a little heavy is healthy; one explained, "Culturally, we don't look like little toothpicks." Being overweight may also be more acceptable to older Hispanics.

Clinical Implications

- Younger and more highly educated Hispanics may be more knowledgeable about and open to lifestyle changes than are older adults.
- Assess cultural norms when prescribing lifestyle changes for adult Hispanics who have hypertension. For example, exercise, stress reduction, and diet modification strategies may have significant cultural barriers.
- Social interactions are highly valued. Exercise and stress reduction can capitalize on this cultural value by building on another cultural value—dancing.
- Public health campaigns should emphasize that modifying traditional foods to make them healthy is appropriate, not only for regular meals but also for parties and social events.

Reference: Aroian, K. J., Peters, R. M., Rudner, N., & Waser, L. (2012). Hypertension prevention beliefs of Hispanics. *Journal of Transcultural Nursing*, 23(2), 134–142.

through schooling and they learn cultural characteristics through that association. The need to work outside the household often exposes women from traditional cultures to others of the majority culture; thus, they learn English more quickly than if they remain isolated at home. When individuals from other cultures seek health care in their host country, they become familiar with its health care system. This does not necessarily mean that they comply with all health advice, but contact with the system decreases anxiety and confusion, and individuals are more likely to seek care again. In addition, if individuals or groups have distinguishing ethnic characteristics, such

as skin color, they may be more isolated because of discrimination and thus retain traditional values, beliefs, and practices over a longer time. Some factors that influence the likelihood that clients, families, and communities will maintain traditional health beliefs and practices are shown in Box 11-2.

Access to Health and Nursing Care for Diverse Cultural Groups

Members of diverse cultural groups, especially those who are poor and without health insurance, face special problems in accessing health and nursing care. Access to care is often determined by economic and geographic factors. Certain cultural groups have faced discrimination and poverty, and their ability to access care has been compromised. Sensitivity to cultural factors has often been lacking in the health care of traditional communities and identified minority groups.

In addition to economic status and discriminatory factors that limit access to care, geographic location plays an important role in health care. Many of these medically underserved areas lack medical personnel and the variety of health facilities and services that are available to urban populations. For example, Native Americans living in sparsely settled and isolated reservations in the western part of the United States must travel long distances, sometimes over primitive roads, to obtain health care services. Individuals who live on the Navajo or Hopi reservations in Northern Arizona and have type 2 diabetes or kidney failure requiring dialysis must travel long distances for care. They may be picked up as early as 4 AM by a shuttle van that takes them into Tuba City, AZ for renal dialysis; the van takes them home later in the afternoon. Depending on the route the van takes and the weather conditions, some individuals may arrive home as late as 5 or 6 PM and spending up to 8 hours per day in travel time. This arduous routine may take place as often as 3 days each week.

Other factors may also limit access to care. Many clients from culturally diverse backgrounds

Box 11-2 Factors Influencing Traditional Beliefs and Practices

1. Length of time in the new host country.
2. Size of the ethnic or cultural group with which an individual identifies and interacts.
3. Age of the individual. As a general rule, children acculturate more rapidly than do adults or seniors.
4. Ability to speak English and communicate with members of the majority culture. Language spoken in the home among family members.
5. Economic status. For example, if the family economic situation necessitates that a Salvadoran woman work outside the home, she may learn English more quickly than if she remains within the household and speaks only Spanish with her family members.
6. Educational status. In general, higher levels of education lead to faster acculturation.
7. Health status of family members. If individuals and their families seek health care in their host country, they begin to "learn the system." This does not mean that they comply with all of the health advice, but contacts with the system should decrease anxiety and confusion.
8. Distinguishing ethnic characteristics, such as skin color. These individuals may be more isolated because of discrimination and thus may retain traditional values related to health beliefs and behavior.
9. Intermarriage. Ethnic intermarriage is associated with a greater loss of traditional ethnic identity.
10. Rigidity or flexibility of the host society. This refers to the extent to which the host society is willing to allow members of different ethnic groups, along with their traditions, beliefs, and practices, into their structure, culture, and identity.

Box 11-3 Factors to Consider in the Nursing Care of Culturally Diverse Groups

1. Employment opportunities and insurance coverage or the financial ability to pay for health care services
2. Different traditional belief systems as well as different norms and values
3. Lack of cultural sensitivity on the part of social service and health care workers
4. Lack of bilingual personnel or staff members or the lack of interpreters to assist clients and care providers
5. Rapid changes in the US health care system, where clients are "lost" in the gaps between agencies and services
6. Inconvenient locations or hours of health and social services that preclude clients from accessing care
7. Lack of understanding, trust, and commitment on the part of health care providers

seek the services of health care professionals who speak their language. When this is not possible, they are reluctant to seek care or may not understand the importance of following medical advice. Undocumented persons may be reluctant to seek health care because they are afraid of revealing their immigration status. Women from traditional Muslim cultures will be reluctant to seek care from male health care providers. Another common and significant factor that limits access to health services is a lack of understanding by clients of how to use health resources. This lack of understanding may be due in part to cultural factors. Often, this lack of understanding means that members of diverse cultural groups are less able to adequately cope with health problems than are other members of the community. Nurses can develop sensitivity to diverse groups within communities and reach out to them with culturally specific health programs. Box 11-3 lists some important factors that nurses must take into account for culturally appropriate community-based care.

Assessment of Culturally Diverse Communities

A **cultural assessment** is the process used by nurses to assess cultural needs of individual clients (Leininger, 1991, 1995; see also Appendix A).

In general, the purpose of all successful cultural assessments is to collect information that helps health professionals better understand and address the specific health needs and interests of their target populations. Individual cultural assessments are accomplished through the use of a systematic process. In community health nursing, the community is considered the client, and several models have been proposed to help nurses assess the community (Stanhope & Lancaster, 2012), including the Andrews/Boyle Transcultural Nursing Assessment Guide for Groups and Communities (Appendix B). A community nursing assessment requires gathering relevant data, interpreting the data (including problem analysis and prioritization), and identifying and implementing intervention activities for community health (Stanhope & Lancaster, 2012). The community nursing assessment often focuses on a broad goal, such as improvement in the health status of a group of people. It is often the characteristics of people that give each community its uniqueness, and these common characteristics, which influence norms, values, religious practices, educational aspirations, and health and illness behaviors, are frequently determined by shared cultural experiences. Thus, including the cultural component to a community nursing assessment strengthens the assessment base. Box 11-4 provides basic principles underlying all cultural assessments.

Box 11-4 Basic Principles of Cultural Assessments

1. **All cultures must be viewed in the context in which they have developed.** Cultural practices develop as a "logical" or understandable response to a particular human problem, and the setting as well as the problem must be considered. This is one reason why environmental and/or contextual data are so important.

2. **The meaning and purpose of the behavior must be interpreted within the context of the specific culture.** For example, the Hispanic client's refusal to take a "hot" medication with a cold liquid is understandable if the nurse is aware that many Hispanic patients adhere to hot/cold theories of illness causation. There is often a range or spectrum of illness beliefs, with one end encompassing illnesses defined within the biomedical model and the other end firmly anchored within the individual culture

(Huff & Kline, 2007). The more widely disparate the differences between the biomedical model and the beliefs within the cultural group, the greater the potential for encountering resistance to biomedical interventions.

3. **There is such a phenomenon as intracultural variation.** Not every member of a cultural group displays all the behaviors that are associated with that group. For instance, not every Hispanic client will adhere to hot/cold theories of illness, and not every Hispanic mother will have a close personal relationship with her son. It is only by careful appraisal of the assessment data, and validation of the nurse's assessment with the client and family, that culturally competent care can be provided.

Cultural Competence in Health Maintenance and Health Promotion

Leininger (1978, 1995) suggested that cultural groups have their own culturally defined ways of maintaining and promoting health. Nursing interventions to improve the health of individuals, groups, and communities can best be planned and implemented by considering persons within their social, cultural, and environmental contexts.

Community nurses, who have direct access to clients in the context of their daily lives, should be especially aware of the importance of cultural knowledge in promoting and maintaining health, because the promotion and maintenance of health occurs in the context of everyday lives rather than in the doctor's office or in a hospital. The range of cultural influences on health maintenance and promotion is considerable. Major cultural issues and considerations must be addressed before health maintenance and promotion programs are implemented for culturally diverse groups. Evidence-Based Practice 11-4 describes a study that sought to understand parental perceptions of

rural African American parents about the human papillomavirus (HPV) vaccine and how HPV vaccination rates among children in rural minority communities might be increased.

Cultural competence in community settings begins with anticipatory planning. In addressing cultural issues, it is important to involve local community leaders or "elders" who are members of the cultural group being targeted to promote the acceptance of health promotion programs. Such a leader, for example, might be the pastor of an African American church in the rural south or a member of the tribal council for a Native American tribe. The nurse must also be sensitive to cultural differences in leadership styles. For example, the African American pastor may not speak in favor of the health education program from his or her pulpit, choosing instead to work through more informal networks. Numerous nurse researchers (Abrums, 2004; Shambley-Ebron & Boyle, 2006) have found that many African Americans rely on spirituality and/or religious practices when they are ill, and in

Rural African American Parents' Knowledge and Decisions About Human Papillomavirus Vaccination

Identifying those cultural factors or predictors of preventive health behaviors is an important activity in community health. The National Cancer Institute advises that certain strands of the human papillomavirus (HPV) are responsible for nearly 99% of cervical cancer cases and at least 20% of cancers of the head, neck, and anogenital areas (National Cancer Institute, 2012). The HPV vaccine can prevent many of these cancers if given to children (both girls and boys) at the age of 11 to 12 years. Previous research has shown that African American women are often skeptical about the HPV vaccine and that African American men are not knowledgeable about HPV or the HPV vaccine.

Understanding parental perceptions about the HPV vaccine is key to increasing vaccine rates, which are significantly lower for children from minority groups living in rural areas. The study sought to find culturally specific points of intervention that would increase HPV vaccination rates among children in rural African American communities. The researchers used a descriptive cross-sectional design and quantitative methods to collect data in three rural communities in Georgia. Four hundred parents participated in the study. Findings imply three major points of intervention: culture, religious affiliation, and parent education:

- *Culture:* Findings describe rural communities with low income, geographic challenges to access care, and large numbers of self-reported religious affiliation (Baptist). Local culture shapes people's perceptions of risk or perceived vulnerability. People assign value (either positive or negative) to an issue on the basis of their experience, and they trust experts who have a similar background to their own.
- *Religious affiliation:* Among participants in this study, religious affiliation had a correlation with vaccinating or planning to vaccinate a child. This is a significant finding since religion and spirituality are integral components of sociodemographics (rural culture) and influence perceived vulnerability to HPV infection and perceived severity of HPV infection and subsequent HPV-related cancer.

The study found a "disconnect" between people's attitudes about faith and healing and their actual choice to vaccinate their children. In other words, those that designated themselves as "Baptist," a reportedly "conservative" religion, reported high rates of HPV vaccination and intent to vaccinate.
- *Parent education:* The findings suggest that in this population of rural African American parents, both low knowledge of HPV vaccination and low level of perceived barriers could be attributed to the lack of knowledge about the connection between persistent HPV infection and HPV-related cancer.

This study reveals several intervention points: educating parents or caregivers about HPV-related cancers, HPV transmission, and HPV vaccination. Other possible interventions include increasing access to health care, reducing the cost of vaccination, and implementing school-based vaccine programs.

Clinical Implications

- Use culturally relevant interventions to educate both parents and youth about HPV. For rural African Americans, sensitivity and respect for the tenets of their faith are important. These tenets include but are not limited to belonging to the church family, giving problems over to God, and recognizing the human body as a temple of God.
- Access to care, cost, and availability of the vaccine influence HPV vaccination rates.
- Advocate for access to health care for rural residents and their children.
- Parental perceptions about the HPV vaccine are key to increasing vaccine rates among African American children in rural communities.
- Direct community interventions to minority families, communities, and the larger systems in which social injustice and racial discrimination have occurred.

Reference: Thomas, T. L., Strickland, O. L., DiClemente, R., Higgins, M., & Haber, M. (2012). Rural african american parents' knowledge and decisions about Human Papillomavirus vaccination. *Journal of Nursing Scholarship, 44*(4), 358–367.

general, a health program that has the support of the church pastor would be viewed favorably by the church community. In addition to local community and religious leaders, it is important to involve those who are most affected by the health-related problem in the planning process. Those involved in planning and participating in the program's activities should likewise participate in its evaluation. Collaboration between the planner and the participants is often the key to success in community-based health programs (Stanhope & Lancaster, 2012).

Second, family members, churches, employers, and community worksites need to be involved in supporting health promotion/education programs through the use of networks that already exist. For example, a health education program about the importance of having a routine screening such as a mammography can be established at a worksite that employs mostly women. A display could be set up in the cafeteria, dining room, or other accessible site. Women could view the educational material during breaks or after lunch. Providing information about sites where women could obtain a mammography would be an important component of such a program.

Third, health messages are more readily accepted if they do not conflict with existing cultural beliefs. If the nurse plans to talk about prevention of teenage pregnancy to mothers and daughters at a local church, he or she should be sensitive to the group's religious values and norms. The nurse could discuss these plans in advance with some of the mothers and the pastor and ask for ways to strengthen the church's position, such as the support of abstinence programs. This is the time to be sensitive to the group's religious values.

Fourth, language barriers and cultural differences are very real problems in many large cities as well as rural areas. For example, in the US–Mexico border areas, *promotoras* (community health workers) are used to disseminate messages in Spanish and to help organize and present information that is culturally appropriate and understood by community members. Many Native American tribes make use of community health representatives (CHRs)

to assist individuals to improve their health and/or access care. The health care professional should not be afraid to ask for help and suggestions and should make it a point to find educational material such as brochures or videos in the appropriate language and with a culturally acceptable message.

Lastly, **cultural sensitivity**, that ability to be aware of the needs and emotions of others, is essential to meeting health needs that exist within diverse cultural groups. For example, HIV/AIDS is spreading rapidly in some Hispanic and African American populations and is associated with intravenous drug use, violence, and the use of crack cocaine (Shambley-Ebron, Dole, & Karikari, 2014). In addition, the root causes of poverty and unemployment should be examined, and programs that improve overall economic status of culturally diverse communities should be developed. Culturally relevant treatment programs should be implemented. Many minority women who seek treatment programs for cocaine addiction encounter barriers that seem insurmountable. Treatment programs are not available in many areas, and child care facilities are not provided—even in day-treatment programs. Thus, a young mother living in a rural area with children would not be able to find a treatment center that meets her needs. If she seeks admittance to a residential treatment program, she might have to agree to place her children in foster care.

Cultural competence to promote and maintain health in families requires knowledge about family systems, including relationships between family members, and how family members individually and collectively cope with health issues and challenges. Promoting and maintaining health also requires that the nurse understand cultural lifeways or practices within the family. Culturally competent nursing care in health maintenance and promotion is guided by four principles (American Academy of Nursing Expert Panel on Culturally Competent Health Care, 1992):

1. Care is designed for the specific client.
2. Care is based on the uniqueness of the client's culture and includes cultural norms and values.

3. Care includes self-empowered strategies to facilitate client decision making in health behavior.
4. Care is provided with sensitivity and is based on the cultural uniqueness of the client.

Family Systems

Because the family is the basic social unit, it provides the context in which health promotion and maintenance are defined and carried out. The nurse can recognize and use the family's role in altering the health status of a family member and in supporting lifestyle changes. This requires an appreciation of the role of the family in diverse cultural groups. African American families, for example, may demonstrate interchangeable roles for their male and female members, extended ties across generations, and strong social support systems for the family such as the African American church, all of which can be tapped by a community health nurse to activate health and wellness in families (Campinha-Bacote, 2013; Giger, Appel, Davidhizar, & Davis, 2008). Immigrant and refugee families also tend to have strong extended ties with their kin, and changes in lifestyle, diet, and other established patterns of daily life that influence health status will need the understanding and support of all family members.

Coping Behaviors

Clients often have distinct, culturally based behaviors to cope with illness as well as to maintain and promote health. These behaviors may be traced to the health–illness paradigms discussed in Chapter 4. Beliefs about hot and cold, yin and yang, and harmony and balance may underlie actions to prevent disease and maintain health. Community nurses who understand their clients' cultural values and beliefs can assess their understanding of health and illness. These assessment data serve as the basis for planning health guidance and teaching strategies that focus on incorporating cultural beliefs and practices in the nursing care plan. It seems likely that clients in the process of coping with illness and seeking help may involve a network of persons, ranging from family members and select laypersons to health care professionals.

Seeking social support is often seen as a means of coping. Social support varies widely across people, cultural groups, and circumstances. An individual's coping behaviors during an illness of a family member may differ remarkably at any one time during the illness, depending on intrapersonal, interpersonal, and environmental factors. Nurses working with diverse cultural populations will want to learn and understand how coping styles are used by individuals and family members as well as how these coping styles change over time as these factors are often influenced by culture.

Lifestyle Practices

Lifestyle is the typical way of life of an individual, group, or culture. Cultural influences that shape lifestyles have a significant impact on such health-promoting practices as diet, exercise, and stress management. Community health nurses should assess the implications of diet planning and teaching to clients and family members who adhere to culturally prescribed practices concerning foods. Some cultural groups believe that certain foods maintain or promote health. Specific foods often are restricted or promoted during illness, for example, the proverbial chicken soup. Cultural preferences determine the style of food preparation and consumption, the frequency of eating, the time of eating, and the eating utensils. Milk is not always considered a suitable source of protein for Native Americans, Hispanics, Blacks, and some Asians because of their relatively high incidence of lactose intolerance.

Nurses who work with culturally different clients must evaluate patterns of daily living as well as culturally prescribed activities before they suggest forms of physical activity or exercise to clients. Not everyone has access to a tennis court or a gym, and many individuals would not feel comfortable in such surroundings, or in aerobics classes regardless of the setting. Helping

clients plan physical activities that are culturally acceptable is an important first step in implementing a program of physical activity for clients in diverse cultures. For example, traditional tribal dancing has become popular on some reservations for Native Americans. Running remains popular for members of the Hopi tribe. Running is deeply rooted in Hopi traditions as a way to carry messages from village to village and is also prominent in Hopi ceremonies. In the past, men of the Hopi tribe were superb distance runners, and the tribe still sponsors running events for its members. Hopi High School in Arizona has earned 23 state cross-country titles in a row and is well known throughout the state for its excellent track teams (Fonseca, 2013).

Another aspect of lifestyle that must be understood for the successful promotion of health and wellness is the manner in which culturally different clients manage stress. Stress management is learned from childhood through our parents, our social group, and our cultural group. Smoking and chewing tobacco, although not healthy habits, are often used to manage stress. Although lifestyle practices such as chewing tobacco and smoking are not associated with a group's culture per se, they are often found in groups whose members do not have appropriate options and/or alternatives and who are poor and unable to access other options.

Evidence-Based Practice 11-5 describes how cardiovascular disease is defined and how Aboriginal women in certain tribal communities in Canada deal with such a diagnosis. Aboriginal women believed that they had taken on many responsibilities within their families and communities and that they could not manage any more lifestyle changes, not even to improve cardiac health. Providing culturally competent nursing care to heal their "broken hearts" requires an understanding of Aboriginal history in Canada and cultural knowledge about how the women made meaning out of their diagnosis and treatment programs.

The presence of large numbers of families with altered family processes and unhealthy lifestyles within any community may create problems for all members of the larger community or society. The nurse who works in **community settings** will frequently encounter these families and is in an ideal position to act as their advocate, to refer them to appropriate care, and, in effect, to improve the health of the community at large. This often requires understanding the individual's or family's lifestyle.

The nurse may find that in some cultural groups, such as Mexican Americans, traditional healers, such as *curanderos*, can be helpful for persons with some emotional or psychological disorders. It has been a tradition for many Mexican Americans to seek care from traditional healers. This lifestyle practice or health seeking behavior seems "appropriate" and the right thing to do, whereas seeking care from a psychiatrist for this particular occasion or situation would be highly unlikely behavior. In some aggregate ethnic settings, such as the Chinatown area in San Francisco, there are practitioners of traditional Chinese medicine as well as Western medicine, acupuncturists, neighborhood pharmacies, and herbalists, all of which are available to meet the diverse needs of that particular neighborhood. Lifestyle is about the parts of our lives that make us feel comfortable and "right with the world." It's how we make our homes, relate to our loved ones, raise our children, and manage our health and the well-being of those around us. Feeling comfortable with a health care provider's office may depend on the health care provider sharing the same ethnic heritage or at least speaking the language of the client.

Cultural Competence in Primary, Secondary, and Tertiary Preventive Programs

Nurses working in community settings use health-related concepts that are identified with the practice of community health nursing. Concepts such as "community as client" and "population-focused practice" were discussed briefly in the first sections of this chapter. Another important concept

Broken Heart Stories: Understanding Aboriginal* Women's Cardiac Problems

The morbidity associated with heart disease is significantly higher in Aboriginal than non-Aboriginal Canadians with Aboriginal women showing the highest rate. Cardiovascular disease is commonly viewed as "White man's sickness." It is important to understand how individuals attribute meaning to cardiac health, healing, and overall life under complex social and cultural conditions. The role of colonialism is not only a historical fact but is a reality of today that serves to maintain health inequalities. Colonialism served to destroy traditional community structures that supported the role of the grandmother and that of women in general. Along with Aboriginal communities becoming more patriarchal, colonialism has altered the responsibilities and identities of women with particular consequences for women's health and also for that of their families and communities.

Cardiovascular disease is highly defined by biomedical terms; thus, the diagnosis of such a disease means introducing a highly medicalized "Western" sickness into a new cultural setting where there are few traditional healing options. The authors used a narrative–discursive approach in their study to capture subtle meaning-making processes that reflected the interplay between the individual and the culture. Sixteen women, all with various heart problems, volunteered for the study. Three major narratives were identified in the findings: problems of the heart, healing, and sociocultural context:

- *Problems of the heart:* While the participants described an illness genealogy of cancer, stroke, and diabetes, they reported that they were shocked to learn that they had heart problems. The women tried to downplay their symptoms and worries while struggling with fear and anxiety, afraid that a racing heart might be the precursor of another cardiac episode. Many of the participants were unaware that there are unique heart symptoms for women and for Aboriginal people.
- *Healing:* Many of the women relied on their Christian beliefs and turned to prayers and reading the Bible. Only one woman practiced traditional alternatives to Western medicine. All were willing to take pharmaceutical medications, believing that taking pills required very little effort on their part. There was great ambivalence and even hostility toward the typically recommended heart-healthy lifestyle changes such as diet management, increasing exercise, and quitting smoking. Generations of White people had told Aboriginal people how to live in the name of "civilization," now health care providers were telling them how to live, this time in the name of "health."
- *Sociocultural context:* The mainstay of the women's narratives focused on the care and attention they gave to others, providing a backdrop to understand why living a heart-healthy lifestyle was so difficult for them. Aboriginal women take care of children and grandchildren, as well as foster and/or adopted children, many of whom had developmental difficulties due to fetal alcohol syndrome. The women made it clear that they often took on extra responsibilities in their families and communities with little or no support from men. Heart problems were not positioned as major concerns. It seemed the women intended to not burden others with what they called their "broken hearts."

Clinical Implications

- Aboriginal women need additional information about the unique symptoms of cardiovascular problems in women and in Aboriginal people. They also need information about the dangers of high blood pressure and the close relationship between anxiety and heart disease; panic attacks can be heart problems in disguise in postmenopausal women.
- Health messages need to focus on positive and achievable goals. Taking prescribed medications can be an achievable goal that has positive results for women's health. Downplay the diet

and exercise regimens. Talk about healthy eating and enjoyable activities.

- Traditional healing practices, such as sharing circles, sweat lodges, smudging, and artwork, include family and community and have repeatedly been associated with positive health outcomes. Health promotion activities that are less "top-down" would create more interest and support and less negativity.
- Consider how heart-healthy messages could be tied into the rich storytelling traditions of First Nations or Native Americans.

- Become knowledgeable and sensitive to First Nations/Native Americans cultures, belief systems, lifeways, and traditions as a first step in developing culturally competent care.

Aboriginal or First Nations are the terms used by Canadians to refer to Native Peoples of Canada

Reference: Medved, M. I., Brockmeier, J., Morach, J., & Chartier-Courchene, L. (2013). Broken heart stories; Understanding Aboriginal women's cardiac problems. *Qualitative Health Research, 23*(2), 1613–1625.

for community nurses is **levels of prevention**. Preventive care, consisting of primary, secondary, and tertiary activities, is directed toward high-risk groups or aggregates within a community setting. **Primary prevention** is composed of activities that prevent the occurrence of an illness, disease, or health risk. The preventive actions take place before the disease or illness occurs. **Secondary prevention** involves the early diagnosis and appropriate treatment of a condition or disease. **Tertiary prevention** focuses on rehabilitation and the prevention of recurrences or complications.

The major aim of community-based preventive programs is to reduce the risk for the population at large, rather than to prevent illnesses in specific individuals. As long as preventive actions are directed toward a given population rather than toward individuals, there is a chance of altering the general balance of forces so that even if not all individuals benefit, many will have a chance to avoid illness. Evidence-Based Practice 11-6 *Yellow Dirt* documents the impact of uranium mining on the Navajo reservation and is an account of the tragic failure of preventive programs at all levels.

Primary Prevention

In their daily practice, community nurses are often involved in activities related to all three levels of prevention. Primary prevention is aimed at individuals and groups who are susceptible to

disease or injury but have no discernable pathology or illness. The example of primary prevention used here is prenatal health services in Mexican American communities. Prenatal services serve as primary preventive measures for both the mother and her infant.

Overview of the Health Concern

When viewed as a group, racial and ethnic minorities suffer from worse health compared to White counterparts. Differences in the incidence, prevalence, mortality, and burden of diseases and other adverse health conditions exist among ethnic population groups in the United States (Minority Health: Quick Facts about Health Disparities, 2009). For many years, public health agencies have tried to improve maternal and infant services to high-risk populations. In 1985, a special government report on minority health reported that many minority women do not begin prenatal care during the first trimester (Heckler, 1985a, 1985b) and that this has serious consequences for mothers and infants. In response to this report, there was a considerable national effort to provide prenatal services to all pregnant women, but especially minority women and teenagers, and to reach them early in their pregnancy. Many communities now have broad-based coalitions that facilitate a comprehensive approach, especially for pregnant teenagers.

Yellow Dirt by Judy Pasternak

Yellow Dirt is a book that documents the impact of uranium mining on the land and the people of the Navajo Nation. During World War II, the Navajo Nation, wanting to support America's role in the war, permitted uranium mining on reservation land. The project was originally kept secret under the guise of national security. As early as 1952, the Public Health Service warned of cancer risks associated with uranium exposure. The Navajo cancer rate doubled between the 1970s and 1990s.

The initial case of *Navajo Neuropathy* was diagnosed in 1959; but it was only a matter of time before other Navajo children were diagnosed with the same syndrome. Scarce research monies were focused solely on genetics as the probable cause, ignoring the role of uranium exposure.

Hodgins and Hodgins (2013) describe the high incidence of severe combined immunodeficiency syndrome (SCIDS) among the Navajo, which results in a failure of the antibody response and cell-mediated immunity. In 2006, SCIDS was "discovered" to be the result of a mutation of the MPV17 gene.

Pasternak describes corporate and government actions, as well as the portrayal of the personal anguish experienced by many Navajo. *Yellow Dirt* is a compelling account that demonstrates the socio-economic, political, cultural, and policy factors that facilitated the exploitation of the Navajo Nation.

Clinical Implications

- Advocacy and education are important roles in community health nursing.
- Nurses can also play a role in community empowerment.
- Become knowledgeable about environmental concerns and their impact on health.
- Become familiar with local, state, and national agencies that are responsible for protecting the environment.
- Identify environmental concerns in your own community. How are they being dealt with?

References:
Hodgins, O., & Hodgins, D. (2013). American indians and Alaskan natives. In L. D. Purnell (Ed.). *Transcultural health care: A culturally competent approach* (pp. 451–449). Philadelphia, PA: F. A. Davis Company.
Pasternak, J. (2010). Yellow dirt. New York, NY: Free Press.
Prengaman, M. V. (2013). Review of Yellow Dirt by Judy Pasternak. *Journal of Transcultural Nursing, 24*(4), 417.

The risk factors of pregnancy include age (both extremes), parity, low socioeconomic status, and other factors such as diabetes and alcohol and tobacco use. In addition, numbers of children within the family (need for child care), transportation problems, and less assistance from a support system influence use of prenatal care and other health services. Many Mexican American women fall in these categories. Furthermore, an infant with health concerns is at risk for further problems; there may be negative and long-term consequences for the child and the mother, as well as other family members. Obtaining early and regular prenatal care greatly enhances a young woman's chance of delivering a healthy, full-term baby.

A program of primary prevention would focus on preventing infant morbidity and mortality and other health problems in Mexican American mothers and their infants. Early prenatal care may enhance pregnancy outcome and maternal health by assessing risk, providing health advice, and managing chronic and pregnancy-related health conditions (McKenzie, Pinger, & Kotecki, 2012). Nurses are in a unique position to advocate for polices that increase women's access to services for prenatal care. Nursing care must be broadly focused,

providing some specific services but also helping clients access other resources in the community.

Access to Care. There are various reasons why Mexican American women might not seek care during pregnancy. Cost is often a factor, and in many areas of the country, Mexican Americans have tended to belong to poorer socioeconomic groups. Twenty-three percent of Mexican American families in the United States live below the poverty level, and many are headed by a single female parent (U.S. Census Bureau, 2010). Mexican Americans are concentrated in blue-collar jobs, farm work, domestic work, and service occupations; lower status jobs translate into lower income and higher poverty rates (Ayón, 2009). In 2005, the Pew Hispanic Center estimated that nearly 11 million undocumented immigrants live in the United States, 6 million of whom are from Mexico (Passel, 2009).

The value of routine prenatal visits to a health care provider should be repeatedly emphasized by nurses; some Mexican American women may stop regular visits if they are feeling well, because they are not accustomed to seeing a health care provider unless they are ill. The community health nurse can provide information about community resources and help clients access care early in pregnancy by referral to appropriate agencies. Nearly all states now offer programs that provide funds and services for low-income pregnant women, although in the recession that began in the 2000s, funding for many of these services was reduced or eliminated in some states. Although not a health program specifically, the Women, Infants, and Children (WIC) Program provides nutritious food and nutrition education to low-income pregnant and breast-feeding mothers, their infants, and their children under age 5 who are found at nutritional risk. WIC also provides health care referrals (U.S. Department of Agriculture, Food and Nutrition Service, 2014). The rate of low birth weight babies among infants born to women on WIC is 25% lower than for infants born to similarly situated women not receiving WIC benefits. WIC is an example of one

of the most popular, successful, and cost-effective public health programs (U.S. Department of Agriculture, Food and Nutrition Service, n.d.). Referring pregnant women to WIC services is a strong primary prevention intervention by community nurses.

Many Mexican Americans are more comfortable accessing health educational services in a setting that is known to them and where they feel comfortable. Neighborhood churches or neighborhood centers are excellent settings for health education; women know where they are located and are familiar with them in contrast to a hospital or clinic setting away from their neighborhood. Often, churches can provide child care so that mothers can leave their children in a safe place while they are attending prenatal classes.

Cultural Views About Modesty. Any prenatal program that serves Mexican American women may be underused unless consideration is given to some Mexican American women's modesty and reluctance to be examined by male health care providers. The use of female nurse practitioners and midwives is ideal for this population. In addition, consideration should be given to incorporation of the traditional *parteras* (lay midwives) or *promotoras* (health workers) in the preventive educational services. *Promotoras,* community health workers who speak Spanish, are especially effective in delivering primary health care services to expectant mothers either in community settings or in the client's home.

Language Barriers. It is absolutely essential in a prenatal program for a Mexican American population that the majority of health care professionals in the program be bilingual. If that is not possible, interpreters must be employed to facilitate the professional services. All prenatal classes should be offered in Spanish and English. This sometimes means that two classes must be offered concurrently; many Mexican American women speak predominantly either Spanish or English and choose the class with the language

they understand best. The availability of health education material in Spanish is critical to reinforce teaching and anticipatory guidance. Videos may be more effective than brochures or other written material. In some border communities, such as Nogales, Arizona, the Hispanic population is high (93.6%), and most residents speak Spanish in their homes (Arizona Department of Health Services, Office of Health Systems Development, 2005). Nurses working in community settings must always be aware of language barriers and plan accordingly.

Cultural Views of Motherhood and Pregnancy. Some evidence indicates that women of Mexican American heritage may adhere to slightly different value orientations and cultural views of motherhood and pregnancy than do those found in mainstream American culture (Zoucha & Zamarripa, 2013). The Mexican American culture traditionally values motherhood, and young women are encouraged to prepare themselves for this role. Community health nurses, nurse practitioners, and professional midwives are in important positions to help pregnant women prepare for motherhood and its associated responsibilities. Understanding and reinforcing cultural

views of pregnancy will be helpful for clients, because trust and mutual goal setting can develop more rapidly. All nursing interventions should incorporate family members, especially mothers and sisters, for support of the pregnant woman. Emphasizing the responsibility for the mother to be healthy for her baby's health and welfare is appropriate for this cultural group.

Traditional Pregnancy-Related Folk Beliefs. Many Mexican Americans adhere to some traditional beliefs and practices related to pregnancy and childbirth. Traditionally, children are greatly valued and are desired soon after marriage. Census data from the 2000 and 2010 census indicate that Mexican Americans tend to marry and have children at earlier ages (Raley, Durden, & Wildssmith, 2004; Zoucha & Zamarripa, 2013). As in many other cultures, Mexican Americans consider pregnancy, birth, and the immediate postpartum period as a time of great vulnerability for women and their newborns. Box 11-5 shows selected beliefs and practices of pregnancy and childbirth in traditional Mexican American culture. Each generation of childbearing women perceives pregnancy and birth differently (Kemp, 2005). It is important for the nurse to assess

---

Box 11-5 Selected Beliefs and Practices of Pregnancy and Childbirth in Traditional Mexican American Culture

- Avoid strong emotions such as anger and fear during pregnancy.
- Cool air is dangerous during pregnancy and should be avoided.
- Bathe often during pregnancy; be active so that the baby will not grow too big and hinder delivery.
- Eat a nutritious diet; "give in" to food cravings.
- Massage is helpful to place the baby in the right position for birth.
- Don't raise your arms above your head or sit with your legs crossed during pregnancy because these actions will cause knots in the umbilical cord.

- Moonlight should be avoided during pregnancy, especially during an eclipse, because it will cause a birth defect.
- After delivery, a 40-day period known as *la diet* or *la cuarentena* is observed. Certain activities and foods are restricted during this time.
- Chamomile tea will relieve nausea and vomiting in pregnancy.
- Heartburn can be treated with baking soda.
- Laxatives and purges may be used to "clean" the intestinal tract.

the views of members of the pregnant mother's support system, especially her mother, who belongs to an earlier generation and may adhere to more traditional values. It is always necessary to assess intracultural variation; not every member of any given culture adheres to the same beliefs and behaviors typical of that culture.

Mexican American Cultural Networks. Traditionally, the family is very important in Mexican American culture, and nursing care should be family focused. The most important social structural factor in the Mexican American culture is family and kinship ties. These ties often go beyond the family to a wide network of kin and fictive kin, such as godparents. If nursing care is to be effective, nurses must tap these kinds of cultural networks to ensure the support of family members, neighbors, or friends.

Using Cultural Competence at the Primary Level of Prevention

The community health nurse should target certain high-risk behaviors for change during pregnancy, such as smoking, using drugs, consuming alcohol, and maintaining poor nutritional habits. A Mexican American mother-to-be may respond well to suggestions for change if she is convinced that her current behavior will cause harm to her baby. Family and social support groups in Mexican American culture can also be helpful and supportive to expectant mothers wishing to make lifestyle changes. With the exception of Puerto Rican women, Hispanic women in general have low rates of smoking during pregnancy (American Lung Association, 2010).

Prenatal services should include information about breast-feeding and family planning and reproductive health services. Traditionally, some health care professionals have assumed that family-planning services will not be accepted in a Mexican American population because of religious opposition and *machismo*—the need of the man to prove his manhood by having children or to believe in the biologic superiority of men. However, Mexican American men

and women may indeed be interested in family planning, particularly if they are concerned about the number of children they can support. This issue should be validated with individual clients and their spouses. During *la cuarentena*, the 40 days after the birth of the baby, women kin of the new mother often help with infant care, household tasks, and preparation of special foods for the mother (Zoucha & Zamarripa, 2013). Many Hispanic families believe that chili and other spicy foods should be avoided during and immediately after pregnancy.

Strategies for promoting breast-feeding should be identified and encouraged. Educational levels, family experiences with breast-feeding, the husband's attitude, the need to return to work, and feelings of embarrassment are all associated with infant-feeding choices among Mexican American women as well as other groups. These factors need to be explored with individual women to help them make the best choices for themselves and their babies. Breast-feeding is becoming more common in the United States as mothers become more educated about the advantages that breast-feeding can provide for a new baby.

Traditionally, Hispanic mothers may bind their own abdomen and also may place a cotton band around the baby's umbilicus (*ombligero*) to prevent the navel from protruding when the baby cries. The nurse can show the mother how to remove the *ombligero*, clean the umbilicus, and put on a clean *omgligero*. Many traditional customs should be supported by nurses who work with postpartum Mexican American women and their babies.

Secondary Level of Prevention

Secondary prevention involves interventions designed to diagnose a disease at a stage when treatment is likely to result in a cure. Nurses often use health education interventions when caring for individuals with a diagnosed health problem with the aim of preventing further complications or exacerbations. For example, at the individual and family level, teaching a patient with diabetes

and his or her family members about eating healthy foods and incorporating physical activities into daily activities could be considered secondary prevention.

Overview of the Health Concern

Type 2 diabetes is seen commonly among many Native Americans, and certain tribes have extremely high rates of the disease. The American Diabetes Association recently indicated that American Indians and Alaska Natives are 2.2 times more likely to have diabetes compared with non-Hispanic Whites. In addition, there has been a 68% increase in diabetes from 1994 to 2004 in American Indian and Alaska Native youth aged 15 to 19 years (American Diabetes Association, 2013). By all accounts, the high rate of diabetes in Native Americans is a leading health concern; diabetes is a leading cause of outpatient visits at Indian Health Service facilities. Although Native

---

Box 11-6 Beliefs and Practices Related to Diabetes of Some Native Americans

Nutritional Practices

- Diets are high in calories, carbohydrates, and fats.
- Sharing communal meals is a common and valued cultural practice.
- Some tribes have a high incidence of obesity and type 2 diabetes.
- Food preparation often adds fats and calories.
- Snack foods (potato chips, carbonated beverages, prepackaged pastries) are common.
- Alcohol abuse is often a concern. High intake of alcohol seriously compromises the treatment of diabetes.

Activity Levels/Fitness Practices

- Sedentary lifestyles have become common.
- Many reservations lack recreational facilities.
- Sometimes, formal exercise activities are associated with the White man's culture and are thought to be inappropriate for Native Americans. This is changing as Native youth excel at sports, and more tribes use "casino" money (funds generated from casinos) to build recreational and exercise facilities on tribal lands.

Beliefs and Values Related to Diabetes

- Ideal body image favors a heavier physique, and weight gain is considered normal; thinness is a cause for worry and concern.
- Concept of "control of one's body," that is, weight, glucose levels, blood pressure, may conflict with values and norms of Native American culture. For example, Native American clients may be uncomfortable with comparison of individual performance against others or against the norms and standards of biomedical care.
- Many Native Americans are uncomfortable with discussing or exposing private body functions, such as providing urine samples or participating in blood testing in a public situation.
- Illness is a personal and unpleasant topic, and Native American clients may be uncomfortable when asked to talk about it.
- Diabetes is a "White man's disease"; Native Americans did not have diabetes until Whites came to this continent.
- The term "diabetic" may be offensive to some, and the label "diabetic clinic" may discourage clients from seeking health care services.
- White health professionals may be viewed with some suspicion and distrust, given the history of cultural contact between Whites and Native Americans.
- Because diabetes is so common in some tribal groups, there is a fatalism about the disease, especially if a family member already has diabetes.
- Beliefs and health practices surrounding diabetes may vary according to the Native American tribe.

Americans make up just 1.5% of the US population, they have the highest rate of diabetes in the world and one of the highest rates of end-stage renal disease (ESRD) (Native Americans and Chronic Kidney Disease, n.d.). Type 2 diabetes has become an epidemic and a national tragedy among many Native peoples.

The reasons for the epidemic of type 2 diabetes among some Native Americans are not clear. It has long been believed that some Native North American tribes have an underlying genetic propensity for the disease that is triggered by major changes in dietary practices, a sedentary lifestyle, and increasing obesity (Neel, 1962; Young, 1994). These factors have been complicated by social conditions, such as poverty and inadequate access to health care, as well as by problems of compliance or lack of adherence to medical regimens. Because of the high rate of diabetes on some reservations, numerous secondary preventive services that focus on early diagnosis and treatment have been initiated. Box 11-6 shows beliefs and practices about diabetes of some Native Americans that could influence the success of secondary preventive programs for diabetes. Validation of beliefs and practices should always take place with individual clients and families, and stereotyping (thinking that all Native Americans are the same) should be avoided.

Using Cultural Competence at the Secondary Level of Prevention

Nursing interventions at the secondary level of prevention should focus on the implementation of healthful lifestyle changes that will ultimately decrease the complications of diabetes. Most of these are related to what health professionals call diet and exercise, but what is appropriate for Native North American culture is an emphasis on health and a healthy lifestyle. Nurses should emphasize health and a healthy lifestyle rather than negative factors such as control of diabetes, prevention of complications, weight reduction, and exercise. The choice of words, as well as the emphasis, is important.

For example, when teaching the client and family about diabetic diets, the nurse can substitute the word "nutrition" for "diet," removing the negative perceptions and leading to a nursing plan that emphasizes substitution of healthy foods rather than deprivation of unhealthy foods. Substituting fruits for candy bars and packaged pastries; whole grains for French fries, potato chips, or doughnuts; and vegetables for sugared snacks will improve the client's nutritional status and lead to a healthier lifestyle. Special traditional foods, even fried bread, can be eaten on special occasions, and other types of bread can be substituted during regular meals. Some reservations have restaurants or cafes that serve traditional foods such as tepary beans, squash, and Indian corn (Figure 11-6). Many Native Americans are interested in eating traditional foods that are more beneficial for a healthy lifestyle.

Health education should be oriented toward the individual client and his or her family as well. Often health education is more effective in a home situation rather than an impersonal clinic. Physical activities that are culturally relevant, such as traditional dancing or even basketball, can be encouraged. Many Native American high schools now have basketball teams for boys and girls, and the competition is significant; games are avidly watched by the entire community. The value of health and a healthy lifestyle should be stressed over exercise and weight reduction. Physical activities that are congruent with overall lifestyle and cultural context will be easier to incorporate into daily living situations.

The Native American family system is typically an extended family that includes several households of closely related kin. Family members become exceedingly important during times of crisis because they are a source of support, comfort, assistance, and strength. The importance of cultural ties with kin and other members of the reservation community must always be considered in planning for early diagnosis and treatment programs. It is in this context (family and community) that clients are encouraged and supported, not only to seek care but also to institute

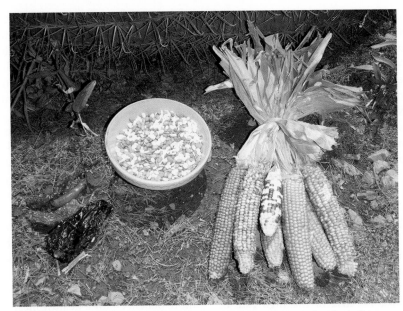

Figure 11-6. These colorful ears of Indian corn were named after the indigenous people of North America who had been cultivating corn for years when they introduced it to the Europeans who arrived in the New World in the 15th century. Unlike the typical niblets of corn on the cob, Indian corn is not sweet. It also has a starchy texture when cooked. The tepary beans are the preferred beans of the Tohono O'odham (the people of the desert). They have a slightly sweet flavor and a firm texture.

lifestyle changes that are congruent with cultural practices and that will enhance the health status of all members of the family and, ultimately, the tribal community.

The increasing rates of type 2 diabetes are of great concern to Native American communities. Introducing preventive health programs requires great sensitivity to cultural traditions and to the past experiences that native communities have had with health care and health research. Understanding the needs of community members is essential for the development of culturally appropriate programs, and each Native American community has its own cultural traditions and beliefs that make up the details of daily life. Understanding the needs of Native communities begins by asking them what they want and need from preventive programs, rather than imposing ideas upon them. The best way to find out what matters to people is to get out into the community and talk to them. In Native American communities, it is wise to begin with respected and esteemed members of the tribal council.

Appendix D, Components of a Cultural Assessment: Traditional Native American Healing provides a framework that can be used to assess traditional healing beliefs and practices in Native communities.

Tertiary Level of Prevention

Tertiary prevention includes interventions aimed at limiting disability and rehabilitation from disease, injury, or disability. Sometimes, the distinction between primary, secondary, and tertiary levels of prevention can blur; tertiary prevention usually includes compliance with long-term treatment and provision of aftercare services. The following example focuses on African Americans who have high rates of hypertension,

often leading to heart disease and stroke. African Americans are a highly heterogeneous group and display considerable variation in health beliefs and behaviors. For the most part, this section discusses a more traditional, rural African American culture; always validate beliefs and behaviors with individual clients and communities.

Overview of the Health Concern

Hypertension is a major risk factor for heart disease and stroke. Mean blood pressure levels are higher in Blacks than in White Americans, with a marked excess in Blacks. In a government study on minority health conducted in the mid-1980s, the chairperson pointed out improvements in the treatment of hypertension in Blacks. In reviewing the data, she stated, "Hypertensive Blacks were at least as likely as Whites of the same sex to be treated with antihypertensive medication and nearly as likely to have their blood pressure controlled" (Heckler, 1985a, p. 110). However, the prevalence of hypertension in Blacks in the United States is still among the highest in the world (Ferdinand & Armani, 2007). It is critical that efforts to treat hypertension in African American populations be continued, because hypertension affects African Americans in unique ways. African Americans develop high blood pressure at younger ages than other groups in the United States. In addition, they are more likely to develop complications associated with high blood pressure. These problems include stroke, kidney disease, blindness, dementia, and health disease (High Blood Pressure in African-Americans, 2015).

Unfortunately, appropriate care often has been complicated by discrimination, poverty, and limited access to care. Poverty is often a problem in rural African American communities and African Americans often experience severe economic deprivation. In 2014, 35% of all African Americans were living below the national poverty level (Poverty Rate by Race/Ethnicity, 2014). Some researchers believe that high blood pressure in African Americans may be due to factors that are unique to the experiences of Blacks in the United States. To date, researchers do not know

exactly why high blood pressure is more common in African Americans. However, we do know that increased age, excessive weight, diabetes, inactivity, diet, and smoking are some risk factors for developing high blood pressure.

The goal of tertiary prevention is to reduce disability and prevent complications from developing further. Weight management; increased physical activities; appropriate diet, such as decreasing dietary salt and fat; and smoking cessation are all amenable to tertiary preventive measures. A major aim of nursing care in the implementation of tertiary activities is to help clients adjust to limitations or changes in daily living, to increase their coping skills, to control symptoms, and in general to minimize the complications of disease by reducing the rate of residual damage in a given population. Cultural factors that should be considered in tertiary prevention programs for African Americans are shown in Box 11-7.

Using Cultural Competence at the Tertiary Level of Prevention

Community nurses have demonstrated competence in the management of community hypertension programs. Although these programs are vital to the early diagnosis and management of hypertension, they also include a component that focuses on helping clients manage a chronic disease—an aspect of tertiary prevention. Numerous studies have shown that African American churches are excellent sites for community-based health programs such as hypertension clinics. The African American community should be involved in every aspect of community-based programs. The goals, objectives, and interventions of the services should reflect the expressed needs of the community target group, as well as their values, beliefs, and interests.

Community health nurses are in the advantageous position of assessing clients and families in their own homes and neighborhoods. This provides an understanding of the daily life situation faced by clients that other health care professionals often lack. Community health nurses can bring this understanding to bear on helping

Box 11-7 Cultural Factors to Consider in Planning Tertiary Prevention for a Traditional African American Population

Language
African American communication concepts and patterns can be identified and used in community education programs.

Cultural Health Beliefs
Good health comes from good luck.
Health is related to harmony in nature.
Illnesses are classified as "natural" or "unnatural."
Illness may be God's punishment.
Maintenance of health is associated with "reading the signs," for example, phase of the moon, season of the year, position of the planets.

Cultural Health Practices
The use of herbs, oils, powders, roots, and other home remedies may be common.
Prayers, reading the Bible, and attending church services will promote health and help cure diseases.

Cultural Healers
Older woman ("old lady") in the community who has knowledge of herbs and healing
Spiritualist who is called by God to heal disease or solve emotional or personal problems
Voodoo priest/priestess who is a powerful cultural healer who uses voodoo, bone reading, and so on to heal or to bring about desired events
Root doctor who uses roots, herbs, oils, candles, and ointments in healing rituals

Time Orientation
May be present-time oriented, which makes preventive care more difficult to implement and maintain

Nutritional Practices
Soul food takes its name from a feeling of kinship among Blacks and may be served at home, provided at church dinners, or served at home-style restaurants.
Diets may reflect traditional rural Southern foods such as fried chicken, collard greens cooked with bacon or ham, grits with butter, corn bread, and chickpeas. Dessert may be peach cobbler.

With the exception of chickpeas, the other foods have a high caloric and fat content.

Economic Status
In 2014, 35% of African Americans were living below the national poverty level (Poverty Rate by Race/Ethnicity, 2014). This has a very negative impact on health status.

Educational Status
High aspirations for education but socioeconomic status and other complex factors limit educational opportunities

Family and Social Networks
Often strong extended family networks with a sense of obligation to relatives

Self-Concept
The importance of race has been a continual issue for the self-identity of African Americans.

Impact of Racism
Unfortunately, racism is still present, and a negative perception of the African American's skin color by health professionals will seriously interfere with efficacious health care.

Religion
African American churches have tremendous influence on the daily lives of their members because they serve as a source of spiritual and social support.
The African American church acts as a caretaker for the cultural characteristics of Black culture.

Biologic Variations
There is a high incidence of lactose intolerance and lactase deficiency; this has implications for diet planning if Black clients cannot tolerate milk or milk products.
There is a higher prevalence of hypertension among African Americans than among Americans of European heritage. Sickle cell anemia is more common among African Americans.

References: Andrews, M. M., & Bolin, L. (1993). The African American Community. In J. M. Swanson & M. Albrecht (Eds.), *Community health nursing: Promoting the health of aggregates* (pp. 443–458). Philadelphia, PA: W.B. Saunders; Campinha-Bacote, J. (2013). People of African American heritage. In L. D. Purnell (Ed.), *Transcultural health care: A culturally competent approach* (pp. 91–114). Philadelphia, PA: F. A. Davis Company.

clients with tertiary preventive activities. African American clients who have been diagnosed with hypertension can be encouraged to lose weight by eating healthier foods, eliminating dietary salt and fat from their diets, and increasing their intake of potassium. If an African American client has diabetes, the nurse can encourage him or her to incorporate healthy eating habits and increase physical activities in their lifestyle as appropriate. Clients who smoke can be encouraged to join smoking cessation programs; nurses can work with family members to encourage and support healthy activities that will keep high blood pressure from further damaging the health of African Americans. Tertiary preventive measures often involve long-time lifestyle changes, and clients can become discouraged when they see no immediate signs of improvement. Encouraging clients and families to continue with tertiary preventive measures requires the nurse to establish rapport by listening and attending to what the client is saying and doing. Mutual goal setting is important, and support for the individual client and family though change provides support and motivation to continue with the tertiary preventive activities.

Summary

Cultural concepts related to community health nursing practice serve as a guide or framework for nurses who work with diverse populations. A guide or framework for providing culturally competent nursing care helps nurses and other health professionals provide care to individuals and groups with diverse cultural backgrounds. Nurses use cultural knowledge in assessing, planning, implementing, and evaluating nursing care. This chapter addressed cultural diversity of clients, families, and communities. Various subcultures, including refugees, asylees, and immigrants, were described to help nurses understand and become comfortable working with these groups in community settings. In-depth information about the Dinka from South Sudan who have been resettled

in the United States will assist nurses in providing culturally competent care to groups such as the Dinka, as well as other refugee and various immigrant groups.

Cultural concepts as they relate to the community at large will help nurses plan care for diverse individuals, families, and communities. A cultural assessment is as an integral component of a community nursing assessment. Culturally competent nursing interventions are an integral part of the nurse's role and ensure health maintenance and health promotion at a community level. Preventive care in the community is of particular importance to community health nursing. The use of cultural knowledge will help nurses in primary, secondary, and tertiary levels of prevention. Examples of cultural diversity and levels of prevention illustrate how cultural knowledge can be used in community health nursing practice.

REVIEW QUESTIONS

1. Describe four cultural concepts, and discuss how they can be used to provide transcultural nursing care to families and community aggregates.
2. Describe an example of how cultural factors influence the health of an aggregate group within the community.
3. List the major cultural considerations in implementing preventive programs for culturally diverse groups. How can cultural considerations be used to identify barriers and facilitators for preventive programs?
4. Identify special health considerations in immigrant groups within the community.
5. Describe an approach to primary preventive health care for the Dinka refugee group from South Sudan.
6. Describe secondary and tertiary programs targeting hypertension for elderly Chinese Americans living in San Francisco's Chinatown.
7. Describe similarities and differences between folk and scientific health care systems. Give an example of each.

CRITICAL THINKING ACTIVITIES

1. Describe sociocultural factors and their impact on health care for a cultural group within your community. Evaluate the access to, availability of, and acceptability of various health care services. Is this cultural group at risk? Why?

2. Conduct a community cultural assessment of a group within your community. Critically analyze the cultural knowledge and/or information that should be considered when planning care for the group. Use Appendix B to identify and collect cultural assessment data—family and kinship, social life, political systems, language, worldview, religious behaviors, health beliefs and practices, and health concerns.

Compare and contrast the assessment of other groups in your community.

3. For a cultural group in your community, develop a program plan or intervention that has components of primary, secondary, and tertiary prevention.

4. Attend religious services at a church, temple, mosque, synagogue, or place of worship to learn about a religion different from your own. How does the church meet the unique needs of its congregation?

5. Identify alternative health care practitioners within your community. Which subcultures do they serve? Describe the kinds of care that they offer to residents.

REFERENCES

Abrums, M. (2004). Faith and feminism: How African American women from a storefront church resist oppression in healthcare. *Advances in Nursing Science, 27*(3), 187–201.

Al-Tohami, K. (2011). Migration in Sudan: A Country Profile 2011. Khartoum: International Organization for Migration. Retrieved 2012 from http://publications.iom.int/bookstore/free/mp_sudan.pdf

American Academy of Nursing Expert Panel on Culturally Competent Health Care. (1992). Culturally competent health care. *Nursing Outlook, 40*, 277–283.

American Diabetes Association. (2013). Native American Programs. Retrieved from http: //www.diabetes.org/community-events/programs/native-american-programs

American Lung Association. (2010). Key facts about smoking among Hispanics. Retrieved from http://www.lung.org.stop-smoking/about-smoking/facts-figurers/hispanics-and-tobacco-use.html

American Psychiatric Association. (2013). *Diagnostic and statistical manual of mental disorders: DSM-5* (5th ed.). Arlington, VA: American Psychiatric Association.

Andrews, M. M., & Bolin, L. (1993). The African American community. In J. M. Swanson & M. Albrecht (Eds.), *Community health nursing: Promoting the health of aggregates* (pp. 443–458). Philadelphia, PA: W.B. Saunders.

Arizona Department of Health Services, Office of Health Systems Development. (2005). Nogales primary care area statistical profile. Arizona primary care area program. Retrieved from http://www.azdhs.gov/index.htm

Aroian, K. J., Peters, R. M., Rudner, N., & Waser, L. (2012). Hypertension prevention beliefs of Hispanics. *Journal of Transcultural Nursing, 23*(2), 134–142.

Ashford, M. W., & Huet-Vaughn, Y. (1997). The impact of war on women. In B. S. Levy & V. W. Sidel (Eds.). *War and Public Health*. New York, NY: Oxford University Press, Inc.

Ayón, D. R. (2009, March 27). *Developing the U.S.-Mexico border region for a prosperous and secure relationship: The impact of Mexican migration on border proximity on local communities*. Houston, TX: James A. Baker III Institute for Public Policy, Rice University. Retrieved from http://bakerinstitute.org/media/files/Research/f5522ada/LAI-pub-BorderSecAyon-032709.pdf

Baird, M. B. (2009). Resettlement transition experiences among Sudanese refugee women. (Ph.D. dissertation, The University of Arizona, United States, Tucson, Arizona). Retrieved from Dissertations & Theses. University of Arizona (Publication No. AAT 3352364).

Baird, M. B., & Boyle, J. S. (2012). Well-Being in Dinka refugee women of Southern Sudan. *Journal of Transcultural Nursing, 23*(1), 14–21.

Baird, M. B., Domian, E. W., Mulcahy, E. R., Mabior, R., Jemutai-Tanui, G., & Filippi, M. K. (2015). Creating a bridge of understanding between two worlds: Community-based collaborative-action research with Sudanese refugee women. *Public Health Nursing, 1–9.* doi: 10.1111/phn.12172

Barnes, D. M., Harrison, C., & Heneghan, R. (2004). Health risks and promotion behaviors in refugee populations. *Journal of Health Care for the Poor and Underserved, 15*, 347–356.

Bixler, M. (2006). *The lost boys of Sudan: The American story of the refugee experience*. Athens, GA: The University of Georgia Press.

Brown, H. (2004, August 21–27). Disease and hunger in Sudan. *Lancet, 364*, 654.

Campinha-Bacote, J. (2013). People of African American heritage. In L. D. Purnell (Ed.). *Transcultural health care: A culturally competent approach*. Philadelphia, PA; F. A. Davis Company.

Canales, M. K., & Drevdahl, D. J. (2014). Community/public health nursing: Is there a future for the specialty? *Nursing Outlook, 62*(6), 448–458.

Degazon, C. E. (2012). Cultural Diversity in the community. In M. Stanhope & J. Lancaster (Eds.). *Public health nursing; population–centered health care in the community* (8th ed., pp. 141–162). Maryland Heights, MO: Mosby.

Deng, F. M. (1984). *The dinka of Sudan*. Prospect Heights, IL: Waveland Press.

DeSantis, L. (1997). Building healthy communities with immigrants and refugees. *Journal of Transcultural Nursing, 9*, 20–31.

Dreachslin, J. L., Gilbert, M. J., & Malone, B. (2013). *Diversity and cultural competence in health care: A systems approach*. San Francisco, CA: Jossey-Bass/A Wiley Imprint.

Eggers, D. (2006). What is the what? New York: Vintage Books.

Ferdinand, K. C., &Armani, A. M. (2007). The management of hypertension in African Americans. *Critical pathways in cardiology. 6*(2), 67–71.

Fonseca, F. (2013, November 2). Championships run deep at Hopi HS. *Arizona Daily Star.*

Gettleman, J. (2011, July). Sudan movement's mission is secured: Statehood. *The New York Times online*. Retrieved from http://www.nytimes.com/2011/07/09/world/africa/09sudan.html?ref=opinion

Giger, J. N., & Davidhizar, R. E. (1991). *Transcultural nursing: Assessment and intervention*. St. Louis, MO: C. V. Mosby.

Giger J. N., Appel, S. J., Davidhizar, R., & Davis, C. (2008, October). Church and spirituality in the lives the African American community. *Journal of Transcultural Nursing, 19*(4), 375–383.

Heckler, M. M. (1985a). *Report of the secretary's task force on black and minority health, Vol. I: Executive summary*. Washington, DC: U.S. Department of Health and Human Services.

Heckler, M. M. (1985b). *Report to the secretary's task force on black and minority health, Vol.2: Crosscutting issues in minority health*. Washington, DC: U.S. Department of Health and Human Services.

High Blood Pressure in African-Americans (2015). Retrieved from https://www.webmd.com/hypertension-high-blood-pressure/guide/hypertension-in-african-americans

Hodgins, O., & Hodgins, D. (2013). American Indians and Alaskan natives. In Purnell, L. D. (Ed.). *Transcultural health care: A culturally competent approach* (pp. 451–449). Philadelphia, PA: F. A. Davis Company.

Huff, R. M., & Kline, M. V. (2007). *Promoting health in multicultural populations*. Thousand Oaks, CA: Sage.

Jaranson, J. M., Butcher, J., Halcon, L., Johnson, D. R., Robertson, C., Savik, K., & Spring, M. (2004). Somali and Oromo refugees: Correlates of torture and trauma history. *American Journal of Public Health, 94*(4), 591–612.

Kemp, C. (2005). *Mexican & Mexican Americans: Health beliefs and practices*. Retrieved from https://bearspace.baylor.edu/Charles_Kempt/www/hispanic_health.htm#top

Leininger, M. (1978). *Transcultural nursing: Concepts, theories and practices*. New York, NY: John Wiley & Sons.

Leininger, M. (1991). Leininger's acculturation health care assessment tool for cultural patterns in traditional and nontraditional lifeways. *Journal of Transcultural Nursing, 2*(2), 40–42.

Leininger, M. (1995). *Transcultural nursing: Concepts, theories, research and practice*. New York, NY: McGraw-Hill.

Lipson, J., & Meleis, A. (1983). Issues in health care of Middle Eastern patients. *Western Journal of Medicine, 139*(6), 854–861.

Luckinbill, T., Grazer, B., Smith, M., Hofmeyr, G., Howard, R., Luckinbill, T., … & Falardeau, P. (Director). (2014). The Good Lie [Motion picture]. (2014). USA: Alcon Entertainment, Imagine Entertainment, Reliance Entertainment. Retrieved on January 4, 2015 from http://www.thegoodliemovie.com/

McEwen, M., & Boyle, J. S. (2007). Resistance, health and latent tuberculosis infection: Mexican immigrants at the U.S.-Mexico border. *Research and Theory for Nursing Practice: An International Journal, 21*(3), 185–197.

McEwen, M. M., Baird, M. B., Pasvogel, A., & Gallegos, G. (2007). Health-illness transition experiences among Mexican immigrant women with diabetes. *Family and Community Health, 30*(3), 201–212.

McGuire, S. (2014). Borders, centers and margins: Critical landscapes in migrant health. *Advances in Nursing Science, 37*(3), 197–212.

McKenzie, J. F., Pinger, R. R., & Kotecki, J. E. (2012). *An Introduction to Community Health* (7th ed.). Sudbury, MA: Jones & Bartlett Learning, LLC

Medved, M. I., Brockmeier, J., Morach, J., & Chartier-Courchene, L. (2013). Broken heart stories; Understanding Aboriginal women's cardiac problems. *Qualitative Health Research, 23*(2), 1613–1625.

Minority Health: Quick Facts About Health Disparities. (December 1, 2009). Retrieved from http://www.familiesusa.org/issues/minority-health/facts/minority-health-health-quick-facts

National Cancer Institute. (2012). Retrieved from http://www.cancer.gov/cancertopics/factsheet/Risk/HPV

National Institute of Nursing Research. (September, 2007). Specialized community interventions. Retrieved from http://www.docstoc.com/docs/7131604/Specialized-Community-Interventions

National Institute of Nursing Research. (2014). Retrieved from http://www.ninr.hih.gov

Native Americans and Chronic Kidney Disease. (n.d.). Retrieved from http://www.davita.com/kidney-disease/causes/assessing-your-risk/diabetes-high-blood-pressure-and-kidney-disease/e/5005

Neel, J. V. (1962). Diabetes mellitus: A "thrifty" genotype rendered detrimental by progress. *American Journal of Human Genetics, 14,* 353–362.

Passel, J. S. (2009). A portrait of unauthorized immigrants in the U.S. Pew Research Center Publications. Retrieved from http://pewresearch.org/pubs/1190/portrait-unauthorized-immigrants-states

Pasternak, J. (2010). *Yellow Dirt.* New York, NY: Free Press.

Pavlish, C., & Ho, A. (2009). Human rights as barriers for displaced persons in Southern Sudan. *Journal of Nursing Scholarship, 41,* 284–292.

Pavlish, C. P., & Pharris, M. D. (2011). *Community-based collaborative action research: A nursing approach.* Sudbury, ON: Jones & Bartlett Learning.

Pinto, A., Saeed, M., El Sakka, H., Rashford, A., Colombo, A., Valenciano, M., & Sabatinelli, G. (2005). Setting up an early warning system for epidemic-prone diseases in Darfur: A participative approach. *Disasters, 29*(4), 310–322.

Poverty Rate by Race/Ethnicity. (2012). Retrieved from http://www.kff.org/other/state-indicator/poverty-rate-by-raceethnicity/

Prengaman, M. V. (2013a). Review of Yellow Dirt by Judy Pasternak. *Journal of Transcultural Nursing, 24*(4), 417.

Prengaman, M. V. (2013b). Review of Yellow Dirt by Judy Pasternak. *Journal of Transcultural Nursing, 24*(4), 417.

Purnell, L. D. (Ed.) (2013). *Transcultural health care: A culturally competent approach* (4th ed.) Philadelphia, PA: F. A. Davis Company.

Raley, R. K., Durden, T. E., & Wildssmith, E. (2004). Understanding Mexican-American marriage patterns using a life-course approach. *Social Science Quarterly, 85*(4), 872–890.

Shambley-Ebron, D., & Boyle, J. S. (2006). Self-care and the cultural meaning of mothering in African American women with HIV/AIDS. *Western Journal of Nursing Research, 28*(1), 42–60.

Shambley-Ebron, D., Dole, D., & Karikari, A. (2014). Cultural preparation for womanhood in urban African American girls: Growing strong women. *Journal of Transcultural Nursing.* doi: 10.1177/1043659614531792

Simich, L., Beiser, M., & Mawani, F. N. (2003). Social support and the significance of shared experience in refugee migration and resettlement. *Western Journal of Nursing Research, 25*(7), 872–891.

Simon, B. (Writer), Mihailoviich, D. (Producer) (2013). Our amazing 12-year journey with the Lost Boys. [Television Series Episode]. In J. Fagar (Executive producer), *60 Minutes Overtime.* New York, NY: CBS Interactive Inc.

Spector, R. E. (2012). *Cultural diversity in health and illness* (8th ed.). New York, NY: Appleton-Century-Crofts.

Stanhope, M., & Lancaster, J. (2012). *Public health nursing: Population-centered health care in the community* (8th ed.). St. Louis, MO: C.V. Mosby/Elsevier.

The UN Refugee Agency (UNHCR). (1966). Convention and protocol relating to the status of refugees. Retrieved from http://www.unhcr.org

The UN Refugee Agency (UNHCR). (2014). Escaping war, time and again. Retrieved January 3, 2015 from: http://tracks.unhcr.org/2014/12/escaping-war-time-and-again/#_ga=1.213054748.925313257.1332254682

The UN Refugee Agency (UNHCR). (2015). 2015 UNHCR country operations profile-Sudan. Retrieved January 4, 2015 from http://www.unhcr.org/cgi-bin/texis/vtx/page?page=49e483b76&submit=GO

Thomas, T. L., Strickland, O. L., DiClemente, R., Higgins, M. & Haber, M. (2012). Rural African American parents' knowledge and decisions about human papillomavirus vaccination. *Journal of Nursing Scholarship, 44*(4), 358–367.

U. S. Census Bureau. (2012). *The foreign-born population in the United States: 2010 American Community Survey reports.* Washington, DC: U. S. Department of Commerce. Retrieved from http://www.census.gov/population/foreign

U. S. Department of Agriculture, Food and Nutrition Service. (2014). Women, Infants, and Children (WIC). Retrieved from http://www.fns.usda.gov/wic/women-infants-and-children-wic

U. S. Department of Agriculture, Food and Nutrition Service. (n.d.). About WIC-How WIC helps. Retrieved from http://www.fns.usda.gov/wic-how-wic-helps

U.S. Census Bureau. (2010). Facts for features. Retrieved from http://www.census.gov/newsroom/releases/archives/facts_for_features_special_editions/cb10-ff08.html

U.S. Department of Health and Human Services. (1990). *Healthy people 2000 review.* Washington, DC: U.S. Government Printing Office.

U.S. Department of Health and Human Services. (2000). *Healthy people 2010 review.* Washington, DC: U.S. Government Printing Office.

U.S. Department of Health and Human Services. (2010). About healthy people, 2020. Retrieved from http://www.healthypeople.gov/2020/about/default.aspx

Vickers, J. (1993). *Women and War.* London & New Jersey: Zed Books.

Williams, C. (2012). Population-focused practice: The foundation of specialization in public health nursing. In M. Stanhope & J. Lancaster (Eds.). *Public health nursing: Population-centered health care in the community.* (pp. 3–21). Maryland Heights, MO: Elsevier/Mosby.

World Health Organization (WHO). (2012). Mental health of refugees, internally displaced persons and other populations affected by conflict. Retrieved from WHO http://www.who.int/hac/techguidance/pht/mental_health_refugees/en/

Young, K. (1994). *The health of Native Americans.* New York, NY: Oxford University Press.

Zoucha, R. & Zamarripa, C. (2013). People of Mexican heritage. In Purnell, L. (Ed.), *Transcultural health care: A culturally competent approach* (pp. 374–390). Philadelphia, PA:. F. A. Davis Company.

Cultural Diversity in the Health Care Workforce

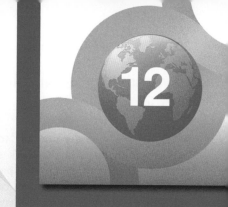

● Margaret M. Andrews

Key Terms

Affirmative Action
Barriers
Bigotry
Concordance
Conflict
Corporate culture
Cross-cultural communication
Cultural diversity
Cultural self-assessment

Cultural values
Diversity management
Dress code
Employment equity
Ethnoviolence
Etiquette
Facilitators
Family obligations
Generational cohort
Hatred
Hygiene

Intergenerational conflict
Multicultural workforce
Multiculturalism
Organizational climate
Organizational cultural
  self-assessment
Organizational inclusion
Positive action
Reservation
Social amnesia
Workplace diversity

Learning Objectives

1. Analyze diversity trends in the nursing and health care workforce.
2. Compare and contrast barriers to diversity in health care organizations and strategies to increase organizational diversity.
3. Compare and contrast diversity management and organizational inclusion in health care.
4. Critically analyze the cultural differences in values and behaviors in the multicultural health care workforce.
5. Examine the process and content of cultural self-assessment for health care organizations, institutions, and agencies.

This chapter examines diversity in the nursing workforce, including the advantages of diversity, demographic and societal trends, legal perspectives, barriers, and strategies to increase diversity in health care organizations and agencies. Cultural differences in workplace perspectives, values, and behaviors are analyzed. And a **cultural self-assessment** of health care organizations, institutions, and agencies is outlined.

Diversity in the Nursing Workforce

∙∙∙∙∙∙∙∙∙∙∙∙∙∙∙∙∙∙∙∙∙∙∙∙∙∙∙∙∙∙∙∙∙∙∙∙

Workplace diversity refers to differences between individuals in the work setting in any attribute that may evoke the perception that another person is different from oneself (Dijk & van Engan, 2013; Guillaume, Dawson, Woods, Sacramento, & West, 2013). One person may differ from another on a number of different attributes including demographic characteristics such as race, ethnicity, national origin, age, gender, and marital status. People also may differ on the basis of sexual orientation, religion, education, expertise, skills, work experience, profession, job title, socioeconomic background, political affiliation, ability/disability, tenure or length of service to an organization, and other characteristics (American Academy of Nursing, 2012; American Association of Colleges of Nursing, 2014a). Workplace diversity is the collective, all-inclusive mixture of human differences and similarities that provides an organization with a large pool of people with knowledge, skills, and abilities required for the accomplishment of organizational goals and objectives (Ewoh, 2013; Sabharwal, 2014).

Advantages

Diversity in the workplace is important because it contributes to the organization's collective decision making, effectiveness, and responsiveness to societal health care needs. Individuals from diverse populations have expectations, insights, approaches, and values from which emerge different points of view, perspectives, and alternative approaches to problem solving and the arrival at alternative solutions to problems. Furthermore, diversity enhances the organization's ability to evaluate the intended and unintended consequences of decisions by examining them through the lens of multiple perspectives. Diversity also enhances rational decision making and organizational efficiency and effectiveness (Ewoh, 2013; Singh, Winkel, & Selvarajan, 2013).

Hospitals, medical centers, community health agencies, rehabilitation and other long-term care facilities, psychiatric and mental health facilities, home care agencies, and related organizations exist to serve people seeking health care services regardless of their cultural, racial, ethnic, and related backgrounds. As the composition of contemporary societies becomes increasingly diverse, there is evidence that creating a more diverse health care workforce has value for the people being served and the health care organization from the perspective of its employees and leaders (Flores & Combs, 2013).

Concordance, matching the demographics of employees to the community served, is tied to better patient outcomes (Flores & Combs, 2013; Georges, 2012; Mittman & Sullivan, 2012; Sabharwal, 2014). People tend to seek care from professionals with ethnic, racial, and linguistic backgrounds that are similar to their own. Minority health care professionals, including nurses, are likely to work in underserved communities leading to improved access among underrepresented groups. There is research that links increasing workforce diversity to better health outcomes, reduction of health disparities, increased patient or client satisfaction, improved employee productivity, retention, satisfaction, and more cost-effective care delivery (Health Resources and Services Administration, 2013; Hedlund, Esparza, Calhoun, & Yates, 2012; Jackson & Gracia, 2014; LaVeist & Pierre, 2014; Mittman & Sullivan, 2012; Williams et al., 2014).

Demographic and Societal Trends

During the past three decades, the registered nurse workforce has undergone gradual changes in its composition. What was once a demographically homogeneous workforce dominated by young, white women prepared primarily in diploma schools of nursing has now become increasingly diverse in age, gender, race, ethnicity, national origin, and educational preparation.

Nursing is in the midst of a period of substantive transformation that is influenced by the following three trends: (1) an aging population of baby boomers (those born between 1946 and 1964) who are now experiencing manifestations of the aging process such as chronic illnesses and retirement from the health care and other workforces; (2) the passage of the Affordable Care Act (ACA) of 2010 that provides health insurance to millions of people in the United States who previously were uninsured; and (3) increased educational preparation for nurses, including greater emphasis on the bachelor of science in nursing (BSN) degree for entry into professional nursing practice, the Doctor of Nursing Practice (DNP) degree for RNs who seek preparation in advanced practice nursing (midwifery, nurse anesthesia, and nurse practitioner), and specialty credentialing (American Association of Colleges of Nursing, 2014; American Nurses Credentialing Center, 2015; Fineberg & Lavizzio, 2013). For minority and other traditionally underrepresented populations in nursing, the demographic and societal changes bring a variety of benefits and challenges. With the aging of the baby boomers, for example, there is expected to be a plethora of new nursing jobs that could lead to higher wages, increased job security, and greater variety in the types of positions available. On the other hand, the infusion of new patients into the health care system could lead to higher patient-to-nurse ratios and more emphasis on work productivity as large numbers of people access the health care system as a result of the ACA (Page, 2015).

Diversity is a requirement for many national nursing organizations, hospital associations, the U.S. Department of Health and Human Services Division of Nursing, philanthropic organizations, and other stakeholders within the health care community whose leaders agree that the recruitment of people from underrepresented groups into nursing is a priority for the nursing profession in the United States (American Association of Colleges of Nursing, 2014). Individuals from racial and ethnic minority groups account for 37% of the US population, with projections indicating that the minority populations will become the majority by 2043 (U.S. Census Bureau, 2012). By comparison, findings from a 2013 survey conducted by the National Council of State Boards of Nursing and the Forum of State Nursing Workforce Centers reveal that nurses from minority backgrounds account for 19% of the RN workforce. When asked about their racial and ethnic background, responses indicated 6% African American, 6% Asian, 3% Hispanic, 1% American Indian/Alaska Native, 1% Native Hawaiian/Pacific Islander, 83% White, and 1% self-identified as "others" (Budden, Zhong, Moulton, & Cimiotti, 2013). Racial and ethnic minorities are markedly underrepresented in the nursing profession, despite numerous initiatives to remedy the lack of concordance (American Association of Colleges of Nursing, 2014).

Another type of diversity in the nursing workforce relates to gender. Women constitute 93.4% of the nation's 3 million RNs, whereas men represent 9.6% of the nursing workforce in the United States. When examining gender differences in nursing roles, the highest representation by men is in the nurse anesthetist position (41%)—the highest paid nursing specialty. As in many female-dominated fields, men in nursing enjoy higher wages and faster promotions than do women. Women working full-time in nursing earn 93 cents for every dollar men earn as registered nurses, 89 cents to the dollar among nurse anesthetists, and 87 cents to the dollar among nurse practitioners (American Community Survey, 2013; Health Resources and Services Administration, 2014). After earning a bachelor's degree in nursing, the RN in Figure 12-1 matriculated into a Doctor of Nursing Practice Family Nurse practitioner program where he will earn credentials that make him highly competitive in the health care workforce.

In contrast to the United States, the total supply of RNs in Canada is 292,883. As in the United States, most Canadian nurses are female (94%).

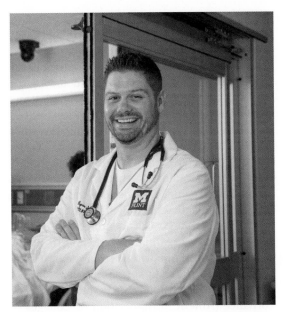

Figure 12-1. After completing his bachelor's degree in nursing, this RN is continuing his studies in a Doctor of Nursing Practice Program to prepare him as a family nurse practitioner.

As indicated in Evidence-Based Practice 12-1, US and Canadian men face challenges as minorities in a female-dominated profession. Historically, women constituted the majority of personnel in nursing and in many allied health disciplines.

Diversity in the age of nurses is another factor that warrants consideration. The average age of the RN population has been rising over the past two decades, and continues to be of concern. A large cohort of currently employed RNs is nearing or has exceeded retirement age. "Over the next 10 to 15 years, the nearly 1 million RNs older than 50—about one-third of the current workforce— will reach retirement age" (Health Resources and Services Administration, 2013, p. 24). The loss of a large number of experienced nurses at a time of rapid increase and complexity in health care is of concern. There are fewer RNs between the ages of 36 and 45 working today, which also indicates that their level of expertise will be lacking as younger, newly educated RNs enter the workforce (Health Resources and Services Administration, 2013). In

Canada, the average age of nurses is 45.1 years. The largest increases in the RNs in Canada are those younger than 30 and those over 60 (Canadian Institute for Health Information, 2014).

In a classic report on diversity in the health care workforce, former U.S. Secretary of Health and Human Services Louis Sullivan refers to underrepresented minorities as "missing persons" in US health professions and notes that, historically, racial and ethnic minorities consistently were underrepresented in key health professions (Mittman & Sullivan, 2012; Sullivan, 2004).

The growing diversity in the US nursing workforce is projected to continue in the foreseeable future. The largest gains for most culturally diverse groups, however, occurred during the mid- to late 1970s. Since that time, with the exception of Asians and Hispanics, racial and ethnic diversity in nursing and other health professions has been relatively stable (American Association of Colleges of Nursing, 2014a; Bureau of Labor Statistics, U.S. Department of Labor, 2014; Harris, Lewis, & Calloway, 2012; Health Resources and Services Administration, 2013).

The majority of health care administrators and leaders in health professions education currently acknowledge that increasing the diversity of the workforce will improve the quality of care, decrease racial disparities in health, and result in the delivery of more culturally congruent and competent care (Flores & Combs, 2013; Hedlund, Esparza, Calhoun, & Yates, 2012; Kirch & Nivet, 2013; Mittman & Sullivan, 2012; Mixer, Lasater, Jenkins, et al., 2013). There is widespread belief among the majority of hospital administrators and members of accrediting bodies that the nursing workforce should reflect the diversity found in the population it serves (Gates & Mark, 2012; Joint Commission, 2010).

Legal Perspectives

Affirmative action, a legal term used in the United States, refers to mandatory and voluntary programs intended to *affirm* the civil rights of designated classes of individuals by taking positive *action* to protect them from discrimination in education, training, employment, and

Recruitment, Retention, and Work Satisfaction of Men Working as Nurses in Acute Care Settings

Although they find meaning in the nursing, men working as nurses in acute care settings in Canada report a variety of challenges as members of a profession that is dominated by women. These challenges include gender discrimination, sexual stereotyping, paucity of male role models, fewer full-time job opportunities, and higher job dissatisfaction than women who are nurses in the same settings. The investigators studied 16 men, ages 21 to 44 years (mean 37.3 years) and having experience in nursing for an average of 9.6 years, using focus groups in four locations in Southern Ontario Province. The majority of the participants report that they became interested in a career in nursing due to the encouragement by a relative (either gender), media portrayal of nursing as exciting and fast-paced, or as a result of prior personal experience with a serious personal illness requiring prolonged hospitalization. The participants reported the following ways in which nursing fails to meet their expectations for a satisfying career: *stressful transitioning from nursing school into practice*; negative aspects of the work environment such as *paucity of full-time positions* in desired area, thus necessitating multiple part-time jobs; *feeling underappreciated* and not listened to by hospital managers; *fear of burnout* from physical and psychological stressors; *prejudice and discrimination* as a result of being a visible minority; and difficulty with colleagues who give them *assignments requiring the most physical strength* or discourage men from carrying out *"mixed gender procedures"* or treatments, ostensibly out of concern for legalities. Lastly, some colleagues and patients don't think that men should be nurses and their repeated use of the redundant "male nurse," rather than simply "nurse."

Clinical Implications

To recruit, retain, and increase the satisfaction of men in nursing, the study participants recommend the following:

- Recruit men into nursing at a younger age, for example, in high school or earlier grades.
- Degender care and caring (viewed as a female trait) and challenge "hegemonic masculinity." (*Hegemony* refers to the social, cultural, ideological, or economic influence exerted by a dominant group.)
- Challenge gender stereotypes of men in nursing by highlighting the significant historical contributions of men and by positive media images of men in nursing, for example, military images of men saving lives in combat situations.
- Replace the label "male nurse" with "nurse." The term "male nurse" serves to highlight the minority status of a man who is a nurse and also to convey the unexpectedness of a man in nursing.
- Change stereotypes associated with the nursing profession, specifically the notion that nursing is "women's work."
- Stop using expressions such as "the nurse..... she."
- Increase full-time employment opportunities for men and women, particularly during the first few years of their career.

Reference: Rajacich D., Kane, D., Williston, M. A., & Cameron, S. (2013). If they do call you a nurse, it is always a "male nurse": Experiences of men in the nursing profession. *Nursing Forum, 48*(1), 71–80.

contract awards. Federal statutes and regulations are designed to remedy discriminatory practices on the basis of race, color, sex, creed, or age. Affirmative action is designed to (1) eliminate existing and continuing discrimination, (2) remedy the effects of past discrimination, and (3) create systems and procedures to prevent future discrimination. The systems and procedures are commonly based on population percentages of minority groups in a particular area. Similar initiatives are known as **employment equity** in Canada, **reservation** in India

and Nepal, and **positive action** in the United Kingdom. The nature of the antidiscrimination policies varies from one location to another. Some countries, such as India, use a quota system, whereby a certain percentage of jobs or school vacancies must be set aside for members of a certain group. In some other regions, specific quotas do not exist. Rather, members of minority groups are given preference in selection processes. The U.S. Equal Employment Opportunity (EEO) laws prohibit specific types of job discrimination in certain workplaces. The Department of Labor has two agencies that deal with EEO monitoring and enforcement: the Civil Rights Center and the Office of Federal Contract Compliance Programs (U.S. Department of Labor, n.d.).

Historically, legal approaches were necessary to rectify workplace discrimination against particular groups such as women, physically and mentally disabled people, veterans, and persons who self-identify as being gay, bisexual, lesbian, or transgendered. Mandatory and voluntary programs continue to be used to protect the civil rights of those same vulnerable populations. For example, federal, state, and local policy initiatives have required health care organizations to develop diversity programs to address problems such as sexual harassment; illiteracy; racial, ethnic, and religious discrimination; and accommodation for disabled persons (Ewoh, 2013; Lauring & Selmer, 2013; U.S. Department of Labor, n.d.). However, the leaders and administrators in many health care organizations have moved from simply upholding legal mandates to genuinely valuing, embracing, and managing diversity.

Title V of the Affordable Care Act (ACA) of 2010 funds scholarships and loan repayment programs to increase the number of primary care physicians, nurses, physician assistants, mental health providers, and dentists in the areas of the country that need them most. With a comprehensive approach focusing on retention and enhanced educational opportunities, the ACA combats the critical nursing shortage. Due to new incentives and recruitment strategies, the ACA increases the supply of public health professionals so that the United States is prepared for health emergencies. The Affordable Care Act also provides state and local governments flexibility and resources to develop health workforce recruitment strategies. Lastly, the Affordable Care Act helps to expand critical and timely access to care by funding the expansion, construction, and operation of community health centers throughout the United States (U.S. Department of Health and Human Services, 2014).

Barriers to Diversity

There are numerous barriers to diversity in nursing and other health professions, beginning with road blocks in the education pipeline that prevent students from traditionally underrepresented and minority groups from gaining admission to nursing, medical, pharmacy, and other health professions schools. The barriers keeping racial and ethnic minorities, men, and other groups from entering nursing include educational deficiencies that are complex and interconnected with inadequate K-12 education systems for students from minority and economically disadvantaged populations who frequently attend poorly funded schools, often in neighborhoods characterized by crime and drugs.

Other barriers relate to the failure of colleges and universities to reach out to students from diverse backgrounds with recruitment and retention services that promote academic, clinical, and career success, as well as their failure to provide application assistance to students who are the first in their family to apply to college (Flores & Combs, 2013; Harris, Lewis, & Calloway, 2012; Mittman & Sullivan, 2012). The cost of higher education is rising, and there is insufficient financial aid available. The majority of entry-level BSN students find it necessary to work full- or part-time while in school as they struggle to pay for educational costs and household expenses. In 2013, the average total debt for undergraduate students upon completion of college was $35,200, and 85% of new graduates reported plans to return home to live after graduation in order to repay student loans (Ellis, 2014).

Faculty shortages at nursing schools across the country are limiting student capacity at a time when the need for nurses is high. US nursing schools turned away 789,089 qualified applicants from baccalaureate and graduate nursing

programs in 2013 due to an insufficient number of faculty, clinical sites, classroom space, clinical preceptors, and budget constraints. Nearly two-thirds of schools of nursing surveyed by the American Association of Colleges of Nursing identify nursing faculty shortages as among the top reason for turning away qualified applicants seeking admission into baccalaureate nursing programs (American Association of Colleges of Nursing, 2014b, 2015). Faculty from traditionally underrepresented backgrounds are in short supply due to barriers that prevent them from experiencing educational mobility, that is, earning their master's and doctoral degrees, credentials that prepare them to be nursing faculty, researchers, and leaders in nursing educational administration and in health care organizations and agencies. For example, in the U.S. nursing school deans and faculty are primarily female and white. Men are represented by only 3.5% of faculty and 2.4% of deans. Minorities represent only 8.7% of faculty and 6.8% of deans (American Association of Colleges of Nursing, 2013, 2014a, 2014b, 2015) (Figure 12-2).

Within health care organizations, nursing positions serve as pipelines for advancement to managerial and leadership positions. There are many reasons why men and minority group members do not pursue careers in nursing or leadership roles. These include role stereotypes, economic barriers, paucity of mentors, gender biases, lack of direction from authority figures, and increased, more lucrative opportunities in other fields. Societal stereotypes are sometimes woven into the social fabric of organizations, becoming part of their unique culture. Supervisors tend to select individuals for leadership positions based on stereotypical organizational norms, making it difficult for individuals who are identified as "different" to be hired and promoted. People tend to associate with others who are similar to themselves; therefore, when filling managerial, supervisory, or leadership positions, those already in power tend to select applicants whom they perceive as similar to themselves. In health care organizations, it becomes increasingly difficult for traditionally underrepresented minorities to be considered for

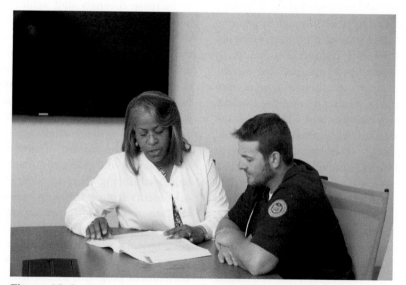

Figure 12-2. Two-thirds of US nursing schools responding to a survey by the American Association of Colleges of Nursing report faculty shortages as one of the top reasons for not accepting qualified applicants into baccalaureate nursing programs. Faculty and students from traditionally underrepresented populations, such as racial and ethnic minorities and men, are in high demand and short supply in nursing education and in the nursing workforce.

leadership or policy-making positions (Flores & Combs, 2013). The impact of perceived organizational marginalization by minorities in health professions is noteworthy. A study of Black nurses found that 12% had filed allegations of racial discrimination against their employer (Seago & Spetz, 2008), and a study of Latino physicians revealed that 20% left at least one job for reasons of discrimination, compared to 9% of White physicians (Nunez-Smith, 2009). Barriers to diversity include homogeneity in the composition of key organizational leaders, and print and electronic messages that fail to recognize the importance of diversity, for example, websites and job postings that fail to value diversity, and other subtle and overt communications that indicate lack of commitment to diversity (Flores & Combs, 2013; Harris, Lewis, & Calloway, 2012; Mittman & Sullivan, 2012).

Negative attitudes and behaviors in the workplace also serve as barriers to diversity. Negative attitudes and behaviors include **hatred**, prejudice, **bigotry**, discrimination, racism, and ethnoviolence. In some organizations, the use of racial, ethnic, sexual, and other derogatory remarks signals a disturbing underlying problem in the workplace. Why does hatred exist in the workplace? Although the reasons are complex and interconnected, some contributing factors include the early socialization of children to cultural and gender stereotypes, personal experiences (or lack of them) with people from diverse backgrounds, and exposure to negative societal attitudes. Negative attitudes and behaviors in the workplace are exacerbated during times of rapid immigration, periods of economic recession or depression, and high unemployment. Competition for sexual partners also is cited as a cause for hatred. Hatred can be the cause of tremendous hostility in the workplace. In some organizations, technology is used to transmit derogatory remarks electronically to individuals or targeted groups by e-mail or social media. Sites on the Internet that allow free expressions of hatred have proliferated. Those responsible justify their actions by citing either the Canadian Charter of Rights and Freedoms or the U.S. Constitution's First Amendment rights to freedom of expression (Este et al., 2013; Krawiec, Conley, & Broome, 2014; Lowe, 2013).

Although not all hatred leads to violence, the number of reported attacks on gays, Muslims, and Jews has increased significantly. **Ethnoviolence** is increasing, not only in the United States and Canada but worldwide. Homosexual men, Muslims, and Jews are the primary targets of hate crimes, some of which occur in the workplace. Although it is impossible to protect all employees and patients or clients from violence in health care settings, reasonable steps must be taken to protect those believed to be at risk. Verbal threats and/or assaults by or against staff members should not be tolerated, nor should offensive jokes, e-mails, or other verbal, written, or electronic communications that reflect hatred, prejudice, and/or discrimination and/or create a hostile work environment. Don't expect the problem to go away unless the perpetrator(s) are identified and punished (New York Employment Law, 2014).

Strategies to Increase Diversity

In addition to the establishment and enforcement of laws, there are other approaches being used to increase diversity and achieve concordance between the cultural composition of the community and the health care workforce that serves the community. Researchers are investigating the influence of corporate culture and organizational climate on increasing diversity and examining two major approaches for increasing diversity with documented success: diversity management and organizational inclusion.

Although the number of minority students in baccalaureate and graduate nursing programs has increased during the past 10 years, the percent of students from racially and ethnically diverse backgrounds did not grow in proportion to the large infusion of funding from federal and state governments, private foundations, schools, and professional associations. Despite funding for enrichment programs in mathematics, sciences, prenursing, career preparation, prematriculation interventions, tutoring, research programs, school partnerships, and faculty development programs, only 29% of generic or entry-level baccalaureate students, 30% of masters students, and

28.4% of research-focused doctoral students in nursing are racial or ethnic minorities (American Association of Colleges of Nursing, 2013). Well-funded federal initiatives, such as the Nursing Workforce Development Program, Centers of Excellence, and the National Health Services Corps (Mittman & Sullivan, 2012), and the use of the military training to facilitate the educational mobility of veterans (e.g., the HRSA-funded veterans to BSN Project) are approaches that have been used with much success to increase the number of underrepresented minorities in the health professions pipeline (Harris, Lewis, & Calloway, 2012). Table 12-1 provides an overview

Table 12-1: Strategies for Increasing Diversity in Nursing

Strategies	Schools of Nursing	Professional Nursing Organizations	Federal/State Governments, Foundations, Corporations	The Media
K-12 Pipeline				
Present a positive, exciting, and inclusive image of nursing	X	X	X	X
Develop print, broadcast, and social media communications portraying men and traditionally underrepresented minorities in nursing in positive ways	X	X	X	X
Provide scholarships, grants, stipends, low-interest loans for tuition, fees, books, and living expenses	X	X	X	
Encourage boys and girls to consider a career in nursing by collaborating with parents, principals, teachers, guidance counselors, and coaches at schools, scouting organizations, sports teams	X	X	X	X
Encourage high school students from diverse backgrounds to join future nurses clubs, volunteer at hospitals, long-term care facilities, and other health care organizations	X	X	X	X
Create nursing mentoring programs that include men and traditionally underrepresented minorities as mentors and mentees	X	X	X	
College/University				
Review admissions criteria, promotional materials, websites, and other communications viewed by prospective nursing students through the lens of applicants from diverse backgrounds	X			
Assist students from diverse backgrounds with the application process	X			
Encourage current students from diverse backgrounds to volunteer at recruitment events, in local schools, health fairs, open houses, and related events	X	X		X
Hire recruiters, academic advisors, faculty, deans, and others who mirror the diversity of the community served	X			

continued

Table 12-1: Strategies for Increasing Diversity in Nursing (continued)

Strategies	Schools of Nursing	Professional Nursing Organizations	Federal/State Governments, Foundations, Corporations	The Media
Involve parents, siblings, and other family members in admission, orientation, white coat/induction, pinning, and related activities	X			
Encourage students to take advantage of student success opportunities, e.g., writing center; review sessions for math, science, and nursing courses; and NCLEX preparation	X			
Establish peer mentoring, tutoring, NCLEX review, and related programs for nursing students	X	X	X	
Prior to graduation, provide assistance with resume preparation, interviewing skills, and networking to obtain the top jobs and salaries	X	X		X
Provide development programs that educate nursing faculty about strategies for promoting the academic success of students from diverse backgrounds (e.g., eliminating cultural bias from assignments and exams) and advising and mentoring them	X	X	X	
Health Care Organizations				
Hire and promote people from traditionally underrepresented backgrounds to mirror the diversity in the community served for positions from grassroots to senior executive-level positions, thus making an institutional commitment to diversity				
Communicate the many advantages and benefits of diversity to all stakeholders (students, staff, and others)				
Use recruiters from diverse backgrounds to attract the diversity being sought in the nursing workforce				
During job interviews, introduce applicants to employees from diverse backgrounds as interviews are two-way processes				
As budget permits, offer internships and summer employment to nursing students from diverse backgrounds				
Develop partnerships between and among health care organizations and schools of nursing, professional organizations, federal/state government agencies, foundations, corporations, and the media to promote mutual diversity goals				
Provide cultural competence training for health care staff to develop cross-cultural communication skills, awareness of respect for and knowledge about diversity in the multicultural workplace	X	X	X	X

Table created using data from American Association of Colleges of Nursing (2014, 2015), Flores and Combs (2013), Jackson and Gracia (2014), Mittman and Sullivan (2012), Mixer, Lasater, Jenkins, et al. (2013).

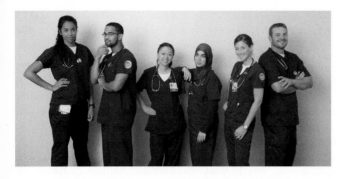

Figure 12-3. Nursing students representing diversity in race, ethnicity, religion, age, and gender.

of selected strategies for increasing diversity in nursing used by schools of nursing, professional organizations, government, foundation, and corporate organizations and the broadcast, print, and social media (National Institute on Minority Health and Health Disparities, 2014; Urban Universities for Health, 2014). Figure 12-3 shows nursing students from diverse racial, ethnic, and religious backgrounds who have matriculated into a BSN nursing program at a Midwestern university in the United States.

Corporate Culture and Organizational Climate

Health care organizations are minisocieties that have their own distinctive patterns of culture and subculture. One organization may have a high degree of cohesiveness, with staff working together like members of a single family toward the achievement of common goals. Another may be highly fragmented, divided into groups that think about the world in very different ways or that have different aspirations about what their organization should be. Just as individuals in a culture can have different personalities while sharing much in common, so can groups and organizations. This phenomenon is referred to as corporate culture. **Corporate culture** is a process of reality construction that allows staff to see and understand particular events, actions, objects, communications, or situations in distinctive ways. These patterns of understanding help people cope with the situations they encounter and provide a basis for making behavior sensible and meaningful.

Shared values, beliefs, meaning, and understanding are components of the corporate culture. The corporate culture is established and maintained through an ongoing, proactive process of reality construction. It is an active, living phenomenon through which staff members jointly create and recreate their workplace and world. One of the easiest ways to appreciate the nature of corporate culture is to observe the day-to-day functioning of the organization. Observe the patterns of interaction among individuals, the language that is used, the images and themes explored in conversation, and the various rituals of daily routine. Historical explanations for the ways things are done will emerge in discussions of the rationale for certain aspects of the culture.

The corporate culture metaphor is useful because it directs attention to the symbolic significance of almost every aspect of organizational life. Structures, hierarchies, rules, and organizational routines reveal underlying meanings that are crucial for understanding how organizations function. For example, meetings carry important aspects of organizational culture, which may convey a sense of conformity and order or of causal informality. The environment in which the meetings are held reflects the formality or informality of the organization.

Box 12-1 contains questions to consider when determining the corporate culture of a health care organization, institution, or agency. The answers to the questions will provide a beginning understanding of the corporate culture of the organization and the ways in which it supports diversity. Health care

Box 12-1 Determining Corporate Culture

The following questions are helpful in determining the corporate culture of an organization.

- Does the person presiding over the group stand or sit?
- Does the presider encourage discussion among group members or engage in a monologue?
- Are group members encouraged to express opinions freely, or is there pressure to silence those who express opposing points of view?
- How do group leaders and members dress?

- What message does the institutional dress code convey about the acceptance of cultural diversity?
- Do policies allow for cultural expressions in clothing, accessories, hairstyle, and related areas?
- Although most institutions require employees to wear identification badges or name tags, what flexibility does the individual have for self-expression and expression of cultural identity and affiliation?

work environments are social settings that encompass many elements of a social system. It is useful to distinguish between the organizational climate of the work environment and the corporate culture. The **organizational climate** usually measures perceptions or feelings about the organization or work environment. The corporate or organizational culture, on the other hand, is what its members share—their beliefs, values, assumptions, and rituals—often unconsciously. Culture provides the community, the sameness, and the consensus that makes those people unique and special.

In the contemporary health care industry, nurse managers, administrators, and executive-level leaders sometimes focus their time and energy on issues such as cost–benefit outcomes, downsizing, territorial struggles with members of other disciplines, appropriate use of technology, and other important topics. With increasing frequency, nurses in key leadership positions are realizing the critical importance of transculturally based administrative practices that recognize, value, and promote the advantages of diversity in the multicultural workplace.

Diversity Management and Organizational Inclusion

Diversity management is a historically situated concept that gained momentum in the United States in the mid-1980s when political forces threatened to overturn equality and affirmative action laws. Proponents of affirmative action and equality legislation successfully argued that diversity should be promoted, not because it is a legal mandate but because it is good for business, including health care businesses. R. Roosevelt Thomas, Jr., President of the American Institute for Managing Diversity, first introduced diversity management as a way of creating an environment that enables employees to reach their full potential in pursuit of organizational goals and objectives (Thomas, 1990). A complex, multifaceted concept, **diversity management** refers to the systematic and planned commitment by organizations to recruit, retain, reward, and promote a heterogeneous mix of employees. There is consensus among senior leaders of health care organizations that diversity management needs to move from a passive (valuing diversity) to an active approach. This active approach includes mentoring programs, alternative work arrangements (e.g., flextime, telework), family-friendly programs (e.g., organizations that provide child care), ongoing development and training programs for staff, a psychologically safe work environment, accountability, and succession planning that allows all qualified individuals, regardless of background, to compete for and be appointed

to key leadership positions within the organization (Sabharwal, 2014; Singh & Winkel, 2012; Singh, Winkel, & Selvarajan, 2013).

Diversity management requires that there is senior-level support for ongoing educational development programs that increase cultural awareness and competence (Lowe, 2013). Caution must be exercised so employees making use of work/life balance programs or alternative work arrangements are not singled out as receiving preferential treatment by coworkers or subject to backlash. For example, there is evidence that single mothers taking advantage of alternative work arrangements are sometimes pejoratively labeled as being on the "mommy track," are not taken as seriously as other employees, and are passed over for promotion because they are perceived as being less committed to the organization (Sabharwal, 2014).

Simply hiring employees from diverse backgrounds for the sake of increasing representation within an organization is insufficient, and may actually be counterproductive unless leaders in the organization devise strategies to eliminate systemic barriers and create avenues for all employees to contribute to their fullest potential (Bendick et al., 2010; Sabharwal, 2014). For maximum productivity and job satisfaction, employees in health care and other organizations need to feel that the groups they belong to are a source of self-esteem and make them feel that they are accepted, fit in, belong, and feel secure. At the same time, the employee needs to feel unique. These basic human needs form the foundation for **organizational inclusion**, which is defined as the degree to which individuals feel that they are part of critical organizational processes as indicated by work group involvement, ability to express ideas and opinions, access to information and resources, ability to influence decision making, and a sense of psychological safety and job security (Gates & Mark, 2012; Sabharwal, 2014; Singh & Winkel, 2012; Singh, Winkel, & Selvarajan, 2013).

In inclusive organizations, leaders recognize that employees and their ideas need to be valued and utilized. Employees partner in a collegial, collaborative, and cooperative manner within and across departments, and employees feel that they are an integral part of the organization. Prospective employees are attracted to the organization because of its respect for and commitment to diversity and an inclusive work environment. People feel connected to each other and to the organization and its goals. Lastly, the organization continuously fosters flexibility, open communication, choice, and diversity. When senior leaders support these principles and administer them in a transparent, equitable manner, there is increased employee productivity, organizational commitment, and greater job satisfaction (van Djik & van Engan, 2013; Gates & Mark, 2013; Ewoh, 2013 Sabharwal, 2014; Singh, Winkel, & Selvarajan, 2013).

The Challenges and Opportunities of a Multicultural Health Care Workforce

A significant number of the US and Canadian national health goals for the current decade and beyond involve specific objectives for improving the health status of members of minority groups identified by both countries' federal governments, particularly those with low incomes. Meanwhile, culturally diverse cohorts of children, women of childbearing age, and the elderly are expected to grow, exacerbating the need for culturally competent providers of health care.

Since 1972, there has been an explosion in the numbers of people migrating to the United States and Canada, both with and without legal documentation. In 2013, the total population of the United States was over 316 million, including 40.1 million foreign-born people, representing 12.9% of the total population. These immigrants come from Europe (12%), North America (2%), Latin American (53%), Asia (28%), and other

areas of the world (U.S. Census Bureau, 2014). The majority of Canada's 265 million immigrants come from China, India, Philippines, U.S., Pakistan, and South Korea (Statistics Canada, 2014)

Cultural Perspectives on the Meaning of Work

The earliest recorded ideas about work refer to it as a curse, a punishment, or a necessary evil needed to sustain life. People of high status did not work; slaves, indentured servants, and peasants worked. In contemporary society, the concept of work must be considered in its historical and cultural context. Cultural views about caring for the sick also must be considered, because such care may be perceived as a divine calling for those with supernatural powers (some African tribes), a religious vocation (some ethnic Catholic groups), or an undignified occupation for lower-class workers (some Arab groups such as Kuwaitis and Saudi Arabians).

Cultural norms influence a staff member's consideration of group interest as opposed to individual interests in the multicultural workplace. Scholars have identified two major orientations embraced by people: individualism and collectivism. With individualism, importance is placed on individual inputs, rights, and rewards. Individualists emphasize values such as autonomy, competitiveness, achievement, and self-sufficiency. Most English-speaking and European countries have individualist cultures. Collectivism entails the need to maintain group harmony above the partisan interests of subgroups and individuals. In collectivist cultures, values such as interpersonal harmony and group solidarity prevail. A staff member whose ethnic heritage is Asian or South American is likely to be influenced by collectivism. Amish and Mennonite groups also are considered collectivist cultures.

One of the most notable distinctions between people from individualist and collectivist cultures is the meaning of work. Individualists work to earn a living. People are expected to work; they need not enjoy it. Leisure or recreational activities frequently are pursued to alleviate the monotony of work. People from individualist cultures tend to dichotomize work and leisure. Individualist concepts of work reflect an orientation toward the future. People from collectivist cultures value group relationships, workplace cooperation, and collaborating as a team. They tend to emphasize shared objectives and long-term, ongoing relationships with coworkers and supervisors in the organization. People from collectivist cultures are more concerned with harmonious, group relationships in the present than self-promotion and getting ahead in the organization.

It also is useful to understand cultural differences about appropriate and desired behavior in the workplace. People from most individualist cultures are typically achievement oriented. Stereotypically, they want to do better, accomplish more, and take responsibility for their actions. They tend to develop personality traits such as assertiveness and competitiveness that facilitate these goals. In many collectivist cultures, however, qualities such as commitment to relationships, gentleness, cooperativeness, and indirectness are valued.

Cultural Values in the Multicultural Workplace

Cultural values frequently lie at the root of cross-cultural differences in the multicultural workplace. Values form the core of a culture. As indicated in Figure 12-4, cultural values exert an influence on (or inform) workplace factors, which in turn influence each other: time orientation, **family obligations**, etiquette, communication patterns, space/distance, touch, meaning of work, and work ethic.

What is the importance of learning about the values of people from diverse cultural groups? Values exert a powerful influence on how each person behaves, reacts, and feels. In the multicultural workplace, values affect people's lives in four

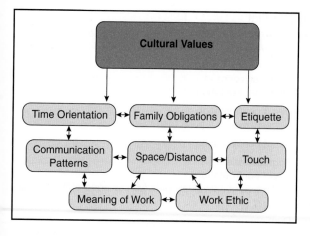

Figure 12-4. Influence of cultural values on the multicultural workplace.

major ways: values underlie *perceived needs, what is defined as a problem, how conflict is resolved,* and *expectations of behavior.* When cultural values of individual staff members conflict with the organizational values or those held by coworkers, challenges, misunderstandings, and difficulties in the workplace become inevitable. You must use these inevitable conflicts as opportunities to foster cross-cultural understanding among staff members from diverse backgrounds and to enhance cross-cultural communication.

Cultural Perspectives on Conflict

The term **conflict** is derived from Latin roots (*configere,* "to strike against") and refers to actions that range from intellectual disagreement to physical violence. Frequently, the action that precipitates the conflict is based on different cultural perceptions of the situation. According to some social scientists, when participants in a conflict are from the same culture, they are more likely to perceive the situation in the same way and to organize their perceptions in similar ways.

By examining proverbs used by members of various cultural groups, it is possible to better understand differences in the way conflict is viewed. Table 12-2 summarizes selected proverbs that relate to conflict and its resolution. The US culture's proverbs emphasize assertive behavior and dealing with conflict through direct

confrontation. Other cultures—particularly collectivist groups—may promote avoidance of confrontation and emphasize harmony (e.g., Native North Americans, Alaskan Natives, Amish, and Asians). The culture-based choices that lead people in these opposite directions are a major source of conflict in the workplace.

Many people from individualist cultures view conflict as a healthy, natural, and inevitable component of all relationships. People from many collectivist cultures, on the other hand, have learned to internalize conflict and to value harmonious relationships above winning arguments and "being right." To many people of Native North American and Asian descent, conflict is not healthy, desirable, or constructive. In the Arab world, mediation is critical in resolving disputes, and confrontation seldom works. Mediation allows for saving face and is rooted in the realization that all conflicts do not have simple solutions.

The assertive, confrontational, direct style of communicating is characteristic of people from individualistic cultures, whereas the cooperative, conciliatory style is a more collectivist or Eastern mode of managing conflict. When attempting to influence others during a disagreement, for example, nurses from China, Japan, and other collectivist cultures may use covert conflict prevention strategies to minimize interpersonal conflicts. Nurses from individualistic cultures are

Table 12-2: Selected Proverbs Related to Conflict

Proverb	Value
United States	
The squeaky wheel gets the grease.	Aggressiveness Direct confrontation
Tell it like it is.	Direct confrontation Honesty even if it hurts the other
Take the bull by the horns.	Direct confrontation
Shoot first, ask questions later.	Aggressiveness Direct confrontation Protection of individual rights (versus good of the group)
Might makes right.	Aggressiveness Dominance
Japanese	
The nail that sticks out gets hammered.	Not calling attention to oneself Going along with the group Harmony and balance
Senegalese	
Misunderstandings do not exist; only the failure to communicate does.	Strive to understand the other's point of view Harmony and balance is normal state, not conflict and confrontation.
Zen	
He who knows does not speak, and he who speaks does not know.	Listen to the other's side during conflict Silence
Arab	
The hand of Allah is with the group.	Primacy of group good (versus individual)
Haste comes from the devil.	Patience Conflict resolution takes time.
Navajo Indian	
If the horse falls, get off.	Practicality and common sense

more likely to rely on the overt confrontation of ideas and argumentation by reason.

The origins of cultural conflict result from influences on the organization and on individuals. As indicated in Figure 12-5, political, economic, legal, technological, and, for organizations owned and operated by religious groups, religious factors influence organizations and their corporate culture and organizational climate. Educational background, socioeconomic factors, family obligations, political factors, economic factors, cultural factors, moral and religious beliefs, and personal traits influence individuals and affect the corporate culture and organizational climate as well. Staff members contribute to the perception that values are in conflict. Although there are many conflicting values that underlie problems, the following areas will be explored here: family obligations; personal hygiene; communication; touch; etiquette; clothing and accessories; intergenerational relationships; relationships with authority figures, peers, subordinates, and patients; national and ethnic rivalries; gender and sexual orientation; moral and religious beliefs; and national origin.

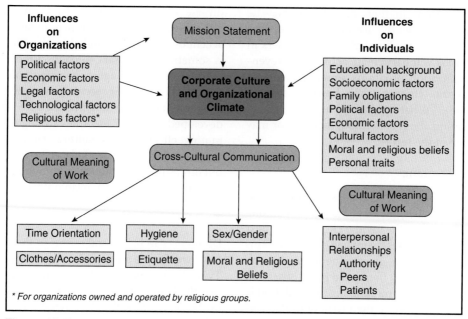

Figure 12-5. Origins of conflict in the multicultural health care setting.

Family Obligations

Although family is important in all cultures, the constellation (e.g., nuclear, single parent, extended, same sex), emotional closeness among members, social and economic commitments among members, and other factors vary cross-culturally.

Independence from the family is highly valued by many from the dominant cultural groups in the United States and Canada, but it ranks very low in the hierarchy of people from most Middle Eastern and Asian cultures. In the latter groups, the family is highly valued, and the individual's lifelong duties toward the family are explicit. Thus, absence from work for family-related reasons may be considered legitimate and important by workers from some cultures, but may be perceived as an unnecessary inconvenience to the supervisor. For example, a Mexican American staff member may submit a last-minute request for vacation time to visit with a distant cousin who has unexpectedly arrived in town after traveling a great distance. The Mexican American staff member thinks, "What a great opportunity to develop a stronger relationship with a distant member of my mother's family. How nice that cousin Juan has traveled so far to see me. I've been thinking about making a trip to Mexico next year, so perhaps I can stay with Juan during my visit. Surely my nurse manager understands how important it is for me to spend time with my family and will be able to rearrange the unit schedule to accommodate my request." The nurse manager may think, "What's wrong with these Mexican Americans? Don't they want to work? This vacation request means that I'll have to redo the schedule for the entire unit. If I permitted everyone to submit last-minute vacation requests, I'd go crazy. What's the big deal about a distant cousin coming to visit, anyway?"

Ideas about the importance of anticipating and controlling the future vary significantly from culture to culture. Whereas some staff members place a high priority on planning for retirement, accumulating sick days, and purchasing insurance, others, particularly recent immigrants with

family obligations in their homelands, may be more concerned with current obligations and living in the present. Similarly, some workers in high-risk jobs will participate actively in preventive immunization programs aimed at hepatitis and influenza, whereas others bewilder managers by saying, "What will be, will be. I can't spend time worrying about something that may or may not happen in the future."

Personal Hygiene

Personal hygiene can be a sensitive topic, and views on personal hygiene can vary greatly among cultures. For some, the saying "cleanliness is next to godliness" describes their view of hygiene. This proverb highlights the great value some place on cleanliness and can be illustrated by an obsession with eliminating or minimizing natural bodily odors—as evidenced by the plethora of deodorants, douches, body lotions, mouthwashes, and related products with hundreds of different fragrances. Others, however, are not unduly bothered by body odors and see no reason to mask natural odors. Some members of the health care workforce may come from a country in which water is scarce and bathing is restricted. Others may be following religious or cultural practices that prohibit bathing during certain times, such as while a woman is menstruating, after the delivery of a baby, and at other times.

Communication

Underlying the majority of conflicts in the multicultural health care setting are issues related to verbal and nonverbal **cross-cultural communication**. Even when interacting with staff members from the same cultural background, it requires administrative skill to decide whether to speak with someone face to face, send an electronic or paper memorandum, contact the person by telephone, send a text message, or opt not to communicate about a particular matter at all. Nurses must exercise considerable judgment when making decisions about effective methods for communicating with staff members and patients from

diverse cultural backgrounds. Communication difficulties caused by differences in language and accent become compounded on the telephone. It is sometimes necessary to counsel recent immigrants from non–English-speaking countries to refrain from giving or receiving medical orders by telephone until their English language skills have developed. Box 12-2 identifies strategies for promoting effective cross-cultural communication in the multicultural workplace. In Figure 12-6, nursing students practice communication and team work in a simulation laboratory.

Touch

Differences in behavioral norms in the **multicultural workforce** are often inaccurately perceived. Typically, people from Asian cultures are not as overtly demonstrative of affection as are Whites or Blacks. Generally, they refrain from public embraces, kissing, and loud talking or laughter. Affection is expressed in a more reserved manner. In some cases, staff members from different cultures may send messages through their use of touch that are not intended. Special attention to male–female relationships is warranted in the multicultural workplace. In general, it is best to refrain from touching staff members of either gender unless necessary for the accomplishment of a job-related task, such as the provision of safe patient care.

Etiquette

Values frequently underlie cultural expectations of behavior, including matters of **etiquette**, the conventional code of good manners that governs behavior. For example, some people from Hispanic, Middle Eastern, and African cultures expect the nurse manager to engage in social conversation and to establish personal and social rapport before giving assignments or orders for the day's work. In developing interpersonal relationships, a high value is placed on getting to know about a person's family, personal concerns, and interests before discussing job-related business. A nurse manager's reluctance to engage in

Box 12-2 Strategies to Promote Effective Cross-Cultural Communication in the Multicultural Workplace

- Pronounce names correctly. When in doubt, ask the person for the correct pronunciation.
- Use proper titles of respect: "Doctor," "Reverend," "Mister." Ask permission to use first names, or wait until you are given permission to do so.
- Be aware of gender sensitivities. If uncertain about the marital status of a woman or her preferred title, it is best to refer to her as Ms. initially, and then ask how she prefers to be addressed at the first opportunity.
- Be aware of subtle linguistic messages that may convey bias or inequality, for example, referring to a White man as Mister while addressing a Black female by her first name.
- Refrain from Anglicizing or shortening a person's given name without his or her permission. For example, calling a Russian American "Mike" instead of Mikhael or shortening the Italian American Maria Rosaria to Maria. The same principle applies to the last name, or surname.
- Call people by their proper names. Avoid slang such as "girl," "boy," "honey," "dear," "guy," "fella," "babe," "chief," "mama," "sweetheart," or similar terms. When in doubt, ask people if they are offended by the use of a particular term.
- Refrain from using slang, pejorative, or derogatory terms when referring to persons from ethnic, racial, or religious groups, and convey to all staff that this is a work environment in which there is zero tolerance for the use of such language. Violators should be counseled immediately.
- Identify people by race, color, gender, and ethnic origin only when appropriate.
- Avoid using words and phrases that may be offensive to others. For example, "culturally deprived" or "culturally disadvantaged" imply inferiority, and "non-White" implies that White is the normative standard.
- Avoid clichés and platitudes such as "Some of my best friends are Mexicans" or "I went to school with Blacks."
- Use language in communications that includes *all* staff rather than excludes some of them.
- Do not expect a staff member to know all the other employees of his or her background or to speak for them. They share ethnicity, not necessarily the same experiences, friendships, or beliefs.
- Communications describing staff should pertain to their job skills, not their color, age, race, sex, or national origin.
- Refrain from telling stories or jokes demeaning to certain ethnic, racial, age, or religious groups. Also, avoid those pertaining to gender-related issues or persons with physical or mental disabilities. Convey to all staff that there will be zero tolerance for this inappropriate behavior. Violators should be counseled immediately.
- Avoid remarks that suggest to staff from diverse backgrounds that they should consider themselves fortunate to be in the organization. Do not compare their employment opportunities and conditions with those people in their country of origin.
- Remember that communication problems multiply in telephone communications because important nonverbal cues are lost and accents may be difficult to interpret. Be patient.
- Provide staff with opportunities to explore diversity issues in their workplace; celebrate the strength that differences bring, and constructively resolve conflicts.

self-disclosure about personal matters may leave the impression that he or she is uncaring and is not interested in the staff member. Such behaviors by a manager are not conducive to building productive, harmonious relationships and may be misunderstood by staff members from diverse backgrounds. Similarly, some cultures, such as the Igbo in Nigeria and other African tribes, value formal greetings at the start of the day or whenever the first encounter of the day

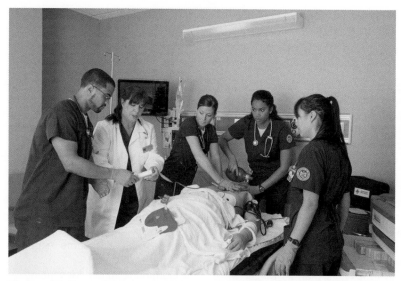

Figure 12-6. Nursing students learn to communicate effectively and work together as members of an interprofessional team to effectively manage life-threatening emergencies such as cardiopulmonary arrest.

occurs—a practice found even among close family members. For example, it is important to say, "Good morning, Mr. Okoro. There has been a change in your patient's insulin orders," rather than immediately "getting to the point" without recognizing by name the person to whom you are speaking.

Clothing and Accessories

Most health care institutions have a **dress code** or policy statement about clothing and accessories worn by staff in various parts of the facility (e.g., delivery room, operating room, specialty units). It is important to review these documents periodically from a cultural perspective. For example, modification of the dress code may be necessary to accommodate Hindu women dressed in saris, Sikh men who wear turbans, Muslim women and Roman Catholic nuns who cover their heads with veils, and Arab men who wear kaffiyehs. Special consideration may need to be given to some Blacks and others who wear jewelry and other accessories in their hair, particularly when the hair is braided.

Intergenerational Relationships

The nursing workforce is composed of a mixture of generational cohorts. A **generation** is defined as an identifiable group of people who share birth years, age, location, and experience the same significant events within a given period of time. The term generation is sometimes used interchangeably with term **generational cohort** (Hendricks & Cope, 2013). Scholars agree that there are four major generational cohorts in the United States, Canada, and Australia that go by the following names: veterans, baby boomers, generation X, and millennials. Evidence-Based Practice 12-2 provides an overview of each of the four cohorts and highlights some of their characteristics.

Interpersonal Relationships

There are cultural differences in interpersonal relationships involving authority figures, peers, subordinates, and patients. To examine these cultural differences, consider the following example. Dr. Kelly, an Irish American physician, gives an order for vital signs to Kim Li, a Chinese American nurse. The nurse perceives the order

Intergenerational Diversity: What Nurse Managers Need to Know

An electronic search of MEDLINE, PubMed, and CINAHL databases was completed using the words *generational diversity, nurse managers*, and *workforce* between 2000 and 2012, with the purpose of examining generational differences and their impact on the nursing workforce and their effect on the work environment. Four generational cohort groups were identified in the literature according to the nurse's date of birth:

The Veterans (1925–1945)

Description: Nurses who lived through the great world wars, experienced economic hardship; hierarchical; remain in the workforce after normal retirement age due to government incentives to prevent a brain drain

Characteristics: Loyal, disciplined, value teamwork, respect for hard work and authority; most hold senior-level health management positions rather than more physically demanding direct care positions

Baby Boomers (1946–1964)

Description: Grew up during period of economic prosperity and free expression; believe they are "entitled"; "Living to work" is the motto of this driven and dedicated cohort

Characteristics: Look to external sources for validation of their worth; equate work with personal fulfillment; competitive, strong willed; seek immediate gratification; want to be noticed and valued for their contribution through work-related perks or recognition, for example, salary increases, promotions, titles, office with a window, and reserved parking

Generation X (1965–1980)

Description: Individualistic in their approach to work, do not value team work; value outcomes more than process

Characteristics: Like to manage their own time, set their own limits, and complete their work without supervision; familiar with ambiguity, uncertainty, and flexibility; cohort values balance between work and personal or family life; well suited to a job market that is characterized by a great deal of change and little stability

Millennials (1980–present)

Description: Thrive on maintaining a balance between home and work; seamless in the way they play and work; adaptable to change; technology dependent; like to challenge assumptions

Characteristics: Enjoy strong peer support and team work; good at synthesizing large amounts of information quickly; job portability and lateral career moves are important to this cohort; rapid technology change sometimes results in the neophyte to the workforce being expert in the critical skill of information gathering and management

Clinical Implications

When working with generational diversity in the nursing workforce, nurse managers need to

- Recognize and value each generation's unique contribution to the provision of safe, culturally congruent, and competent patient care
- Respect the different ways in which nurses from each generation are instrumental in creating a cohesive workplace
- Be aware that each generation of nurses manifests differences in the 3 C's—communication, commitment, and compensation
- Promote collaboration and productivity among nurses from different generations
- Keep the patient as the focal point of all communications and nursing actions
- Highlight mutual team goals
- Encourage nurses from different generations to support one another and resolve conflicts amicably among themselves

When nurse managers acknowledge generational characteristics, they're able to develop strategies that focus on effective communication techniques, mentoring, motivation, appropriate technologies, and ethics of nursing to bridge the gap between generations of nurses and increase nursing workforce cohesion.

Reference: Hendricks, J. M., & Cope, V. C. (2013). Generational diversity: What nurse managers need to know. *Journal of Advanced Nursing, 69*(3), 717–725.

as unnecessary (but not harmful) to the patient; that is, she thinks the physician is requesting vital signs more frequently than is warranted by the patient's condition. Nurse Li refrains from questioning the physician or negotiating with him out of respect for his position of authority and the value she places on maintaining harmony in the relationship. Nurse Li says nothing and carries out the physician's order. At the change of shift, the charge nurse becomes angry because she concurs with the assessment that Dr. Kelly is ordering vital signs too frequently and believes that Nurse Li should have confronted the physician about the order. Nurse Li intentionally chose to avoid questioning Dr. Kelly's order. In her cultural value system, causing conflict through direct confrontation would be perceived negatively. She would have experienced lowered self-esteem and "loss of face" if she had been responsible for causing disharmony in the nurse–physician relationship. The charge nurse, on the other hand, perceives the physician as a colleague whose respect would be earned by assertive, direct communication with him.

National and Ethnic Rivalries

The global media is filled with news, documentaries, human interest stories, and related programs pertaining to nations with long-standing historic rivalries. Within nations, there is also intergroup conflict, such as the rivalries and civil war involving the Sunni and Shia Islamic groups throughout the Middle East, Asia, and Africa. Islamic extremists now live in many parts of the world—the United States, Canada, Australia and the Pacific Rim, Western and Eastern Europe, Latin America, and elsewhere in the world. At any given moment, there are numerous armed conflicts between two or more nations or factions. On occasion, the multicultural workplace becomes a battleground, where long-standing historic rivalries and more recent geopolitical differences are reenacted in the form of interpersonal conflict between two or more staff members. After ruling out other potential sources of conflict, it may be

worth examining the ethnic heritage and national origins of staff members for possible reasons. For example, the nurse manager may observe a pattern of strained relationships between an Israeli physician and Palestinian physicians, nurses, laboratory technicians, physical therapists, and other health care providers. Similar observations may be made concerning staff members from countries known to be rivals, such as North and South Korea, Russia and Afghanistan, Iran and Iraq, India and Pakistan, and other national rivalries.

Cues that may signal underlying historic rivalries include (1) the expression of high levels of emotional energy when a staff member is interacting with a person from a rival group and the topic does not seem to warrant it; (2) sudden, uncharacteristic behavior changes when the staff member is in the presence of a person from the rival group, for example, an ordinarily cordial staff member unexpectedly becomes acrimonious for no apparent reason; (3) the repeated expression of strong opinions about historical, political, and current events involving rival nations or factions; and (4) inappropriate attempts to persuade others to adopt the staff member's partisan views about the rivalry.

Gender and Sexual Orientation

Women have historically constituted the majority of personnel in nursing and in many allied health disciplines. The complex interrelationship between gender and culture has been studied extensively. In the health care setting, nurses of both genders may face the biases and preconceptions of physicians, fellow nurses, and other health care providers. The issue is further complicated by cultural beliefs about relationships with authority figures and cross-national perspectives on the status of various health care disciplines. For example, in many less developed nations, nursing is a low-status occupation. In some oil-rich Arab countries (e.g., Saudi Arabia, Kuwait), care for the sick is carried out by health care providers who are hired from abroad for the purpose

of caring for the bodily needs of the sick—an activity that is considered unacceptable in its cultural context. In the multicultural health care workplace, both men and women face the gender biases that exist in society. These issues frequently emerge in verbal and nonverbal communication and in interpersonal relationships. Our language also betrays covert gender biases and preconceptions. For example, the expression "male nurse" is sometimes used, but seldom does one hear about the "female nurse" because that term is considered redundant and unnecessary. An extensive analysis of workplace issues concerning gay, lesbian, bisexual, and transgendered staff members is beyond the scope of this text, but these types of diversity must be considered in the multicultural workplace.

Moral and Religious Beliefs

In some circumstances, moral and religious beliefs may underlie conflicts in the multicultural workplace. Consider the following dilemmas:

- A nurse who believes that it is morally wrong to drink alcohol refuses to carry out a physician's order for the therapeutic administration of alcohol as a sedative–hypnotic or to administer medicines with an alcohol base (e.g., cough syrup).
- A nurse who philosophically believes that humankind should not unleash the power of nuclear energy refuses to care for cancer patients undergoing irradiation.
- A Roman Catholic nurse working in the operating room refuses to scrub for abortions, tubal ligations, vasectomies, and similar procedures because of religious prohibitions.
- A Jehovah's Witness nurse refuses to hang blood or counsel patients concerning blood or blood products.
- A Seventh-Day Adventist nurse who cites biblical reasons for following a vegetarian diet is unwilling to conduct patient education involving diets that contain meat.
- Muslim and Jewish staff members express concern that the hospital cafeteria fails to

serve foods that meet their religious dietary requirements.

These philosophical, moral, and religious issues reflect the diversity that characterizes staff members in the health care workplace. The challenge is to balance the health care needs and rights of patients with the moral and religious beliefs of health care providers. In some instances, it may be impossible to provide the services demanded by the organization's mission statement if all nurses refuse to engage in a particular activity. There may be legal implications for refusing to provide patients with certain services, for example, those related to reproductive health. In the clinical world, the options available to accommodate the diverse moral and religious beliefs of staff members frequently depend on the size of the organization, the moral and religious proclivities of workers, the attitudes and beliefs of managers, the organizational climate, fiscal constraints, and other factors. The challenge faced by nurse managers is to balance the conflicting moral and religious beliefs of diverse groups with the achievement of organizational goals. This must be accomplished in a manner that is respectful of the moral and religious beliefs of staff members (Newton, Pillay, & Higginbottom, 2012).

National Origin

Another form of diversity in the workplace is the national origin of nurses and the country in which nurses are educated. The current number of internationally educated RNs licensed in the United States is approximately 6,000 (HRSA, 2013). Internationally educated RNs licensed in the United States are most frequently from the Philippines, Canada, India, South Korea, and Nigeria (U.S. Department of Health and Human Services, Health Resources and Services Administration, 2013). The proportion of foreign-educated nurses working in Canada, 8.4%, is higher than in the United States (Canadian Institute for Health Information, 2014).

Nurses entering the United States or Canada from a similar culture and with English as the

primary language, for example, nurses from Australia or the United Kingdom, are likely to experience less difficulty with cultural adjustment than do nurses from the Near and Middle East, Asia, or Africa, where language, religion, dress, and many other components of culture may be markedly different. Although social scientists speculate that people from similar cultures are more readily able to relate to one another, health care providers must be able to transcend cultural differences and to recognize that there are differences in role expectations.

Discrepancies in role expectations tend to create intrapersonal and interpersonal conflict. For example, nurses in Taiwan, the Philippines, and many African nations expect the families of patients to participate significantly in caregiving during hospitalization. Family members, who may be encouraged to remain with the patient around the clock, provide all aspects of personal hygiene, often sleeping on the floor or in chairs. This may result in conflict, as families are less involved in the care of hospitalized patients in the United States.

In many countries, nurses have considerably expanded roles, and their scope of practice is correspondingly broader. For example, in Nigeria, it is clearly stated by the Board of Nursing and Midwifery that nurses diagnose and treat common illnesses such as malaria, typhoid, cholera, tetanus, and similar maladies. To graduate from a nursing program in the Philippines, nursing students must deliver a minimum of 25 babies unassisted and also assist at major and minor surgical procedures. In Haiti, nurses routinely perform episiotomies and repair lacerations. In the mastery of technical skills, recent graduates of many international nursing programs have logged a considerable number of hours of clinical experience, often as apprentices mentored by experienced nurses who serve as their clinical faculty.

Some British and Irish nurses perceive US and Canadian nurses as "junior physicians," second-guessing and anticipating therapy. Some nurses perceive that counterparts in Great Britain and Ireland have greater freedom in ordering nursing modalities without a physician's orders. For example, decubitus ulcer care, ambulation, dressings, and nutritional therapy are all nurse-initiated activities based on nursing assessment. British and Irish nurses also expect that the nursing role includes activities that are defined by US and Canadian nurses as nonnursing activities. For example, in many British hospitals, nurses are expected to clean patient rooms after discharge and prepare them for the next admission.

In many nations, nurse midwives are primarily responsible for obstetric care. In some ways, the United States and Canada are anomalous with so much emphasis on the medically dominated specialty of obstetric medicine. Viewing childbirth as a medical problem, rather than a normal physiologic process, reveals an underlying philosophic difference between the US and Canadian health care delivery systems and those in other nations. Some nurses who have been educated abroad are both nurses and midwives; thus, the transition to the medically dominated US and Canadian models may leave them feeling underutilized and confused about the roles of the obstetrician and the maternal–child nurse or nurse midwife.

Because of the shortage of qualified health care providers in many less developed countries, there usually are fewer interdisciplinary differences about the nature and scope of practice for various health care disciplines. There are also various categories of licensed and unlicensed health care providers who contribute to the overall health and well-being of people in countries around the world. For example, there are feldshers in the former Soviet Union, barefoot doctors in China, and herbalists in nearly every nation.

Cultural Self-Assessment of Health Care Organizations, Institutions, and Agencies

Organizational   cultural   self-assessment should be part of the strategic planning process for medical centers, hospitals, public and

community health organizations, home health care agencies, psychiatric/mental health institutions, and related facilities. Organizational cultural self-assessment may focus on the entire health care organization, institution, or agency or a particular unit or division of the organization. A variety of tools may be used to assess organizational culture.

Box 12-3 provides an instrument to use when assessing an entire organization or a particular

---

Box 12-3 Cultural Assessment of an Organization, Institution, or Agency

Demographics/Descriptive Data

- What types of cultural diversity are represented by clients, families, visitors, and others significant to the clients? Indicate approximate numbers and percentages according to the conventional system used for reporting census data.
- What types of cultural diversity are represented? What types of diversity are present among patients, physicians, nurses, x-ray technicians, and other staff? Indicate approximate numbers and percentages by department and discipline.
- How is the organization, institution, or agency structured? Who is in charge? How do the administrators support cultural diversity and interventions to foster multiculturalism?
- How many key leaders/decision makers within the organization, institution, or agency come from culturally diverse backgrounds?
- What languages are spoken by patients, family members or significant others, and staff?

Assessment of Strengths

- What are the cultural strengths or positive characteristics and qualities?
- What institutional resources (fiscal, human) are available to support multiculturalism?
- What goals and needs related to cultural diversity already have been expressed?
- What successes in making services accessible and culturally appropriate have occurred to date? Highlight goals, programs, and activities that have been successful.
- What positive comments have been given by clients and significant others from culturally

diverse backgrounds about their experiences with the organization, institution, or agency?

Assessment of Community Resources

- What efforts are made to use multicultural community-based resources (e.g., community organizations for ethnic or religious groups, anthropology and foreign languages faculty and students from area colleges and universities, and similar resources)?
- To what extent are leaders from racial, ethnic, and religious communities involved with the institution (e.g., invited to serve on boards and advisory committees)?
- To what extent is there political and economic support for multicultural programs and projects?

Assessment of Weakness/Areas for Continued Growth

- What are the organization's weaknesses, limitations, and areas for continued growth?
- What could be done to better promote multiculturalism?

Assessment from the Perspective of Clients and Families

- How do clients (and families/significant others) evaluate the multicultural aspects of the organization, institution, or agency? Do patient satisfaction data indicate that clients from various cultural backgrounds are satisfied or dissatisfied with care? How are the quality outcomes the same and different for individuals of various races and ethnicities?

(continued)

- How adequate is the system for translation and interpretation? What materials are available in the client's primary language (in written and other forms such as audiocassettes, videotapes, computer programs)? How is the literacy level of clients assessed?
- Are educational programs available in the languages spoken by clients?
- Are cultural and religious calendars used in determining scheduling for preadmission testing, procedures, educational programs, follow-up visits, or other appointments?
- Are cultural considerations given to the acceptability of certain medical and surgical procedures (e.g., amputations, blood transfusions, disposal of body parts, and handling various types of human tissue)?
- Are cultural considerations a factor in administering medicines? How familiar are nurses, physicians, and pharmacists with current research in ethnopharmacology?
- If a client dies, what cultural considerations are given during postmortem care? How are cultural needs associated with dying addressed with the family and others significant to the deceased? Does the roster of religious representatives available to nursing staff include traditional spiritual healers such as shamans and medicine men/women as well as rabbis, priests, elders, and others?

Assessment from an Institutional Perspective

- To what extent do the philosophy and mission statement support, foster, and promote multiculturalism and respect for cultural diversity? Is there congruence between philosophy/mission statement and reality? How is this evident?
- To what extent is there administrative support for multiculturalism? In what ways is support present or absent? Provide evidence to support this.
- Are data being gathered to provide documentation concerning multicultural issues? Are there missing data? Are data disseminated to appropriate decision makers and leaders within the institution? How are these data used?

- Are opportunities for continuing professional education and development in topics pertaining to multiculturalism provided for nurses and other staff?
- Are there racial, ethnic, religious, or other tensions evident within the institution? If so, objectively and nonjudgmentally assess their origins and nature in as much detail as possible.
- Are adequate resources being allocated for the purpose of promoting a harmonious multicultural health care environment? If not, indicate areas in which additional resources are needed.
- What multicultural library resources and audiovisual and computer software are available for use by nurses and other staff?
- What efforts are made to recruit and retain nurses and other staff from racially, ethnically, and religiously diverse backgrounds? What other types of diversity (e.g., sexual orientation) are fostered or discouraged?
- How would you describe the cultural climate of the institution? Are ethnic/racial/religious jokes prevalent? Are negative remarks or comments about certain cultural groups permitted? Who is doing the talking and who is listening to negative comments/jokes?
- Are human resources initiatives pertaining to advertising, hiring, promotion, and performance evaluations free from discrimination?
- Are cultural and religious considerations reflected in staff scheduling policies for nursing and other departments?
- Are policies and procedures appropriate from a multicultural perspective? What process is used for reviewing them for cultural appropriateness and relevance?

Assessment of Need and Readiness for Change

- Is there a need for change? If so, indicate who, what, when, where, why, and how.
- Who is in favor of change? Who is against it?
- What are the anticipated obstacles to change?
- What financial and human resources would be necessary to bring about the recommended changes?

unit or division. For example, staff in the operating room, specialty units, home health care division, ambulatory care area, and so forth may perceive a need to engage in an organizational self-assessment because of changing demographics in populations served or concerns with quality of care for diverse patients.

The Process of Cultural Self-Assessment by Organizations, Institutions, and Agencies

Although the manner in which the cultural self-assessment is carried out will vary for each institution, organization, or agency and for different units or divisions within it, the process remains fundamentally the same. After identifying key staff members to lead the institutional cultural self-assessment process, the leaders should communicate the purpose of the cultural self-assessment to those who will be participating in it. It is important to involve grassroots members of the staff and to solicit input from the patient population served through interviews, focus groups, written surveys, or other methods. The process of cultural self-assessment by organizations, institutions, and

agencies (Figure 12-7) involves collecting and analyzing demographic and descriptive data, assessing strengths and weaknesses or limitations, assessing the need and readiness for change, implementing change, evaluating the effectiveness of changes, and implementing any necessary revisions.

Demographic and Descriptive Data

As with any assessment, begin by gathering demographic and descriptive data. It is highly likely that some of these data have already been collected and stored centrally. If reports containing the necessary data are available, the group should review and discuss them as part of the cultural assessment process. Data such as types and numbers of diverse patients and staff members should be determined. There should be an assessment of the predominant languages spoken and of the effectiveness of the system being used for translation and interpretation. After the data have been gathered, a team of key leaders should convene to critically review and analyze them. Because this will be an active working group, membership should be limited to approximately 12 people. If the group is larger, consideration should be given to division into smaller subgroups.

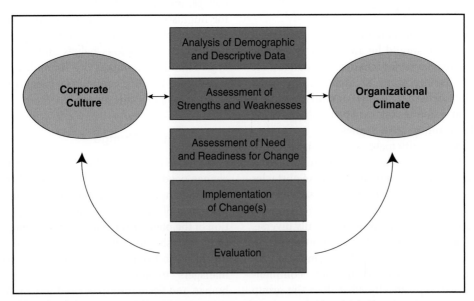

Figure 12-7. Cultural self-assessment of a health care organization, institution, or agency.

Strengths and Limitations

The purpose of the review is to assess the strengths, limitations, and areas for continued growth in terms of promoting a harmonious multicultural environment for patients and staff members of diverse backgrounds. It is important to identify strengths and limitations from both an emic (insider) and an etic (outsider) perspective. This incorporates the viewpoints of health care providers (insiders) and patients, those significant to them, and visitors (outsiders). For example, although the staff may believe the system is structured adequately to meet the needs of linguistically diverse persons, it would be important to compare that perception with the patients' point of view. From their perspective, examine the ways in which cultural aspects are part of the care provided. From the institutional perspective, critically examine the infrastructure for philosophic, fiscal, and human resources that reflect a commitment—or lack of one—to promoting harmony in the multicultural workplace. Throughout the process, comparative analyses are made between input from staff members and that from patients to identify strengths and limitations.

Need and Readiness for Change

Once the strengths and limitations have been identified, there should be an assessment of the need and readiness for change. If changes are needed, it is important to identify why, who, what, when, where, and how. Identify the fiscal and human resources that will be needed to bring about the recommended change(s).

Be sure to anticipate staff **resistance to change**. Determine who is likely to favor and oppose the proposed change, anticipate obstacles to it, and develop contingency plans. Different people will see different meanings in activities by organizations to become more culturally diverse. Depending on the nature of the recommendation and the corporate culture of the organization, an action plan should accompany the recommendation, that is, specifically what does the group believe ought to be done? Although most staff members will support the change, it is insufficient for nurse managers and supervisors to say, "A new law has been passed mandating diversity" or "Hospital policy requires diversity." Resistance can be expected to increase to the degree that staff members influenced by the changes have pressure on them to change, and it will decrease to the degree they are actively involved in planning diversity activities. Resistance can be expected if the changes are made on personal grounds rather than as requirements, sanctions, or policies. Finally, resistance can be expected if the organizational culture is ignored. There are informal as well as formal norms within every organization. An effective change will neither ignore old customs nor abruptly create new ones. As with most change, timing is important.

In developing an action plan for change, be sure to assess the community resources available to assist with goal achievement. For example, it may be possible to invite leaders from ethnic communities to provide staff in-service programs aimed at increasing understanding of the health care needs of persons from diverse backgrounds. A second example might be to involve foreign language faculty and students from area colleges and universities to assist with translation for linguistically diverse patients and clients. A final example might be to invite clergy to discuss health-related religious beliefs and practices. If organizational resources are limited, it may be possible to identify community-based resources that are available at low cost.

Implementing Change

Once those responsible for determining whether change needs to be made decide that change will occur, an implementation committee composed of key stakeholders is established. The implementation of the plan for the purpose of creating desired change(s) should involve key members of the organization from the grassroot level to midlevel managers to senior executives. The requisite human and fiscal resources need to be integral to the budgeting and strategic planning process.

Box 12-4 Promoting Harmony in the Multicultural Workplace

Facilitators

Identification of cultural values of the organization, institution, or agency
Mission statement and policies about diversity
Zero tolerance for discrimination
Effective cross-cultural communication
Skill with conflict resolution involving diversity
Commitment to multiculturalism at all levels of management

Barriers

Hatred
Prejudice
Bigotry
Racism
Discrimination
Negative attitudes or behaviors based on race, ethnicity, religion, gender, sexual orientation, national origin, class, handicap/disability

---

Evaluation

After implementation of the recommended changes, an evaluation of their effectiveness should be conducted, and revisions should be made as needed. In recognition of the rapid pace of change in contemporary health care, the process of institutional cultural self-assessment should be repeated at periodic intervals. Although significant fiscal and human resources are expended by organizations in diversity initiatives, there is a need to be more diligent in monitoring and evaluating outcomes. It may be useful to develop a grid that articulates goals, diversity initiatives, and outcome measures.

Promoting Harmony in the Multicultural Workplace

After conducting a cultural assessment of the health care organization, institution, or agency, the nurse will have data about the strengths and weaknesses; fiscal, human, and community resources; areas in which to pursue change; and readiness of the staff to engage in change.

As indicated in Box 12-4, there are **facilitators** and **barriers** to promoting harmony in the multicultural workplace. Facilitators include

identification of the cultural values of the organization, institution, or agency; clear articulation of the mission statement and policies about diversity; zero tolerance for discrimination; effective cross-cultural communication; skill with conflict resolution involving diversity; and commitment to multiculturalism at all levels of management. The barriers that must be overcome include hatred, prejudice, bigotry, racism, discrimination, and ethnoviolence. Negative behaviors aimed at employees, patients, their families, others significant to them, and other visitors, based on race, ethnicity, religion, gender, sexual orientation, national origin, class, or handicap/disability, should not be tolerated. All employees should understand that there will be zero tolerance for those who engage in negative behaviors, and management staff at all levels should be given the authority to impose sanctions when violations occur.

Summary

Given the demographic composition of the contemporary health care workforce, nurses will continue to find both challenges and opportunities as they practice nursing in multicultural

health care settings. Microcosms of society at large, health care organizations, institutions, and agencies consist of staff members from increasingly diverse backgrounds. It is important to remember that culture influences the manner in which people perceive, identify, define, and solve problems in the workplace.

Understanding cultural differences in the workplace and developing skill in conflict resolution will continue to be needed in transcultural nursing administration in the new millennium. The successful transcultural nurse administrator will behave respectfully toward others from diverse backgrounds and will implement policies that promote cultural understanding, knowledge, and skill in the workplace. Nurses in leadership and management positions will apply the principles of transcultural nursing to the multicultural workplace, just as they have done in the past to provide culturally competent and congruent care for patients. Lastly, nursing leaders and managers in health care organizations, institutions, and agencies will use the process of cultural self-assessment identified to collect and analyze demographic and descriptive data, assess strengths and weaknesses or limitations, assess the need and readiness for change, implement change, evaluate the effectiveness of change(s), and implement any necessary revisions.

REVIEW QUESTIONS

1. Define diversity in your own words.
2. What are the key advantages or benefits of a diverse health care workforce?
3. What are some barriers to diversity in the nursing profession?
4. What strategies might be used to increase diversity in a) the nursing profession? and b) a health care organization?
5. Compare and contrast corporate culture and organizational climate.
6. Compare and contrast diversity management and organizational inclusion.

7. Discuss cultural perspectives on the meaning and value of work.
8. What are the key components of an organizational cultural self-assessment?

CRITICAL THINKING ACTIVITIES

1. Reflect on your personal experience(s) with hatred, prejudice, bigotry, racism, discrimination, and/or ethnoviolence. Were you the victim or the perpetrator? How did you feel during the incident(s)? Discuss your reflections with someone from a different cultural background than your own.

2. From a cultural perspective, critically examine the dress code or policy statement about clothing and accessories that are permitted for staff at a health care organization, agency, or institution. How effectively does the code or policy address the widespread diversity that characterizes the health care workforce? Identify the strengths and limitations of the dress code or policy statement. What modifications or changes would you recommend to accommodate the attire worn by staff from diverse cultures?

3. As the nurse manager at a community hospital with a mission statement that embraces diversity and an inclusive workplace, you encounter the following situation:

Rachel Goldberg, the laboratory technician assigned to your floor, asks to speak with you concerning an urgent matter. Rachel reports that while drawing blood on Mrs. Silverstein, a patient who had a cholecystectomy earlier in the day, the patient comments that her nurse refuses to give her any pain medication. When Rachel goes to the Nurses' Station to find Mrs. Silverstein's nurse, she overhears Margarett Schwartz, a Lutheran nurse of German heritage, comment to a fellow nurse, "Mrs. Silverstein is just a Jewish princess who complains about pain all the time. I'm going to make her wait another half-hour before I

give her any medication." Rachel exchanges angry words with Margarett, then approaches you demanding to know what you intend to do about the "blatant anti-Semitism" on the unit.

How would you handle this situation?

4. You are the Operating Room Supervisor. A slightly built African American male nurse, Robert, asks to meet with you about a neurosurgeon who had recently emigrated from Russia. Robert complains, "Dr. Ivanovich keeps asking me why I became a nurse. He asks very personal questions about my sexual orientation and wants to know if I'm 'queer.' I consider this a hostile work environment and refuse to scrub for his surgical cases any more." How would you handle this situation?

5. You are the supervisor of the emergency department at a large academic health science center. After receiving a report on a critically ill victim of a motor vehicle accident, Dr. Juan Valdez-Rodriguez, the physician on call, asks for the patient's name. You hear the nurse, who admitted the patient, reply, "I don't know. Martinez,

Hernandez, something like that. You'll recognize him when you see him—just another drunk Mexican who ran his pickup truck into a tree." Upon entering the examination room, the physician immediately recognizes the victim as his cousin. What do you say to Dr. Valdez-Rodriguez? What do you say to the nurse?

6. As a staff nurse on a medical–surgical unit, you enter into a conversation with a Chinese American food service worker. Ms. Chin remarks that for the past 4 days, your nurse manager has asked her to be the interpreter for an elderly Chinese man for whom she delivers food. "I don't want to offend the nurse manager who asked me to interpret, but it is not right for a younger woman to speak for an older man about his bowel movements. It is not our custom. Besides, my supervisor scolded me for being so slow to do my work. She thinks I have become lazy. Would you talk to the nurse manager for me?" What would you say to Ms. Chin? Would you become part of the triangle of communication and speak with the nurse manager on behalf of Ms. Chin? Why or why not?

REFERENCES

American Academy of Nursing. (2012). Diversity and inclusivity statement. Retrieved from http://www.aannet.org/assets/docs/diversity%20and%20inclusivity%20statement_2.13.2012.pdf

American Association of Colleges of Nursing. (2014a). Enhancing diversity in the workforce. Retrieved from http://www.aacn.nche.edu/media-relations/fact-sheets/enhancing-diversity

American Association of Colleges of Nursing. (2014b). Policy brief. The changing landscape: Nursing student diversity on the rise. Retrieved from http://www.aacn.nche.edu/government-affairs/Student-Diversity-FS.pdf

American Association of Colleges of Nursing. (2014c). The changing landscape: Nursing student diversity on the rise. Retrieved from http://www.aacn.nche.edu/government-affairs/Student-Diversity-FS.pdf

American Association of Colleges of Nursing. (2015). Effective strategies for increasing diversity in nursing programs. Retrieved from http://www.aacn.nche.edu/aacn-publications/issue-bulletin/effective-strategies

American Community Survey. (2013). Men in nursing occupations. American Community Survey Highlight Report 2013. Retrieved from http://www.census.gov/people/io/files/Men_in_Nursing_Occupations.pdf

American Nurses Credentialing Center. (2015). ANCC certification center. Retrieved from http://www.nursecredentialing.org/default.aspx

Brown, I. C. (1973). *Understanding race relations*. Englewood Cliffs, NJ: Prentice-Hall.

Budden, S., Zhong, E. H., Moulton, P., & Cimiotti, J. P. (2013). The National Council of State Boards of Nursing and the Forum of State Nursing Workforce Centers 2013 National Workforce Centers 2013 survey of registered nurses. *Journal of Nursing Regulation, 4*(2), S1–S72.

Bureau of Labor Statistics, U.S. Department of Labor. (2014). Occupational Outlook Handbook, 2014-15 Edition, Registered Nurses, on the Internet at http://www.bls.gov/ooh/healthcare/registered-nurses.htm

Canadian Institute for Health Information. (2014). Canada's nursing workforce continues to grow: Regulated Nurses,

2013. Retrieved from http://www.cihi.ca/CIHI-ext-portal/internet/EN/Home/home/cihi000001

Davis, P. D. (1995). Enhancing multicultural harmony. *Nursing Management, 26*(7), 32D–32E.

Ellis, B. (2014). Class of 2013 grads average $35,200 in total debt. CNN Money. Retrieved from http://money.cnn.com/2013/05/17/pf/college/student-debt/index.html

Este, D., Bernard, W. T., James, C. E., Benjamin, A., Lloyd, B., & Turner, T. (2013). African Canadians: Employment and racism in the workplace. *Seeing ourselves: Exploring race, ethnicity and culture.* Ottawa, ON: Association for Canadian Studies.

Ewoh, A. I. E. (2013). Managing and valuing diversity: Challenges to public managers in the 21st century. *Public Personnel Management, 42*(2), 107–122.

Fineberg, H. V., & Lavizzio, R. (2013). A look back at the landmark Institute of Medicine report. Institute of Medicine, National Academy of Sciences. Retrieved from http://www.iom.edu/~/media/Files/Perspectives-Files/2013/Commentaries/EO-Nursing.pdf

Flores, K., & Combs, G. (2013). Minority representation in healthcare: Increasing the number of professionals through focused recruitment. *Hospital Topics, 91*(2), 25–36.

Gates, M. G., & Mark, B. A. (2012). Demographic diversity, value congruence, and workplace outcomes in acute care. *Research in Nursing & Health, 35,* 265–276.

Georges, C. (2012). Project to expand diversity in the nursing workforce. *Nursing Management, 19*(2), 22–26.

Government of Canada. (2012). Immigration and ethnocultural diversity in Canada. Retrieved from http://www12.statcan.gc.ca/nhs-enm/2011/as-sa/99-010-x/99-010-x2011001-eng.cfm#a2

Grainger, K. (2006). Equal access to training for black and minority ethnic nurses. *Nursing Standard, 20*(42), 41–49.

Guillaume, Y. R. F., Dawson, J. F., Woods, S. A., Sacramento, C. A., & West, M. A. (2013). Getting diversity to work at work: What we know and what we still don't know. *Journal of Occupational and Organizational Psychology, 86*(2), 123–141.

Harris, G. L. A., Lewis, E. L., & Calloway, M. (2012). A call to action: Increasing health providers in underrepresented populations through the military. *Journal of Health and Human Services Administration, 35*(3), 356–412.

Health Resources and Services Administration. (2014). The future of the nursing workforce: National- and state-level projections, 2012-2025. U.S. Department of Health and Human Services, Health Resources and Services Administration, Bureau of Health Workforce, National Center for Health Workforce Analysis. Retrieved from http://bhpr.hrsa.gov/healthworkforce/supplydemand/nursing/workforceprojections/nursingprojections.pdf

Hedlund, N., Esparza, A., Calhoun, E., & Yates, J. (2012). Importance of staff diversity to address disparity. *Physician Executive Journal, 9,* 6–12.

Henderson, G. (1994). *Cultural diversity in the workplace.* Westport, CT: Praeger.

Hendricks, J. M., & Cope, V. C. (2013). Generational diversity: What nurse managers need to know. *Journal of Advanced Nursing, 69*(3), 717–725.

Immigration and Ethnocultural Diversity in Canada. (2014). Immigration. Retrieved from http://www12.statcan.gc.ca/nhs-enm/2011/as-sa/99-010-x/99-010-x2011001-eng.cfm#a2

Jackson, C. S., & Gracia, J. N. (2014). Addressing health and health-care disparities: The role of a diverse workforce and the social determinants of health. *Public Health Reports, 129*(Suppl. 2), 57–61.

Joint Commission. (2010). *Advancing effective communication, cultural competence, and patient- and family-centered care: A roadmap for hospitals.* Oakbrook Terrace, IL: The Joint Commission. Retrieved from http://www.jointcommission.org/assets/1/6/ARoadmapforHospitalsfinalversion727.pdf

Jung, C. A. (1968). In G. Adler (Ed.). *The collected works of Carl Jung* (Vol. 10). Princeton, NJ: University Press.

Kirch, D. G., & Nivet, M. (2013). Increasing diversity and inclusion in medical school to improve the health of all. *Journal of Healthcare Management, 58*(5), 311–313.

Krawiec, K. D., Conley, J. M., & Broome, L. L. (2014). A difficult corporate conversation: Corporate directors on race and gender. *Pace International Law Review Symposium, 26*(1), 13–22.

Lauring, J., & Selmer, J. (2013). International language management and diversity climate in multicultural organizations. *International Business Review, 21,* 156–166.

LaVeist, T. A., & Pierre, G. (2014). Integrating the 3-Ds-social determinants, health disparities, and health-care workforce diversity. *Public Health Reports, 129*(Suppl. 2), 9–14.

Lowe, F. (2013). Keeping leadership white: Invisible blocks to black leadership and its denial in white organizations. *Journal of Social Work Practice, 27*(2), 149–162.

Mittman, I. S., & Sullivan, L. W. (2012). Forming state collaborations to diversify the nation's health workforce: The experience of the Sullivan alliance to transform the health professions. *Journal of Best Practices in Health Professions Diversity: Education, Research, and Policy, 5*(1), 757–773.

Mixer, S. M., Lasater, K. M., Jenkins, K. M., & Burk, R. C. (2013). Preparing a culturally competent nursing workforce. *Online Journal of Cultural Competence in Nursing and Healthcare, 3*(4), 1–14. doi: 10.9730/ojccnh,org/v3n4a1

Modern Language Association. (March 2006). Number and percentage of speakers per language in the entire U. S. http://www.mla.org/map_single. Accessed March 6, 2010.

National Institute on Minority Health and Health Disparities. (2014). New study finds holistic admissions benefit health professions schools. Retrieved from http://nimhd.nih.gov/news/holisticStudy.html

New York Employment Law. (2014). Better late than never: Stop long-simmering racial hostility as soon as you find it. *New York Employment Law, 9*(9), 2–3.

Newton, S., Pillay, J., Higginbottom, G. (2012). The migration experiences of internationally educated nurses: A global perspective. *Journal of Nursing Management, 20,* 534–550.

Nunez-Smith, M. (2009). Health care workplace discrimination and physician turnover. *Journal of the National Medical Association, 101,* 1274–1282.

Page, L. (2015). Baby boomers and beyond: The evolution of Nursing. *Minority Nurse, Winter 2015, 22–27.*

Health Resources and Services Administration. (2013). The U.S. nursing workforce: Trends in supply and demand. Retrieved from http://bhpr.hrsa.gov/healthworkforce/supplydemand/nursing/nursingworkforce/nursingworkforcefullreport.pdf

Sabharwal, M. (2014). Is diversity management sufficient? Organizational inclusion to further performance. *Public Personnel Management, 43*(2). 197–217.

Samovar, L. A., Porter, R. E., & McDaniel, E. R. (2006). *Intercultural communication: A reader.* Belmont, CA: Thomson/Wadsworth.

Seago, J. A., & Spetz, J. (2008). Minority nurses' experiences on the job. *Journal of Cultural Diversity, 15,* 16–23.

Singh, B., & Winkel, D. E. (2012). Racial differences in helping behaviors: The role of respect, safety, and identification. *Journal of Business Ethics, 106,* 467–477.

Singh, B., Winkel, D. E., & Selvarajan, T. T. (2013). Managing diversity at work: Does psychological safety hold the key to racial differences in employee performance? *Journal of Occupational and Organizational Psychology, 86,* 242.

Statistics Canada. Statistics Canada. (2014).

Sullivan, L. W. (2004). Missing persons: Minorities in the health professions: A report of the Sullivan commission on diversity in the healthcare workforce. Retrieved from http://depts.washington.edu/ccph/pdf_files/Sullivan_Report_ES.pdf

Thomas, R. R. (1990). From affirmative action to affirming diversity. *Harvard Business Review, 68,* 107–117.

U.S. Census Bureau. (2012). U.S. Census Bureau projections show a slower growing, older, more diverse nation a half-century from now. Retrieved from http://www.census.gov/newsroom/releases/archives/population/cb12-243.html

U.S. Census Bureau. (January 2014). Foreign-born population in the US. Retrieved from http://www.census.gov/library/infographics/foreign_born.html

U.S. Department of Health and Human Services. (2014). Key features of the Affordable Care Act. Retrieved from http://www.hhs.gov/healthcare/facts/timeline/index.html

U.S. Department of Labor. (n.d.). Equal employment opportunity. Retrieved from http://www.dol.gov/dol/topic/discrimination/

Urban Universities for Health. (2014). Holistic admissions in the health professions: Findings from a national survey. National Institute on Minority Health and Health Disparities. Retrieved from http://urbanuniversitiesforhealth.org/media/documents/Holistic_Admissions_in_the_Health_Professions.pdf

van Djik, H., & van Egen, M. L. (2013). A status perspective on the consequences of work group diversity. *Journal of Occupational and Organizational Psychology, 86*(2), 223–241.

Williams, S. D., Hansen, K., Smithey, M., Burnley, J., Koplitz, M., Koyama, K., … Bakos, A. (2014). Using social determinants of health to link health workforce diversity, care quality and access, and health disparities to achieve health equity in nursing. *Public Health Reports, 129* (Suppl. 2), 32–36.

Part Four

Contemporary Challenges in Transcultural Nursing

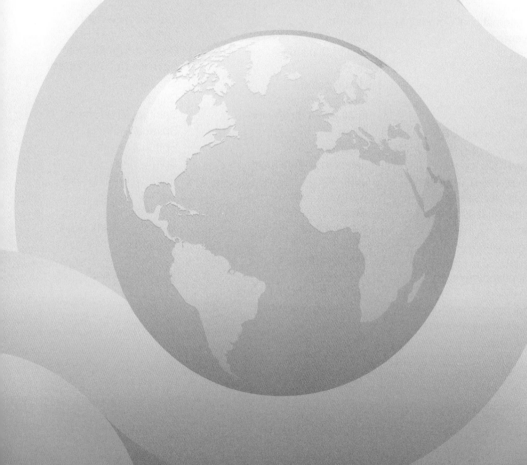

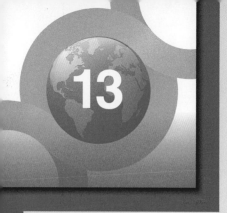

13

Religion, Culture, and Nursing

● Patricia A. Hanson and Margaret M. Andrews

Key Terms

Allah
Amish
Anointing of the Sick
Bad death
Baha'i International Community
Bereavement
Brahman
Brit milah
Buddha
Buddhism
Caste system
Catholic Charities USA
Catholic
Christian Science
Church of Jesus Christ of
    Latter-Day Saints
Consequential dimension
Curandero
Ethnoreligion
Eucharist
Experiential dimension
Faith healing
Fasting
Five core characteristics of
    the Amish

Four Noble Truths
Friendscraft
Funeral
Garment
Good death
Grief
Hadith
Halal
Health Ministries
Hindu
Home going
Ideologic dimension
Intellectual dimension
Islam
Jehovah
Jehovah's Witnesses
Judaism
Karma
Kosher
Mennonites
Mohel
Moslem/Muslim
Mourning
Native American Church
    (Peyote Religion)
Nirvana
Noble Eightfold Way

Ordinances
Pillars of Faith
Principle of totality
Protestantism
Qur'an (Koran)
Reincarnation
The Relief Society
Religion
Ritualistic dimension
Seventh-Day Adventists
Shema
Shiva
Spiritual assessment
Spiritual distress
Spiritual health
Spirituality
Spiritual nursing care
Talmud
Torah
Unitarian Universalist
Vedas
Wake
Word of Wisdom

Learning Objectives

1. Explore the meaning of spirituality and religion in the lives of clients across the lifespan.
2. Identify the components of a spiritual needs assessment for clients from diverse cultural backgrounds.
3. Examine the ways in which spiritual and religious beliefs can be incorporated into the nursing care of clients from diverse cultures.
4. Discuss cultural considerations in the nursing care of dying for bereaved clients and families.
5. Describe the health-related beliefs and practices of selected religious groups in North America.

As an integral component of culture, religious and spiritual beliefs may influence a client's explanation of the cause(s) of illness, perception of its severity, decisions about healing intervention(s), and choice of healer(s). In times of crisis, such as serious illness and impending death, religion and spirituality are often a source of consolation for the client and family and may influence the course of action believed to be appropriate by the nurse involved in the person's care and the care of their family.

The first half of this chapter discusses dimensions of religion, religion and spiritual nursing care, religious trends in North America, and contributions of religious groups to the health care delivery system. The second half highlights the health-related beliefs and practices of selected religions, which are presented in alphabetical order.

Dimensions of Religion

Religion is complex and multifaceted in both form and function. Religious faith and the institutions derived from that faith become a central focus in meeting the human needs of those who believe. The majority of faith traditions address the issues of illness and wellness, disease

and healing, and caring and curing (Leonard & Carlson, 2010; Touhy & Jett, 2011).

Religious Factors Influencing Human Behavior

First, it is necessary to identify specific religious factors that may influence human behavior. No single religious factor operates in isolation, but rather exists in combination with other religious factors and the person's ethnic, racial, and cultural background. When religion and ethnicity combine to influence a person, the term **ethnoreligion** is sometimes used. Examples of ethnoreligious groups include the Amish; Russian Jews; Lebanese Muslims; Italian, Irish, and Polish Catholics; Tibetan Buddhists; American Samoan Mormons; and so forth.

In their classic work, Faulkner and DeJong (1966) proposed five major dimensions of religion: experiential, ritualistic, ideologic, intellectual, and consequential. The **experiential dimension** recognizes that every religious person will experience religious emotion and/or feeling about their purpose in life and their connection with a higher power. The **ritualistic dimension** refers to religious practices, such as prayer, attending worship services, participating in sacraments, and reading religious literature. The **ideologic dimension**

consists of the shared beliefs that members of a religion must adhere to in order to be considered members. The **intellectual dimension**, which is closely related to the ideologic dimension, consists of the cognitive understanding of the basic tenets or beliefs of the religion and its sacred writing or scriptures. Finally, the **consequential dimension** consists of how closely members adhere to the prescribed standards of conduct and/or attitudes as a consequence of belonging to a religion, such as political beliefs, attitudes about sex, and observing holy days.

Religious Dimensions in Relation to Health and Illness

Each religious dimension has a different significance when related to matters of health and illness. Different religious cultures may emphasize one of the five dimensions to the relative exclusion of the others. Similarly, individuals may develop their own priorities related to the dimensions of religion. This affects the nurse providing care to clients with different religious beliefs in several ways.

First, it is the nurse's role to determine from the client, or from significant others, the dimension or combinations of dimensions that are important so that the client and nurse can have mutual goals and priorities. Second, it is important to determine what a given member of a specific religious affiliation believes to be important by asking the client or, if the client is unable to communicate this information personally, a close family member. Third, the nurse's information must be accurate. Making assumptions about clients' religious belief systems on the basis of their cultural, racial, ethnic, or even religious affiliation is imprudent and may lead to erroneous inferences. Our Lady of Lourdes is a Catholic shrine, yet people from many different Christian and non-Christian faiths visit Lourdes each year seeking peace and healing from illnesses and injuries (Figure 13-1).

The following example illustrates the importance of verifying assumptions with the client: Observing that a patient was wearing a Star of

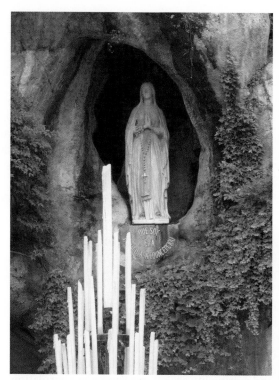

Figure 13-1. Our Lady of Lourdes statue in Lourdes, France, commemorates the site of a Marian apparition in 1858. Four to six million people visit the shrine each year, seeking peace and healing from physical and mental afflictions.

David on a chain around his neck and had been accompanied by a rabbi upon admission, a nurse inquired whether he would like to order a kosher diet. The patient replied, "Oh, no. I'm a Christian. My father is a rabbi, and I know it would upset him to find out that I have converted. Even though I'm 40 years old, I hide it from him. This has been going on for 15 years now." The key point in this anecdote is that the nurse validated an assumption with the patient before acting. Furthermore, not all Jewish persons follow a kosher diet nor wear a Star of David.

Fourth, even when individuals identify with a particular religion, they may accept the "official" beliefs and practices in varying degrees. It is not the nurse's role to judge the religious virtues of clients, but rather to understand those aspects

related to religion that are important to the client and family members. When religious beliefs are translated into practice, they may be manipulated by individuals in certain situations to serve particular ends; that is, traditional beliefs and practices are altered. Thus, it is possible for a Jewish person to eat pork or for a Catholic to take contraceptives to prevent pregnancy. Homogeneity among members of any religion cannot be assumed. The nurse should be open to variations in religious beliefs and practices and allow for the possibility of change in an individual's views. Individual choices frequently arise from new situations, changing values and mores, and exposure to new ideas and beliefs. Few people live in total social isolation, surrounded by only those with similar religious backgrounds.

Fifth, ideal norms of conduct and actual behavior are not necessarily the same. The nurse is frequently faced with the challenge of understanding and helping clients cope with internal conflict, which can occur when the patient faces differences between their own behaviors and the norms of their religion. Sometimes, conflicting norms are manifested by guilt or by efforts to minimize or rationalize inconsistencies, which may impact their health and desires regarding health care.

Sometimes, norms are vaguely formulated and filled with discrepancies that allow for a variety of interpretations. In religions having a lay organization and structure, moral decision making may be left to the individual without the assistance of members of a church hierarchy. In religions having a clerical hierarchy, moral positions may be more clearly formulated and articulated for members. Individuals retain their right to choose, regardless of official church-related guidelines, suggestions, or laws; however, the individual who chooses to violate the norms may experience the consequences of that violation, including social ostracism, public removal from membership rolls, or other forms of censure. Social ostracism is especially problematic for those clients experiencing mental illness (Fayard, Harding, Murdoch, & Brunt, 2007; Yurkovick & Lattergrass, 2008).

Religion and Spiritual Nursing Care

For many years, nursing has emphasized a holistic approach to care in which the needs of the total person are recognized. Most nursing textbooks emphasize the physical and psychosocial needs of clients rather than ways to address spiritual needs (Fayard et al., 2007; Touhy & Jett, 2011; Yurkovick & Lattergrass, 2008). Recently, more has been written about guidelines for providing spiritual care to clients from diverse cultural backgrounds (Andrews, 2013; Cates, 2014; Friedman, 2013; Jeffers, Nelson, Barnet, & Brannigan, 2013; Sorajjakool, Carr, & Nam, 2010; Tuell, 2011). Because nurses endeavor to provide holistic health care, addressing spiritual needs becomes essential.

Religious concerns evolve from and respond to the mysteries of life and death, good and evil, and pain and suffering. Although the religions of the world offer various interpretations of these phenomena, most people seek a personal understanding and interpretation at some time in their lives. Ultimately, this personal search becomes a pursuit to discover a Supreme Being, God, gods, or some unifying truth that will give meaning, purpose, and integrity to existence (Ebersole et al., 2008; Leonard & Carlson, 2010; Touhy & Jett, 2011; Yurkovick & Lattergrass, 2008).

An important component in discussing spiritual care for culturally diverse patients is the distinction between religion and spirituality. *Religion* is an organized system of beliefs about the cause, nature, and purpose of the universe, often including the belief in or worship of a Supreme Being (Leonard & Carlson, 2010). According to Pattison (2013), religion can be defined in many different ways depending upon the individual. For adherents to a particular religion, it is a "system for responding to the reality of the transcendent in their lives" (p. 198). Specific religious activities are dependent on ethnoreligious beliefs and can include praying (Figure 13-2), reading scriptures, and participating in individual and/or communal worship (Leonard & Carlson, 2010).

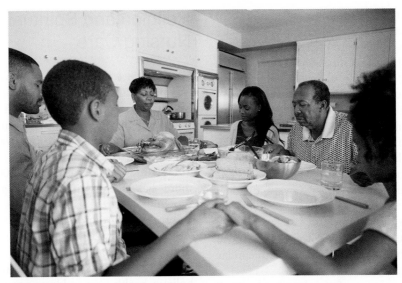

Figure 13-2. Prayer before meals is prevalent in many families, religions, and cultures around the world (Monkey Business Images/Shutterstock.com).

Spirituality, on the other hand, is a person's personal effort to find meaning and purpose in his or her life. It is more focused on individual growth, more subjective, more emotionally based, and rising from personal experience (Jeffers et al., 2013). According to Leonard and Carlson (2010), spirituality can include "embracing, celebrating and voicing all the connections with the ultimate/mystery/divine, within me and beyond me, in experiences that give meaning, purpose, direction, and values for my daily journey" (Leonard & Carlson, 2010).

While religion and spirituality have similarities and overlapping concepts, they are separate and distinct from one another (Pattison, 2013). In general, religion addresses questions related to what is true and right and helps individuals determine where they belong in the scheme of their life's journey. Spirituality emphasizes the pursuit of meaning, purpose, direction, and values.

Spiritual Nursing Care

In 2001, The Joint Commission (TJC) included an accreditation standard that required a brief spiritual assessment to be conducted with all patients in health care settings. This standard was revised in November 2008. It is nonprescriptive, but states that each organization will define what **spiritual assessment** means for them and how it will be evaluated. Suggestions include such items as "who or what provides the patient/client with strength and hope, how does the patient express their spirituality, what kind of religious/spiritual support does the patient desire, etc." (Standard FAQ details, 2008). Given that pastoral services may be limited, the responsibility of obtaining this brief spiritual assessment may fall to the nurse. This assessment is the beginning of providing spiritual nursing care.

The goal of spiritual nursing care is to assist clients in integrating their own religious beliefs about a Supreme Being or a unifying truth into the ultimate reality that gives meaning to their lives. This is especially meaningful when people face a serious health challenges or crisis that precipitated the need for nursing care in the first place. Spiritual nursing care promotes clients' physical and emotional health as well as their **spiritual health**. When providing care, the nurse must remember that the goal of spiritual intervention is not, and should not be, to impose his or

her own religious beliefs and convictions on the client (Taylor, 2012).

Although spiritual needs are recognized by many nurses, spiritual care is often neglected. There are many reasons why nurses fail to provide spiritual care, including the following:

1. They view religious and spiritual needs as a private matter concerning only an individual and his or her Creator.
2. They are uncomfortable about their own religious beliefs or deny having spiritual needs.
3. They lack knowledge about spirituality and the religious beliefs of others.
4. They mistake spiritual needs for psychosocial needs.
5. They view meeting the spiritual needs of clients as a family or pastoral responsibility, not a nursing responsibility.

Spiritual intervention is as appropriate as any other form of nursing intervention and recognizes that the balance of physical, psychosocial, and spiritual aspects of life is essential to overall good health. Nursing is an intimate profession, and nurses routinely inquire without hesitation about very personal matters such as hygiene and sexual habits. The spiritual realm also requires a personal, intimate type of nursing intervention (Daly & Fahey-McCarthy, 2014; Ramezani, Ahmadi, Mohammed, & Kazemnejad, 2014).

In North America, efforts to integrate spiritual care and nursing have been under way since the early 1970s. In 1971, at the White House Conference on Aging, the spiritual dimension of care was defined as those aspects of individuals pertaining to their inner resources, especially their ultimate concern, the basic value around which all other values are focused, the central philosophy of life that guides their conduct, and the supernatural and nonmaterial dimensions of human nature. The spiritual dimension encompasses the person's need to find satisfactory answers to questions about the meaning of life, illness, or death (Jett & Touhy, 2010; Raffay, 2014; Touhy & Jett, 2011).

In 1978, the Third National Conference on the Classification of Nursing Diagnoses recognized the importance of spirituality by including "spiritual concerns," "spiritual distress," and "spiritual despair" in the list of approved diagnoses. Because of practical difficulties, these three categories were combined at the 1980 National Conference into one category, **spiritual distress**, which is defined as disruption in the life principle that pervades a person's entire being and that integrates and transcends the person's biologic and psychosocial nature. Pattison (2013) acknowledges the multidimensional nature of spiritual concerns and defines them as the human need to deal with sociocultural deprivations, anxieties and fears, death and dying, personality integration, self-image, personal dignity, social alienation, and philosophy of life.

Assessment of Ethnoreligious and Spiritual Issues

As discussed in Chapters 3 and 11, cultural assessment includes assessment of religious and spiritual issues as they relate to the health care status of clients. In the integration of health care and religious/spiritual beliefs, the focus of nursing intervention is to help the client maintain his or her own beliefs in the face of a serious health challenge or crisis and to use those beliefs to strengthen the client's coping patterns. Box 13-1 includes guidelines for assessing spiritual needs in clients from diverse cultural backgrounds.

Spiritual Nursing Care for Ill Children and Their Families

Any hospitalization or serious illness can be viewed as stressful and, therefore, has the potential to develop into a crisis. Religion may play an especially significant role when a child is seriously ill and in circumstances that include dying, death, or bereavement.

Illness during childhood may be an especially difficult clinical situation. Children have spiritual needs that vary according to their developmental

Box 13-1   Assessing Spiritual Needs in Clients from Various Ethnoreligious Backgrounds

What Do You Notice About the Client's Surroundings?

- Does the client have religious objects, such as the Qur'an (Koran) Bible, prayer book, devotional literature, religious medals, rosary or other type of beads, photographs of historic religious persons or contemporary religious leaders (e.g., Catholic Pope, Dalai Lama, or image of another religious figure), paintings of religious events or persons, religious sculptures, crucifixes, objects of religious significance at entrances to rooms (e.g., holy water founts, a mezuzah, or small parchment scroll inscribed with an excerpt from scripture), candles of religious significance (e.g., Paschal candle, menorah), shrine, or other items?
- Does the client wear clothing that has religious significance (e.g., head covering, undergarment, uniform)? Does the hairstyle connote affiliation with a certain ethnoreligious group, for example, earlocks worn by Hasidic Jewish men?
- Are get well greeting cards religious in nature or from a representative of the client's church, mosque, temple, synagogue, or other religious congregations?

How Does the Client Act?

- Does the client appear to pray at certain times of the day or before meals?

- Does the client make special dietary requests (e.g., kosher diet, vegetarian diet, or refrain from caffeine, pork or pork derivatives such as gelatin or marshmallows, shellfish, or other specific food items)?
- Does the client read religious magazines or books?

What Does the Client Say?

- Does the client talk about God, Allah, Buddha, Yahweh, Jehovah, prayer, faith, or other religious topics?
- Does the client ask for a visit by a clergy member or other religious representatives?
- Does the client express anxiety or fear about pain, suffering, dying, or death?

How Does the Client Relate to Others?

- Who visits? How does the client respond to visitors?
- Does a priest, rabbi, minister, elder, or other religious representatives visit?
- Does the client ask the nursing staff to pray for or with him/her?
- Does the client prefer to interact with others or to remain alone?

---

level and the relative importance of religion and spirituality in the lives of their primary providers of care. Parental perceptions about the illness of their child may be partially influenced by religious beliefs. For example, some parents may believe that a transgression against a religious law has caused a congenital anomaly in their offspring. Other parents may delay seeking medical care because they believe that prayer should be tried first.

The nurse should be respectful of parents' preferences regarding the care of their child. If the nurse determines that parental beliefs or practices threaten the child's well-being and health, he or she is obligated to discuss the matter with the parents. It may be possible to reach a compromise in which parental beliefs are respected and necessary care is provided. On rare occasions, it may become a legal matter. Religion may be a source of consolation and support to parents, especially those facing the unanswerable questions associated with life-threatening illness in their children.

Spiritual Nursing Care for the Dying or Bereaved Client and Family

While all people mourn, all people do not mourn alike. Mourning is a form of cultural behavior, and it is manifest in a multicultural society. Mourning customs help people cope with the loss of loved ones. Nurses inevitably focus on restoring health or on fostering environments in which the client returns to a previous state of health or adapts to physical, psychological, or emotional changes. However, one aspect of care that is often avoided or ignored, although it is every bit as crucial to clients and their families, is death and the accompanying dying and grieving processes.

Death is indeed a universal experience, but one that is highly individual and personal. Although each person must ultimately face death alone, rarely does a person's death fail to affect others. There are many rituals, serving many purposes, that people use to help them cope with death. These rituals are often determined by cultural and religious orientation. Situational factors, competing demands, and individual differences are also important in determining the dying, bereavement, and grieving behaviors that are considered socially acceptable.

The role of the nurse in dealing with dying clients and their families varies according to the needs and preferences of both the nurse and client as well as the clinical setting in which the interaction occurs. By understanding some of the cultural and religious variations related to death, dying, and bereavement, the nurse can individualize the care given to clients and their families (Kisvetrova, Klugar & Kableka, 2013; Wynne, 2013).

Nurses are often with the client through various stages of the dying process and at the actual moment of death, particularly when death occurs in a hospital, nursing home, extended care facility, or hospice. The nurse often determines when and whom to call as the impending death draws near. Knowing the religious, cultural, and familial heritage of a particular client, as well as his or her devotion to the associated traditions and practices, may help the nurse determine whom to call when the need arises.

Death Practices

Universally, people want to die with dignity. Historically, this was not a problem when individuals died at home in the presence of their friends and families. Now, when more and more people are dying in institutions (hospitals, hospices, and extended care facilities), with a variety of technological advances available that may prolong life but decrease dignity, ensuring dignity throughout the dying process is more complex. When death is seen as a problem requiring professional management, instead of a natural process, the hospital displaces the home, and specialists with different kinds and degrees of expertise take over for the family (Sherwen, 2014).

Preparation of the Body

A nurse may or may not actually participate in the rituals associated with death. When people die in the United States and Canada, they are usually transported to a mortuary, where the preparation for burial occurs.

In many cultural groups, preparation of the body has traditionally been very important. Whereas members of many cultural groups have now adopted the practice of letting the mortician prepare the body, there are some, particularly new immigrants, who want to retain their native and/or religious customs. For example, for certain Asian immigrants, it is customary for family and friends of the same sex to wash and prepare the body for burial or cremation. In other situations, the family or religious representatives may go to the funeral home to prepare the body for burial by dressing the person in special religious clothing.

If a person dies in an institution, it is common for the nursing staff to "prepare" the body according to standard policy and procedure. Depending on the ethnoreligious practices of the family, this may be objectionable—the family members may view this washing as an infringement on a special task that belongs to them alone. If the family is present, it is important to ask family members about their preference. If ritual washings will

eventually take place at the mortuary, it may be necessary to carry out the routine procedures and reassure the family that the mortician will comply with their requests, if that has in fact been verified.

The initial preparation of the body, as commonly practiced in North America, has been described in a classic work by Kalish and Reynolds (1981) in the following way:

"After delivery to the undertaker, the corpse is in short order sprayed, sliced, pierced, pickled, trussed, trimmed, creamed, waxed, painted, rouged and neatly dressed...transformed from a common corpse into a beautiful memory picture. This process is known in the trades as embalming and restorative art, and is so universally employed in North America that the funeral director does it routinely without consulting the corpse's family. He regards as eccentric those few who are hardy enough to suggest it might be dispensed with. Yet no law requires it, no religious doctrine commends it, nor is it dictated by considerations of health, sanitation or even personal daintiness. In no part of the world but in North America is it widely used. The purpose of embalming is to make the corpse presentable for viewing in a suitably costly container, and here too the funeral director routinely without first consulting the family prepares the body for public display" (Kalish & Reynolds, 1981, p. 65).

This extensive preparation and attempt to make the body look "alive," "just as he used to," or "just as if she were asleep" may reflect the fact that North Americans have come into contact with death and dying less than other cultural groups.

Funeral Practices

By their very nature, people are social beings who need to develop social attachments. When these social attachments are broken by death, people need to bring closure to the relationships. The **funeral**, a formal commemoration of the person's life, and the wake/viewing are an appropriate and socially acceptable time for the expression of sorrow and grief. Although there are some mores that dictate acceptable behaviors associated with the expression of grief, such as crying and sobbing, the funeral and wake/viewing are generally viewed as times when members of the living social network can observe and comfort the grieving survivors in their mourning. It is important to keep in mind that even the terms used for the wake and the funeral may vary according to religious and cultural beliefs. What is called a wake in many North American religions may be called a viewing or **home going** by others. Whether it is called a wake, viewing, or home going, it serves the same function: allowing the survivors to mourn together, comfort each other, and say a last goodbye.

Customs for disposal of the body after death vary widely. Muslims have specific rituals for washing, dressing, and positioning the body as well as time constraints regarding how soon the person is to be buried. In traditional Judaism, cosmetic restoration is discouraged, as is any attempt to hasten or retard decomposition by artificial means. As part of their lifelong preparation for death, Amish women sew white burial garments for themselves and for their family members (Cates, 2014; Sharpnack, Griffin, Benders & Fitzpatrick, 2010). For the viewing and burial, faithful Mormons are dressed in white temple garments. Burial clothes and other religious or cultural symbols may be important items for the funeral ritual. If such items are present in the hospital or long-term care facility, ensure that they are taken by the family or sent to the funeral home.

Believing that the spirit or ghost of the deceased person is contaminated, some Navajos are afraid to touch the body after death. In preparation for burial, the body is dressed in fine apparel, adorned with expensive jewelry and money, and wrapped in new blankets. After death, some Navajos believe that the structure in which the person died must be burned. There are specific members of the culture whose role is to prepare the body and who must be ritually cleansed after contact with the dead.

Funeral arrangements vary from short, simple rituals to long, elaborate displays. Among the Amish, family members, neighbors, and friends are relied on for a short, quiet ceremony. Many Jewish families use unadorned coffins and stress simplicity in burial services. Some Jews fly the body to Jerusalem for burial in ground considered to be holy. Regardless of economic considerations, some groups believe in lavish and costly funerals.

Taboos

In some cultures, people believe that particular omens, such as the appearance of an owl or a message in a dream, warn of approaching death. Breaking a taboo, for example, removing an object believed to have healing powers, is also believed by some to cause death. Nurses should take care to avoid moving or removing any objects of religious or spiritual significance without first consulting the client or family members.

Voodoo beliefs and practices are present in North America. Incidents of sudden death or minor injuries after hexing have been attributed to the power of suggestion and to total social isolation, which have been thought to trigger fatal physiologic responses and sensitization of the autonomic nervous system.

Unexpected and Violent Death

Acceptance of sudden, violent death is difficult for family members in most societies. For example, suicide is strictly forbidden under Islamic law. In the Filipino culture, suicide brings shame to the individual and to the entire family. Many Christian religions prohibit suicide and may impose sanctions even after death for the "sin." For example, a Roman Catholic who commits suicide may be denied burial in blessed ground or in a Catholic cemetery. In some religions, a church funeral is not permitted for a suicide victim, requiring the family to make alternative arrangements. This imposition of religious law can further add to the grief of surviving family members and friends.

The Northern Cheyenne believe that suicide, or any death resulting from a violent accident, disturbs the individual's spiritual balance. This disharmony is termed **bad death** and is believed to render the spirit earthbound in its wanderings, thus preventing it from entering the spirit world. A good death among the Tohono O'odham comes at the end of a full life, when a person is prepared for death. A bad death, by contrast, occurs unexpectedly and violently, leaving the victim without a chance to settle affairs or to say good-bye. "A 'bad death' is 'bad' because evil caused it, which leaves the soul of the dead unrestful, unfulfilled, and desirous of returning to the living out of a longing for what has been taken away. The soul returns to the living, although not out of malevolence, to visit loved ones. It is on these visits, that the dead can bring a form of ka:cim mumkidag (staying–Indian–sickness), to the living—hence their dangerousness" (McIntyre, 2008).

The categories of "good" and "bad" deaths among the Tohono O'odham have implications for research on excess deaths. Accidents, homicide, and suicide produce bad deaths; in Tohono O'odham view, these are deaths that should not occur, deaths that should be avoided if possible. "Bad" deaths are excess deaths. If the medical community's concern is with eliminating excess deaths, it must also be concerned with the larger cultural, social, and economic context in which these deaths occur. Other causes of death, while still important, may affect a people to a much lesser degree. Diabetes mellitus, for example, most often affects people of more advanced years and, because of its slow progress, allows them to prepare for death. This is still an excess death by Western medical standards, but it is not a "bad" death (Yurkovick & Lattergrass, 2008).

Death memorials provide a place for the dead to go without bringing harm to the living and a place for the living to go to help the dead to a proper afterlife. Among the Tohono O'odham, there has been a notable increase in violent deaths, particularly for young males. The majority of these violent deaths are the result of motor

vehicle accidents and are marked by roadside death memorials or shrines. Suicides and homicides are also sometimes commemorated with death memorials.

Deaths resulting from nonviolent but untimely causes can be equally difficult for the client, family, and friends. Cancers and chronic diseases may give the client and family time to "prepare" for the death, but the death still occurs and must receive attention. A good death to the elderly Japanese American often means to not have been a burden to others (Hattori & Ishid, 2012).

The Death of a Child

Although a great deal has been written about children's conceptions of death, cross-cultural studies have not yet been reported. Children develop a concept of death through innate cognitive development, which has significant cultural variations, and through acquired notions conveyed by the family, which vary according to the family's cultural beliefs. Thus, it is unsafe to assume that all children, regardless of family culture, will develop parallel concepts of and reactions to death.

Most children's initial experiences with death occur with the loss of a pet rather than a person. Because of reduced childhood mortality and delayed adult mortality, children in the United States and Canada are now much less exposed to death in family than they used to be, and they tend to be sheltered from the experience. The current lack of direct exposure of children to death is both a class phenomenon and a cultural phenomenon.

In many Western societies, children are considered precious, valued, and vulnerable; they are protected and often the first to be saved in emergencies. In less developed societies, by contrast, parents are less likely to see most of their children grow into adulthood because of a high infant mortality rates. As a result, a child's life may be viewed as less valued and precious than an adult's, although the child is still viewed as valuable to the parents and other loved ones. Regardless of the sociocultural situation, each society has a special view of the significance of children and their death as it affects the bereaved family.

Bereavement, Grief, and Mourning

Bereavement is a sociologic term indicating the status and role of the survivors of a death. **Grief** is an affective response to a loss, whereas **mourning** is the culturally patterned behavioral response to a death. What differs between cultural groups is not so much the feelings of grief but their forms of expression or mourning.

Different family systems may alleviate or intensify the pain experienced by bereaved persons. In the typical nuclear North American family, the death of a member leaves a great void because the same few individuals fill most of the roles. By contrast, cultural groups in which several generations and extended family members commonly reside within a household may find that the acute trauma of bereavement is softened by the fact that the familial role of the deceased is easily filled by other relatives. It should be noted, however, that the loss is experienced and mourned irrespective of the person's cultural background.

Although nurses frequently encourage clients and their families to express their grief openly, many people are reluctant to do so in the institutional setting. The nurse often sees family members when they are still in shock over the death and are responding to the situation as a crisis rather than expressing their grief. When asked who would be sought for comfort and support in a time of bereavement, most frequently named were a family member or a member of the clergy. In an institutional setting, a nurse who has been with the patient and family throughout the dying process may be surprised at the time of death when the grieving persons turn to other family, and the nurse is "left out."

Contemporary bereavement practices of various cultural and religious groups demonstrate the wide range of expressions of bereavement. Each group reflects practices that best meet its members' needs. The nurse can help promote a culturally appropriate grieving process; hindering

or interfering with practices that the client and family find meaningful can disrupt the grieving process. Bereaved people can experience physical and psychological symptoms, and they may succumb to serious physical illnesses, leading even to death. Although bereavement is regarded as a universal stressor, the magnitude of the stress and its meaning to the individual vary significantly cross-culturally. For example, one Western misconception is that it is more stressful to mourn the death of a child than the death of an older or more distant relative. Yet, cross-cultural studies show that emotional attachments to relatives vary significantly and are not based on Western concepts of kinship.

Although traditional funeral and postfuneral rituals have benefited both bereaved persons and their social groups in their original settings, the influence of the contemporary Western urban setting is unknown. It is likely that in North America, most individuals have assimilated US and Canadian practices in varying degrees. The role of the nurse is to obtain information from individual clients in a caring manner, explaining that you wish to provide culturally appropriate nursing care.

Religious Trends in the United States and Canada

The United States and Canada are cosmopolitan nations to which all of the major and many of the minor faiths of Europe and other parts of the globe have been transplanted (Figure 13-3). Religious identification among people from different racial and ethnic groups is important because religion and culture are interwoven. Table 13-1 details the statistical breakdown of major religious affiliations of the United States and Canada.

As discussed, a wide range of beliefs frequently exists within religions—a factor that adds complexity. Some religions have a designated spokesperson or leader who articulates, interprets, and applies theological tenets to daily life experiences, including those of health and illness. These leaders include, but are not limited to, Jewish rabbis, Catholic priests, Lutheran ministers, and Muslim imams. Some religions rely more heavily on individual conscience, whereas others entrust decisions to a group of individuals or to a single

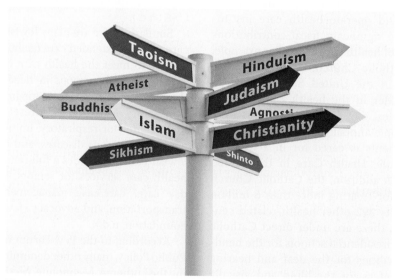

Figure 13-3. Multiple religions are present in all societies, and this diversity enhances opportunities for nurses to encounter multiple belief systems and to adjust their care accordingly (Ryan DeBerardinis/Shutterstock.com).

Table 13-1: Major Religious Affiliations of the United States and Canada (%)

	United States	Canada	World
Christianity	78.5	57.9	33
Atheism, Agnosticism, no affiliation	17.3	23.9	12.7 5
Judaism	1.7	1.0	0.22
Islam	0.7	3.2	19.6
Buddhism	0.6	1.1	5.9
Hinduism	0.7	1.5	13.4
Major Christian Faith Groups			
Roman Catholic	23.9	38.7	32.3
Protestant	44.4	19.2	9.2

Sources: Pewforum.org/affiliations; 2011 National household Survey.

person vested with ultimate authority within their religious tradition.

Contributions of Religious Groups to the Health Care Delivery System

In the United States and Canada, many denominations own and operate health care institutions and make significant fiscal contributions that help control health care costs. For example, the Roman Catholic Church, the largest single denomination in the United States, is also a major stakeholder in the health care field. In the United States, 642 Catholic hospitals treat 5.4 million people annually, meaning that 1 out of every 6 patients is cared for in a Catholic hospital (Catholic Health Care in the United States, 2014). In addition, the Catholic Church is responsible for treating more than 6 million individuals at its 392 other health-related centers. Moreover, there are under direct Catholic auspices 79 nonresidential schools for the handicapped; 14 facilities for the deaf and hearing impaired; 4 centers for the blind and visually impaired; 517 facilities for the aged; 72 facilities for abused, abandoned, neglected, and emotionally disturbed children; 116 centers for those

with developmental disabilities; 2 residences for the orthopedically and physically handicapped; 8 cancer hospitals; and 11 substance abuse centers (Catholic Health Care in the United States, 2014). **Catholic Charities USA**, an umbrella agency that oversees nonhospital work, reports that its agencies serve more than 1,046 million people each year, often functioning as a centralized referral source for clients ultimately treated in non-Catholic agencies (Catholic Charities USA, n.d.).

Similarly, there are many Jewish hospitals, day care centers, extended care facilities, and organizations to meet the health care needs of Jewish and non-Jewish persons in need. For example, the National Jewish Center for Immunology and Respiratory Medicine is a research and treatment center for respiratory, immunologic, allergic, and infectious diseases, and the Council for Jewish Elderly provides a full range of social and health care services for seniors, including adult day care, care/case management, counseling, transportation, and advocacy (Jewish Healthcare Foundation, n.d.).

According to the Pew Forum on Religion and Public Policy, many other denominations, including the Lutheran, Mennonite, Methodist, Muslim, and Seventh-Day Adventist groups, also own and operate hospitals and health care organizations (Extending Christ's Ministry, n.d.).

In Canada, hospital care, outpatient care, extended care, and medical services have been publicly funded and administered since the Medical Care Act of 1966. However, before the Medical Care Act and into the present, religious organizations have made important contributions to the health and well-being of Canadians at individual, community, and societal levels. For example, countless church-run agencies, charities, and facilities offer care and social support to individuals and families coping with such conditions as chronic illness, disability, poverty, and homelessness. At the national level, church-run organizations, such as the Catholic Health Association of Canada, are committed to addressing social justice issues that affect the health system and offer leadership through research and policy development regarding health care ethics, spiritual and religious care, and social justice.

Health-Related Beliefs and Practices of Selected Religions

Some of the world's religions fall into major branches or divisions, such as Vaishnavite and Shaivite Hinduism; Theravada and Mahayana Buddhism; Orthodox, Reform, and Conservative Judaism; Roman Catholic, Orthodox, and Protestant Christianity; and Sunnite and Shi'ite Islam. There also are subdivisions into what are often called denominations, sects, or schools of thought and practice.

Health-related beliefs and practices of select religions are important to understand, especially considering the diverse religious groups in the United States and Canada. Evidence-Based Practice 13-1 provides information regarding other research done on this topic. Box 13-2 summarizes some of the religious and nonreligious holidays covered in this chapter. A brief overview of selected religious groups and their health-related beliefs and practices follows.

Amish

The term **Amish** refers to members of several ethnoreligious Christian groups who choose to live separately from the modern world through manner of dress, language, family life, and selective use of technology. There are four major orders or affiliating groups of Amish: (1) *Old Order Amish*, the largest group, whose name is often used synonymously with "the Amish"; (2) the ultraconservative *Swartzentruber* and *Andy Weaver Amish*, both more conservative than the Old Order Amish in their restrictive use of technology and shunning of members who have dropped out or committed serious violations of the faith; (3) the less conservative *New Order Amish*, which emerged in the 1960s with more liberal views of technology but with an emphasis on high moral standards in restricting alcohol and tobacco use and in courtship practices; and (4) the *Liberal Beachy Amish*, more commonly known as Mennonites, who maintain many of the same features as the more conservative Amish, but allow electricity and use of automobiles.

The Amish are direct descendants of a branch of Anabaptists (which means "to be rebaptized"), which emerged during the Protestant Reformation and resided in Switzerland, the Netherlands, Austria, France, and Germany. Anabaptists stressed adult baptism, separation from and nonassimilation with the dominant culture, conformity in dress and appearance, marriage to others within the group, nonproselytization, nonparticipation in military service, and a disciplined lifestyle with an emphasis on simple living. These basic tenets remain today.

A former Catholic priest from the Netherlands named Menno Simmons (1496–1561) wrote down the beliefs and practices of the Anabaptists, who became known as **Mennonites**. In 1693, under the leadership of a church elder named Jacob Ammann (1656–1730), a more conservative group broke away and formed the group currently known as the Amish. The total population of Amish is estimated at 261,000, spread throughout more than 220 settlements in 21 states and one Canadian province.

Four Studies on Religion and Health Care Practices

The Adventist Health Study-2 studied the relationship of vegan, lactoovovegetarian, pescovegetarian, semivegetarian, and nonvegetarian dietary patterns of 97,000 members of the Seventh-Day Adventist church exploring the relationship of those dietary patterns to health outcomes, specifically obesity, metabolic syndrome, hypertension, type 2 diabetes mellitus, osteoporosis, cancer, and mortality. While the data regarding cancer have yet to be analyzed in depth, the data showed that "vegetarian diets in the AHS-2 population studied are associated with lower BMI values, lower prevalence of hypertension & metabolic syndrome and lower prevalence and incidence of type 2 diabetes as well as lower all-cause mortality" (p. 357S). While there has long been a concern that vegetarian diets put the person at risk for osteoporosis, it appears from this study that when plant sources of protein are consumed, the risk is decreased.

Reference: Orlich, M.J., & Fraser, G. E. (2014). Vegetarian diets in the Adventist health study 2: A review of initial published findings. _American Journal of Clinical Nutrition, 1000_ (suppl), 353S–358S.

In this study, the researchers divided 999 consenting participants into two groups (490 controls, 509 intervention receivers), one that received intercessory prayer from an established prayer group in a congregation distant to the institution and one that did not. All subjects were blinded as to their group. The researchers were exploring whether intercessory prayer made an impact on spiritual well-being and quality of life. Subjects received prestudy questionnaires as well as repeated poststudy questionnaires at the end of 6 months. There was an overall 66.6% rate for completion of the study. The data showed a small but statistically significant improvement in spiritual well-being in the intervention group. The clinical significance of this finding was not able to be determined. The control group showed a decreased functional well-being over the 6-month period, while the intervention group showed improvement.

Reference: Oliver, I. N., & Dutney, A. (2012). A randomized, blinded study of the impact of intercessory prayer on spiritual well-being in patients with cancer. _Alternative Therapies, 18_(5), 18–27.

In this study, the researchers explored whether Hispanics, in general, and Catholic Hispanics, in particular, follow a "cultural belief" called "fatalism," which precludes the person from participating in cancer screening practices. Sixty-seven participants (33 men, 34 women) attended one of eight focus groups with 8 to 10 participants per group. Men and women attended separate groups. The intent was to explore the "participants' cultural explanatory models of cancer, including their cultural beliefs, attitudes, personal life experiences and their understanding of both biomedical and population explanations of health and illness" (p. 841). Contrary to the stereotype of "fatalism," this group "expressed few fatalistic beliefs with regard to cancer" and instead indicated a general belief that cancer was preventable if caught early. This group reported that their religion supported them in their search for health, including cancer screening. They also indicated that there is a role for faith and calling upon God and saints in the face of illness.

Reference: Leyvam, B., Allen, J. D., Tom, L.S., Ospino, H., Torres, M. I., & Abraido-Laza, A. F. (2014). Religion, fatalism and cancer control: A qualitative study among Hispanic Catholics. _American Journal of Health Behavior, 38_(6), 839–849.

This exploratory study examined the cancer screening practices of 100 Arab Muslim women (AMW) using a mailed questionnaire. The final response rate was 50%. Results showed that mammography screening for women greater than age 40 was 86.7%. Barriers for not obtaining a mammogram included not knowing where to go, concerns about insurance, time, and modesty. Transportation and childcare, though anticipated, were not identified as barriers. Cervical cancer screening (Pap test) was completed by 50% of the respondents. This was an anticipated finding because of the expectation of virginity for unmarried AMW; thus, most providers

would not have recommended this screening for them. Proficiency with the English language, embarrassment, and modesty were found to be the primary barriers for obtaining cervical screening.

Reference: Salman, K. F. (2012). Health beliefs and practices related to cancer screening among Arab Muslim Women in an urban community. *Health Care for Women International,* 33(45–74).

Clinical Implications

What questions might you consider after thinking about the evidence provided in these studies?

How might this information impact your care of patients who are not from any of the ethnic backgrounds found in these studies?

What other evidence might you want to explore to seek answers to clinical questions that you have faced?

Box 13-2 Religious and Nonreligious Holidays in the United States and Canada

This calendar is a guide to religious and nonreligious holidays that are celebrated in the United States and Canada. The list is not exhaustive but reflects major holidays and festivals of religious and ethnic groups in North America.

B = Buddhist

Ba = Baha'i

C = Christian (general)

Ci = Civic holiday

H = Hindu

I = Islam

J = Jewish

Ja = Jain

M = Mormon

O = Eastern Orthodox Christian

P = Protestant

RC = Roman Catholic

S = Sikh

January
1 New Year's Day (Ci)
1 Feast of St. Basil (O)
6 Epiphany (C)
7 Nativity of Jesus Christ (O)
3rd Monday Martin Luther King, Jr. Birthday Observance (Ci)

February
Black History Month (United States)
8 Scout Day (Ci)
14 Valentine's Day (Ci)
Mid-month President's Day (United States; Ci)
Other holidays that often fall in February according to the lunar calendar:
Chinese New Year
Ramadan (30 days; I)
Nehan-e (Death of Buddha; B)
Vasant Panchami (Advent of Spring; H, Ja)

Ash Wednesday (RC, P)
Purim (J)

March
Women's History Month (United States)
17 St. Patrick's Day (C)
25 Annunciation (C)
Other holidays that often occur in March according to the lunar calendar:
Eastern Orthodox Lent begins (O)
Higan-e (First Day of Spring; B)
Naw-Ruz (Baha'i and Iranian New Year)
Palm Sunday (RC, P)
First Day of Passover (8 days; J)
Holi (Spring Festival; H, Ja)
Maundy Thursday (The Thursday prior to Easter; RC, P)
Good Friday (The Friday prior to Easter; RC, P)
Easter (C, RC, P, M)
Mahavir Jayanti (Birth of Mahavir; Ja)

(continued)

April

16 Yom Ha'atzmaut (Israel Independence Day; J)
Holidays that often occur in April according to the lunar calendar:
Hana-Matsuri (Birth of Buddha; B)
Yom HaShoah (Holocaust Remembrance Day; J, Ci)
Baisakhi (Brotherhood; S)
Huguenot Day (P)
Ramavani (Birth of Rama; H)
Palm Sunday (O)
Holy Friday (O)
Easter (O)

May

5 Cinco de Mayo (Ci)
23 Victoria Day (Canada)
30 Memorial Day (Ci)
Holidays that often occur in May according to the lunar calendar:
Shavuot (J)
Idul-Adha (Day of Sacrifice; I)
Ascension Day (RC, P)
Pentecost (RC, P)

June

12 Anne Frank Day
14 Flag Day (United States; Ci)
24 Nativity of St. John the Baptist (RC, P, O)
Holidays that often occur in June according to the lunar calendar:
Ratha-Yatra (H)
Ascension Day (O)
Muharram (I)
Pentecost (O)
Islamic New Year (I)
Hindu New Year (H)

July

1 Canada Day (Canada; Ci)
4 Independence Day (United States; Ci)
24 Pioneer Day (M)
Holidays that often occur in July according to the lunar calendar
Obon-e (B)

August

6 Transfiguration (C)
15 Feast of the Blessed Virgin Mary (RC, O)

September

First Monday Labor Day (United States; Ci)
15 National Hispanic Heritage Month (30 days; Ci)
17 Citizenship (US Constitution; Ci)
19 San Gennaro Day (RC)
25 Native American Day (Ci)
Holidays that often occur in September according to the lunar calendar:
Higan-e (First Day of Fall; B)
Rosh Hashanah (Jewish New Year, 2 days; J)

October

12 Columbus Day (United States, Ci)
Thanksgiving Day (Canada, Ci)
24 United Nations Day (Ci)
31 Reformation Day (P)
31 Halloween (RC, P, Ci)
Holidays that often occur in October according to the lunar calendar:
Dussehra (Good over Evil; H, JA)
Yom Kippur (Atonement; J)
Sukkot (Tabernacles; J)
Shemini Atzeret (End of Sukkot; J)
Diwali, or Deepavali (Festival of Lights; H, Ja)

November

1 All Saints Day (RC, P)
11 Veterans Day (Ci)
25 Religious Liberty Day (Ci)
First Tuesday Election Day (United States; Ci)
4th Thursday Thanksgiving Day (United States; Ci)
Holidays that often occur in November according to the lunar calendar:
Baha'u'llah Birthday (Ba)
Guru Nanak Birthday (S)

December

6 St. Nicholas Day (C)
8 Feast of the Immaculate Conception (RC)
10 Human Rights Day (Ci)
12 Festival of Our Lady of Guadalupe (Mexico-Hispanic)
25 Christmas (C, RC, P, M, Ci)
Holidays that often occur in December according to the lunar calendar:
Bodhi Day (Enlightenment; B)
Hanukkah (8 days; J)
Kwanzaa (7 days)

General Beliefs and Religious Practices

The imperative to remain separate is the common theme of the nearly 500-year history of the Amish. There are **five core characteristics of the Amish** (Graham & Cates, 2013): subculture, ordnung, meidung/shunning, selective use of technology, and gelassenheit.

First, the Amish are a *subculture*: a group with beliefs, values, and behaviors that are distinct from the greater culture of which the group is a part. The Amish maintain their separateness and distinctiveness from US and Canadian societies in a variety of ways. Geographically, the Amish live close together in areas referred to as settlements and rely primarily on the horse and buggy or bicycles for transportation (Kraybell, 2014).

The Amish continue to practice their faith in the tradition of Anabaptism, which includes small church districts of a few dozen families led by a bishop, church services that rotate from house to house of each family (there is no separate church building), the practice of adult baptism, communion twice a year, and shunning. Church leaders are chosen through a process of nomination and drawing by lot, and they serve for life. All but a few Amish marry, extended family remains important, and divorce is rare. The Amish dress in distinctive clothing (plain colors and mostly without buttons and zippers). They speak a form of German among themselves known as Pennsylvania Dutch or High German, and they sometimes refer to non-Amish as the "English."

The second core feature of the Amish is the *ordnung*, the guiding principles for Amish life, which is used for passing on religious values and way of life from one generation to the next. Parts of the ordnung are based on specific biblical passages, but much of it consists of rules for living the Amish way.

The third characteristic of the Amish is *meidung*, the practice of shunning members who have violated the ordnung. After all members of the church district have discussed the case and agreed to impose meidung, the individual is separated from the rest of his or her community.

It is the church's method of enforcing the ordnung. Meidung is an important way of maintaining both a sense of community among Amish and a sense of separation from the rest of the world. In most cases, when *meidung* is applied, it is for a limited time. Meidung applies only to Amish adults who have been baptized, not to their unbaptized children. Children of Amish who choose not to be baptized often become members of neighboring Mennonite congregations and maintain contact with their Amish relatives.

With less serious violations of the ordnung, a member is visited privately by the deacon and a minister, and the matter is resolved quietly. For more serious offenses, the punishment is carried out publicly during a church service. A few offenses, such as adultery and divorce, are automatically conditions of excommunication. By displaying deep sorrow and repentance for an offense, excommunicated members can be allowed back, but this is not easily accomplished.

The fourth core characteristic is the *selective use of technology*. The Amish selectively use many modern technologies, but only if this does not threaten their ability to maintain a community of believers. The Amish restrict the use of electricity in their homes and farms, and they limit their use of telephones. Although they may ride in automobiles, trains, and airplanes, they do not operate them (Figure 13-4). Tractors for farm field work might reduce the opportunity for sons and daughters to help parents with farm chores, and the farm would become larger, reducing the number available for future generations, so typically, gasoline-powered tractors are not used by the Amish. Thus, technology is not inherently bad, but when its consequences result in destruction of family and community life, it is avoided.

The fifth and final core characteristic of the Amish is *gelassenheit*. This term means "submission," or yielding to a higher authority, and it represents a general guide for behavior among Amish members. I represents the high value that the Amish place on maintaining a sense of

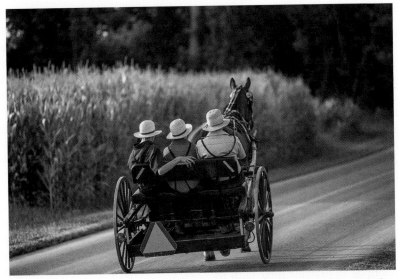

Figure 13-4. Amish use of horse and buggy transportation can be a health/safety hazard in heavily motor trafficked areas (hutch photography/Shutterstock.com).

community, which is accomplished by not drawing too much attention to one's self. Amish cite gelassenheit as the reason they avoid having their photographs taken and prohibit mirrors in their homes.

Holy Days, Rites, and Rituals

Amish hold church services every other Sunday on a rotating basis in the homes or barns of church district members. The church services last several hours with hymns, scriptures, and services in High German or Pennsylvania Dutch. The family hosting the service is expected to provide a meal for all in attendance. Christmas celebrations include family dinners and exchange of gifts. Weddings last all day and include eating and singing. An important part of Amish life is informal visiting. Families often visit one another without advance notice, and it is common for unexpected visitors to stay for a meal. Amish observe adult baptism and communion twice a year.

Social Activities

The Amish strive for high standards of conduct in both their private and public lives. This includes chastity before marriage and humility in dress,

language, and behavior. The function of dating is to afford individuals an opportunity to become acquainted with each other's character. Couples contemplating marriage may engage in a practice called bundling, in which they lie together in bed, fully clothed, without having sexual contact.

Substance Use

Once baptized, alcoholic beverages and drugs are forbidden unless prescribed by a physician. Teenagers and unmarried young adults may experiment with cigarettes, alcohol, and sometimes other chemical substances. It is important to assess persons in this age group for substance abuse.

Health Care Practices

Illness is seen as the inability to perform daily chores; physical and mental illness are equally accepted. Health care practices within the Amish culture are varied and include folk, herbal, homeopathic, and biomedicine. Unlike the use of episodic biomedicine, however, preventive medicine may be seen as against God's will. The use of the biomedical health care system is largely episodic and crisis oriented. If biomedicine fails,

there is no hesitancy in visiting an herb doctor, pow-wow doctor (a practitioner of a folk healing art, known as *brauche*, in which touch is used to heal), or a chiropractor. Folk, professional, and alternative care are often used simultaneously. Cost, access, transportation, and advice from family and friends are the major factors that influence healing choices. The Amish are at risk for a variety of genetic diseases due to frequent intermarriage among close relatives. Farming accidents are also a common reason for seeking health care service (Graham & Cates, 2013).

Medical and Surgical Interventions

The use of narcotic drugs is prohibited. There are no restrictions against the use of blood or blood products, if advised by health care providers. Vaccinations are acceptable, especially for children, but may not be accepted for adults or elderly individuals.

Practices Related to Reproduction

The Amish believe that the fundamental purpose of marriage is procreation, and couples are encouraged to have large families. Children are an economic asset to the family because they assist their parents with housework, farm chores, gardening, and family business. Women are expected to have children until menopause. If situations arise that justify sterilization (e.g., removal of cancerous reproductive organs), those called upon to make the decisions would rely on the best medical advice available and the council of the church leaders. Although the Amish family structure is patriarchal, the grandmother is often a key decision maker concerning reproductive and other health-related issues.

Abortion is inconsistent with Amish values and beliefs. Artificial insemination, genetics, eugenics, stem cell research, and in vitro fertilization are also inconsistent with Amish values and beliefs.

Religious Support System for the Sick

Individual members of local and surrounding communities assist and support one another in times of need. From birth to death, each person knows that he or she will be cared for by those in the community. **Friendscraft** is a unique three-generational extended family support network inherent in the Amish community that provides informal support, emotional and financial assistance, and advice. The extended family consists of aunts, uncles, cousins, and grandparents, who usually live only a few miles away and can be counted on to assist in times of illness.

The Amish do not use religious titles. So, a nurse may call any visitor by typical titles of Mr. or Mrs. There are approximately 1,931 Amish church districts in the United States and Canada, each representing about 20 to 35 families, and a minimal hierarchy of church leaders (a bishop, deacon, and two ministers). The bishop is the spiritual head; the deacon assists the bishop and is responsible for donations to help members with medical bills and other expenses; and the ministers help the bishop with preaching at church services and providing spiritual direction for the church district and its members. Although bishops meet periodically, there is no church hierarchy above the level of the church district. Because the Amish are surrounded by US and Canadian societies, which continuously exert strong economic and cultural pressures that are incompatible with Amish values, the Amish represent a subculture that is among the most "self-consciously engineered of all societies" (Donnermeyer, 1997, p. 9).

Individual members of local church districts look after the needs of the sick person and his or her family. When an Amish person is hospitalized, there will likely be a large number of visitors. Since they will not want to be in the way, asking them to step out when necessary is acceptable. Physical touch should be limited except for direct care. Parents will likely stay with children. Home health care is acceptable and often welcomed. While most will speak both English and Pennsylvania Dutch, in times of stress, they may revert to their Pennsylvania Dutch dialect and interpreters may be necessary.

Practices Related to Death and Dying

Advanced directives are uncommon. With a fatalistic view of life (God's will), there may be resistance to extensive procedures, tests, and life-prolonging interventions. Decisions are made on a family-by-family basis. When death is imminent, the bishop may perform an anointing, which is usually silent. Space and privacy needs to be provided. Prolongation of life (right to die) and euthanasia are personal matters that may be discussed with the bishop, ministers, and/or family members. Autopsy is acceptable in the case of medical necessity or legal requirement, but is seldom performed on the Amish. Although there is no specific prohibition, the Amish usually prefer to bury the intact body and generally do not donate body parts for medical research. Organ and tissue donation will require consultation with church leaders. While not expressly forbidden, it is a matter that is determined on an individual basis. Bodies are buried in small cemeteries in Amish communities on private property. Cremation is not acceptable.

Additional Considerations

The Amish beliefs of self-sufficiency, separation from the world, and mutual aid have resulted in their rejection of formal assistance from outside the Amish community. For example, the Amish obtained exemption for self-employed workers from Social Security, including Medicare, in 1965 on religious grounds and received exemption for all Amish workers from these programs in 1988. The Amish have also been exempted from the stipulations of the Affordable Care Act (As US Struggles with Health Care reform, Amish go their own way, October 5, 2013). Amish seldom purchase commercial health insurance; instead, they have traditionally relied on personal savings and various methods of mutual assistance within the immediate and larger Amish community to meet their medical expenses. It is expected that each family has planned for future health care needs (e.g., childbirth and minor illness), but it is recognized that catastrophic illnesses resulting in extensive medical expenses do sometimes occur. In these instances, the Amish community provides assistance, usually through participation in one of the Amish Hospital Aid plans.

Changing occupational patterns among the Amish have resulted in shifting views toward commercial health insurance. Data on the Amish are limited. The most recent study on the Amish use of commercial health insurance was conducted in the late 1990s in Holmes County, Ohio, where only 32.9% of Amish breadwinners earn their living as farmers: 24.5% are active farmers, 4% are retired farmers, and 3.4% hold dual occupations (both farm and nonfarm). Similar trends have been reported among other Amish settlements, where 30% to 80% of adult men work in nonfarm wage labor jobs in construction, factories, and home-based shops (e.g., cabinetmaking, harness making, blacksmithing, and so forth). The underlying reasons for the change are attributed to two factors: population growth and difficulty finding sufficient farmland for the growing numbers of Amish (Donnermeyer, 1997).

Baha'i International Community

The Baha'i Faith (pronounced Buh-high) is an independent world religion. It has members in approximately 340 countries and localities and represents 1,900 ethnic groups and tribes. North American membership is 753,423, and worldwide membership is approximately 6 million (Top 10 Largest International Bodies, n.d.)

General Beliefs and Religious Practices

The writings that guide the life of the **Baha'i International Community** comprise numerous works by Baha'u'llah, prophet–founder of the Baha'i Faith. Central teachings are the oneness of God, the oneness of religion, and the oneness of humanity. Baha'u'llah proclaimed that religious truth is not absolute but relative, that Divine Revelation is a continuous and progressive process, that all the great religions of the world are divine in origin, and that their missions represent

successive stages in the spiritual evolution of human society.

For Baha'is, the basic purpose of human life is to know and worship God and to carry forward an ever-advancing civilization. To achieve these goals, they strive to fulfill certain principles:

1. Oneness of God (all religions derive their inspiration from one heavenly source), oneness of religion (all religions of the world are one), and oneness of mankind (there is just one race—the human race).
2. Fostering of good character and the development of spiritual qualities, such as honesty, trustworthiness, compassion, and justice.
3. Eradication of prejudices of race, creed, class, nationality, and sex.
4. Elimination of all forms of superstitions that hamper human progress and achievement of a balance between the material and spiritual aspects of life. An unfettered search for truth and belief in the essential harmony of science and religion are two aspects of this principle.
5. Development of the unique talents and abilities of every individual through the pursuit of knowledge and the acquisition of skills for the practice of a trade or profession.
6. Full participation of both sexes in all aspects of community life, including the elective, administrative, and decision-making processes, along with equality of opportunities, rights, and privileges of men and women.
7. Fostering of the principle of universal compulsory education.

Baha'is may not be members of any political party, but they may accept nonpartisan government posts and appointments. They are expected to obey the government in their respective countries and, without political affiliation, may vote in general elections and participate in the civic life of their communities.

The Baha'i administrative order has neither priesthood nor ritual; it relies on a pattern of local, national, and international governance, created by Baha'u'llah. Institutions and programs are supported exclusively by voluntary contributions from members.

The Baha'i International Community has consultative status with the United Nations Economic and Social Council and with the United Nations Children's Fund. It is also affiliated with the United Nations Environment Program and with the United Nations Office of Public Information.

The World Center of the Baha'i Faith is in Israel, established in the two cities of Haifa and Akka. The affairs of the Baha'i world community are administered by the Universal House of Justice, the supreme elected council, in Haifa.

Holy Days, Rites, and Rituals

Extending from sunset to sunset are Baha'i holy days, feast days, and days of fasting. These holy days are not contraindications to medical care or surgery.

Although the Baha'i Faith does not have sacraments in the same sense that Christian churches do, it does have practices that have similar meanings to members. These practices include the recitation of obligatory prayers and participation in the observance of holy days and the Nineteen-Day Fast, abstaining from food between sunrise and sunset from March 2nd until March 20th, which is mandatory for all Baha'is between the ages of 15 and 70 years. Exceptions are made for illness, travel away from home, and pregnancy. **Fasting** occurs from sunrise to sunset for an entire Baha'i month, which consists of 19 days.

Social Activities

Baha'is strive for high standards of conduct in both their private and public lives; this includes chastity before marriage; moderation in dress, language, and amusements; and complete freedom from prejudice in their dealings with peoples of different races, classes, creeds, and orders.

The Baha'i Faith forbids monastic celibacy, noting that marriage is fundamental to the growth and continuation of civilization. The function of dating is to afford individuals an opportunity to become acquainted with each other's character. Those contemplating marriage are encouraged

to engage in some form of work and service together—a practice intended to promote assessment of their own maturity and readiness for marriage as well as to improve their knowledge of the character and values of the prospective marriage partner.

Substance Use

Alcoholic beverages and drugs are forbidden unless prescribed by a physician. Tobacco use is strongly discouraged.

Health Care Practices

With an attitude of harmony between religion and science, Baha'is are encouraged to seek out competent medical care, to follow the advice of those in whom they have confidence, and to pray.

Medical and Surgical Interventions

The use of narcotic drugs is prohibited except by prescription. There are no restrictions against the use of blood, blood products, or vaccines if advised by health care providers. Amputations, organ transplantation, biopsies, and circumcision are permitted if advised by health care providers.

Practices Related to Reproduction

Baha'i teachings state that the human soul comes into being at conception. Birth control is allowed as long as it does not involve aborting a conceptus: Members are discouraged from using methods of contraception that produce abortion after conception has taken place (e.g., intrauterine device). Abortion and surgical operations for the purpose of preventing the birth of unwanted children are forbidden unless circumstances justify such actions on medical grounds. In this case, the decision is left to the consciences of those concerned, who must carefully weigh the medical advice they receive in the light of the general guidance given in the Baha'i writings.

Advanced directives are encouraged and at the discretion of the individual.

Amniocentesis is permitted if advised by health care providers.

Although there are no specific Baha'i writings on artificial insemination, Baha'is are guided by the understanding that marriage is the proper spiritual and physical context in which the bearing of children must occur. Couples who are unable to bear children are not excluded from marriage, because marriage has other purposes besides the bearing of children. The adoption of children is encouraged.

Circumcision is not a religious practice; therefore, it is at the discretion of the parents.

No specific guidelines exist from the Baha'i Faith regarding in vitro fertilization. Nor do specific guidelines exist at this time regarding stem cell research. Since there are many sources for stem cells, a decision may come in the future.

The Baha'is view scientific advancement as a noble and praiseworthy endeavor of humankind. Baha'i writings do not specifically address eugenics and genetics.

Religious Support System for the Sick

Individual members of local and surrounding communities assist and support one another in time of need. Religious titles are not used. Individual members of local communities look after the needs of the sick.

Practices Related to Death and Dying

Because human life is the vehicle for the development of the soul, Baha'is believe that life is unique and precious. The destruction of a human life at any stage, from conception to natural death, is rarely permissible. The question of when natural death has occurred is considered in the light of current medical science and legal rulings on the matter.

Decisions are left to the individual regarding whether to withdraw or withhold life support. Consulting the opinion of a competent physician is recommended. Autopsy is acceptable in the case of medical necessity or legal requirement. Baha'is are permitted to donate their bodies for medical research or for restorative purposes. Local burial laws are followed. Unless required by state law, Baha'i law states that the body is not to

be embalmed. Cremation is forbidden. The place of burial must be within 1-hour travel from the place of death. This regulation is always carried out in consultation with the family, and exceptions are possible (McAteen & Edalati, 2013).

Buddhist Churches of America

Buddhism is a general term that indicates a belief in Buddha and encompasses many individual churches. There are approximately 2.7 million Buddhists in North America (Buddhism Canada on the Move, n.d.; Buddhist Churches of America, n.d.), and the worldwide membership is greater than 350 million (Number of Buddhists worldwide, n.d.).

The Buddhist Churches of America is the largest Buddhist organization in mainland United States. There are numerous Buddhist sects in the United States and Canada, including Indian, Sri Lankan, Vietnamese, Thai, Chinese, Japanese, and Tibetan.

Buddhism was founded in the 6th century BC in northern India by Gautama Buddha. In the 3rd century BC, Buddhism became the state religion of India and spread from there to most of the other Eastern nations. The term **Buddha** means "enlightened one."

At the beginning of the Christian era, Buddhism split into two main groups: Hinayana, or southern Buddhism, and Mahayana, or northern Buddhism. Hinayana retained more of the original teachings of Buddha and survived in Sri Lanka (formerly Ceylon) and southern Asia. Mahayana, a more social and polytheistic Buddhism, is strong in the Himalayas, Tibet, Mongolia, China, Korea, and Japan.

General Beliefs and Religious Practices

Buddha's original teachings included Four Noble Truths and the Noble Eightfold Way, the philosophies of which affect Buddhist responses to health and illness. The **Four Noble Truths** expound on suffering and constitute the foundation of Buddhism. The truths consist of (1) the truth of dissatisfaction and suffering, (2) the truth of the origin of dissatisfaction and suffering, (3) the truth

that dissatisfaction and suffering can be destroyed, and (4) the way that leads to the cessation of pain.

The **Noble Eightfold Way** gives the rule of practical Buddhism, which consists of (1) right views, (2) right intention, (3) right speech, (4) right action, (5) right livelihood, (6) right effort, (7) right mindfulness, and (8) right concentration. **Nirvana** or **Enlightenment**, a state of greater inner freedom and spontaneity, is the goal of all existence. When one achieves Nirvana, the mind has supreme tranquility, purity, and stability.

Although the ultimate goals of Buddhism are clear, the means of obtaining those goals are not religiously prescribed. Buddhism is not a dogmatic religion, nor does it dictate any specific practices. Individual differences are expected, acknowledged, and respected. Each individual is responsible for finding his or her own answers through awareness of the total situation.

Religious Objects

Prayer beads and images of Shakyamuni Buddha and other Buddhist deities may be utilized for specific prayer or meditation practices (Sorajjakool & Naewood, 2010; Stanford, 2013, Toneatto, 2012).

Holy Days

The major Buddhist holy day is Saga Dawa (or Vesak), which is the observance of Shakyamuni Buddha's birth, Enlightenment, and parinirvana. This holiday falls during the months of May or June. It is based on a lunar calendar, and therefore, the actual date varies from year to year (Figure 13-5). Although there is no religious restriction for therapy on this day, it can be highly emotional, and a Buddhist client should be consulted about his or her desires for medical or surgical intervention. Some Buddhists may fast for all or part of this day.

Rites and Rituals

Buddhism does not have any sacraments that need to be taken into consideration for a hospitalized member of the Buddhist faith. A ritual that symbolizes one's entry into the Buddhist faith is the expression of faith in the Three Treasures (Buddha, Dharma, and Sangha).

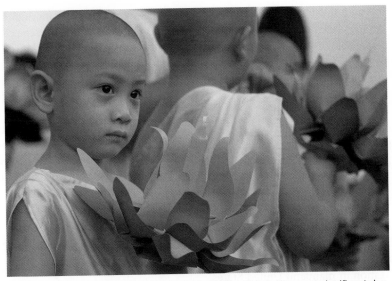

Figure 13-5. A young boy celebrates Vesak Day. This is the most significant day of the Buddhist calendar and a time when Buddhists engage in community service activities and make donations to charities (yuanann/Shutterstock.com).

Diet

Moderation in diet is encouraged. Specific dietary practices are usually interconnected with ethnic practices. Some branches of Buddhism have strict dietary regulations, for example, vegetarianism, while others do not. It is important to inquire about the client's preferences.

Health Care Practices

Buddhists do not believe in healing through a faith or through faith itself. However, Buddhists do believe that spiritual peace and liberation from anxiety by adherence to and achievement of awakening to Buddha's wisdom can be important factors in promoting healing and recovery.

Medical and Surgical Interventions

There are no restrictions in Buddhism for nutritional therapies, medications, vaccines, and other therapeutic interventions, but some individuals may refrain from alcohol, stimulants, and other drugs that adversely affect mental clarity. Buddha's teaching on the Middle Path may apply here: He taught that extremes should be avoided. What may be medicine to one may be poison to another, so generalizations are to be avoided. Medications should be used in accordance with the nature of the illness and the capacity of the individual. Whatever will contribute to the attainment of Enlightenment is encouraged. Treatments such as amputations, organ transplants, biopsies, and other procedures that may prolong life and allow the individual to attain Enlightenment are encouraged.

Practices Related to Reproduction

The immediate emphasis is on the person living now and the attainment of Enlightenment. If practicing birth control or having an amniocentesis or sterility test will help the individual attain Enlightenment, it is acceptable.

Buddhism does not condone the taking of a life. The first of Buddha's Five Precepts is abstention from taking lives. Life in all forms is to be respected. Existence by itself often contradicts this principle (e.g., drugs that kill bacteria are given to spare a patient's life). With this in mind, it is the conditions and circumstances surrounding

the client that determine whether abortion, therapeutic or on demand, may be undertaken.

Religious Support System for the Sick
Support of the sick is an individual practice in keeping with the philosophy of Buddhism, but Buddhist priests often render assistance to those who become ill.

Practices Related to Death and Dying
If there is hope for recovery and continuation of the pursuit of Enlightenment, all available means of support are encouraged. If life cannot be prolonged so that the person can continue to search for Enlightenment, conditions might permit euthanasia. If the donation of a body part will help another continue the quest for Enlightenment, it might be an act of mercy and is encouraged. The body is considered a shell; therefore, autopsy and disposal of the body are matters of individual practice rather than of religious prescription. Burials are usually a brief graveside service after a funeral at the temple. Cremations are common.

Catholicism According to the Roman Rite

Roman **Catholic** membership in North America includes approximately 85 million people; worldwide membership is more than 1.2 billion (How many catholics are there in the World? March 14, 2013).

General Beliefs and Religious Practices

The Roman Catholic Church traces its beginnings to about 30 AD, when Jesus Christ is believed to have founded the church. Catholic teachings, based on the Bible, are found in declarations of church councils and Popes and in short statements of faith called creeds. The Apostle's Creed and the Nicene Creed are forms of the Profession of Faith, which is recited during the central act of worship, the Mass. The creeds summarize Catholic beliefs concerning the Trinity and creation, sin and salvation, the nature of the church, and life after death.

Holy Days
Catholics are expected to observe all Sundays as holy days. Sunday or holy day worship services may be conducted any time from 4:00 PM on Saturday (a vigil mass celebrated on Saturday evening) until Sunday evening. Other days set aside for special liturgical observance include the Solemnity of Mary, Mother of God (January 1st), Ascension Thursday (the Lord's ascension bodily into Heaven, observed 40 days after Easter), Feast of the Assumption (August 15th), All Saints Day (November 1st), the Feast of the Immaculate Conception (December 8th), and Christmas (December 25th). Other days that may be particularly important to the observant Roman Catholic include the Easter Triduum (Holy Thursday, Good Friday, and Easter Sunday).

Rites and Rituals
The Roman Catholic Church recognizes seven sacraments: Baptism, Reconciliation (or Penance or Confession), Holy Communion (or the **Eucharist**) (Figure 13-6), Confirmation, Matrimony, Holy Orders, and Anointing of the Sick (or Extreme Unction).

Religious Objects
Rosaries, prayer books, and holy cards are often present and may be of great comfort to the client and their family. They should be left in place and within the reach of the client whenever possible.

Diet
The goods of the world have been given for use and benefit. The primary obligation people have toward food and beverages is to use them in moderation and in such a way that they are not injurious to health. Fasting in moderation is recommended as a valued discipline. Additionally, Catholics have an obligation to fast on Ash Wednesday and Good Friday. When fasting, a person is permitted to eat one full meal. Two smaller meals may also be taken, but not to equal a full meal. Abstinence from meat is also required on these days and on all of the Fridays of Lent. The sick are never bound by this prescription

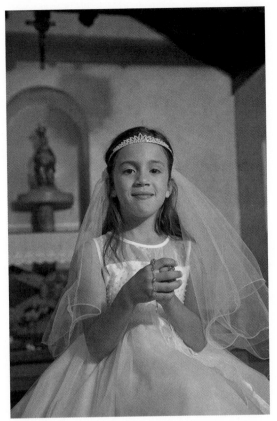

Figure 13-6. In the Roman Catholic tradition, when children reach the age of reason (7 years), they continue the ongoing initiation into their religion by making their First Communion, usually during 2nd grade. In addition to the religious ritual, there are sometimes cultural traditions surrounding this event, many of which involve a family celebration after the religious services have concluded (Golden Pixels LLC/Shutterstock.com).

of the law. Healthy persons between the ages of 18 and 59 are encouraged to engage in fasting as described; abstinence applies to those over the age of 14.

Social Activities

The major principle is that Sunday is a day of rest; therefore, unnecessary servile work is prohibited. The holy days of obligation are also considered days of rest, although many persons must engage in routine work-related activities on some of these days.

Substance Use

Alcohol and tobacco are not evil per se. They are to be used in moderation and not in a way that would be injurious to one's health or that of another party. The misuse of any substance is not only harmful to the body but also sinful.

Health Care Practices

In time of illness, the basic rite is the sacrament of **Anointing of the Sick**, which is performed by a priest and includes reading of scriptures, prayers, communion if possible, and anointing with oil. Prayers are frequently offered for the sick person and for members of the family. The Eucharistic wafer (a small unleavened wafer made of flour and water) is often given to the sick as the food of healing and health. Other family members may participate if they wish to do so.

Medical and Surgical Interventions

As long as the benefits outweigh the risk to the individuals, judicious use of medications is permissible and morally acceptable. A major concern is the risk of mutilation. The Church has traditionally cited the **principle of totality**, which states that medications are allowed as long as they are used for the good of the whole person. Blood, blood products, and amputations are acceptable if consistent with the principle of totality. Biopsies and circumcision are also permissible.

The transplantation of organs from living donors is morally permissible when the anticipated benefit to the recipient is proportionate to the harm done to the donor, provided that the loss of such an organ does not deprive the donor of life itself or of the functional integrity of his or her body.

Practices Related to Reproduction

The basic principle is that the conjugal act should be one that is love-giving and potentially life-giving. Only natural means of contraception, such as abstinence, the temperature method, and the ovulation method, are acceptable. Ordinarily, artificial aids and procedures for permanent sterilization are forbidden. Birth control

(anovulants) may be used therapeutically to assist in regulating the menstrual cycle.

Amniocentesis in and of itself is not objectionable. However, it is morally objectionable if the findings of the amniocentesis are used to lead the couple to decide on termination of the pregnancy or if the procedure injures the fetus.

Direct abortion is always morally wrong. Indirect abortion may be morally justified by some circumstances (e.g., treatment of a cancerous uterus in a pregnant woman). Abortion on demand is prohibited. The Roman Catholic Church teaches the sanctity of all human life from the time of conception.

The use of sterility tests for the purpose of promoting conception, not misusing sexuality, is permitted. Although artificial insemination has been debated heavily, traditionally, it has been looked on as illicit, even between husband and wife.

Research in the fields of eugenics and genetics is objectionable. This violates the moral right of the individual to be free from experimentation and also interferes with God's right as the master of life and human beings' stewardship of their lives. Some genetic investigations to help determine genetic diseases may be used, depending on their ends and means. There is support for research using adult stem cells, but opposition to the use of embryonic stem cells.

Religious Support System for the Sick

Although a priest, deacon, or lay minister usually visits a sick person alone, the family or other significant people may be invited to join in prayer. In fact, that is most desirable, since they too need support.

The priest, deacon, or lay minister will usually bring the necessary supplies for administration of the Eucharist or Anointing of the Sick. The nursing staff can facilitate these rites by ensuring an atmosphere of prayer and quiet and by having a glass of water on hand (in case the patient is unable to swallow the host). Consecrated wine can be made available but is usually not given in the hospital or home. The nurse may wish to join in the prayer. Candles may be used if the patient is not receiving oxygen. The priest, deacon, or lay minister will usually appreciate any information pertaining to the patient's ability to swallow. Any other information the nurse believes may help the priest or deacon respond to the patient with more care and effectiveness would be appreciated, but HIPPA laws must be remembered and information that violates privacy must not be divulged.

Catholic lay persons of either gender may visit hospitalized or homebound elderly or sick persons. Although they may not administer the sacraments of Anointing of the Sick or Reconciliation, they may bring Holy Communion (the Eucharist).

The titles of religious representatives include Father (priest), Mr. or Deacon (deacon), Sister (Catholic woman who has taken religious vows), and Brother (Catholic man who has taken religious vows).

Privacy is most conducive to prayer and the administration of the sacraments. In emergencies, such as cardiac or respiratory arrest, medical personnel will need to be present. The priest will use an abbreviated form of the rite and will not interfere with the activities of the health care team.

Most major cities have outreach programs for the sick, handicapped, and elderly. More serious needs are usually handled by Catholic Charities and other agencies in the community or at the local parish level. Organizations such as the St. Vincent de Paul Society may provide material support for the poor and needy as well as some counseling services, depending on the location. In the United States, the Catholic Church owns and operates hospitals, extended care facilities, orphanages, maternity homes, hospices, and other health care facilities. Although the majority of tertiary care facilities in Canada are publicly owned, many such institutions are strongly influenced by the leadership of the Catholic Church and its members. It is usually best to consult the pastor or chaplain in specific cases for local resources.

Practices Related to Death and Dying

The Catholic Church endorses the use of advanced directives and recommends that its members prepare these documents and review them periodically.

Members are obligated to take ordinary means of preserving life (e.g., intravenous medication) but are not obligated to take extraordinary means. What constitutes extraordinary means may vary with biomedical and technological advances and with the availability of these advances to the average citizen. Other factors that must be considered include the degree of pain associated with the procedure, the potential outcome, the condition of the patient, the economic factors, and the patient's or family's preferences.

Direct action to end the life of patients is not permitted. Extraordinary means may be withheld, allowing the patient to die of natural causes.

Autopsy is permissible as long as the corpse is shown proper respect and there is sufficient reason for doing the autopsy. The principle of totality suggests that organ donation is justifiable, being for the betterment of the person who does the giving.

Ordinarily, bodies are buried. Cremation is acceptable in certain circumstances, such as to avoid spreading a contagious disease. Because life is considered sacred, the body should be treated with respect. Any disposal of the body should be done in a respectful and honorable way (Dysinger, 2012; Spencer, 2013).

Christian Science

Christian Science accepts physical and moral healing as a natural part of the Christian experience. Members believe that God acts through universal, immutable, spiritual law. They hold that genuine spiritual or Christian healing through prayer differs radically from the use of suggestion, willpower, and all forms of psychotherapy, which are based on the use of the human mind as a curative agent. In emphasizing the practical importance of a fuller understanding of Jesus' works and teachings, Christian Science believes healing to be a natural result of drawing closer to God in one's thinking and living. The church does not keep specific membership data; however, they report that there are between 150,000 and 400,000 adherents and approximately 3,000 congregations worldwide (Christian Science Fast Facts, n.d.).

General Beliefs and Religious Practices

Christian Science beliefs and practices rely on the individual's faith and a reliance on prayer to achieve health when disease is present. Christian Science is based on the teachings of Christ Jesus, who said, "He that believeth on me, the works that I do shall he do also..." (John 14:12). Mary Baker Eddy said, "these mighty works are not supernatural, but supremely natural..." (*Science and Health*, p.xi:14). This can mean resolving difficult challenges with health, relationships, employment, and other personal and global issues through prayer. People who practice Christian Science are free to make their own choices about what to think and do in each situation, including health care. But Christian Science is more than a system of self-help or health care. Ultimately, it is a way to draw closer to our loving Father–Mother, God, as well as all of humanity.

Holy Days

Besides the usual weekly day of worship (Sunday), other traditional Christian holidays are observed on an individual basis. Worldwide, Wednesday evenings are observed as times for members to gather for testimony meetings.

Rites and Rituals

Although sacraments in a strictly spiritual sense have deep meaning for Christian Scientists, there are no outward observances or ceremonies. Baptism and holy communion are not outward observances but deeply meaningful inner experiences. Baptism is the daily purification and spiritualization of thought, and communion is finding one's conscious unity with God through prayer.

Social Activities and Substance Use

Members are encouraged to be honest, truthful, and moral in their behavior. Although every effort is made to preserve marriages, divorce is recognized. The Christian Science Sunday School teaches young people how to make their religion practical in daily life as related to school studies, social life, sports, and family relationships.

Members abstain from alcohol and tobacco; some abstain from tea and coffee.

Health Care Practices

Viewed as a by-product of drawing closer to God, healing is considered proof of God's care and one element in the full salvation at which Christianity aims. Christian Science teaches that faith must rest not on blind belief but on an understanding of the present perfection of God's spiritual creation. This is one of the crucial differences between Christian Science and **faith healing**. The practice of Christian Science healing starts from the Biblical basis that God created the universe and human beings "and made them perfect." Christian Science holds that human imperfection, including physical illness and sin, reflects a fundamental misunderstanding of creation and is therefore subject to healing through prayer and spiritual regeneration.

An individual who is seeking healing may turn to Christian Science practitioners, members of the denomination who devote their full time to the healing ministry in the broadest sense. In cases requiring continued care, nurses grounded in the Christian Science faith provide care in facilities accredited by the mother church, the First Church of Christ, Scientist, in Boston, Massachusetts. Individuals may also receive such care in their own homes. Christian Science nurses are trained to perform the practical duties a patient may need while also providing an atmosphere of warmth and love that supports the healing process. No medication is given, and physical application is limited to the normal measures associated with hygiene. The *Christian Science Journal*, a monthly publication, contains a directory of qualified Christian Science practitioners and nurses throughout the world.

Before they can be recognized and advertised in *The Christian Science Journal*, practitioners must have instruction from an authorized teacher of Christian Science and provide substantial evidence of their experience in healing. There are approximately 4,000 Christian Science practitioners throughout the world. Practitioners who speak other languages may also be listed in appropriate editions of *The Herald of Christian Science,* which is published in 12 languages.

The denomination has no clergy. Practitioners are thus lay members of the Church of Christ, Scientist, and do not conduct public worship services or rituals. Their ministry is not an office within the church structure but is carried out on an individual basis with those who seek their help through prayer. Both members and non-members are welcome to contact practitioners by telephone, by letter, or in person for help or for information.

Christian Science practitioners are supported not by the church but by payments from their patients. Their ministry is not restricted to local congregations but extends worldwide. Many insurance companies include coverage of payments to practitioners and Christian Science nursing facilities in their policies. In spite of such superficial resemblances to the health care professions, the work of Christian Science practitioners involves a deeply religious vocation, not simply alternative health care. Practitioners do not use medical or psychological techniques.

The term *healing* applies to the entire spectrum of human fears, grief, wants, and sin as well as to physical ills. Practitioners are called upon to give Christian Science treatment not only in cases of physical disease and emotional disturbance but also in family and financial difficulties, business problems, questions of employment, schooling problems, theological confusion, and so forth. The purpose of prayer, or Christian Science treatment, is to deal with these interrelated and complex problems of establishing God's law of harmony in every aspect of life. When healings are accomplished through perception and living of spiritual truth, they are effective and permanent. Physical healing is often the manifestation of a moral and spiritual change.

Ordinarily, a Christian Science practitioner and a physician are not employed in the same case, because the two approaches to healing differ so radically. During childbirth, however, an

obstetrician or qualified midwife is involved. Since bone setting may be accomplished without medication, a physician is also employed for repair of fractures if the patient requests this medical intervention. In cases of contagious or infectious disease, Christian Scientists observe the legal requirements for reporting and quarantining affected individuals. The denomination recognizes public health concerns and has a long history of responsible cooperation with public health officials.

Christian Scientists are not necessarily opposed to doctors. They are always free to make their own decisions regarding treatment in any given situation. They generally choose to rely on spiritual healing because they have seen its effectiveness in the experience of their own families and fellow church members—experience that goes back over 100 years and in many families for three or four generations. Where medical treatment for minor children is required by law, Christian Scientists strictly adhere to the requirement. At the same time, they maintain that their substantial healing record needs to be seriously considered in determining the rights of Christian Scientists to rely on spiritual healing for themselves and their children. They do not ignore or neglect disease, but they seek to heal it by the means they believe to be most effective.

Medical and Surgical Interventions

Christian Scientists ordinarily do not use medications. Immunizations and vaccines are acceptable only when required by law. Ordinarily, members do not use blood or blood products. A Christian Scientist who has lost a limb might seek to have it replaced with a prosthesis. Christian Scientists are unlikely to seek transplants and are unlikely to act as donors. Christian Scientists do not normally seek biopsies or any sort of physical examination. Circumcision is considered an individual matter.

Practices Related to Reproduction

Matters of family planning (i.e., birth control) are left to individual judgment. Because abortion involves medication and surgical intervention, it is normally considered incompatible with Christian Science. Artificial insemination is unusual among Christian Scientists. Christian Scientists are opposed to programs in the field of eugenics and genetics.

Religious Support System for the Sick

Christian Scientists have their own nurses and practitioners. No special religious titles are used. Organizations to assist the sick include Benevolent Homes, staffed by Christian Science nurses, and visiting home nurse services.

Practices Related to Death and Dying

A Christian Science family is unlikely to seek medical means to prolong life indefinitely. Family members pray earnestly for the recovery of a person as long as the person remains alive. Euthanasia is contrary to the teachings of Christian Science. Most Christian Scientists believe that they can make their particular contribution to the health of society and of their loved ones in ways other than donation of the body. Disposal of the body is left to the individual family to decide. The individual family decides the form of burial and burial service (Committee on Publication, 2013).

Additional Considerations

A wide variety of books and journals are published by the Christian Science Publishing Society, Boston, Massachusetts. Most major cities have Christian Science Reading Rooms, which carry these publications and are staffed by church members, who are available to provide additional information (Church of Christ, Scientist, n.d.).

The Church of Jesus Christ of Latter-day Saints

The **Church of Jesus Christ of Latter-day Saints**, commonly known as **Mormonism**, is a Christian religion established in the United States in the early 1800s. North American membership is approximately 7 million, and worldwide membership is approximately 15 million.

General Beliefs and Religious Practices

Latter-day Saints (members of the Church of Jesus Christ of Latter-day Saints) believe in Christianity as preached by Jesus Christ. They believe that church was lost shortly after the death of Christ and was restored in the early 1800s by Joseph Smith. As a consequence, Latter-day Saints hold that God the Father is an embodied being, yet the roles Latter-day Saints ascribe to members of the Godhead largely correspond with the views of others in the Christian world. Latter-day Saints believe that God is omnipotent, omniscient, and all-loving, and they pray to Him in the name of Jesus Christ. They acknowledge the Father as the ultimate object of their worship, the Son as Lord and Redeemer, and the Holy Spirit as the messenger and revealer of the Father and the Son.

Religious Objects

Copies of scriptures are often found at the bedside of members of this church. Reading these scriptures often brings comfort during times of illness. Scriptures sacred to members of the Church of Jesus Christ of Latter-day Saints include the Bible (Old and New Testament), the Book of Mormon, Doctrine and Covenants, and Pearl of Great Price.

Holy Days

Sunday is the day observed as the Sabbath in the United States. In other parts of the world, the Sabbath may be observed on a different day; in Israel, for example, members observe the Sabbath on Saturday.

Rites and Rituals

Within the Church of Jesus Christ of Latter-day Saints, an **ordinance** is a formal, sacred act representing a commitment of the person to the beliefs of the church.

The Ordinances of Salvation include the following:

1. Baptism at the age of accountability (8 years or after); never performed in infancy or at death; always by immersion

2. Confirmation at the time of baptism to receive the gift of the Holy Ghost
3. Partaking of the sacrament of the Lord's Supper at weekly Sunday sacrament meetings
4. Endowments
5. Celestial marriage
6. Vicarious ordinances

Endowments, celestial marriage, and vicarious ordinances occur in temples. Temples are sacred places of worship that are accessible only to observant Mormons, who are "worthy" to enter them as deemed by their local religious leaders.

The Ordinances of Comfort, Consolation, and Encouragement include

1. Blessing of babies
2. Blessing of the sick
3. Consecration of oil for use in blessing of the sick
4. Patriarchal blessings
5. Dedication of graves

After being deemed worthy to go to a temple, a member of the Church of Jesus Christ of Latter-day Saints will wear a special type of underclothing, called a **garment**. In a health care setting, the garment may be removed to facilitate care. As soon as the individual is well, he or she is likely to want to wear the garment again. An elderly person may not wish to part with the garment in the hospital. The garment has special significance to the person, symbolizing covenants or promises the person has made to God.

Diet

Members of this church have a strict dietary code called the **Word of Wisdom**. This code prohibits all alcoholic beverages (including beer and wine), hot drinks (e.g., tea and coffee, although not herbal tea), tobacco in any form, and any illegal or recreational drugs.

Fasting to a member means no food or drink (including water), usually for 24 hours. Fasting is required once a month on the designated fast Sunday. Pregnant women, the very young, the very old, and the ill are not required to fast.

The purpose of fasting is to bring oneself closer to God by controlling physical needs. The person is expected to donate the price of what has not been eaten to the church to be used to care for the poor.

Social Activities

The Church of Jesus Christ of Latter-day Saints has a wide variety of activities for its youth and encourages group activities until young people are at least 16. Young men are highly encouraged to perform missions for the church for 2 years at their own expense, beginning at the age of 18. Women may go on missions when they are 19, but marriage is more strongly emphasized for them.

Substance Use

Alcohol, caffeinated beverages (such as tea, coffee, and soda), and tobacco are forbidden. In recent years, "recreational drugs" and nonmedically indicated sedatives and narcotics have also been considered forbidden substances.

Health Care Practices

The members of the Church of Jesus Christ of Latter-day Saints believe that the power of God can be exercised on their behalf to bring about healing at the time of illness. The ritual of blessing the sick consists of one member (Elder) of the priesthood (male) anointing the ill person with oil and a second Elder "sealing the anointing with a prayer and a blessing." Commonly, both Elders place their hands on the individual's head. Faith in Jesus Christ and in the power of the priesthood to heal, requisite to the healing use of priesthood, does not preclude medical intervention but is seen as an adjunct to it. Mormons believe that medical intervention is one of God's ways of using humans in the healing process.

Medical and Surgical Interventions

There is no restriction on the use of medications or vaccines. It is not uncommon to find many members using herbal folk remedies, and it is wise to explore in detail what an individual may already have done or taken. There is no restriction on the use of blood or blood components.

Surgical intervention is a matter of individual decision in cases of amputations, transplants, and organ donations (both donor and recipient). Biopsies and resultant surgical procedures are also a matter of individual choice. The circumcision of infants is viewed as a medical health promotion measure and is not a religious ritual.

Practices Related to Reproduction

According to church doctrine, one of the major purposes of life is procreation; therefore, any form of prevention of the birth of children is contrary to church teachings. Exceptions to this policy include ill health of the mother or father and genetic defects that could be passed on to offspring. The decision of how many children to have and when to have them is extremely intimate and private, and the position of the church is that it should be left between the couple and the Lord.

Amniocentesis is a matter of individual choice. However, even if the fetus is found to be deformed, abortion is not an option unless the mother's life is in danger.

Abortion is forbidden in all cases except when the mother's life is in danger or when a competent physician determines that the fetus has severe defects that will not allow the baby to survive birth. Even in these circumstances, abortion is looked upon favorably only if the local priesthood authorities, after fasting and prayer, receive divine confirmation that the abortion is acceptable. In the event of pregnancy resulting from rape or incest, the church encourages that the child should be born and put up for adoption if necessary, rather than be aborted. The final decision rests with the mother. No official church sanction is used if she chooses to abort the child. Abortion on demand is strictly forbidden.

Because bearing children is so important, all measures that can be taken to promote having children are acceptable. Artificial insemination is acceptable if the semen is from the husband.

Religious Support System for the Sick

The Church of Jesus Christ of Latter-day Saints has a highly organized network, and many church representatives are likely to visit a hospitalized member, including the bishop and two counselors (leaders of the local congregation), home teachers (two men assigned to visit the family each month), and visiting teachers (two women assigned to visit the female head of household each month). Friends within the local congregation can also be expected to visit.

Various titles are used for members of this church's hierarchy. For men, the term *Elder* is generally acceptable, regardless of the man's position; the term Sister is acceptable for women.

To perform a blessing of the sick, the Elders performing the blessing need privacy and, if possible, silence. They generally bring a vial of consecrated oil with which to anoint the person. If they plan to perform a Sacrament of the Lord's Supper, they usually bring what they need with them. Bread and water are used for this ordinance.

The Relief Society is the organization for helping members. It is organized by the women of the church, who work closely with priesthood leaders to determine the general needs of members, including use of the church-run welfare organization. Church members who are in need may receive local help, such as child care when parents are ill or hospitalized and money for medical expenses or food when the family is in need.

Practices Related to Death and Dying

Whenever possible, medical science and faith healing are used to reverse conditions that threaten life. When death is inevitable, the effort is to promote a peaceful and dignified death. The church teaches that life continues beyond death and that the dead are reunited with loved ones; death is another step in eternal progression.

Euthanasia is not acceptable because the church teaches that life and death are in the hands of God, and humans must not interfere in any way. Autopsy is permitted with the consent of the next of kin and within local laws. Organ donation is permitted; it is an individual decision. Cremation is discouraged but not forbidden; burial is customary. A local priesthood member dedicates the graves (The Public Affairs Department of The Church of Jesus Christ of Latter Day Saints, 2013; Top & Callister, 2012; What do mormons believe?, n.d.).

Hinduism

The **Hindu** religion may be the oldest religion in the world. There are over 900 million Hindus worldwide, with a North American following of approximately 1 to 1.3 million members (How many Hindus are there in the World?, n.d.).

General Beliefs and Religious Practices

Hindus may be monotheistic, polytheistic, or atheistic; the basis of Hindu belief is the unity of everything. The major distinguishing characteristic is the social caste system.

Hinduism is founded on sacred, written scripture called the **Vedas**. **Brahman** is the principle and source of the universe and the center from which all things proceed and to which all things return. **Reincarnation** is a central belief in Hinduism. The law of **karma** determines life. According to karma, rebirth is dependent on moral behavior in a previous stage of existence. Life on earth is transient and a burden. The goal of existence is liberation from the cycle of rebirth and redeath and entrance into what in Buddhism is called nirvana (a state of extinction of passion).

The practice of Hinduism consists of roles and ceremonies performed within the framework of the **caste system**, a social order determined by birth. These rituals focus on the main ethnoreligious events of birth, marriage, and death. Hindu temples are dwelling places for deities to which people bring offerings. There are numerous places for religious pilgrimage.

Holy Days

The following holy days follow the lunar calendar:

1. Purnima (day of full moon)
2. Janmashtami (birthday of Lord Krishna)

3. Ramnavmi (birthday of Rama)
4. Shivratri (birth of Lord **Shiva**)
5. Naurate (nine holy days occurring twice a year; in about April and October)
6. Dussehra
7. Diwali
8. Holi

Social Activities, Diet, and Substance Use

Social activities are strictly limited by the caste system.

The eating of meat is forbidden because it involves harming a living creature. Most will not eat beef and many are vegetarian. At different stages of one's life, one may change one's dietary habits. For instance, in old age, a person who has been vegetarian may begin to eat fish or chicken.

Substance use is not restricted.

Religious Objects

A small picture of a deity may be found at the bedside. Prayer is often accompanied by the use of a "mala" (prayer beads) and a mantram (a sound representing an aspect of the divine). Facing North or East during prayer is preferable, but not required.

Health Care Practices

Some Hindus believe in faith healing; others believe illness is God's way of punishing people for their sins.

Medical and Surgical Interventions

The use of medications, blood, and blood components is acceptable. Persons who lose a limb are not outcasts from society. Loss of a limb is considered to be caused by "sins of a previous life." Organ transplantations are acceptable for both donors and recipients. Women may prefer to be examined by a female health care practitioner. Both men and women may retain their own clothes underneath a hospital gown.

Practices Related to Reproduction

All types of birth control are acceptable. Amniocentesis is acceptable, although not often available. Abortion, except for medical reasons, is discouraged. Artificial insemination is not restricted, but it is not often practiced because the technology to perform artificial insemination is not readily available, especially in rural areas.

Noting the exact time of a baby's birth is very important because it is used to determine the baby's horoscope. Males are not circumcised. Breast-feeding is expected. The infant is traditionally given a name on the 10th day following the birth, although in American hospitals, the child is sometimes named at birth.

Religious Support System for the Sick

Religious representatives use the title of priest. Church organizations to assist the sick do not exist; family and friends within the caste provide help.

Practices Related to Death and Dying

No religious customs or restrictions related to the prolongation of life exist. Life is seen as a perpetual cycle, and death is considered as just one more step toward nirvana. Euthanasia is not practiced. Autopsy is acceptable. The donation of body or parts is also acceptable.

Cremation is the most common form of body disposal. Ashes are collected and disposed of in holy rivers. The fetus or newborn is sometimes buried (Bhattacharyya, 2013).

Islam

Islam is a monotheistic religion founded between 610 and 632 AD by the prophet Muhammad. Derived from an Arabic word meaning "submission," Islam literally translated means "submission to the will of God." A follower of Islam is called Moslem or Muslim, which means "one who submits." The current North American membership is approximately 6 to 7 million, with a worldwide membership of between 2.8 and 3 billion (World's muslim population is more widespread than you think, June 7, 2013).

Muhammad, revered as the prophet of **Allah** (God), is seen as succeeding and completing both

Judaism and Christianity. Good deeds will be rewarded at the last judgment, whereas evil deeds will be punished in hell.

General Beliefs and Religious Practices

Islam has five essential practices, or **Pillars of Faith**. These are:

1. The profession of faith (*Shahada*), which requires bearing witness to one true God and acknowledging Muhammad as his messenger
2. Ritual prayer five times daily—at dawn, noon, afternoon, sunset, and night—facing Mecca, Saudi Arabia, Islam's holiest city (*salat*)
3. Almsgiving (*zakat*) to the needy, reflecting the Koran's admonition to share what one has with those less fortunate, including widows, orphans, homeless persons, and the poor
4. Fasting (*sawm*) from dawn until sunset throughout Ramadan during the 9th month of the Islamic lunar calendar
5. Making a pilgrimage to Mecca at least once during one's lifetime (*Hajj*) (Figure 13-7)

The sources of the Islamic faith are the **Qur'an (Koran)**, which is regarded as the uncreated and eternal Word of God, and **Hadith** (tradition), regarded as sayings and deeds of the prophet Muhammad. All Muslims recognize the existence of the sharia and the five categories into which it divides human conduct: required, encouraged, permissible, discouraged, and prohibited.

Various sects of Islam have developed. When Muhammad died, a dispute arose over the leadership of the Muslim community. One faction, the *Sunni*, derived from the Arabic word for "tradition," felt that the caliph, or successor of Muhammad, should be chosen as Arab chiefs customarily are by election. Therefore, they supported the succession of the first four (the "rightly guided") caliphs who had been Muhammad's companions. The other group maintained that Muhammad chose his cousin and son-in-law, Ali, as his spiritual and secular heir and that succession should be through his bloodline. In 680 AD, one of Ali's sons, Hussein, led a band of rebels against the ruling caliph. In the course of the

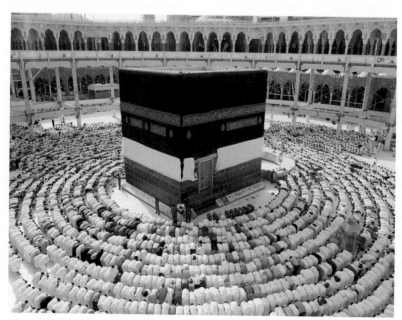

Figure 13-7. Pilgrims in prayer at Kaaba, the Holy mosque in Mecca (2013) (Zurijeta/Shutterstock.com).

battle, Hussein was killed, and with his death began the *Shi'a* (sometimes called the *Shi'ite*) movement, whose name comes from the word meaning "partisans of Ali." The Shi'a and the Sunni are the two major branches of Muslims; the Sunni constitute about 85% of the total. The Sunni are found in Lebanon, the West Bank, Jordan, and throughout Africa; the Shi'a are in Iran, Iraq, Yemen, Afghanistan, and Pakistan. The Shi'a and the Sunni also have different rituals, practices, and structural and political orientations.

Holy Days

Days of observance in Islam are not "holy" days but days of celebration or observance. The Muslims follow a lunar calendar, so the days of observance change yearly.

Each Muslim observance has its own significance. They are listed here in the same order in which they occur in the Muslim lunar calendar, and their standard Arabic names are used. However, the Arabic spellings for the names of the holidays may vary, or local names may be used.

- Muharram 1 Rasal-Sana (or New Year): The first day of the first month, celebrated much the same as the first day of the year, is celebrated throughout the world.
- Muharram 10 Ashura (the 10th of the first month): A religious holiday through which pious Muslims may fast from dawn to sunset. For Shi'ite Muslims, this is a special day of sorrow commemorating the assassination of the prophet's grandson, Hussein.
- Rabi'i 12 Mawlid al-Nabi: The birthday of the prophet Muhammad. In some regions, this holiday goes on for many days; it is a time of festivities and exchanging of gifts.
- Rajab 27 Lailat al-Isra wa al Miraj (literally, "The Night of the Journey and Ascent"): Commemorates Muhammad's night journey from Mecca to the Al-Aqsa mosque in Jerusalem and his ascent to heaven and return on the same night.
- Sh'ban 14: This is the 14th night of the 8th month of Sh'ban. It is widely celebrated by pious

Muslims and is sometimes called the Night of Repentance. It is treated in many parts of the Muslim world as a New Year's celebration.
- Ramadan (the 9th month of the Muslim year): This entire month is devoted to meditation and spiritual purification through self-discipline. It is a period of abstinence from eating, drinking, smoking, and sexual relations. The fast is an obligation practiced by Muslims throughout the world unless they are old, infirm, traveling, or pregnant. The fast is from sunup to sundown, at which time a meal (*Iftar*) is taken (Rauf Mir & Qazwini, 2013).
- Ramadan 27 Lailat al-Qadir (next to the last night of the fasting month): This is called the Night of Power and Greatness, and it is by custom a very special holy time. It commemorates the time when revelation was first given to Muhammad.
- Shawwal 1 "Id ad-Fitr": This is called the Lesser Feast because it begins immediately after the month-long Ramadan feast. It is perhaps Islam's most joyous festival, marking as it does the month of abstinence and the cleansing of the believer. It usually lasts for 2 or 3 days. Families and friends visit one another's homes, new clothes and presents are exchanged, and sweet pastries are a favorite treat.
- Dhu al-Hijjah 1 to 10: Muslims, if they are able, are obliged to undertake a pilgrimage to Mecca at least once in their lifetime. This journey, called the Hajj, is performed during the last month of the Muslim calendar, Dhu al-Hijjah.
- Dhu al-Hijjah 10: All Muslims, whether they are on the pilgrimage or at home, participate in the feast of the sacrifice, Id al-Adha, which marks the end of the Hajj on the tenth of Dhu al-Hijjah. The feast is the Feast of the Sacrifice, called the Greater Feast, and is observed by the slaughtering of animals and the distribution of the meat. In some places, this is done individually. The meat is shared equally among the family and the poor. Sometimes, the slaughtering takes place in public areas, and the meat is then distributed.

Diet and Substance Use

Eating pork and drinking alcoholic or other intoxicating beverages are strictly prohibited. In all cases, moderation in one's life is expected. Some Muslims consume meat that has been ritually slaughtered by the process called **halal**, which means "the lawful or that which is permitted by Allah." A patient may inquire if the food received is "halal." If it is not, the client may request that food be brought from home by family or friends.

Fasting during the month of Ramadan is one of the pillars of Islam. Children (boys 7 years old, girls 9 years old) and adults are required to fast. Fasting means to abstain from food from dawn until dusk. Pregnant women, nursing mothers, the elderly, and anyone whose physical condition is so fragile that a physician recommends not fasting are exempt from fasting but are expected to fast later in the year or to feed a poor person to make up for the unfasted Ramadan days (Rauf Mir & Qazwini, 2013).

Religious Objects

A prayer rug and the Koran are often present with a Muslim patient and should not be handled or touched by anyone who is ritually unclean. Nothing should be placed on top of these items. Some Muslims may wear an amulet, which is a black string or a silver or gold chain, on which sections of the Koran are attached. If worn by the patient, it should not be removed and should remain dry.

Health Care Practices

Muslim women typically prefer to have female physicians and health care providers, while men prefer male physicians and health care providers (Rauf Mir & Qazwini, 2013). Faith healing is not acceptable unless the psychological health and morale of the patient are deteriorating. At that time, faith healing may be used to supplement the physician's efforts. Vaccinations are encouraged. Touching between men and women is discouraged, another reason why health care providers of the same sex are preferred (Rauf Mir & Qazwini, 2013).

Medical and Surgical Interventions

There are no restrictions on medications. Even items normally forbidden (e.g., pork derivatives) are permitted if prescribed as medicine, although some Muslims will request medications that don't have a pork derivative, such as insulin. The use of blood and blood components is not restricted. Amputations are not restricted. Organ transplantations are acceptable for both donor and recipient. Biopsies are acceptable. No age limit is fixed, but circumcision is practiced on boys at an early age. For adult converts, circumcision is not obligatory, although it is sometimes practiced.

Practices Related to Reproduction

All types of birth control are generally acceptable in accordance with the law of "what is harmful to the body is prohibited." The family physician's advice on method of contraception is required. The husband and wife should agree on the method.

Amniocentesis is available in many Islamic countries. "Progressive" doctors and expectant parents use amniocentesis only to determine the status of the fetus, not the sex of the child; this is left in the hands of God.

There is a strong religious objection to abortion, which is based on Muhammad's condemnation of the ancient Arabian practice of burying unwanted newborn girls alive. If in vitro fertilization takes place, the destruction of fertilized eggs would be considered an abortion and not allowed (Rauf Mir & Qazwini, 2013).

Artificial insemination is permitted only if from the husband to his own wife. No official policy exists on practices in the fields of eugenics and genetics. Different Islamic schools of thought accept differing opinions.

Religious Support System for the Sick

In Islam, care of the physical body is not regarded highly. In many wealthy, oil-rich Middle Eastern nations, expatriates are hired to staff hospitals and provide for health care. Islamic clerics, called imams, may provide guidance that could be helpful for emotional and psychological disorders.

Formal, organized support systems to assist the sick do not exist; family and friends provide emotional and financial support.

Practices Related to Death and Dying

The right to die is not recognized in Islam. Any attempt to shorten one's life or terminate it (suicide or otherwise) is prohibited. Euthanasia is not acceptable. Autopsy is permitted only for medical and legal purposes. The donation of body parts or body is acceptable, without restrictions.

Withholding of life-sustaining care is acceptable to both Sunni and Shia Muslims; however, withdrawal of care is not acceptable from the Shia perspective. Maintaining a terminal patient on artificial life support is not encouraged in the Sunni tradition, but is encouraged in the Shia tradition.

Burial of the dead, including fetuses, is compulsory. It is important in Islam to follow prescribed burial procedures. Under conditions that cause fragmentation of the body, sections of the burial ritual may be omitted. The burial procedure consists of five steps:

1. Ghasl El Mayyet: Rinsing and washing of the dead body according to Muslim tradition. Muslim women cleanse a woman's body and Muslim men a man's body. At the time of death, the person's eyes are closed, the limbs straightened, and the entire body is covered with a sheet of cloth (Rauf Mir & Qazwini, 2013).
2. Muslin: After being washed three times, the body is wrapped in three pieces of clean white cloth. The Muslim word for "coffin" is the same as that for "muslin."
3. Salat El Mayyet: Special prayers for the dead are required. They are performed by those in attendance for the ritual washing, which prepares the body for burial (Rauf Mir & Qazwini, 2013).
4. The body should be prepared and buried as soon as possible. This must occur within 24 hours of the death. Cremation and embalming are prohibited. The body should always be buried so that the head faces toward Mecca.
5. Burial of a fetus: Before a gestational age of 130 days, a fetus is treated like any other discarded tissue. After 130 days, the fetus is considered a fully developed human being and must be treated as such.

Jehovah's Witnesses

North American membership of the **Jehovah's Witnesses** is 1.3 million (1.2 million in the United States; 112,705 in Canada); worldwide membership is approximately 7.3 million (Interesting Jehovah's Witness statistics, n.d.).

General Beliefs and Religious Practices

Jehovah's Witnesses are Christians and derived their name from the Hebrew name for God (**Jehovah**), according to the King James Bible. Thus, Jehovah's Witness is a descriptive name, indicating that members profess to bear witness concerning Jehovah, his Godship, and his purposes. Every Bible student devotes approximately 10 hours or more each month to proselytizing activities (Jehovah's Witnesses Official Website, n.d.).

Jehovah's Witnesses are opposed to saluting the flag, serving in the armed forces, voting in civil elections, and holding public office. These prohibitions are related to belief in a theocracy that is in harmony with their understanding of New Testament Christianity. Governed by a body of individuals, members united with the theocracy are to dissociate themselves from all activities of the political state and give full allegiance to "Jehovah's organization." This practice is related to the belief that Jesus Christ is King and Priest and that there is no need to hold citizenship in more than one kingdom. Members also refrain from gambling (Pellechia, 2013).

Membership in the Jehovah's Witness faith is difficult to ascertain. A member who fulfills their monthly obligation in proselytizing is known as a "publisher," while those who attend the yearly Memorial service are counted as members only (Interesting Jehovah's Witness statistics, n.d.), and membership data are reported differently according to whether a person is a "publisher" or a "member," which confounds the statistics.

Holy Days

Although Witnesses do not celebrate Christmas, Easter, or other traditional Christian holy days, a special annual observance of the Lord's Supper is held. Witnesses and others may attend this important meeting, but only those numbered among the 144,000 chosen members (Revelation 7:4) may partake of the bread and wine as a symbol of the death of Christ and the dedication to God. This memorial of Christ's death takes place on the day corresponding to Nisa 14 of the Jewish calendar, which occurs sometime in March or April. These elite members will be raised with spiritual bodies (without flesh, bones, or blood) and will assist Christ in ruling the universe. Others who benefit from Christ's ransom will be resurrected with healthy, perfected physical bodies (bodies of flesh, bones, and blood) and will inhabit this earth after the world has been restored to a paradisiacal state.

Social Activities and Substance Use

Youth are encouraged to socialize with members of their own religious background. Members abstain from the use of tobacco and hold that drunkenness is a serious sin. Alcohol used in moderation, however, is acceptable.

Health Care Practices

The practice of faith healing is forbidden. However, it is believed that reading the scriptures can comfort the individual and lead to mental and spiritual healing.

Medical and Surgical Interventions

Vaccinations are encouraged. Use of vaccinations is an individual's choice, even those made from a small fraction of blood (Pellechia, 2013). To the extent that they are necessary, medications are acceptable.

Blood in any form and agents in which blood is an ingredient are not acceptable. Blood volume expanders are acceptable if they are not derivatives of blood. Mechanical devices for circulating the blood are acceptable as long as they are not primed with blood initially. The determination of

Jehovah's Witnesses to abstain from blood is based on scriptural references and precedents in the history of Christianity. Courts of law have often upheld the principle that each individual has a right to bodily integrity, yet some physicians and hospital administrators have turned to the courts for legal authorization to force blood to be used as a medical treatment for an individual whose religious convictions prohibit the use of blood. In some cases, children have been made wards of the court so that they could receive blood when a medical condition mandating blood transfusion was life threatening. This can threaten the standing of the child in the community and must be approached with great care.

Although surgical procedures are not in and of themselves opposed, the administration of blood during surgery is strictly prohibited. There is no church rule pertaining to the loss of limbs or the amputation of body parts. If they are a violation of the principle of bodily mutilation, transplants are forbidden. However, this is usually an individual decision. Biopsies are acceptable. Circumcision is an individual decision.

Practices Related to Reproduction

Sterilization is prohibited because it is viewed as a form of bodily mutilation. Other forms of birth control are left to the individual. Amniocentesis is acceptable. Both therapeutic and on-demand abortions are forbidden. Sterility testing is an individual decision. Artificial insemination is forbidden both for donors and for recipients. Jehovah's Witnesses do not condone any activities in the areas of eugenics and genetics; they are considered to interfere with nature and therefore are unacceptable.

Religious Support System for the Sick

Individual members of a congregation, including elders, visit the ill. Visitors pray with the sick person and read scriptures. Male religious representatives are referred to as "Mr." or "Elder" and females as "Ms." or "Mrs." Religious titles are not generally used. Individuals and members of the congregation look after the needs of the sick.

Practices Related to Death and Dying

The right to die or the use of extraordinary methods to prolong life is a matter of individual conscience. Euthanasia is forbidden. An autopsy is acceptable only if it is required by law. No parts are to be removed from the body. The human spirit and the body are never separated. The donation of a body is forbidden. Disposal of the body is a matter of individual preference. Burial practices are determined by local custom. Cremation is permitted if the individual chooses it.

Judaism

Judaism is an Old Testament religion that dates back to the time of the prophet Abraham. Worldwide, there are approximately 14.5 million Jews. Membership includes approximately 6.7 million members in the United States and 375,000 members in Canada (Vital Statistics: Jewish Population in the World, 2012; Number of adherents of major religions, n.d.).

General Beliefs and Religious Practices

Judaism is a monotheistic religion. Jewish life historically has been based on interpretation of the laws of God as contained in the **Torah** and explained in the **Talmud** and in oral tradition. Ancient Jewish law prescribed most of the daily actions of the people. Diet, clothing, activities, occupation, and ceremonial activities throughout the life cycle are all part of Jewish daily life.

Today, there are at least three schools of theological thought and social practice in Judaism. The three main divisions include Orthodox, Conservative, and Reform. There is also a fundamentalist sect called Hasidism. Hasidic Jews cluster in metropolitan areas and live and work only within their Jewish communities.

Any person born of a Jewish mother or anyone converted to Judaism is considered a Jew. All Jews are united by the core theme of Judaism, which is expressed in the **Shema**, a prayer that professes a single God.

Holy Days

The Sabbath is the holiest of all holy days. The Sabbath begins each Friday 18 minutes before sunset and ends on Saturday, 42 minutes after sunset, or when three stars can be seen in the sky with the naked eye.

Other Holy Days include

1. Rosh Hashanah (Jewish New Year)
2. Yom Kippur (Day of Atonement, a fast day)
3. Sukkot (Feast of Tabernacles)
4. Shemini Atzeret (8th Day of Assembly)
5. Simchat Torah
6. Chanukah (Festival of Lights, or Rededication of the Temple in Jerusalem)
7. Asara B'Tevet (Fast of the 10th of Tevet; Not observed by liberal or Reform Jews)
8. Fast of Esther
9. Purim
10. Passover
11. Shavuot (Festival of the Giving of the Torah)
12. Fast of the 17th of Tammuz
13. Fast of the 9th of Ave (Commemoration of the Destruction of the Temple)

Holy days are very special to practicing Jews. If a condition is not life threatening, medical and surgical procedures should not be performed on the Sabbath or on holy days. Preservation of life is of greatest priority and is the major criterion for determining activity on holy days and the Sabbath. If a Jewish patient is hesitant to receive urgent and necessary treatment because of religious restrictions, a rabbi should be consulted.

Rites and Rituals

Brit milah, the covenant of circumcision, is performed on all Jewish male children on the 8th day after birth. Although circumcision is a surgical procedure, for Jews, it is a fundamental religious obligation. Circumcision is usually performed by a **mohel**, a pious Jew with special training, or by the child's father. Because the severing of the foreskin constitutes the essence of the ritual, the practice of having a non-Jewish or nonobservant physician perform the circumcision in the presence of a rabbi or other person who pronounces

the blessing is not acceptable according to Jewish law. Circumcision may be delayed if medically contraindicated. For example, if the child has hypospadias, a congenital defect of the urethral wall for which surgical repair usually occurs at age 3 years and requires the use of the foreskin in reconstructive plastic surgery, the circumcision may be delayed. At times, Jewish law requires postponement of circumcision, though contemporary medical science recognizes no potential threat to the health of the baby (e.g., for physiologic jaundice). As soon as the jaundice disappears, the brit milah may be performed. In Reform and Conservative traditions, girls mark the 8th day of life with a dedication ceremony in which prayers and blessings are invoked on her behalf.

The bar mitzvah (meaning "son of the commandment") is a confirmation ceremony for boys at age 13 that has been preceded by extensive religious study, including mastery of key Torah passages in Hebrew (Figure 13-8). In Reform and Conservative traditions, the bas (or bat) mitzvah (meaning "daughter of the commandment") is the equivalent ceremony for girls.

Diet

The dietary laws of Judaism are very strict; the degree to which they are observed varies according to the individual. Strictly observant Jews never eat pork or predatory fowl and never mix milk dishes and meat dishes. Only fish with fins and scales are permissible; shellfish and other water creatures are prohibited.

The word **kosher** comes from a Hebrew word *kashrut* that means "proper." All animals must be ritually slaughtered to be kosher. This means that the animal is to be killed by a specially qualified person, quickly, with the least possible pain. More colloquially, many people think that "kosher" refers to a type of food. If a patient asks for kosher food, it is important to determine what he or she means.

Religious Objects

On the Sabbath and on holidays, it is customary to light two candles in candleholders. Many Jewish men and some women wear *kippot* or *yarmulkes* (small head coverings) and *tallit* (prayer shawls) when praying. A *siddur* (prayer book) may also be present.

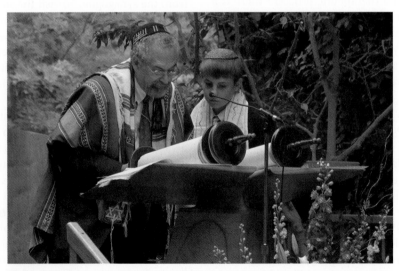

Figure 13-8. A 13-year-old boy recites from the Torah, with the rabbi by his side, during his bar mitzvah.

Social Activities

Like all ethnic groups, Jews tend toward socializing among themselves. Social activities that might lead to marriage outside the faith are discouraged. However, it is recognized that a significant number of individuals in Jewish society will seek partners outside of the Jewish faith. When this occurs, every effort is made to bring the non-Jewish partner into Judaism and to keep the Jewish partner a member and part of Jewish society.

Substance Use

The guideline is moderation. Wine is a part of religious observance and used as such. Historically, Jews well connected with their faith have had a low incidence of alcoholism.

Health Care Practices

Medical care from a physician in the case of illness is expected according to Jewish law. There are many prayers for the sick in Jewish liturgy. Such prayers and hope for recovery are encouraged.

Medical and Surgical Interventions

There are no restrictions when medications are used as part of a therapeutic process. There is a prohibition in Judaism against ingesting blood (e.g., blood sausage, raw meat). However, this does not apply to receiving blood transfusions. Beliefs and practices related to body mutilation (e.g., organ transplantation, amputations) vary widely among Jews. Individual beliefs should be explored with the client before any procedure that involves body mutilation.

Practices Related to Reproduction

It is said in the Torah that Jews should be fruitful and multiply; therefore, it is a *mitzvah* (a good deed) to have at least two children. Since the Holocaust of World War II, it has been increasingly acceptable to have more children to replace those who were lost. It is permissible to practice birth control in traditional and liberal homes. In the past, contraception was limited to the woman;

vasectomy was prohibited. Currently, Judaism permits contraception by either partner, although Hasidic and Orthodox Jews rarely use vasectomy.

Although therapeutic abortion is always permitted if the health of the mother is jeopardized, traditional Judaism regards the killing of an unborn child to be a serious moral offense; liberal Judaism permits it with strong moral admonitions (i.e., it is not to be used as a means of birth control). The fetus, although not imbued with the full sanctity of life, is a potential human being and is acknowledged as such.

Sterility testing is permissible when the goal is to enable the couple to have children. Artificial insemination is permitted under certain circumstances. A rabbi should be consulted in each individual case.

Jews have an understandable aversion to genetic engineering because of the experimentation carried on during the Nazi era. At the same time, eugenic practices are permitted under a limited range of circumstances. The Jewish belief in the sanctity of life is a guiding factor in rabbinical counseling.

Religious Support System for the Sick

The most likely visitors will be family and friends from the synagogue. To visit the sick is a mitzvah of service (an obligation, a responsibility, and a blessing). There are often many Jewish social service agencies to help those in need. The Jewish Federation and Jewish Community Service are two large organizations that provide services to fulfill a variety of needs.

The formal religious representative from a synagogue is the rabbi. A visit from the rabbi may be spent talking, or the rabbi may pray with the person alone or in a minyan, a group of 10 adults (aged 13 years or older). If the patient is male and strictly observant, he may wish to have a prayer shawl (*tallit*), a cap (*kippah*), and *tefillin* (special symbols tied onto the arms and forehead). If the patient's own materials are not at the hospital, it may be necessary to ask that they be brought. Prayers are often chanted. If possible, privacy should be provided.

Practices Related to Death and Dying

A person has the right to die with dignity. If a physician sees that death is inevitable, no new therapeutic measures that would artificially extend life need to be initiated. It is important to know the precise time of death for the purpose of honoring the deceased after the first year has passed.

Euthanasia is prohibited under any circumstances. It is regarded as murder. However, in the administration of palliative medications that carry the calculated risk of overdose, the amelioration of pain is paramount.

Any unjustified alteration of a corpse is considered a desecration of the dead, to be avoided in normal circumstances. When postmortem examinations are justified, they must be limited to essential organs or systems. Needle biopsy is preferred. All body parts must be returned for burial. Jewish family members may ask to consult with a rabbinical authority before signing an autopsy consent form.

Donation of body parts is a complex matter according to Jewish law. If it seems necessary, consultation with a rabbi should be encouraged.

The body is ritually washed at a funeral home after death, if possible by members of the Chevra Kadisha (Ritual Burial Society). The body is then clothed in a simple white burial shroud. Embalming and cosmetic treatment of the body are forbidden. Public viewing of the body is considered a humiliation of the dead. Relatives are forbidden to touch or embrace the deceased, except when involved in preparation for interment. The exact time of burial is significant for sitting shiva, the mourning period. After death in an institution, a nurse may wash the body for transport to the funeral home. Ritual washing then occurs later. Human remains, including a fetus at any stage of gestation, are to be buried as soon as possible. Cremation is not in keeping with Jewish law (Friedman, 2013; Katz, 2013).

Mennonite Church

Mennonites take their name from Menno Simons, an Anabaptist bishop who united a fragmented group of Anabaptists in the early 1500s. Menno had been a Catholic priest in Holland but left the church over theological differences after his brother was killed as an Anabaptist. The word "Anabaptist" comes from the doctrine that baptism to be valid must be upon confessed faith. Membership in North America is 443,918; worldwide membership is 1.25 million (Mennonite Church USA and Worldwide, n.d.).

General Beliefs and Religious Practices

Mennonites believe that each person is responsible before God to make decisions based on his or her understanding of the Bible. For this reason, there are very few official statements or regulations. Those that do exist, for example, the Mennonite Confession of Faith, are perceived by members as guidelines rather than proclamations to supplant individual responsibility. The Mennonite faith encompasses a wide spectrum of cultural circumstances, which are more responsible for variations among individual Mennonites than is the basic theology, which is relatively uniform. It is therefore even more important to ascertain individual preferences among members of the Mennonite faith and to work with patients on a one-to-one basis rather than stereotyping according to assumptions related to religious affiliation.

Holy Days

Mennonites observe the religious days of the traditional Christian churches. Observance places no restrictions on health-related procedures on these days.

Rites and Rituals

Mennonites observe Baptism and Holy Communion as official church sacraments. Patients will request sacraments as necessary. Neither sacrament is believed necessary for salvation.

Health Care Practices

Healing is believed to be a part of God's work in the human body through whatever means He chooses, whether medical science or healing that

comes in answer to specific prayer. There is no religious ritual to be applied unless the patient asks for one in whatever way is personally meaningful. Sometimes, anointing with oil is practiced.

Medical and Surgical Interventions

No specific guidelines or restrictions exist for the administration of medications, blood and blood components, or surgical procedures.

Practices Related to Reproduction

All types of contraception are acceptable. The choice is left to the individual.

Therapeutic abortions are acceptable. Mennonites generally believe that on-demand abortion must be decided according to specifics of individual cases. The church has chosen to avoid making a ruling that must be followed unquestionably. The individual must follow her own conscience and learn to live with the consequences. Some parts of the Mennonite Church have adopted statements opposing abortion on demand.

The church does not have regulations regarding artificial insemination. The individual conscience and point of view of the patient need to be respected. Usually, artificial insemination is sought only if husband and wife are donor and recipient, respectively.

The church accepts scientific endeavor as a valid activity that needs to respect all of God's creation. The concerns of eugenics and genetics in its future potential have not been fully confronted. Mennonites believe that God and human beings work together in caring for and improving the world.

Practices Related to Death and Dying

The church does not believe that life must be continued at all cost. Health care professionals should decide whether to take heroic measures on the basis of the patient's individual circumstances and the emotional condition of the family. When life has lost its purpose and meaning beyond hope of meaningful recovery, most Mennonites feel that relatives should not be censured for allowing life-sustaining measures to be withheld.

Euthanasia as the termination of life by an overt act of the physician is not condoned. Autopsy and the donation of the body are acceptable, without restrictions. Procedures for disposal of body and burial follow local customs and legal requirements (Carlson, 2013).

Native North American Churches

Differentiating Native North American health care practices from their religious and cultural beliefs is much more difficult than with the other religions presented in this chapter. There are 6.2 million Native North Americans, who comprise approximately 566 tribal units. Each group has individual beliefs and practices, yet generally, they maintain a similar nonprescriptive attitude toward health care (American Indians by Numbers, n.d.).

General Beliefs and Religious Practices

The Oklevueha **Native American Church** or **Peyote Religion** encompasses members of many tribes. Its focus is on the revival of Native North American culture, beliefs, and spirituality.

When trying to support a Native American in physical or psychological crisis, the nurse needs to remember several seemingly unrelated facts. First, the non-Westernized Native North American belief about disease is not necessarily based on symptoms. Disease may be attributed to intrusive objects, soul loss, spirit intrusion, breach of taboo, or sorcery. Disease may also be attributed to natural or supernatural causes. Second, the Native North American may embrace an organized, usually Christian religion and still be a member of a particular Native North American tribe and Native American religion. Native North Americans also balance "modern theories of disease" with long-standing tribal beliefs or customs. Therefore, during illness and particularly hospitalization, Native North Americans may ask to see a priest or minister as well as a tribal "medicine man" or *curandero*. Visits from these persons will likely be spiritually supportive, although the form of the support may vary greatly.

Health Care Practices

The spiritual basis for much of Native North American belief and action is symbolized by the number four. This number is seen in the extended hand, which means life, unity, equality, and eternity. The clasped hand symbolizes unity, the spiritual law that binds the universe.

It is this unity on which decisions should be made. Questions about abortion, the use of drugs, giving and receiving blood, the right to life, euthanasia, and so on do not have dogmatic "yes" or "no" answers; rather, answers are based on the situation and the ultimate unity or disunity that a decision would produce.

To the Native North American, everything is cyclical: Communication is the key to learning and understanding, understanding brings peace of mind, peace of mind leads to happiness, and happiness is communicating. Other guidelines also function in groups of four.

Four guidelines toward self-development:

1. Am I happy with what I am doing?
2. What am I doing to add to the confusion?
3. What am I doing to bring about peace and contentment?
4. How will I be remembered when I am gone, in absence, and in death?

The four requirements of good health:

1. Food
2. Sleep
3. Cleanliness
4. Good thoughts

The four divisions of nature:

1. Spirit
2. Mind
3. Body
4. Life

The four divisions of goals:

1. Faith
2. Love
3. Work
4. Pleasure

The four ages of development:

1. Learning age
2. Age of adoption
3. Age of improvement
4. Age of wisdom

The four expressions of sharing:

1. Making others feel you care
2. An expression of interest
3. An expression of friendship
4. An expression of belonging

Unity, the great spiritual law, also can be expressed in four parts:

1. Going into the silence in spirit, mind, and body
2. The union through which all spirituality flows
3. A goal toward communicating with all things in nature
4. Recognized through sense, emotions, and impressions

In concert with the belief in the interconnectedness of all things, natural remedies in the form of herbal medicine are often used. Native North American folk medicine and herbal remedies provided the forerunners of many of today's pharmaceutical remedies. Herbal treatments are still used today and may be requested by Native North American patients in a Western medical setting. A nurse caring for a Native North American client should obtain a careful and complete history, including a list of whatever folk remedies have been tried. The patient may not know the names of herbs used in the treatment, and the tribal medicine man or woman may need to be consulted.

Respecting the concept that religion, medicine, and healing are inseparable to the Native North American, one must be sensitive to the fact that asking for the names of native medicines or descriptions of healing practices tried in an attempt to cure the person before his or her entrance into the Western medical system is not just simply obtaining a history but also entering into the realm of what might be not only private

but also very sacred. The nurse must use care and sensitivity and show deep respect for the information received (Gober, & Kim, 2010; Oklevueha: Native American Church, n.d.).

Protestantism

General Beliefs and Religious Practices

In its broadest meaning, **Protestantism** denotes the whole movement within Christianity that originated in the 16th century with Martin Luther and the Protestant Reformation. Historically and traditionally, the chief characteristics of Protestantism are the acceptance of the Bible as the only source of infallible revealed truth, the belief in the universal priesthood of believers, and the doctrine that Christians are justified in their relationship to God by faith alone, not by good works or dispensations of the church.

It is difficult to accurately categorize Protestant churches and impossible to mention them all; there are more than 30,000 different denominations. Protestantism can be divided into four major forms: Lutheran, Anglican, Reformed, and the free (or independent) church.

The oldest and second largest Protestant religion, *Lutheranism,* began in 1517 with Martin Luther's split from the Roman Catholic Church. Lutherans emphasize theological doctrine and spirituality. Many North American Lutherans are of German or Scandinavian heritage. There are approximately 64 million Lutherans worldwide (Major branches of religions ranked by number of adherents, n.d.).

Anglicanism is represented by the established Church of England and similar churches. Unlike most other Protestant churches, they have an episcopal system of government in which each church or parish is served by a priest who is supervised by a bishop. A bishop supervises a group of churches called a diocese. A bishop, in turn, is responsible to a council of bishops. Anglican churches allow their clergy to marry. The Methodist church was established by followers of John Wesley, an 18th-century Anglican who sought to bring reform to the Church of England.

Wesley's movement spread to the United States and Canada in the 18th century. There are approximately 73 million Anglicans worldwide (Major branches of religions ranked by number of adherents, n.d.).

The *Reformed denominations* include Presbyterianism and are based on the teachings of John Calvin and his followers. These churches are distinguished from Lutheranism and Anglicanism, which maintain symbolic and sacramental traditions that originated before the Protestant Reformation. There are approximately 75 million people who practice one of the reformed denominations (Major branches of religions ranked by number of adherents, n.d.).

Free or *independent churches,* including Baptists, Congregationalists, Adventists, and Churches of Christ, exercise congregational government. Each local denomination is an independent autonomous unit, and there is no official doctrine. With 27 million members of the Baptist faith in the United States and more than 70 million worldwide, The Baptist church makes up more than 10% of the population of the United States. Black and White Baptist church denominations exist separately. The largely White Southern Baptist Convention has about 12 million members, whereas 9 million Blacks (30% of all Blacks in the United States) are members of the National Baptist Conventions.

Health Care Practices

Given the wide diversity that exists within Protestant denominations, it is beyond the scope of this text to identify health-related beliefs and practices for each group.

Seventh-Day Adventists

North American membership of **Seventh-Day Adventists** is approaching 1 million, with worldwide membership now exceeding 17 million (Seventh-Day Adventist Statistics, 2012). Doctrinally, Seventh-Day Adventists are heirs of the interfaith Millerite movement of the late 1840s, although the movement officially adopted

the name Seventh-Day Adventist in 1863. Between 1831 and 1844, William Miller, a Baptist preacher and former army captain in the War of 1812, launched the "great second advent awakening," which eventually spread throughout most of the Christian world. At first, the work was largely confined to North America, but it quickly spread to Switzerland, Africa, Italy, Egypt, and many other nations.

General Beliefs and Religious Practices

Seventh-Day Adventists accept the Bible as their only creed and hold certain fundamental beliefs to be the teaching of the Holy Scriptures. There are official statements by the General Conference of the Seventh-Day Adventists concerning the scriptures, the trinity, creation, nature of man, the great controversy (Christ versus Satan), life, death, resurrection, and other topics.

Holy Days

The seventh day (Saturday) is observed as the Sabbath—from Friday sundown to Saturday sundown. The Sabbath is the day that God blessed and sanctified. It is a sacred day of worship and rest. Worship services are held on Saturday; weekly evening prayer meetings are usually held mid week.

Rites and Rituals

There are three church ordinances: (1) baptism by immersion, (2) the Ordinance of Humility, and (3) the Lord's Supper or Communion. There are no rituals at the time of birth. There is no requirement for a final sacrament at death. If requested by the individual or family member, the dying person might be anointed with oil.

Diet and Substance Use

Seventh-Day Adventists believe that because the body is the temple of God, it is appropriate to abstain from any food or beverage that could prove harmful to the body. Because the first human diet consisted of fruits and grains, the Church encourages a vegetarian diet. Nevertheless, some members choose to eat beef and poultry. Based on a passage in Leviticus 11:3, nonvegetarian members refrain from eating foods derived from any animal having a cloven hoof that chews its cud (e.g., meat derived from pigs, rabbits, or similar animals). Although fish with fins and scales are acceptable (e.g., salmon), shellfish are prohibited. Consumption of some birds is prohibited, but common poultry such as chicken and turkey are acceptable. Fasting is practiced, but only when members of a specific church elect to do so. Practiced in degrees, fasting may involve abstention from food or liquids. Fasting is not encouraged if it is likely to have adverse effects on the individual. Fermented beverages are prohibited. Members should abstain from the use of tobacco products.

Social Activities

Dancing is not encouraged as a form of recreation or social activity. Members are encouraged to date other members or persons holding similar beliefs and values.

Health Care Practices

The church believes in divine healing and practices anointing with oil and prayer. This is in addition to healing brought about by medical intervention. Since 1865, the church has maintained chaplains and physicians as inseparable in its institutions.

Medical and Surgical Interventions

Adventists operate one of the world's largest religiously operated health systems, including a medical school. The **Health Ministries** include 142 hospitals and sanitariums worldwide, with 68 in the United States. Worldwide, there are also 16 nursing home/rehabilitation sites and 27 senior living centers. Worldwide, there are many clinics and dispensaries, orphanages and children's homes, as well as a number of airplanes and medical launches. Physical medicine and rehabilitation are emphasized and recommended, along

with therapeutic diets. There are no restrictions on the use of vaccines. Similarly, there are no restrictions on the use of blood and blood products, amputations, organ transplants, donation of organs, biopsies, and circumcisions (Extending Christ's Ministry, n.d.).

The Seventh-Day Adventist church is opposed to the use of hypnotism in the practice of medicine or under any other circumstance. Clinical implications for psychotherapy from the Seventh-Day Adventist tradition have been addressed by faculty from Loma Linda University School of Medicine (Fayard et al., 2007).

Practices Related to Reproduction

The use of birth control is an individual decision; the church prohibits cohabitation except between husband and wife. There are no restrictions on amniocentesis. Therapeutic abortion is acceptable if the mother's life is in danger and in cases of rape and incest. On-demand abortion is unacceptable because Adventists believe in the sanctity of life. Artificial insemination between husband and wife is acceptable. Although the church views practices in the fields of eugenics and genetics as an individual decision, it upholds the principle of responsibility in dealing with children.

Religious Support System for the Sick

At the request of the sick person or the family, the pastor and elders of the church will come together to pray and anoint the sick person with oil. The religious representative is referred to as Doctor, Pastor, or Elder.

Practices Related to Death and Dying

Although there is no official position, the church has traditionally followed the medical ethics of prolonging life and prohibiting euthanasia. Autopsy and the donation of the entire body or parts are acceptable. No directives or recommendations exist regarding disposal of the body. No specific directives concerning burial exist; this is an individual decision (Johnsson, 2013).

Unitarian Universalist Church

Worldwide, Unitarian Universalist membership is 800,000, with a North American membership of 208,177 (Unitarian Universalist Membership Statistics, 2012).

General Beliefs and Religious Practices

Unitarianism was officially organized in 1774 in England. This organization occurred after a long history of debate and dissension regarding the nature of God, particularly regarding the Trinitarian concept, which existed in various forms in the Catholic and Protestant religions. The Unitarian Universalist Association is the modern institutional embodiment of two separate denominations that grew out of movements and faith traditions extending back to the Christian Reformation era (14th to 16th century CE). Universalist convictions include the belief that all creation will ultimately be drawn back to its divine source and that no person or thing would be ultimately and forever excluded. The Unitarian conviction is reflected in the belief that God is ultimately and absolutely one.

Holy Days, Rites, and Rituals

No religious holy days are celebrated. Members come from various cultural and religious backgrounds and observe special days according to their own heritage and desire.

Typical milestones of life, including birth, marriage, and death, may be celebrated religiously. Although it is uncommon, puberty and divorce may also include religious observances.

Baptism of infants and occasionally of adults is sometimes performed as a symbolic act of dedication. The Lord's Supper is administered in some congregations.

Diet and Substance Use

No restrictions on diet exist. Substances should be used according to reason.

Health Care Practices

Faith healing is considered largely superstitious and wishful thinking. Members believe in the use

of the empirical method, reason, and science to facilitate healing.

Medical and Surgical Interventions

The use of medications is not restricted. The use of blood and blood products is similarly not restricted. Amputations, organ transplants, and biopsies are not restricted. Circumcision is viewed as a health practice, not a religious one.

Practices Related to Reproduction

Unitarian Universalists strongly favor all types of birth control as a human right. Both therapeutic and on-demand abortions are acceptable. Members strongly favor the right of the woman to decide. Amniocentesis is not restricted and is encouraged if medical evaluation deems it necessary. Sterility testing is acceptable; in fact, more research is encouraged. Both donation and receipt of artificial insemination are acceptable and strongly favored as a human right.

Practices Related to Death and Dying

Members favor the right to die with dignity— meaning to die without pain and in the care of those who love and care for them. Personhood is sacred, not the spark of life. Members tend to favor nonaction, including withdrawal of technical aids when death is imminent or when the patient has made a written request in advance, such as a durable power of attorney for health care. Autopsy is recommended. The donation of the body is acceptable. Cremation is most common. Donation to a medical school for study is not uncommon. Burial of a fetus is rare. A memorial service in the church or at home without the body present is customary.

Summary

Religious and cultural beliefs are interwoven and influence a client's understanding of illness and health care practices. In times of serious illness and death, religion may be a source of consolation for the client. Five dimensions of religion influence human behavior, including health-related practices. The goal of spiritual nursing care is to assist clients in integrating their own religious and spiritual beliefs into the ultimate reality that gives meaning to their lives in relation to the health care crisis that has precipitated the need for nursing care. For the nurse providing spiritual nursing care, issues related to death and dying are of particular importance. Health-related beliefs and practices of select religions are important to understand, especially considering the diverse religious groups in the United States and Canada.

REVIEW QUESTIONS

1. When assessing the spiritual needs of clients from diverse cultural backgrounds, what key components should you consider?
2. In providing nursing care for the dying or bereaved client and family, what cultural considerations should the nurse include in the plan?
3. Compare and contrast the religious beliefs and practices concerning diet, medications, and procedures for five of the religious groups discussed in this chapter.
4. Analyze the contributions of religious organizations to the United States and/or Canadian health care delivery system. What effect do health care facilities that are owned and operated by religious groups have on the overall cost and quality of health care in the United States and Canada? Critically analyze concerns about these religiously operated facilities in terms of philosophical, ethical, and legal aspects pertaining to types of services offered to patients.
5. What religious rituals mark significant developmental milestones for children and adolescents? Identify the ritual or ceremony, the approximate age at which the child or adolescent participates in it, and the name of the religion(s) associated with it.

CRITICAL THINKING ACTIVITIES

1. Visit a church or worship center not of your own belief system, and interview a member of the clergy or an official representative about the health-related beliefs of that religion. Discuss with him or her the implications of those beliefs for someone hospitalized for an acute or chronic illness. Inquire about the ways in which nurses can be of most help to hospitalized members of this religion.

2. Interview members of various religions concerning their beliefs about health and illness. Compare these interviews with the published beliefs or official statements from these religions. Discuss the implications of the differences (if any) that you found.

3. Interview fellow students, classmates, or coworkers about what they know of the health beliefs of various religions, especially those religions most often encountered among the patients with whom you work. Make a poster or prepare a presentation comparing the results of your interviews with the official beliefs of those religions. Share this information with your classmates.

4. Interview four or more members of the same religious group who are of various ages (i.e., children, teenagers, young adults, middle aged, and elderly). Ask them about their religious beliefs and how they affect their health. Compare the results, commenting on similarities and differences.

5. Explore the meaning of various unique items of clothing worn by members of different religions.

6. If you have thought about the above exercises in terms of physical health, consider each of the activities from the perspective of mental health and spiritual health.

REFERENCES

American Indians by Numbers. (n.d.). Retrieved from http://www.infoplease.com/spot/aihmcensus1.html

Andrews, J. D. (2013). *Cultural, ethnic and religious reference manual for healthcare providers* (4th ed.). Kernersville, NC: JARARDA Resources, Inc.

As US Struggles with Health Care reform, Amish go their own way. (October 5, 2013). Retrieved from: http://www.reuters.com/article/2013/10/05/usa-healthcare-amish-idUSL1N0HR1IV20131005

Bhattacharyya, A. (2013). Hinduism. In S. L. Jeffers, M. E Nelson, V. Barnet, & M. C. Brannigan (Eds.), *The essential guide to religious traditions and spirituality for health care providers*. New York, NY: Radcliffe.

Buddhism Canada on-the-move. (n.d.). Retrieved from http://buddhismcanada.com/

Buddhist Churches of America. (n.d.). Retrieved from http://buddhistchurchesofamerica.org/

Catholic Charities USA. (n.d.). Retrieved from https://support.catholiccharitiesusa.org/p/salsa/donation/common/public/?donate_page_KEY=9113&iq_id=69647056-VQ6-59488489107-VQ16-c

Catholic health care in the United States. (2014). Retrieved from http://www.chausa.org/docs/default-source/general-files/cha_miniprofile_final.pdf?sfvrsn=0

Cates, J. A. (2014). *Serving the amish*. Baltimore, MD: Johns Hopkins University Press.

Carlson, R. J. (2013). Mennonites. In S. L. Jeffers, M. E. Nelson, V. Barnet, & M. C. Brannigan (eds.). *The essential guide to religious traditions and spirituality for health care providers*. New York, NY: Radcliffe.

Church of Christ, Scientist. (n.d.) Retrieved from http://www.religionfacts.com/a-z-religion-index/christian_science.htm

Christian Science Fast Facts. (n.d.). Retrieved from http://www.religionfacts.com/a-z-religion-index/christian_science.htm

Committee on Publication. (2013). Christian science. In S. L. Jeffers, M. E. Nelson, V. Barnet, & M. C. Brannigan (Eds.), *The essential guide to religious traditions and spirituality for health care providers*. New York, NY: Radcliffe.

Daly, L., & Fahey-McCarthy, E. (2014). Attending to the spiritual in dementia care nursing. *British Journal of Nursing*, 23(14), 788–791.

Donnermeyer, J. F. (1997). Amish society: An overview. *The Journal of Multicultural Nursing and Health*, 3(2), 6–12.

Dysinger, L. (2012). Roman Catholics. In E. J. Taylor (Ed.), *Religion: A clinical guide for nurses*. New York, NY: Springer Publishing.

Ebersole, P., Hess, P., & Luggan, A. S. (2008). *Toward healthy aging* (6th ed.). St. Louis, MO: C.V. Mosby.

Extending Christ's Ministry. (n.d.). Retrieved from http://pew-forum.org/docs; http://www.pewforum.org/2012/10/09/nones-on-the-rise-religion/

Faulkner, J.E. & DeJong, C.F. (1966). Religiosity in 5D: An empirical analysis. *Social Forces*, 45, 246–254.

Fayard, C., Harding, G., Murdoch, W., & Brunt, J. (2007). Clinical implications for psychotherapy from the Seventh-day Adventist tradition. *Journal of Psychology and Christianity*, 26(2), 207–217.

Friedman, D. A. (2013). *Jewish pastoral care: A practical handbook from traditional and contemporary sources* (2nd ed.). Woodstock, VT: Jewish Lights Publishing.

Graham, L. I., & Cates, J. A. (2013). Amish. In S. L. Jeffers, M. E. Nelson, V. Barnet, & M. C. Brannigan (Eds.), *The Essential guide to religious traditions and spirituality for health care providers*. New York, NY: Radcliffe.

Gober, C., & Kim, R. (2010). American Indian religions. In S. Sorajjakool, M. F. Carr, & J. L. Nam (Eds.), *World religions for healthcare professionals*.

Hattori, K., & Ishid, D. N. (2012). Ethnographic study of good death among elderly Japanese Americans. *Nursing & Health Sciences*, 14, 488–494.

How many Catholics are there in the world? (2013). Retrieved from http://www.bbc.com/news/world-21443313

How many Hindus are there in the world? (n.d.). Retrieved from http://www.religioustolerance.org/hinduism5.htm

Interesting Jehovah's Witness statistics. (n.d.). Retrieved from http://www.adherents.com/largecom/com_jw.html

Jeffers, S. L., Nelson, M. E., Barnet, V., & Brannigan, M. C. (Eds.) (2013). *The essential guide to religious traditions and spirituality for health care providers*. London, UK: Radcliffe Publishing Ltd.

Jehovah's Witness official Web site. (n.d.). Retrieved from http://www.jw.org/en/

Jett, K., & Touhy, T. (2010). *Ebersole and Hess' gerontological nursing and healthy aging*. St. Louis, MO: Mosby.

Jewish Healthcare Foundation. (n.d.). Retrieved from http://www.jhf.org/

Johnsson, W. G. (2013). Seventh-day adventist church. In S. L. Jeffers, M. E. Nelson, V. Barnet, & M. C. Brannigan (Eds.), *The essential guide to religious traditions and spirituality for health care providers*. New York, NY: Radcliffe.

Kalish, R. A., & Reynolds, D. K. (1981). *Death and ethnicity: A psychocultural study*. New York, NY: Baywood.

Katz, A. W. (2013). Judaism. In S. L. Jeffers, M. E. Nelson, V. Barnet, & M. C. Brannigan (Eds.), *The essential guide to religious traditions and spirituality for health care providers*. New York, NY: Radcliffe.

Kisvetrova, H., Klugar, M, & Kableka, L. (2013). Spiritual support interventions in nursing care for patients suffering death anxiety in the final stage of life. *International Journal of Palliative Nursing*, 19(12), 599–605.

Kraybill, D. B. (2014). Opting out: How the Amish have survived in America. *Commonweal, March 7*, 13–17.

Leonard, B., & Carlson, D. (2010). Spirituality in health care. Accessed on February 17, 2010 at www.csh.umn.edu/modules/spirituality

Leyvam B, Allen, J. D., Tom, L. S., Ospino, H., Torres, M. I., & Abraido-Laza, A. F. (2014). Religion, fatalism and cancer control: A qualitative study among Hispanic Catholics. *American Journal of Health Behavior*, 38(6), 839–849.

Major branches of religions ranked by number of adherents. (n.d.). Retrieved from http://www.adherents.com/adh_branches.html

McAteen, B., & Edalati, D. (2013). Baha'I Faith. In S. L. Jeffers, M. E. Nelson, V. Barnet, & M. C. Brannigan (Eds.), *The essential guide to religious traditions and spirituality for health care providers*. Totton Hants, UK: Hobbs & Printers.

McIntyre, A. J. (2008). *The Tohono O'odham and Pimeria Alta*. Chicago, IL: Arcadia Publishing.

Mennonite Church USA and Worldwide. (n.d.). Retrieved from http://www.mcusa-archives.org/resources/membership.html

Number of adherents of major religions. (n.d.). Retrieved from http://www.religioustolerance.org/worldrel.htm

Number of buddhists worldwide. (n.d.). Retrieved from: http://www.buddhanet.net/e-learning/history/bud_statwrld.htm

Oklevueha: Native American Church. (n.d.). Retrieved from: http://nativeamericanchurches.org/

Oliver, I. N., & Dutney, A. (2012). A randomized, blinded study of the impact of intercessory prayer on spiritual well-being in patients with cancer. *Alternative Therapies*, 18(5), 18–27.

Orlich, M. J., & Fraser, G. E. (2014). Vegetarian diets in the Adventist health study 2: A review of initial published findings. *American Journal of Clinical Nutrition, 1000* (Suppl):353S–358S.

Pattison, S. (2013). Religion, spirituality and health care: Confusions, tensions, opportunities. *Health Care Analysis, 21*, 193–207. doi: 10.1007/s10728-013-0245-4

Pellechia, J. N. (2013). Jehovah's witnesses. In S. L. Jeffers., M. E. Nelson, V. Barnet, & M. C. Brannigan (Eds.), *The essential guide to religious traditions and spirituality for health care providers*. New York, NY: Radcliffe.

Raffay, J. (2014). How staff and patient experience shapes our perception of spiritual care in a psychiatric setting. *Journal of Nursing Management, 22*(7), 940–950.

Ramezani, M., Ahmadi, F., Mohammed, E., & Kazemnejad, A. (2014). Spiritual care in nursing: A concept analysis. *International Nursing Review, 61*(2), 211–219.

Rauf Mir, A., & Qazwini, H. (Imam). (2013). Islam. In S. L. Jeffers, M. E. Nelson, V. Barnet, & M. C. Brannigan (Eds.), *The essential guide to religious traditions and spirituality for health care providers*. New York, NY: Radcliffe.

Salman, K. F. (2012). Health beliefs and practices related to cancer screening among Arab Muslim Women in an urban community. *Health Care for Women International, 33*, 45–74.

Sharpnack, P. A., Griffin, M. T., Benders, A. M., & Fitzpatrick, J. J.. (2010). Spiritual and alternative healthcare practices of the Amish. *Holistic Nursing Practice, 24*(2), 64–72.

Seventh Day Adventist Statistics. (2012). Retrieved from http://www.adventist.org/information/statistics/article/go/0/seventh-day-adventist-world-church-statistics-2012/

Sherwen, E. (2014). Improving end of life care for adults. *Nursing Standard, 28*(32), 51–57.

Sorajjakool, S., Carr, M. F., & Nam, J. J. (Eds.) (2010). *World religions for healthcare professionals.* New York, NY: Routledge.

Sorajjakool, S., & Naewbood, S. (2010). Buddhism. In S. Sorajjakool, M. F. Carr, & J. J. Nam (Eds.), *World religions for healthcare professionals.* New York, NY: Routledge.

Spencer, J. L. (2013). Roman catholicism. In S. L. Jeffers, M. E. Nelson, V. Barnet, & M. C. Brannigan (Eds.), *The essential guide to religious traditions and spirituality for health care providers.* New York, NY: Radcliffe.

Standard FAQ details. (2008). Retrieved from http://www.jointcommission.org/standards_information/jcfaqdetails.aspx?StandardsFAQId=290

Stanford, C. (2013). Buddhism: General introduction. In S. L. Jeffers, M. E. Nelson, V. Barnet, & M. C. Brannigan (Eds.), *The essential guide to religious traditions and spirituality for health care providers.* New York, NY: Radcliffe.

Taylor, E. J. (Ed.) (2012). *Religion: A clinical guide for nurses.* New York, NY: Springer Publishing.

The Public Affairs Department of the Church of Jesus Christ of Latter Day Saints. (2013). In S. L. Jeffers, M. E. Nelson, V. Barnet, & M. C. Brannigan (Eds.), *The essential guide to religious traditions and spirituality for health care providers.* New York, NY: Radcliffe.

Toneatto, T. (2012). Buddhists. In E. J. Taylor (Ed.), *Religion: a clinical guide for nurses.* New York, NY: Springer Publishing.

Top, B. L. & Callister, L. (2012). Latter-day saints (Mormons). In E. J. Taylor (ed.), *Religion: A clinical guide for nurses.* New York, NY: Springer.

Top 10 Largest International Bodies. (n.d.). Retrieved from: http://www.adherents.com/adh_rb.html#International.

Touhy, T. A., & Jett, K. F. (2011). *Ebersole & Hess' toward healthy aging: Human needs and nursing response* (8th ed.). St. Louis, MO: Mosby.

Tuell, R. S. (2011). *Islamic approaches to patient care.* Beltsville, MD: Amana Publications.

Unitarian Universalist Membership Statistics. (2012). Retrieved from http://www.uua.org/directory/data/demographics/281427.shtml

Vital Statistics: Jewish Population in the World. (2012). Retrieved from https://www.jewishvirtuallibrary.org/jsource/Judaism/jewpop.html

What do Mormons believe? (n.d.). Retrieved from http://beta.mormon.org/mormon101/detail/prayer.php#d

World's Muslim population is more widespread than you think. (June 7, 2013). Retrieved from http://www.pewresearch.org/fact-tank/2013/06/07/worlds-muslim-population-more-widespread-than-you-might-think/

Wynne, L. (2013). Spiritual care at the end of life. *Nursing Standard, 28*(2), 41–45.

Yurkovick, E. E., & Lattergrass, I. (2008). Defining health and unhealthiness: Perceptions held by Native Americans with persistent mental illness. *Mental Health, Religion and Culture, 11*(5), 437–459.

Andrews/Boyle Transcultural Nursing Assessment Guide for Individuals and Families

Joyceen S. Boyle and Margaret M. Andrews

Biocultural Variations and Cultural Aspects of the Incidence of Disease

- Does the client and/or family members relate a health history associated with genetic or acquired conditions that are more prevalent for a specific cultural group (e.g., diabetes, hypertension, cardiovascular disease, sickle cell anemia, Tay–Sachs disease, G-6-PD deficiency, lactose intolerance)? Does the client's family relate such a history?
- Are there socioenvironmental conditions more prevalent among a specific cultural group that can be observed in the client or family members (e.g., lead poisoning, alcoholism, HIV/AIDS, drug abuse, ear infections, family violence, fetal alcohol spectrum disorder [FASD], obesity, respiratory diseases)?
- Are there diseases against which the client has an increased resistance (e.g., skin cancer in darkly pigmented individuals, malaria for those with sickle cell anemia)?
- Does the client have distinctive features characteristic of a particular ethnic or cultural group (e.g., skin color, hair texture)? Do his or her family members have such features? Within the family group, are there variations in anatomy characteristic of a particular ethnic or cultural group (e.g., body structure, height, weight, facial shape and structure [nose, eye shape, facial contour], upper and lower extremities)?
- How do anatomic, racial, and ethnic variations affect the physical and mental examination?

Communication

- What language does the client speak at home with family members? In what language would the client prefer to communicate with you? What other languages does the client speak or read? What other languages do the client's family members speak or read?
- What is the fluency level of the client in English—both written and spoken? What is the fluency level of the client's family members?
- Does the client need an interpreter? Do his or her family members need an interpreter? Does the health care setting provide interpreters? Who would the client and his or her family members prefer to assist with interpretation? Is there anyone whom the client would prefer not to serve as an interpreter (e.g., member of the opposite sex, person younger or older than the client, member of a rival tribe, ethnic group, or nationality)?
- If the client is hearing or visually impaired, how does he or she communicate? Are any assistive devices used to foster communication and/or ensure the client's safety?
- What are the rules and style (formal or informal) of communication? If the client is hearing impaired and requires someone who knows sign language, how will arrangements be made? If the client is blind and requires that communications be made available in braille, how will that be accomplished? How much time will it take to provide the resources needed for hearing and visually impaired clients? How does the client prefer to be addressed? What do his

or her family members prefer? What are the preferred terms for greeting?

- How is it necessary to vary the technique and style of communication during the relationship with the client to accommodate his or her cultural background (e.g., tempo of conversation, eye contact, sensitivity to topical taboos, norms of confidentiality, and style of explanation)? How do these factors vary with family members, if at all?
- What are the styles of individual and family members' nonverbal communication?
- How does the client's nonverbal communication compare with that of individuals from other cultural groups? How does the client's style of nonverbal communication differ from the health care provider's style? How does it affect the client's relationships with you and with other members of the health care team? How does communication with the family influence the care environment?
- How do the client and family members feel about health care providers who are not of the same cultural or religious background (e.g., Black, middle-class nurse; Hispanic of a different social class; Muslim or Jewish care provider)? Does the client prefer to receive care from a nurse of the same cultural background, gender, and/or age? How do family members react to care providers of different cultural backgrounds, age, and gender?

Cultural Affiliations

- With what cultural group(s) does the client report affiliation (e.g., American, Hispanic, Irish, Black, Navajo, American Indian, or combination)? It is becoming increasingly common for Americans to identify with two or more groups, such as Native American and African American. Equally important, to what degree does the client identify with the cultural group (e.g., "we" concept of solidarity or as a fringe member)?
- How do the views of other family members coincide with or differ from those of the client regarding cultural affiliations?

- What is the preferred term that the cultural group chooses for itself? What term does the client choose?
- Where was the client born? Where were his or her parents born? What are the generational similarities and differences in regard to cultural identification, language, customs, values, and so on?
- Where has the client lived (country, city, or area within a country) and when (during what years of his or her life)? If the client has recently immigrated to the United States from another country, knowledge of prevalent diseases in his or her country of origin as well as sociopolitical history may be helpful. If the client is a recent immigrant, did he or she live in countries of transit? For how long? Current residence? Occupation? Occupation in home country?

Cultural Sanctions and Restrictions

- How does the client's cultural group regard expression of emotion and feelings, spirituality, and religious beliefs? How are feelings related to dying, death, and grieving expressed in a culturally appropriate manner?
- How do men and women express modesty? Are there culturally defined expectations about male–female relationships, including the nurse–client relationship?
- Does the client or family express any restrictions related to sexuality, exposure of various parts of the body, or certain types of surgery (e.g., vasectomy, hysterectomy, abortion)?
- Are there restrictions against discussion of dead relatives or fears related to the unknown?

Developmental Considerations

- Are there any distinct growth and development characteristics that vary with the cultural background of the client and family (e.g., bone density, psychomotor patterns of development, fat folds)?
- What factors are significant in assessing children of various ages from the newborn period through adolescence (e.g., male circumcision, female genital mutilation [FGM], expected

growth on standards grid, culturally acceptable age for toilet training, duration of breastfeeding, introduction of various types of foods, gender differences, discipline, and socialization to adult roles)?

- What are the beliefs and practices associated with developmental life events such as pregnancy, birth, puberty, marriage, and death?
- What is the cultural perception of aging (e.g., is youthfulness or the wisdom of old age more valued)?
- How are elderly persons cared for within the cultural group (e.g., cared for in the home of adult children, placed in institutions for care)? What are culturally accepted roles for the elderly?

Economics

- Who is the principal wage earner in the family and what is the income level? Is there more than one wage earner? Are there other sources of financial support? (*Note:* These may be potentially sensitive questions.)
- What insurance coverage does the client and his or her family have? Does the client and/or family members understand the terms/rates/coverage of their health insurance policies?
- What impact does the economic status have on the client and his or her family's lifestyle and living conditions?
- What has been the client and family's experience with the health care system in terms of reimbursement, costs, and insurance coverage?

Educational Background

- What is the client's highest educational level obtained? What values do the family members express regarding educational achievements?
- Does the client's educational level affect his or her knowledge level concerning his or her health literacy—how to obtain the needed care, teaching related to or learning about health care, and any written material that he or she is given in the health care setting (e.g., insurance forms, educational literature, information

about diagnostic procedures and laboratory tests, admissions forms, etc.)? Does the client's educational level affect health behavior? As an example, in the United States, cigarette smoking and obesity have been linked to socioeconomic levels.

- What learning style is most comfortable and familiar? Does the client prefer to learn through written materials, oral explanations, videos, and/ or demonstrations?
- Does the client access health information via the Internet or use social media as a source of health-related information?
- Do the client and family members prefer intervention settings away from hospitals and other clients, which may have negative connotations for them? Are community sites such as churches, schools, or adult day care centers a good alternate choice for the client and his or her family, considering they are informal settings that may be more conducive for open discussion, demonstrations, and reinforcement of information and skills? Are the client and family more comfortable in their home setting?

Health-Related Beliefs and Practices

- To what cause does the client attribute illness and disease or what factors influence the acquisition of illness and disease (e.g., divine wrath, imbalance in hot/cold, yin/yang, punishment for moral transgressions, a hex, soul loss, pathogenic organism, past behavior, growing older)? Is there congruence within the family on these beliefs?
- What are the client's cultural beliefs about ideal body size and shape? What is the client's self-image in relation to the ideal?
- How does the client describe his or her health-related condition? What names or terms are used? How does the client express pain, discomfort, depression, or anxiety? In some cultures, clients may somaticize their emotional feelings, for example, "My heart hurts" rather than say, "I'm feeling sad or depressed about my physical condition."

- What do the client and family members believe promotes health (e.g., eating certain foods, wearing amulets to bring good luck, sleeping, resting, getting good nutrition, reducing stress, exercising, praying or performing rituals to ancestors, saints, or other deities)?
- What is the client's religious affiliation? How is the client actively involved in the practice of religion? Do other family members have the same religious beliefs and practices? Do the client and/or family members incorporate religious practices, such as healing ceremonies or prayer, into health/illness care?
- Do the client and his or her family rely on cultural healers (e.g., curandero, shaman, spiritualist, priest, medicine man or woman, minister)? Who determines when the client is sick and when he or she is healthy? Who influences the choice or type of healer and treatment that should be sought?
- In what types of cultural healing or health-promoting practices does the client engage (e.g., use of herbal remedies, potions, or massage; wearing of talismans, copper bracelets, or chains to discourage evil spirits; healing rituals; incantations; or prayers)? Do family members share these beliefs and practices?
- How are biomedical health care providers perceived? How do the client and his or her family perceive nurses? What are the expectations of nurses and nursing care workers?
- Who will care for the client at home? What accommodations will family members make to provide caregiving?
- How does the client's family and cultural group view mental disorders? Are there differences in acceptable behaviors for physical versus psychological illnesses?

Kinship and Social Networks

- What is the composition of a "typical family" within the kinship network? What is the composition of the client's family?
- Who makes up the client's social network (family, friends, peers, neighbors)? How do they influence the client's health or illness status?

- How do members of the client's social support network define caring or caregiving? What is the role of various family members during health and illness episodes? Who makes decisions about health and health care?
- How does the client's family participate in the promotion of health (e.g., lifestyle changes in diet, activity level, etc.) and nursing care (e.g., bathing, feeding, touching, being present) of the client?
- Does the cultural family structure influence the client's response to health or illness (e.g., beliefs, strengths, weaknesses, and social class)?
- What influence do ethnic, cultural, and/or religious organizations have on the lifestyle and quality of life of the client (e.g., the National Association for the Advancement of Colored People [NAACP], churches, such as African American, Muslim, Jewish, Catholic, and others, that may provide schools, classes, and/or community-based health care programs)?
- Are there special gender issues within this cultural group? Do the client and family members conform to traditional roles (e.g., women may be viewed as the caretakers of home and children, while men work outside the home and have primary decision-making responsibilities)?

Nutrition

- What nutritional factors are influenced by the client's cultural background? What is the meaning of food and eating to the client and his or her family?
- Does the client have any eating or nutritional disorders (e.g., anorexia, bulimia, obesity, lactose intolerance)? Do the client's family members have any similar disorders? How do the client and family view these conditions?
- With whom does the client usually eat? What types of foods are eaten? What is the timing and sequencing of meals? What are the usual meal patterns?

- What does the client define as food? What does the client believe constitutes a "healthy" versus an "unhealthy" diet? Are these beliefs congruent with what the client actually eats?
- Who shops for and chooses food? Where are the foodstuffs purchased? Who prepares the actual meals? How are the family members involved in nutritional choices, values, and choices about food?
- How are the foods prepared at home (type of food preparation, cooking oil[s] used, length of time foods are cooked [especially vegetables], amount and type of seasoning added to various foods during preparation)? Who does the food preparation?
- Has the client chosen a particular nutritional practice such as vegetarianism or abstinence from red meat or from alcoholic or fermented beverages? Do other family members adhere to these beliefs and practices?
- Do religious beliefs and practices influence the client's or family's diet (e.g., amount, type, preparation, or delineation of acceptable food combinations [e.g., kosher diets])? Does the client or client's family abstain from certain foods at regular intervals, on specific dates determined by the religious calendar, or at other times? Are there other food prohibitions or prescriptions?
- If the client or client's family's religion mandates or encourages fasting, what does the term *fast* mean (e.g., refraining from certain types of foods, eating only during certain times of the day, skipping certain meals)? For what period of time are family members expected to fast? Are there exceptions to fasting (e.g., are pregnant women or children excluded from fasting)?
- Are special utensils used (e.g., chopsticks, cookware, kosher restrictions)?
- Does the client or client's family use home and folk remedies to treat illnesses (e.g., herbal remedies, acupuncture, cupping, or other healing rituals often involving eggs, lemons, candles)? Which over-the-counter medications are used?

Religion and Spirituality

- How does the client or family's religious affiliation affect health and illness (e.g., life events such as death, chronic illness, body image alteration, cause and effect of illness)?
- What is the role of religious beliefs and practices during health and illness? Are there special rites or blessings for those with serious or terminal illnesses?
- Are there healing rituals or practices that the client and family believe can promote well-being or hasten recovery from illness? If so, who performs these? What materials or arrangements are necessary for the nurse to have available for the practice of these rituals?
- What is the role of significant religious representatives during health and illness? Are there recognized religious healers (e.g., Islamic Imams, Christian Scientist practitioners or nurses, Catholic priests, Mormon elders, Buddhist monks)?

Values Orientation

- What are the client's attitudes, values, and beliefs about his or her health and illness status? Do family members have similar values and beliefs?
- How do these influence behavior in terms of promotion of health and treatment of disease? What are the client's or family's attitudes, values, and beliefs about health care providers?
- Does culture affect the manner in which the client relates to body image change resulting from illness or surgery (e.g., importance of appearance, beauty, strength, and roles in the cultural group)? Is there a cultural stigma associated with the client's illness (i.e., how is the illness or the manner in which it was contracted viewed by the family and larger culture)?
- How do the client and his or her family view work, leisure, and education?
- How does the client perceive and react to change?

- How do the client and his or her family perceive changes in lifestyle related to current illness or surgery?
- How do the client and his/her family view biomedical health care (e.g., suspiciously, fearfully, acceptingly, unquestioningly, with awe)?

- How does the client value privacy, courtesy, touch, and relationships with others?
- How does the client relate to persons outside of his or her cultural group (e.g., withdrawal, suspicion, curiosity, openness)?

Andrews/Boyle Transcultural Nursing Assessment Guide for Families, Groups, and Communities

● Joyceen S. Boyle and Margaret M. Andrews

Family and Kinship Systems

- Are the families nuclear, extended, or blended? Do family members live in close proximity? What are communication patterns within the distinct community groups? What is the role and status of individual family members? By age and gender?
- How do the family and/or group members relate to the larger community or groups?
- Are there distinct neighborhoods or areas of the community where distinct cultural, ethnic or religious groups, refugees, or immigrants live?
- If working with a refugee community, ask about names of tribes and/or clans.
- What place do the "ancestors" have in the worldview of the group? How is the belief in the power of the ancestors incorporated in the daily life and rituals of the group?
- Is the group now or has it traditionally been matriarchal or patriarchal? Is there a preference for first cousins to marry? Who is permitted to marry whom among those who are related by blood/genetics?

Social Life and Networks

- What are the daily routines of the group? What are the important life cycle events such as birth, marriage, family bearing, family rearing, and death? How are they celebrated or observed?
- How are the educational systems organized? How do they receive and accept input from the community? How do they assist students and their families who are new immigrants or refugees?
- What are the social problems experienced by the group within the community or by the community itself?
- Are there special concerns with a particular ethnic or cultural group such as abuse of alcohol, FASD, gang membership, and polygamy? How does the group view domestic violence and corporal punishment?
- Are newly arrived groups, such as immigrants or refugees, included within the local community or isolated? Who are the group's local leaders?
- Are there centers or organizations that reach out to special groups within the community? What activities or opportunities are available to community members? For example, are General Educational Development (GED) courses, English as a second language classes, and/or work training available to newcomers?
- How does the social environment contribute to a sense of belonging? Do all members of the group belong to a distinct religious group? What are the ways that the group practices its religion? What are the dominant religious groups within the community?
- What are the group's social interaction patterns? Do all members of the group speak a common language?
- Are ethnic grocery stores, restaurants, and churches located within the community?

What foods do members of the cultural group commonly eat? What foods/substances do they commonly avoid (i.e., alcohol, pork products)?

- Are members of the group comfortable moving away from the larger group?
- Where are ethnic groups, immigrants, or refugees located within the larger community?

Political or Government Systems

- Which factors in the political system influence the ways in which the group perceives its status vis-à-vis the dominant culture, that is, laws, justice, and cultural heroes?
- How does the economic system influence control of resources such as land, water, housing, education and technical training, jobs, and opportunities?
- What is the legal status of the group members? Refugee or immigrant visas? Temporary worker permits? Documented or undocumented?
- How does the local government respond to the ethnic and cultural makeup of the group? What are the ways that the local community "embraces its diversity"?

Language and Traditions

- Are there differences in dialects or languages spoken between health care professionals and local groups within the community?
- What is the literacy level of members of the group? Can they read or write in any language(s)?
- Do health care facilities provide educational materials in diverse languages?
- In what ways do the major cultural traditions of history, art, drama, and so on, influence the cultural identity of the group?
- How are local cultures or ethnic traditions embraced during holidays or special celebrations?

Worldviews, Value Orientations, and Cultural Norms

- What are the major cultural values about the relationships of cultural groups to nature and to one another? How can the group's ethical beliefs be described?
- What are the norms and standards of behavior (authority, responsibility, dependability, and competition)?
- Is the group communal or individualistic? How different is their worldview from the dominant worldview of the larger society or culture?
- What are the cultural attitudes about time, family, hospitality, family work, and leisure?
- What are the common values of the group, such as education, work, and so on?
- How are the cultural values reflected in factors such as dress? Do the women cover their hair? Do they prefer skirts or dresses over pants or trousers?
- Are there unique cultural practices within the group that might bring wider community censure, such as the role of women, discipline of children, and relationships between husband and wife?

Religious Beliefs and Practices

- What are the major religious beliefs and practices within the community?
- How do they influence daily life? How do they relate to health practices? What are the practices surrounding major life events such as birth, marriage, and death?
- Does the cultural group have particular practices related to grieving or mourning?

Health Beliefs and Practices

- What are the group's attitudes and beliefs regarding health and illness? Does the cultural group seek care from indigenous (folk) practitioners? Where do group members go to seek care? Who makes the decisions about seeking health care? Accepting treatments? Are there biologic variations that are important to the health of this group? What are the group's expressed health concerns? Are there cultural or ethnic stores in neighborhoods selling medicinal herbs?

- What are the primary health concerns and/or illnesses in this population/cultural group (e.g., malaria, HIV/AIDS, female genital mutilation [FGM], malnutrition, tuberculosis)? How do the group's concerns align with those of the local and state health care systems?

Health Care Systems

- Do community health care facilities provide interpreters? Do physician offices and other health care facilities offer educational materials in languages other than English? Are health facilities located in accessible locations, that is, in ethnic neighborhoods? Do health care providers incorporate aspects of other health care systems, for example, acupuncture and referrals to traditional healers?
- Do members of the group have access to health care? Do they have adequate transportation?

Are the hours of operation of health care facilities and availability of appointment times appropriate for members of the group?

Economic Factors

- Does the group or community own or operate its own clinic, neighborhood health center, child or adult day care center, long-term care facility, or nursing home? How will the group or community pay for health care services?
- Is there a group health care policy on all members? Will key leaders in the community work with members to collectively pay for health care services? For example, although the Amish religious leaders have no health insurance, members pool their resources and often settle a hospital bill in cash at the time of the client's discharge.

Andrews/Boyle Transcultural Nursing Assessment Guide for Health Care Organizations and Facilities

Joyceen S. Boyle, Margaret M. Andrews, and Patti Ludwig-Beymer

Physical Environment

- What is the general environment of the community that surrounds the health care organization? Where is the facility located in proximity to the population that it serves?
- What is the socioeconomic status of the adjacent community? What are race/ethnicity characteristics of residents? What are the identified health disparities?
- What are the community's views on health and illness?
- Is there appropriate and easy access to the facility? Is the signage to the facility easy to understand and follow? Are there adequate parking facilities? Are bus routes nearby?
- Is there access to social services? Where are residential and business districts located? What are the sources of employment near the facility?
- Is there appropriate signage in diverse languages within the facility?
- What is the proximity to other health care facilities?

Language, Communication, and Ethnohistory

- What languages are spoken within the institution? By employees? By patients?
- How formal or informal are the lines of communication within the organization?
- Is the organizational governance hierarchical? What communication strategies are used within the organization?
- What is the history of the organization? What was the original mission of the organization? How does the history influence the current organization? How has it traditionally responded to change?

Technology

- How is technology used in the organization? Who uses it? Do all work stations have access to computers? Do all employees have access to email? Are electronic health records being used? Is new technology in place in the emergency department, critical care areas, labor and delivery, laboratory, and X-ray departments?

Religious/Philosophical Factors

- Does the institution have a religious affiliation? How is this shown in the decor of the institution? How does the religious affiliation influence the philosophy, values, and norms of the agency?
- Is the institution public or private? For profit or not-for-profit?
- Is the Patient's Bill of Rights prominently displayed within the institution? Are such documents displayed in languages to meet the needs of the community?

Social Factors

- What are the working relationships within nursing? Between nursing and ancillary services? Within each nursing unit? Between physicians and nurses? How closely are staff members aligned throughout the organization?
- Is the environment initially "warm and loving"? How do volunteers or staff members at the information desk behave? Do employees get together outside of work?
- Is there a hierarchal distance between ancillary staff, nurses, and administrators?
- How are family members welcomed (or not welcomed) to the unit? Is the waiting room comfortable? Reading materials? Are they appropriate for the visitors?
- Are there public telephones available? Vending machines?
- Is the signage adequate within the units and institution? Is the signage available in appropriate languages other than English? Can visitors easily find their way to a specific unit or room?
- How has the institution tried to be inclusive to visitors or patients?

Cultural Values

- Are values explicitly stated? What is valued within the institution? What is valued as "good" and "bad"? Is there a gap between stated values and what actually happens on a daily basis?
- Are interpreter services readily available? Translated medical literature and educational materials?
- How does the institution value and institutionalize culturally competent care?
- How does the institution recruit and retain minority staff members? How are personnel trained in cultural competencies?
- Is there coordination with traditional healers and use of community health workers?
- How does the organization respond to the community it serves (clinic hours, locations, physical environment, network memberships, and written materials)?
- How do the interior design, decor, and artwork reflect the cultural values of the institution and community at large?

Political/Legal Factors

- Where does the power rest within the institution? With the administration? With the physicians? With the business office? With nursing? Is power shared? How is power divided among competing groups? Is there an active board of directors? What are their responsibilities? What types of legal actions have been taken against the institution? On behalf of the institution?
- How do employees or staff have input? How does the institution encourage or value suggestions or contributions from staff? Is shared governance a value? How is it enacted?

Economic Factors

- What is the financial viability of the institution? Has this changed over the past 10 years? Who makes financial decisions? What values are the basis of financial decisions? How do the salaries and benefits compare with those of competitors in the immediate environment?

Education

- How is education valued within the institution? What type of assistance (financial, scheduling, flexibility) is provided for staff seeking advanced training or degrees? What opportunities are offered to those staff members who are earning advanced degrees? Does the institution pay baccalaureate-prepared nurses more than associate degree nurses?
- Does the institution provide clinical learning experiences for medicine, nursing, and other health professionals? How does the institution demonstrate that it values students?
- Are advanced practice nurses utilized? What is the educational background of staff nurses? Nurse managers? Nursing leaders? How does this compare with the educational levels of staff in competing institutions?

Components of a Cultural Assessment: Traditional Native American Healing

Joyceen S. Boyle

Worldview, Value Orientations, and Cultural Norms

In all Native American cultures, interactions on all levels contain the fundamental element of respect. Respect is how a person presents himself or herself to the world and how a person acts, and it is tied to being Native American. Respect is an essential element of the relationship between the healer and the client. No single Native American worldview or set of beliefs is shared by all Native Americans. However, most Native Americans share universal concepts that differ from those in European American culture.

For Native Americans in the southwest, acculturation is even more complex. Within any one tribe (e.g., Pascua Yaqui or Tohono O'odham), some members may be tribally identified. Others may be Mexican identified and speak primarily Spanish with Mexican traditions. Others may be American identified, speak English, and have a belief system based on the dominant white culture. Historical trauma has been identified as a risk for poor health outcomes in Native Americans. Strengthening native identity and encouraging enculturation (the understanding and valuing of one's own culture), spiritual practices, and traditional healing are positive coping strategies.

- Nature is more powerful than human beings.
- Individual success is not valued as highly as providing security and care to the extended family. Native Americans have a "collectivist culture" as opposed to the White American individualistic culture.
- The integrity of the individual must be respected. There is a respect for the decisions of others. Individuals usually consider the extended family's welfare when making decisions.

Family and Kinship Systems

- Native Americans often have an extended family although the family constellation may be different from those in mainstream America. Some families are "matriarchal" in nature and consist of an older woman and her husband and unmarried children, together with married daughters and their husbands and children. Others live in various kinds of living arrangements including nuclear families.
- Many Native Americans have unique categories of relatives or kinship systems.
- The Navajo trace descent through the mother, and they have a clan system of kinship.
- Traditionally, the head of household was the husband, although the wife had a voice in decision making. Today, many families are "blended," and there are households headed by women with children.
- Children are highly valued and are given responsibility early in life for making decisions about themselves.
- There is a prestige with aging as the elderly are seen as wise and experienced.
- Tribal and family ties are strong. Ties to the reservation remain for the younger generation of Native Americans, drawing them back to the reservation to live or to frequently visit family members.

- It is the extended families who provide care, comfort, and assistance to elderly family members or those who are ill.

Religious Ideology or Philosophical Beliefs

- Religion enters every phase of the traditional American Indian life. It has an important emphasis in curing illness.
- Many important Native American ceremonies (prayers, purification ceremonies, sweat lodge) are used with illness. Theology and medicine are difficult to separate in traditional Native American culture.
- Earth and nature are part of traditional cosmology, and health is viewed as harmony with nature, not just the curing of disease.
- Herbs are often used in Native American healing rituals. These herbs are often potent and can be dangerous if used by unskilled persons. Herbs such as peyote and the sacred datura may be used. The Tohono O'odham have a saying about the sacred datura plant, a hallucinogenic: If you have white skin and blue eyes, then do not use it as you do not have the appropriate relationship with the earth.
- There may be certain individuals who are able to cause sickness in others by practicing witchcraft.

Traditional Beliefs and Practices of Healing

- Health is a reflection of a correct relationship between human beings and the environment. Health is associated with the mind, spirit, and connections with creation and the creator.
- Illness is not an isolated episode in one's life. To make meaning of the illness, you must ask: How do I understand this illness in the trajectory of my life?
- The traditional healer is not technically a healer. Individuals heal themselves. The true healer is a facilitator; the responsibility for healing rests with the patient. The patient must take knowledge and incorporate that knowledge to heal

himself/herself. Remember, healing does not equate with "cure."

- Harmony and balance in one's life are the ultimate goals of healing.
- Many Native Americans use both their traditional health care system, including traditional health care practices, and the modern health care system.
- Different kinds of ceremonies may be used for healing. Sweat lodge, traditional herbs, songs, dances, and prayers are common. The traditional healer may fast before performing ceremonies. Unique ceremonies (for childbirth, for strength, for blessings) are common. The rituals (songs, prayers, dances) create a "healing environment."

Components of Traditional Healing

- An important component of traditional healing is unconditional love that encompasses the body, mind, and spirit as well as the individual's relations with the creator.
- Responsibility for healing rests with the patient. The traditional medicine practitioner is a facilitator. The true healer is the patient. The patient must take the knowledge, incorporate it into his or her life, and heal himself or herself.
- The patient must seek or ask for assistance and play an active role in his or her recovery.
- Every illness is a learning experience for the patient and for the healer. Every healing situation presents an opportunity for teaching or a cultural interpretation to help the patient understand his or her illness within the context of his or her life.
- There are no accidents in healing. An accident might be the spirits talking to you in order to get your attention and make you change your ways.

Use of Herbal Remedies

- Fifty percent of the drugs that are commonly used in Western medicine come from plants.
- Respect Mother Earth and the plants that have healing qualities. Express appreciation to the

creator. Do not "strip" the plant of all of the leaves. Take only what you need.

- Know your plants and know your patients. Traditional healers often remind us that there is a saying that individuals with white skin and blue eyes do not have the same relationships as a native does with Mother Earth. Many herbs are powerful and can be extremely dangerous.
- Many herbs require commitment on the part of the healer and the patient as the effect may disappear quickly and then a little more is given. Western medicine uses the active ingredient in the herb to produce the significant effects. Many traditional herbs "nudge" you along.

- While many plants have healing qualities, they cannot heal the individual without prayers and ceremonies.

What the mind cannot deal with
The body will manifest.
Therefore, to look for the cause
of Disease or disharmony (life
out of balance), look to the Spirit
for the Spirit cannot lie.
Edgar Monetathchi, Jr., 1987
Comanche Medicine Man*

---

*From the Traditional Indian Medicine Workshop presented by the University of Arizona Indians into Medicine Program and the Stoklos Native American Health Education Fund.

REFERENCE

Barnard, A. (2007). Providing psychiatric mental health care to Native Americans. *Journal of Psychosocial Nursing, 45*(5), 30–35.

Boyle/Baird Transcultural Nursing Assessment Guide for Refugees[1]

● Joyceen S. Boyle and Martha B. Baird

Migration Experience

Most refugees arrive in the United States from developing countries, countries with meager economic resources. Thus, refugees are often poor, have low levels of formal education, and have few marketable work skills. Many refugees are women of childbearing age and their children, and many of them are in poor health and have experienced physical and psychological trauma. Refugees usually are settled in urban areas, even though they may have a rural orientation.

- Ask your client how to pronounce his or her name; find out what name he or she wishes to be called. Be sure you're clear on what is the first and last name as in many cultural groups, the children do not share the same surname as their parents. How do they wish to be greeted?
- Ask about the client's primary language and assess his or her ability to communicate in English in both written and oral forms. What other languages does the client speak and write?
- Ask the clients in which language they prefer to receive written health care information.
- How long has your client been in this country? Has he or she lived in other US cities? How did the client travel here from the home country? How many years did the client spend in the diaspora (or the time from leaving the country

of origin to the present day)? What other countries has the client lived in? What were those circumstances like?
- Did the client come to this country with family members? With others from the same village or from the same clan?
- Can the client describe the migration experience? Ask about the events that happened to the client that he or she believes are important.
- What precipitated the client's leaving his or her country?
- Did the client have any major health events prior to arrival in the host country? If so, what? And did the client receive treatment? If so, where, and what were the outcomes?

The US Health Care System

- What were the client's experiences like when seeking health care in the United States? Has the client ever experienced discrimination? What was that experience like for his or her family members?
- What barriers might exist to using the US health care system, such as language difficulties, lack of financial resources, and transportation?
- What provisions, if any, are made for refugee health care within your community?
- Are bilingual health care workers readily available? Is there distrust, suspicion, or unfamiliarity of health care workers and biomedicine? Is there eye contact with the health care professional?

---

[1]Refugees are people who flee one area, usually their home country, to seek shelter or protection from danger, such as war, or escape from famine or other environmental disasters.

- Are health care professionals genuinely interested in learning about the refugees?
- Does your client or others in the refugee community strongly prefer same sex providers?
- What are the difficulties of accessing health and social services for refugees?

Language and Traditions

- What are the differences in dialects or languages spoken by health care professionals and the refugees? Can some of the problems be identified prior to a health care visit?
- What is the literacy level of members of the refugee group? Can they read and write in any language? This may vary within specific refugee groups depending on educational level and social status within home country.
- Do the health care facilities provide educational materials in appropriate languages?
- Are there appropriate numbers and appropriate ages and genders of translators and interpreters available in health care agencies? Are the interpreters/translators trained and/or certified?
- Is there adequate outreach to individual homes and families?

Traditional Beliefs and Practices of Healing

- What is the client's understanding of his or her health problem? The understanding of how a client views his/her condition is extremely helpful information. It facilitates the health care provider's understanding of the social and cultural construction of illness. This information helps us understand the client's beliefs and behavior, facilitates further discussion of an ailment, and guides the course of treatment. It is always helpful to begin this discussion with a statement of respect such as: *"I know different people have very different ways of understanding illness...help me understand how you see things."*

- The following nine questions from Kleinman (1980) can be a useful way to gain the client's perspective about the illness or health condition:

    What do you think has caused your problems?
    What do you call the problem or illness?
    Why do you think it started when it did?
    What do you think your sickness does to you?
    How severe is your sickness? Will it have a long or short course?
    What kind of treatment do you think you should receive?
    What are the most important results you hope to receive from this treatment?
    What are the chief problems your sickness has caused for you?
    What do you fear most about your sickness?

- How do religious beliefs and practices relate to health and illness?
- Do members of the refugee group seek care from indigenous healers and/or folk practitioners? Do they use traditional herbs or medicines? Are there cultural or ethnic stores in the neighborhood that sell herbs and traditional medicines? Or do they purchase any medicines, herbs, or vitamins from their home country?
- What contemporary health care is available for this refugee group? What immunizations has the client received? When? What insurance or payment mechanisms are provided? For how long? Does the client understand how to access care?
- Which individuals in the family and/or in the refugee group make decisions about seeking health care? About the treatment options?
- What are the primary health concerns and/or illnesses in this refugee group (e.g., female genital mutilation [FGM], malnutrition, mental health/trauma issues)? How do the refugees' concerns align with those of the local and state health care systems? For example, FGM can be a significant concern during labor and delivery. In addition, if the procedure is carried out in the United States by relatives of the female child/adolescent, health care providers have ethical and legal reporting obligations.

Family and Kinship Systems

- Are the families extended or nuclear or other? Has the structure of the family changed during or since migration? Do family members live in close proximity? Do they visit often? Where are the members of your client's family?
- What is the role and stature of individual family members? How do family members relate to each other? How have family roles changed since coming to this country?
- Ask if there are tribes and/or clans in the refugee group.
- Do the parents and/or others make arrangements for marriages? Is there a preference for first cousins to marry?
- What is the role of "elders" or "leaders" in this refugee group? How do they function within the community?
- Did the client leave family members behind or lose family members from death in the home country?

Social Life and Networks

- What are the daily routines of this group? How do the routines vary by gender? How have family roles changed? Is the refugee group integrated into the community or fairly isolated? Who are the group's leaders?
- How does the refugee group observe important life cycle events?
- What are the educational aspirations of individual/family refugees? What are the educational experiences of the children?
- Are there special concerns such as abuse of alcohol, domestic violence, gang membership, polygamy, and child marriage? How does this refugee group view these issues?

Religious Beliefs and Practices

- What are the major religious beliefs and practices within the refugee community? Does your client adhere to the predominant beliefs? Is there a special church associated with the refugees? (Churches often serve as a site for social life of the refugee community and are comfortable and acceptable places for health educational programs and other forms of outreach.) How is social life integrated within the church membership?
- How do the religious beliefs and practices influence everyday life? How are they expressed in everyday life?
- Are there special beliefs and practices surrounding major life events such as birth, marriage, and death?
- Are there special "cultural" occasions, such as circumcision rites and *quince años* parties?
- Are there specific beliefs about gender roles? Are these beliefs tied to religious beliefs?

Trauma/Torture

Recently, it has become common practice to integrate trauma assessment into primary care and other health care situations. There are several trauma assessment tools that are available. These tools assess important mental health factors in a refugee, who can be referred to a mental health care provider for further assessment. It is important to note that screening instruments should be administered by health care workers under the supervision and support of a psychiatrist, physician, and/or psychiatric mental health care nurse. These tools were *not* designed to be used as a self-report; they cannot replace the role of a mental health professional.

The Harvard Trauma Questionnaire

The Harvard Trauma Questionnaire (HTQ) is a checklist that inquires about a variety of traumatic events as well as the emotional symptoms considered to be uniquely associated with trauma. Currently, there are six versions of this questionnaire. The Vietnamese, Cambodian, and Laotian versions were written for use with Southeast Asian refugees. The Japanese version was written for survivors of the 1995 Kobe earthquake. The Croatian Veterans' version was written for military personnel who survived the ways in the Balkans; the Bosnian version was written for civilian survivors of that conflict.

Questions focus on (1) subjective descriptions of the most traumatic event(s) that an individual experienced; (2) events that may have led to a head injury; (3) trauma symptoms, including symptoms of post-traumatic stress disorder (PTSD); and, (4) specific refugee trauma, such as violence, rape, starvation, etc. Responses include "Experienced," "Witnessed," "Heard about it," or "No." Other scales include "Not at all," "A little," "Quite a bit," and "Extremely."

The Hopkins Symptom Checklist-25

The Hopkins Symptom Checklist-25 (HSCL-25) is a symptom inventory that measures symptoms of anxiety and depression and has been correlated with DSM-IV-R diagnostic criteria. It consists of 25 items; Part I has 10 items for anxiety symptoms; Part II has 15 items for depression symptoms. Each question includes four categories of responses: "Not at all," "A little," "Quite a bit," and "Extremely," rated 1 to 4, respectively.

The HSCL-25 has been translated into 17 different languages including Arabic, Bosnian, Cambodian, Croatian, Japanese, Laotian, Vietnamese, and Dinka.

REFERENCE

Kleinman, A. (1980). *Patients and healers in the context of culture: An exploration of the borderland between anthropology, medicine and psychiatry.* Berkeley, CA: University of California Press.

Index